THE PITUITARY ADENOMA

THE PITUITARY ADENOMA

Edited by

KALMON D. POST, M.D.
IVOR M.D. JACKSON, M.D.
and
SEYMOUR REICHLIN, M.D., Ph.D.

New England Medical Center Hospital
Boston, Massachusetts

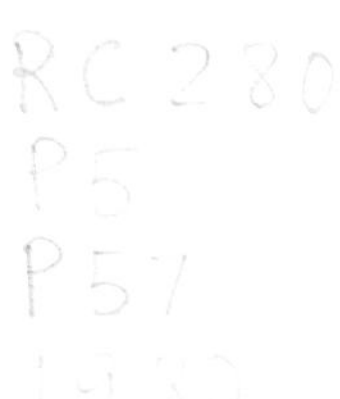

PLENUM MEDICAL BOOK COMPANY
NEW YORK AND LONDON

Library of Congress Cataloging in Publication Data

Main entry under title:

The Pituitary adenoma.

Includes index.
1. Pituitary body—Tumors. 2. Adenoma. I. Post, Kalmon D. II. Jackson, Ivor M.D. III. Reichlin, Seymour.
RC280.P5P57 616.9'93'47 79-24811
ISBN 0-306-40382-X

227 West 17th Street, New York, N.Y. 10011

Plenum Medical Book Company is an imprint of
Plenum Publishing Corporation

Printed in the United States of America

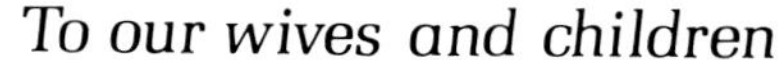

To our wives and children

Contributors

Lester S. Adelman, M.D., Associate Professor of Neuropathology, Tufts University School of Medicine; Neuropathologist, Department of Pathology, Division of Neuropathology, Tufts–New England Medical Center Hospital, Boston, Massachusetts 02111

Bruce J. Biller, M.D., Associate Staff Physician, Department of Medicine, Division of Endocrinology, Tufts–New England Medical Center Hospital, Boston, Massachusetts 02111; Staff Physician, Department of Medicine, Massachusetts Institute of Technology, Cambridge, Massachusetts 02139

Aubrey Boyd III, M.D., Associate Professor of Medicine, Department of Internal Medicine, Division of Endocrinology and Metabolism, Baylor College of Medicine, Houston, Texas 77030

William E. Cobb, M.D., Assistant Clinical Professor of Medicine, Department of Medicine, Division of Endocrinology, Tufts–New England Medical Center Hospital, Boston, Massachusetts 02111; Director of Medical Education, Quincy City Hospital, Quincy, Massachusetts 02169

Bahman Emami, M.D., Assistant Professor of Therapeutic Radiology, Tufts University School of Medicine; Radiotherapist, Department of Therapeutic Radiology, Tufts–New England Medical Center Hospital, Boston, Massachusetts 02111

John W. Gittinger, Jr., M.D., Assistant Professor of Ophthalmology and Assistant Professor of Neurology, Tufts University School of Medicine; Department of Ophthalmology, Division of Neuro-ophthalmology, Tufts–New England Medical Center Hospital, Boston, Massachusetts 02111

Richard H. Goodman, M.D., Ph.D., Fellow in Endocrinology, Tufts University School of Medicine; Department of Medicine, Division of Endocrinology, Tufts–New England Medical Center Hospital, Boston, Massachusetts 02111

Ivor M.D. Jackson, M.D., Associate Professor of Medicine, Tufts University School of Medicine; Physician, Department of Medicine, Division of Endocrinology, Tufts–New England Medical Center Hospital, Boston, Massachusetts 02111

David L. Kasdon, M.D., Major, USAF, Department of Neurosurgery, Wilford Hall Medical Center, Lackland Air Force Base, San Antonio, Texas 78213

Eugene B. Kern, M.D., F.A.C.S., Assistant Professor of Otolaryngology, Department of Otolaryngology, Mayo Medical School, Rochester, Minnesota 55901

Raymond N. Kjellberg, M.D., Associate Professor of Surgery, Harvard Medical School; Visiting Neurosurgeon, Department of Neurosurgery, Massachusetts General Hospital, Boston, Massachusetts 02114

Bernard Kliman, M.D., Associate Professor of Medicine, Harvard Medical School; Associate Physician, Department of Medicine, Massachusetts General Hospital, Boston, Massachusetts 02114

Peter O. Kohler, M.D., Professor of Medicine, University of Arkansas for Medical Sciences, Little Rock, Arkansas 72205; Professor and Chairman of the Department of Medicine, Little Rock Arkansas University Hospital, Little Rock, Arkansas 72201

Edward R. Laws, Jr., M.D., Associate Professor of Neurological Surgery, Department of Neurological Surgery, Mayo Medical School, Rochester, Minnesota 55901

Thomas J. McDonald, M.D., M.S., F.A.C.S., Assistant Professor of Otolaryngology, Department of Otolaryngology, Mayo Medical School, Rochester, Minnesota 55901

Mark E. Molitch, M.D., Assistant Professor of Medicine, Tufts University School of Medicine; Assistant Physician, Department of Medicine, Division of Endocrinology, Tufts–New England Medical Center Hospital, Boston, Massachusetts 02111

Bruce W. Pearson, M.D., F.R.C.S. (C), F.A.C.S., Assistant Professor of Otolaryngology and Anatomy, Department of Otolaryngology, Mayo Medical School, Rochester, Minnesota 55901

Kalmon D. Post, M.D., F.A.C.S., Associate Professor of Neurosurgery, Tufts University School of Medicine; Neurosurgeon, Department of Neurosurgery, Tufts–New England Medical Center Hospital, Boston, Massachusetts 02111

Seymour Reichlin, M.D., Ph.D., Professor of Medicine, Tufts University School of Medicine; Department of Medicine, Chief of Division of Endocrinology, Tufts–New England Medical Center Hospital, Boston, Massachusetts 02111

Samuel M. Wolpert, M.D., Professor of Radiology, Tufts University School of Medicine; Chief of Section of Neuroradiology, Department of Radiology, Section of Neuroradiology, Tufts–New England Medical Center Hospital, Boston, Massachusetts 02111

Preface

The idea for this book developed as an outcome of a multidisciplinary symposium entitled "Pituitary Adenoma Update" that was held at Tufts–New England Medical Center in April 1977. The purpose of that symposium was to put together our current knowledge of the cause of pituitary tumors and discuss the diagnostic evaluation and management that was now appropriate, in light of the rapid advances that had taken place so recently in this area. Those of our colleagues who had presented papers at the symposium, as well as a number of others, were invited to contribute to this volume, which should serve as a presentation of the "state of the art" on all aspects of pituitary tumors. We felt that such a book would be of value to endocrinologists, neurosurgeons, neuroradiologists, and pathologists who are involved in the investigation or care of patients with pituitary disorders.

For a number of reasons, a review of pituitary adenomas seems particularly timely. Rapid advances have taken place coincidentally in the fields of neurosurgery, neuroendocrinology, neuroradiology, neuropathology, and neuropharmacology. Seven major developments in these areas have occurred independently and almost simultaneously that have virtually revolutionized our approach to pituitary adenomas.

1. The first is the refinement of transsphenoidal surgery. Although this route to the pituitary had been utilized by Harvey Cushing and his predecessors, poor illumination and potential for infection limited the application of this procedure, which consequently was little used by a whole subsequent generation of neurosurgeons. The technological advance that allowed the reintroduction of this procedure was the development of the operating microscope along with televised radiofluoroscopic control, which allows microadenomas within the pituitary gland itself to be directly visualized. It thus has become feasible to treat pituitary tumors by neurosurgery without the morbidity and mortality that accompany transfrontal craniotomy.

2. The second development was the remarkable advance that has taken place in radiological diagnosis, which has permitted the detection of microadenomas (<10 mm) of the pituitary by means of pluridirectional tomography. Modern neuroradiology can now define the pituitary tumors that were previously inapparent by conventional X-ray. The neurosurgeon, secure in the preoperative diagnosis of a microadenoma, can now intervene early in its

course and remove it before either tumor or surgery need compromise other parameters of pituitary function. Computed tomography (CT scanning) has enabled the neuroradiologist to define the extrasellar anatomical relationships of a tumor arising from the glandular pituitary without the necessity of resorting to invasive procedures.

3. The development of radioimmunoassay and its application to a hitherto unrecognized human pituitary hormone, prolactin, provides a sensitive tumor marker for many cases of so-called "inactive" pituitary chromophobe adenoma. The application of the prolactin radioimmunoassay to the clinical problem of galactorrhea–amenorrhea, together with the neurosurgical and neuroradiological advances described above, demonstrated that many women with the syndrome of amenorrhea–galactorrhea have microadenomas of the pituitary secreting excess prolactin; some men with impotence and hypogonadism have similarly been shown to harbor pituitary adenomas. Removal of these tumors has been shown to correct the infertility and impotence of these patients.

4. The isolation and synthesis of the hypophysiotropic hormones of the hypothalamus, thyrotropin-releasing hormone (TRH), luteinizing-hormone-releasing hormone (LH-RH), and somatostatin (for which Guillemin and Schally received the Nobel Prize in 1977), can truly be said to have ushered in the modern era of clinical neuroendocrinology. The availability of these substances in pure form has allowed the endocrinologist to directly study the regulation of secretion from the adenohypophysis. The development of assays to measure these materials has radically altered our appreciation of the role of the brain in the control of the pituitary gland.

5. Neuropharmacological studies have led to the development of new therapeutic agents that significantly affect pituitary secretion and allow the physician to reverse many of the ravages of hyperpituitarism. In certain instances, a "medical adenomectomy" can occasionally be obtained. The agent of most interest and widespread application is bromergocryptine, an ergot derivative and dopamine agonist, which is of considerable benefit as an oral therapeutic agent in the treatment of hyperprolactinemia and acromegaly.

6. In neuropathology, the application of the technique of immunohistochemistry has totally altered the designation of pituitary adenomas from the anachronistic eosinophil, basophil, and chromophobe tinctorial designation toward a functional and practical classification of pituitary adenomas. Newer staining techniques can provide a reliable intraoperative frozen-tissue diagnosis by which tumor tissue can be readily separated from normal gland.

7. Finally, the concepts of molecular peptide engineering have been applied to the therapeutic problems of hypothalamic pituitary disease. The potential importance of this approach for the practice of clinical endocrinology is especially illustrated by the development of an analogue of the neurohypophyseal peptide vasopressin, 1-deamino-8-D-arginine vasopressin (dDAVP), which has greatly improved our ability to treat diabetes insipidus, a frequent and often distressing sequela of pituitary disorders and the treatment thereof. We may reasonably predict that dDAVP will turn out to be a prototype of further contributions that can be expected from the protein chemists for the therapy of neuroendocrinological disorders in man.

The fortunate happenstance of these separate but contemporaneous developments has altered in a wholly unexpected and unanticipated manner our approach to hypothalamic–pituitary disorders. Nonetheless, despite much experience garnered through application of these advances, there is still much that we do not know about pituitary adenomas. In these pages, it has been our purpose to place into perspective these recent advances and to recommend an approach to pituitary tumors based on sound physiological principles; when appropriate, we have outlined for the reader those areas that might be designated as future growth points in the field.

Together with our colleagues, mainly, but not exclusively, from Tufts–New England Medical Center in Boston, we have put together a comprehensive review of current concepts into the pathogenesis, diagnosis, and treatment of pituitary adenomas. We have endeavored at all times to present a balanced viewpoint on these different areas, some of which excite much controversy. Our own personal biases have been indicated in circumstances where discordant viewpoints abound. It is our hope that this treatise will be useful to those who deal with neuroendocrine disease.

Our special thanks go to the following people, whose competence and enthusiasm made this project infinitely easier to complete. Sandra Navarroli patiently collated, typed, and retyped the manuscript; Hilary Evans coordinated the overall format of the book; and Nancy Mester and her team edited the completed chapters.

Kalmon D. Post
Ivor M.D. Jackson
Seymour Reichlin

Boston

Contents

I. Pathophysiology of Pituitary Tumors

Chapter 1

Anatomical and Physiological Basis of Hypothalamic–Pituitary Regulation

Seymour Reichlin

Chapter 2

Etiology of Pituitary Adenomas

Seymour Reichlin

Chapter 3

The Pathology of Pituitary Adenomas

Lester S. Adelman

II. Clinical Features of Pituitary Tumors

Chapter 4

Galactorrhea Syndromes

Bruce J. Biller, Aubrey Boyd III, Mark E. Molitch, Kalmon D. Post, Samuel M. Wolpert, and Seymour Reichlin

Chapter 5

Prolactin-Secreting Adenomas in the Male

Richard H. Goodman, Mark E. Molitch, Kalmon D. Post, and Ivor M.D. Jackson

Chapter 6

Growth-Hormone-Secreting Pituitary Adenomas

Ivor M.D. Jackson

Chapter 9

Nonsecreting Adenomas

Mark E. Molitch

Chapter 10

Sellar and Parasellar Lesions Mimicking Adenoma

Kalmon D. Post and David L. Kasdon

III. Clinical Evaluation of Pituitary Tumors

Chapter 11

Diagnostic Tests for the Evaluation of Pituitary Tumors

Ivor M.D. Jackson

Chapter 12

Pituitary Hormone Concentrations in Cerebrospinal Fluid in Patients with Pituitary Tumors

Kalmon D. Post, Bruce J. Biller, and Ivor M.D. Jackson

Chapter 13

Ophthalmological Evaluation of Pituitary Adenomas

John W. Gittinger

Chapter 14

The Radiology of Pituitary Adenomas—An Update

Samuel M. Wolpert

IV. Treatment of Pituitary Tumors

Chapter 15

Medical Therapy of Pituitary Tumors

Mark E. Molitch

Chapter 16

General Considerations in the Surgical Treatment of Pituitary Tumors

Kalmon D. Post

Chapter 21

Conventional Radiotherapy and Pituitary Tumors

Bahman Emami

Chapter 22

Radiosurgery Therapy for Pituitary Adenoma

Raymond N. Kjellberg and Bernard Kliman

Chapter 23

Overview of Pituitary Tumor Treatment

Peter O. Kohler

I

Pathophysiology of Pituitary Tumors

1

Anatomical and Physiological Basis of Hypothalamic–Pituitary Regulation

SEYMOUR REICHLIN

1. Anatomical Overview

The pituitary gland and the hypothalamus are closely related both anatomically[1–9] and embryologically[10] (Figs. 1 and 2).

The pituitary gland is divided into a glandular portion (adenohypophysis, anterior lobe, pars distalis), an intermediate lobe (pars intermedia), and a neural lobe (posterior pituitary, infundibular process) that is a direct downgrowth of tissue from the base of the hypothalamus. The intermediate lobe is rudimentary in man, making up less than 0.8% of total weight. This figure underestimates the mass of intermediate-lobe cells, however, because of the significant number of intermediate-lobe cells that are diffusely distributed in the adenohypophysis and neural lobe of man.[11] The neurohypophysis consists of specialized tissue at the base of the hypothalamus, together with the neural stalk and the neural lobe. The neurohypophyseal portion of the hypothalamus that forms the base of the third ventricle is funnel-shaped, a resemblance that gave rise to the term *infundibulum* and to the hypothesis of Vesalius that animal spirits (cerebrospinal fluid) drained mucus ("pituita") from the brain into the nose via this structure. The central portion of the infundibulum is enveloped from below by the pars tuberalis portion of the anterior pituitary gland and is penetrated by numerous capillary loops of the primary portal plexus of the hypophyseal–portal circulation. This neurovascular complex forms a small but conspicuous structure at the base of the hypothalamus that is termed the *median eminence* of the *tuber cinereum*. Although the median eminence is anatomically classified as part of the neurohypophysis, and is traversed by fibers of the supraoptic and paraventricular neurons, this structure is primarily related to control of the anterior pituitary. In the median emi-

SEYMOUR REICHLIN • Tufts University School of Medicine; Department of Medicine, Division of Endocinology, Tufts–New England Medical Center Hospital, Boston, Massachusetts 02111.

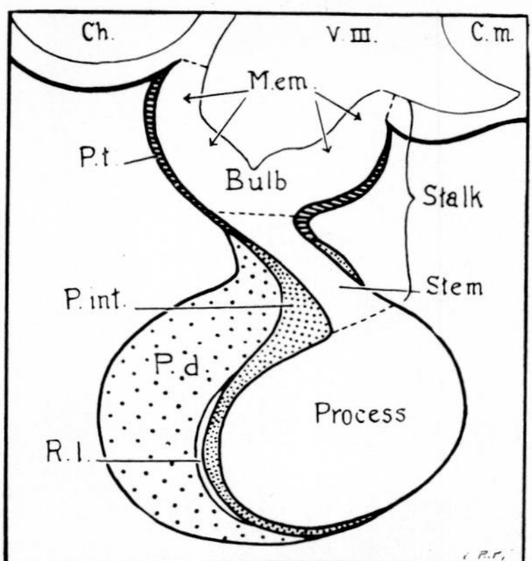

Fig. 1. Diagrammatic outline of the structure and standard nomenclature of the hypothalamic–pituitary unit of the hypophysis of a macaque monkey (*Macaca mulatta*). (Bulb) Infundibular "bulb" of "infundibulum"; (Ch.) optic chiasm; (C.m.) mammillary body; (M.em.) median eminence; (P.d.) pars distalis; (P.t.) pars tuberalis; (P.int.) pars intermedia; (Process) infundibular process (neural); (R.l.) residual lumen; (Stalk) infundibular stalk; (Stem) infundibular stem; (V.III.) third ventricle. Reproduced from Rioch *et al.*[1] with permission of the Association for Research in Nervous and Mental Disease.

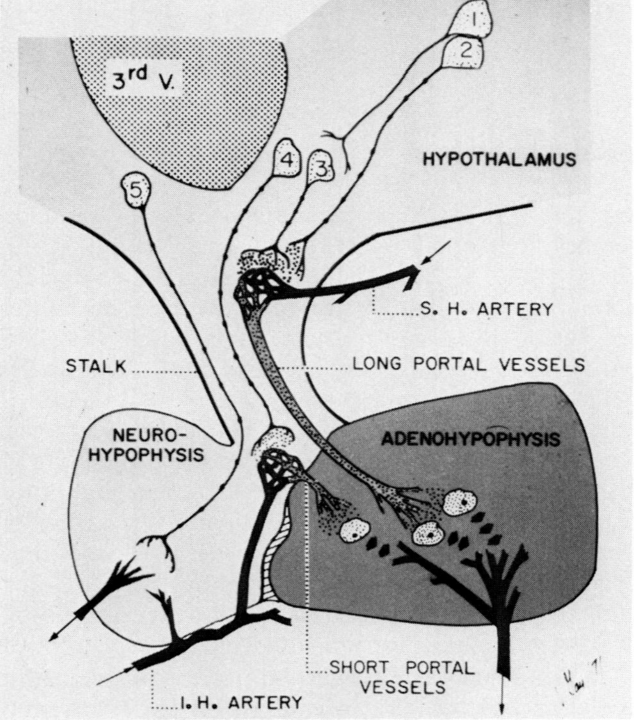

Fig. 2. Neural control of pituitary gland. This figure summarizes the types of neural inputs into pituitary regulation. Neuron 5 represents the peptidergic neurons of the supraoptico–hypophyseal and paraventriculo–hypophyseal tracts, with hormone-producing cell bodies in the hypothalamus and nerve terminals in the neural lobe. Neurons 4 and 3 are the peptidergic neurons of the tubero-hypophyseal tract, which secrete the hypophysiotropic hormones into the substance of the median eminence in anatomical relationship to the primary plexus. Neuron 3 ends in the median eminence. Neuron 4 ends low in the stalk. Neuron 1 represents a monoaminergic neuron ending in relation to the cell body of the peptidergic neuron. Neuron 2 represents a monoaminergic neuron ending on terminals of the peptidergic neuron to give axo–axonic transmission as proposed by Schneider and McCann. Neurons 1 and 2 are the functional links between the remainder of the brain and the peptidergic neuron. From Gay, V.L., The hypothalamus: Physiology and clinical use of releasing factors, *Fertil. Steril.* **23**:50, 1972. Reproduced with the permission of the publisher, The American Fertility Society.

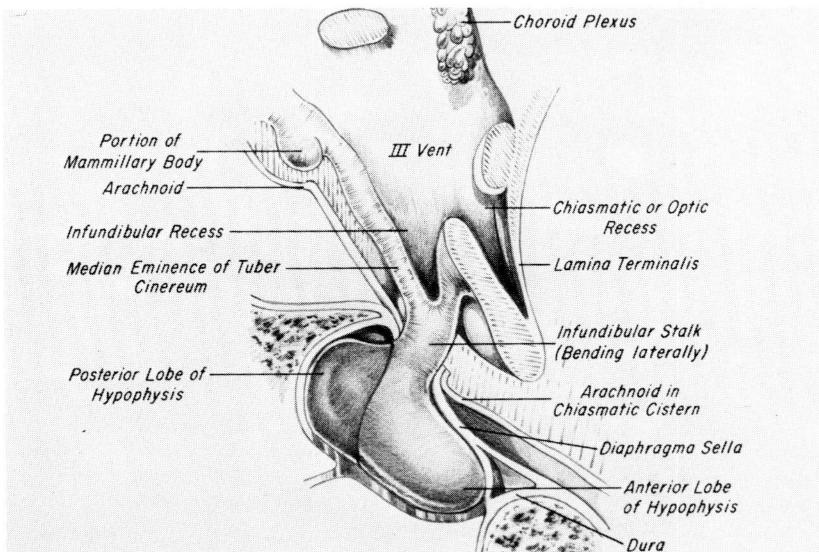

Fig. 3. Sagittal view of the human hypothalamic–pituitary unit illustrating the anatomical relationships between optic chiasm and pituitary stalk.

nence, transfer of neurosecretions of hypophysiotropic neurons of the hypothalamus to the pituitary blood supply takes place.

By gross examination, the hypothalamus is readily outlined by several landmarks (Fig. 3). Anteriorly, it is bounded by the optic chiasm and laterally by the sulci formed with the temporal lobes. The mammillary bodies are the posterior portion of the hypothalamus. The smooth, rounded base of the hypothalamus is termed the *tuber cinereum,* and its central region, from which descends the *pituitary stalk,* is termed the *median eminence.* In fresh specimens (with blood-filled vessels) or India-ink-perfused specimens, the extent of the median eminence can be easily determined because it is coextensive with the distribution of the primary plexus of the hypophyseal–portal circulation. Dorsally, the hypothalamus is delineated from the thalamus by the hypothalamic sulcus.

2. The Neurohypophysis

2.1. Anatomy

The neural lobe develops embryologically as a downgrowth from the ventral diencephalon and retains its natural connections and its neural character in adult life. The dominant features of the neurohypophysis are the supraoptico–hypophyseal and paraventriculo–hypophyseal nerve tracts (Figs. 2 and 4). These unmyelinated nerve tracts descend through the infundibulum and the neural stalk to terminate in the neural lobe.

Cells of origin of these tracts are strikingly large (and hence are called "magnocellular") and are consolidated into well-characterized groups situ-

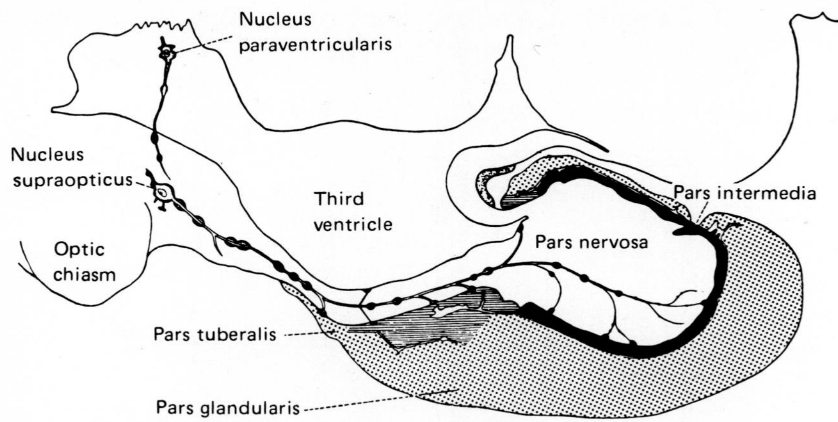

Fig. 4. Course of the neurosecretory substance from the hypothalamic cell body, along the neural stalk, to the neurohypophysis. This diagram illustrates the concept of cell-body formation of oxytocin–vasopressin and passage of the material down the stalk to a storage site in the neural lobe. The dilated areas on the axons have been thought in the past to represent extraneuronal accumulation of neurosecretory material (NSM). Electron microscopy now shows that all the NSM is within the axon itself. Most of the fibers are unmyelinated. Reproduced from Bargmann and Scharrer[51] with permission.

ated in paired nuclei above the optic tract (supraoptic) and on each side of the ventricle (paraventricular). A few small cells of this system are also distributed between the two nuclei. The other nerve cells of the hypothalamus are relatively small (parvicellular) and do not have any obvious distinguishing characteristics by conventional microscopy. Because of the prominence of the neurohypophyseal cell bodies, they have been the subject of study for many years, and have been shown to be richly endowed by capillaries the fenestrated endothelia of which are characteristic of endocrine glands generally.

Specific antisera directed singly against vasopressin, oxytocin, and the two chief classes of neurophysin (the neurohypophyseal carrier protein) have confirmed earlier morphological studies that show that principal projections of the two nuclei terminate in the neural lobe.[9] New specific methods have shown an additional pathway of neurophysin-containing nerve endings within the median eminence in opposition to the primary plexus of the hypophyseal–portal circulation. Thus, the neurohypophyseal neurons may have a role in anterior pituitary regulation, as well as in neural lobe regulation. Direct assays of blood in the portal circulation show high concentrations of neurophysin, vasopressin, and oxytocin, thus confirming the anatomical observations, although more recent work suggests that they may arise by reflux from the pituitary.[12] Most of the cell bodies in the supraoptic nucleus are vasopressin-containing, but some contain oxytocin. A somewhat smaller percentage (but still the majority of stainable cells) in the paraventricular nucleus contain vasopressin. Most cells contain either one or the other peptide, but studies by Defendini and Zimmerman[9] suggest that a given cell may contain both. Because vasopressin and oxytocin release can be dissociated physiologically, the two different types of cells must be regulated individually. Very recently, ACTH-like and β-lipotropin immunoreactivity have also been identified in the supraoptic nuclei as well as in other cells.[13,14]

2.2. Hormone Synthesis, Transport, and Secretion

Vasopressin and oxytocin are synthesized mainly in the cell bodies of the supraoptic and paraventricular neurons. Like all neurosecretions, these hormones are transported in small vesicles, enclosed by a membrane. Secretory vesicles containing the hormones flow down the axons to the neural lobe, where they are stored and later released when stimulated by a propagated action potential originating in the neuronal cell body.

In the neural lobe, the neurosecretory vesicles accumulate in palisade formation in dilated nerve endings, located on delicate basement membranes separated from the basement membranes of capillaries by a narrow perivascular space. This anatomical relationship of nerve ending to capillary wall is characteristic of endocrine cells in general. The posterior-lobe neurons thus present the morphology of a nerve cell modified to act as an endocrine organ. Neuro-secretory cells and cells of this type are called "neuroendocrine transducers." They convert (transduce) neural information to hormone information. They are analogous to the cells of the tuberohypophyseal system that regulate anterior pituitary function by way of the hypothalamic hypophysiotropic factors (releasing hormones) (Fig. 5, neurosecretory neurons).

The function of neurohypophyseal neurons is in turn directly controlled mainly by cholinergic and noradrenergic neurotransmitters, but several neuropeptides may also be important regulators of secretion.[15] Release of vasopressin and oxytocin is *stimulated* by cholinergic impulses, thus explaining the antidiuretic effects of smoking as a nicotinic-receptor stimulator. Adrenergic influences, in contrast, are *inhibitory* to both hormone secretion and electrical activity. Pharmacological analysis has shown that the response is β-adrenergic. It is likely that the stress-induced inhibition of the "milk letdown" reflex, well known from both animal husbandry and human nursing experience, is due to β-adrenergic inhibition of oxytocin release. The same kind of reaction may be responsible for stress-induced diuresis.

The secretion of vasopressin and electrophysiological activation of supraoptic neurons is also stimulated by angiotensin II. This peptide can be synthesized entirely by reactions within the brain as well as by the peripheral renin–angiotension system.[16] Neurohypophyseal neurons are also stimulated by endogenous opiates (endorphins). The well-known antidiuretic action of morphine is due to release of vasopressin, an effect that can be duplicated by the administration of β-endorphin.

2.3. Physiological Regulation of Neurohypophyseal Hormone Release

Plasma osmolarity is the most important determinant of vasopressin secretion, an effect mediated through neural mechanisms. When hypertonic saline is introduced into the carotid artery, the activity of certain neurons in the supraoptic and paraventricular nuclei that project to the neural lobe is accelerated.[15] This neuronal activation—and accompanying release of vasopressin—is functional proof that some type of "osmoreceptor" exists within the perfusion area of the internal carotid artery. Whether the osmoreceptor neuron is distinct from the vasopressin neurosecretory neuron has not been established with certainty, but it has been shown by direct electrical recording that some neurons that project to the neural lobe are immediately activated following exposure to hypertonic saline. Changes in osmolarity most likely alter the electrical properties of the membranes of the osmoreceptor cell, thereby changing its firing rate.

The neurohypophyseal neurons also respond to blood-volume receptors located in the left atrium and in other vascular areas. In addition, the secretion of vasopressin is affected by various parts of the "visceral brain" and the reticular activation system—regions involved in the maintenance of consciousness and in emotional expression.

The influence of "higher" neural centers on vasopressin secretion is evidenced by stress-induced antidiuresis in both man and animals and by the experimental induction of diuresis or antidiuresis by hyponotic suggestion or by psychological conditioning.

When the supraoptico–hypophyseal system is deprived of neural input from other parts of the brain, neurons in this region are electrically more active than normal and vasopressin secretion enhanced.[17] Denervation hyperfunction of the neurohypophysis may provide the explanation for the syndrome of "inappropriate ADH [antidiuretic hormone] secretion," which occurs in certain kinds and locations of brain damage.

The phenomenon of milk "let-down" is another example of neural control of neurohypophyseal function first recognized in animal husbandry and shown to occur in other species including man. Suckling is followed by the appearance of the milk at the nipple after some delay. The young do not begin to obtain milk until after 30 sec or more. A neurogenic reflex is responsible for this effect. The stimulus of suckling, transmitted from afferent nerve endings in the nipple, is conducted through the spinal cord, midbrain, and finally to the hypothalamus, where it triggers the release of oxytocin from the neurohypophysis. The released oxytocin causes contractions of the myoepithelial cells that encircle mammary acini and thence expels the milk into the nipple. In the absence of this reflex contraction, milk cannot be obtained from even a full breast; for example, nursing rats cannot obtain milk from their posterior-hypophysectomized mothers until injections of oxytocin are given. This reflex is accompanied by changes in hypothalamic electrical activity.

Milk "let-down" occurs in women in response to suckling and in some women is a conditioned stimulus to the hungry crying of their babies. Milk "let-down" may be inhibited by emotional stress and triggered by sexual excitement and orgasm.

Secretion of vasopressin and of oxytocin are independent. For example, in lactating women, ADH secretion can be achieved by hypertonic saline infusion without producing "let-down," and the suckling stimulus induces "let-down" without accompanying antidiuresis.

Damage to the neurohypophysis or to its central controlling input leads to diabetes insipidus (see Chapter 20). Excessive secretion by the neurohypophysis can also occur due to an abnormality of the neural regulating system.

Harris and Green were the first to recognize fully the functional significance of the fact that nearly all the blood that reaches the anterior pituitary has first traversed capillary plexuses located in the median eminence and adjoining neural stalk.[5,18,19] Their postulate, now termed the *portal vessel–chemotransmitter hypothesis,* was that these vessels formed part of a neurovascular link by which the hypothalamus, through the mediation of neurohumoral substances, regulated the secretion of the anterior pituitary tropic hormones.

3.1. Anatomy

The median eminence consists of a neural component (the infundibulum of the hypothalamus), a vascular component (the hypophyseal–portal capillaries and veins), and an epithelial component (the pars tuberalis of the adenohypophysis). Electron-microscopic studies show that the infundibulum is composed mainly of densely packed nerve endings, capillaries with conspicuous perivascular spaces, supporting cells resembling neurohypophyseal pituicytes, and specialized ependymal cells (tanycytes) that traverse the median eminence from the lumen of the third ventricle to the outer mantle plexus (Fig. 5). The nerve endings are the terminals of the tuberohypophyseal neurons that arise chiefly in the ventral hypothalamus; the capillaries form the primary plexus of the portal circulation.

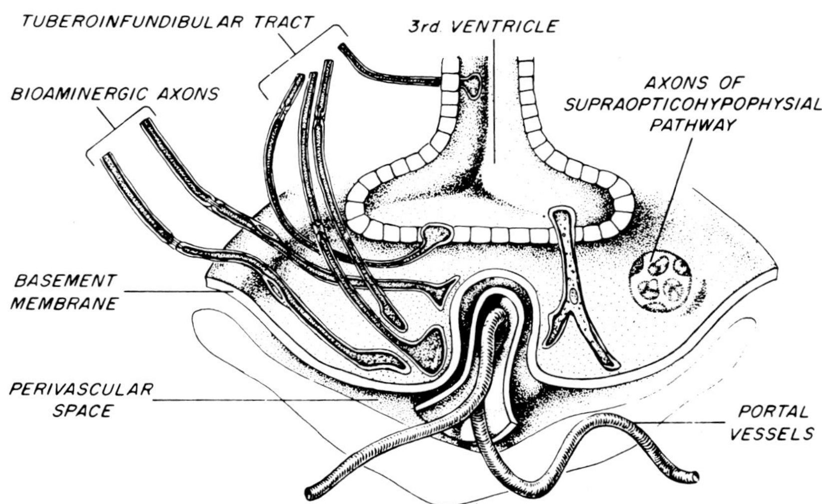

Fig. 5. Schematic diagram of the relationships of nerve endings in the median eminence. Note that the interstitial space of the median eminence is a diffuse region without the usual blood–brain barrier, in which end the nerves of tuberoinfundibular and bioaminergic tracts. Through the median eminence pass the projections of the supraoptico–hypophyseal pathway. Neurotransmitters and neurohormones are free to diffuse from the interstitial space to the primary plexus of the hypophyseal–portal circulation.

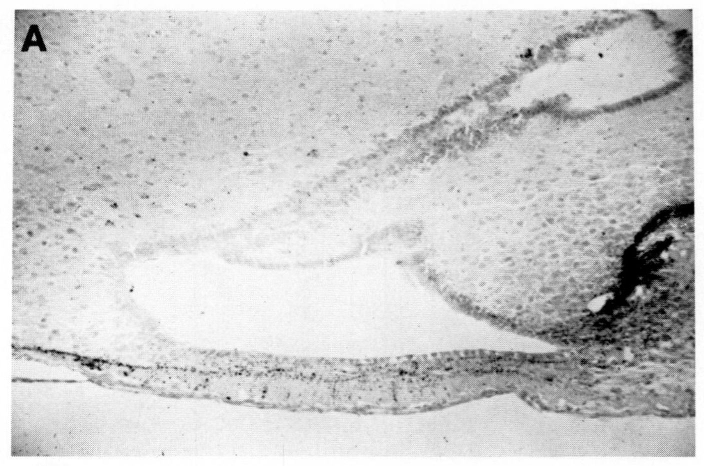
A

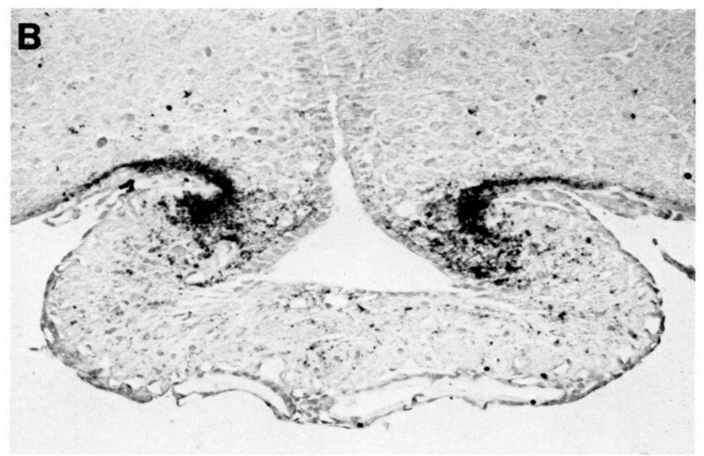
B

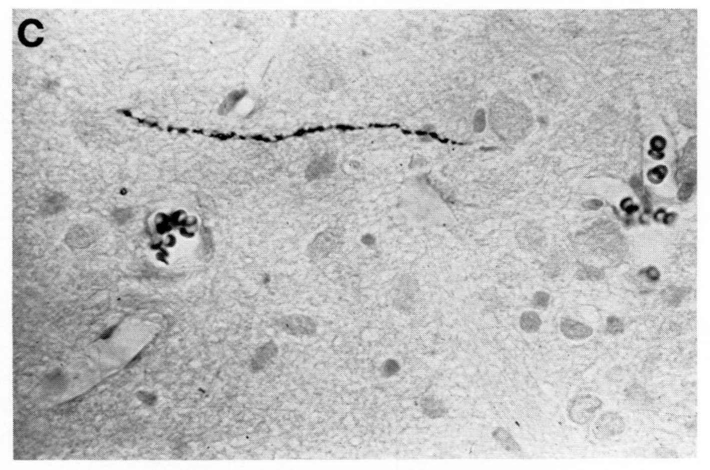
C

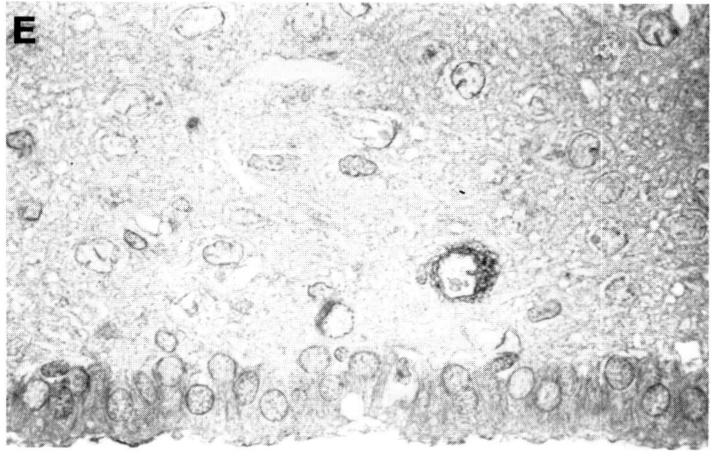

Fig. 6. Demonstration of the LH-RH and somatostatin pathways in rat brain by immunohistochemical staining utilizing antisera directed against the synthetic peptides visualized as dark-staining granules. These "peptidergic" pathways arise for the most part in the anterior hypothalamus and are distributed to the basal median eminence, where they come into contact with the primary plexus of the hypophyseal–portal system. (A) Sagittal section of rat hypothalamus stained with anti-LH-RH. (B) Frontal section of rat hypothalamus stained with anti-LH-RH. (C) LH-RH-containing axons in the anterior hypothalamus of rat. (D) Sagittal section of rat hypothalamus stained with antisomatostatin. (E) Somatostatin-containing cells in rat anterior hypothalamus. From Reichlin.[52] Photographs courtesy of Dr. Lesley Alpert.

Two classes of tuberohypophyseal neurons project to the median eminence. Some are peptidergic (for example, TRH, LH-RH) and somatostatinergic (Fig. 6), and others are bioaminergic, the most important being dopaminergic.

Relationships of nerve ending, basement membrane, interstitial space, and capillary wall are identical in plan to those in the neural lobe, and thus the process of secretion at median-eminence terminals is probably analogous to the stimulus–secretion mechanism of the neurohypophysis. The large perivascular space contact area and the peculiar vessels in this region, which have fenestrations typical of those seen in ordinary endocrine glands, account for the observation that the neurohypophysis including the median eminence, unlike most of the brain, is particularly permeable to molecules such as thyroxine, trypan blue, and growth hormone.

The median eminence contains ten or more biologically active substances including several hypothalamic peptides, neurotransmitters (dopamine, norepinephrine, serotonin, acetylcholine, GABA, histamine), and a variety of other active substances. Most workers believe that there are no morphologically demonstrable synapses or axons in the median eminence. As Joseph and Knigge[7] point out:

> The extracellular and perivascular space of the median eminence would appear to be a medium of remarkable composition. Although some regional topography is emerging, the phenomenon of diffusion occurring after release alone would suggest that large pools of nerve terminals and nonneuronal elements are bathed in an interstitial fluid containing a multitude of hormones, and excitatory and inhibitory neurotransmitters.

In man, capillaries of the median eminence and stalk form loops that are part of spiral structures termed *gomitoli.* These penetrate the infundibulum and stalk. Arterioles of the stalk and median eminence of man have highly muscular walls, suggesting that hemodynamic changes in these vessels might affect pituitary function, but evidence to support this point of view is lacking. Reflex constriction of these vessels following postpartum hemorrhage has been suggested as a factor in the genesis of pituitary infarction. The pattern of distribution of blood to the hypothalamus and pituitary is discussed by Bergland and Page[20] and Daniel.[2]

Although classic studies have demonstrated that the direction of blood flow in the long portal vessels is from the hypothalamus to the pituitary, more recent work indicates that flow of blood from pituitary to median eminence can also occur. One consequence of this circular flow is that the hypothalamus is exposed to exceedingly high concentrations of the secretions of both anterior and posterior pituitary lobes.[12,20]

The epithelial component of the median eminence, the pars tuberalis, is in the form of a thin glandular sheath around the infundibulum and pituitary stalk. In some animals, the epithelial component may make up as much as 10% of the total glandular tissue of the pituitary, and several pituitary tropic hormones have been extracted from this region. Moreover, nerve fibers can be traced to the pars tuberalis. These findings to the contrary, the bulk of studies indicate that the pars tuberalis does not have an important physiological function, but serves merely as the region through which arteries and veins of the hypophyseal–portal circulation are conducted.

3.2. The Portal Vessel–Chemotransmitter Hypothesis and Hypophysiotropic Hormones

The hypophyseal portal–chemotransmitter hypothesis of pituitary control was introduced as an explanation of how the anterior pituitary gland, which is devoid of secretomotor nerve fibers, could be influenced by the nervous system. According to this hypothesis, neurohumoral substances released from nerve endings in the median eminence enter capillaries of the primary plexus of the hypophyseal–portal circulation and are carried by the portal veins of the hypophyseal stalk into the sinusoids of the pituitary.

Definitive proof of this hypothesis came when thyrotropic-hormone-releasing hormone (TRH) and luteinizing-hormone-releasing hormone (LH-RH) were chemically identified and shown to be present in hypophyseal–portal blood. These findings together with the demonstration of neurosecretory tuberohypophyseal neurons permit the conclusion that the portal-vessel chemotransmitter hypothesis has been fully validated. For their work on the elucidation of the chemistry of the hypophysiotropic hormones, Roger Guillemin and Andrew Schally were awarded Nobel Prizes in 1977.

The search for hypothalamic neurohumors with anterior-pituitary-regulating properties focused on extracts of stalk median eminence (SME) and hypothalamus. Hypophysiotropic materials that stimulate the release of pituitary hormones (see Fig. 8) have been called releasing *factors*, after the first description of corticotropin-releasing factor (CRF). At present, the term releasing *factor* is still applied to substances of unknown chemical nature, while those with established chemical identity, such as thyrotropin-releasing hormone (TRH) and luteinizing-hormone-releasing hormone (LRH), have been called releasing *hormones*. Use of the term "hypophysiotropic" or "releasing factor" to describe hypothalamic secretions regulating adenohypophyseal function is too restrictive. One such regulator is somatostatin, which *inhibits* growth hormone (GH) and thyroid-stimulating hormone (TSH) secretion. Another hypothalamic secretion that inhibits pituitary secretion is dopamine. The chemical structures of the three peptide pituitary regulating hormones thus far identified are shown in Fig. 7. Dopamine can also be included in the list of hypothalamic secretions that act directly on the pituitary, since it is present in portal-vessel blood in sufficient concentration to duplicate all its known effects on the pituitary gland.[21] Biological activities in hypothalamic extracts as yet uncharacterized chemically are shown in Table 1.

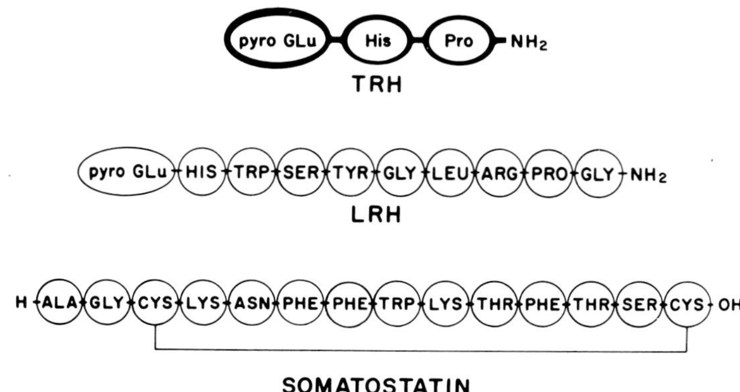

Fig. 7. Structure of established hypothalamic releasing hormones.

TABLE 1. Hypophysiotropic Hormones of Established Function but Unknown Structure (1979)

Name	Function
Corticotropin-releasing factor (CRF)	Releases ACTH[a]
Growth-hormone-releasing factor [(GRF), somatotropin-releasing factor (SRF)]	Releases GH[b]
Prolactin-releasing factor (PRF)	Releases prolactin[c]
Prolactin-inhibitory factor (PIF)	Inhibits prolactin release[d]
Melanocyte-stimulating-hormone-releasing factor (MSH-RF)	Stimulates MSH release[e]
Melanocyte-stimulating-hormone-inhibiting factor (MSH-IF)	Inhibits MSH release[e]

[a] A number of peptides will stimulate release of ACTH under certain conditions *in vivo* or *in vitro*. These include vasopressin and TRH. Neither of these peptides is believed to be an authentic CRF because of inconsistencies of response in several test systems.
[b] A number of amino acids and peptides will stimulate release of GH under certain conditions *in vivo* or *in vitro*. These include glucagon, MSH, β-endorphin, neurotensin, substance P, TRH, LH-RH, and a decapeptide isolated from porcine hypothalamic extracts that is chemically identical with the α-chain of porcine hemoglobin. None is now believed to be an authentic GRF because of inconsistencies of effects in various test systems, and because the GH-release system is relatively easily affected by nonspecific factors.
[c] TRH, a peptide of established structure, is a potent prolactin-releasing factor and has a role in maintenance of normal prolactin secretion, but is not the most potent releaser of prolactin found in hypothalamic extracts.
[d] Hypothalamic extracts contain two or more factors that inhibit prolactin release; one is dopamine, another GABA, and there may also be peptide(s).
[e] The actual status of MSH-regulatory hormones is very much in question. Recent physiological work indicates that the principal control over the intermediate lobe is mediated by inhibitory dopaminergic nerve fibers that end directly as secretomotor nerve terminals. Direct hypophyseal–portal blood supply to the intermediate lobe is relatively sparse.

Certain hypothalamic factors exert significant inhibitory actions on anterior pituitary function. Inhibitory factors interact with the respective releasing factor to exert dual control of secretion of prolactin, GH, TSH, and to a lesser extent the gonadotropins.

Contrary to expectations, the action of each of the hypophysiotropic hormones is not limited strictly to a single pituitary hormone. For example, thyroid-stimulating-hormone-releasing hormone (TRH) is a potent releaser of prolactin, and under some circumstances releases ACTH and GH. LH-RH releases both LH and follicle-stimulating hormone (FSH). Somatostatin inhibits secretion of GH, TSH, and a wide variety of other nonpituitary hormones. The principal inhibitor of prolactin secretion is dopamine, but this potent bioamine acting directly on the pituitary is also inhibitory to TSH and gonadotropin secretion, and under some circumstances is also inhibitory to GH secretion.

3.2.1. Thyrotropin-Releasing Hormone (TRH)

The chemical structure of TRH was elucidated by investigators working in association with Drs. Roger Guillemin and Andrew Schally. Their work, which was the culmination of more than a decade of effort to identify the nature of the thyrotropin-releasing activity of crude hypothalamic extracts, made neuroendocrinology credible to the general scientific and clinical community. It also made possible the introduction of TRH into clinical medicine, vastly widened the scope of understanding of TRH in other biological systems, and gave a powerful incentive to efforts to identify other biological activities in hypothalamic extract.

TRH is a relatively simple substance, a tripeptide amide, (pyro)Glu-His-Pro-NH_2 (Fig. 7). TRH is chemically stable, but is rapidly degraded in plasma by enzymatic action. Following injection in the human or in the rat, blood TSH levels rise rapidly and dramatically, a change being detected within 3 min; peak values are attained between 10 and 20 min after injection in normal individuals (Fig. 8), somewhat later in patients with pituitary or hypothalamic hypothyroidism. The standard clinical dose commonly administered as a bolus is 500 μg. Transient mild nausea, a sense of urinary urgency, and mild decreases or increases in blood pressure occur as side effects of injection in an appreciable number of patients, but no serious or life-threatening complications have been reported. The surge of TSH release induced by TRH injection leads to a readily detected rise in plasma triiodothyronine and an increase in thyroxine release that may not be large enough to produce significant increase in plasma levels of this hormone. The clinical applications of TRH testing are covered in detail in Chapter 11, and its role in neuroendocrine regulation of TSH secretion is discussed below.

One of the most important aspects of TRH action on the pituitary is that its effects are blocked by prior treatment with thyroid hormone. In fact, it is the interaction of the negative-feedback action of thyroxine on the pituitary with the stimulating effects of TRH that is the basis of the integrated neuroendocrine control system of TSH secretion. For this reason, TRH cannot be used as a diagnostic agent in patients receiving thyroid hormone replacement.

In addition to bringing about TSH release, TRH is also a potent prolactin-releasing factor (Fig. 8). The time course of response of blood prolactin levels to TRH, dose–response characteristics, and suppressibility by thyroid hormone pretreatment (all of which parallel changes in TSH secretion) make it seem likely that TRH is involved in the regulation of prolactin secretion.

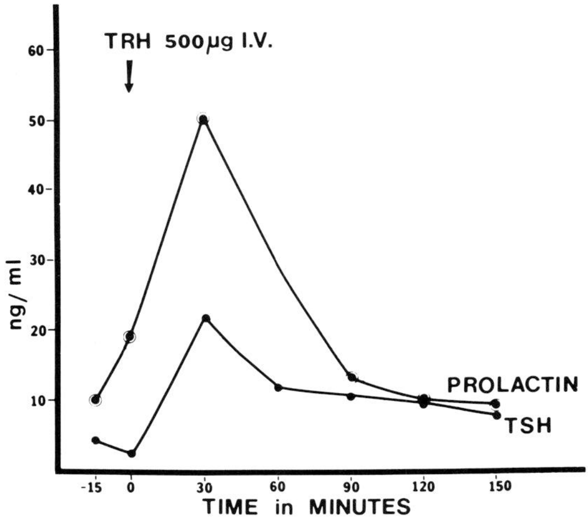

Fig. 8. Effect of TRH on plasma TSH and plasma prolactin levels.

However, despite these striking overlapping effects, the evidence suggests that TRH plays no more than a modulator role in prolactin regulation under normal circumstances.

TRH has no influence on pituitary hormones other than TSH and prolactin in normal individuals. However, under special circumstances, it exerts a number of other effects on pituitary secretion including the release of ACTH in some patients who have Cushing's disease[22] and of GH in some acromegalics (cf. Müller *et al.*[23,24]). These responses are thought to be due to the presence on pituitary cell membranes of TRH receptors ordinarily obscured by the normal regulatory processes of the pituitary or appearing as a consequence of "derepression" of the adenoma to a more primitive cell resembling an ancestral pituitary stem cell. TRH also releases GH in some patients with anorexia nervosa, in children with hypothyroidism, and in patients with psychotic depression.[23,24] TRH also inhibits sleep-induced GH release through a central nervous system mechanism and has other central nervous system effects (see below).

Extrahypothalamic Distribution and Function of TRH. One of the most surprising consequences of the development of specific methods for detection of TRH was its demonstration in brain tissue outside the classic "thyrotropic area" of the hypothalamus. TRH has been found by immunoassay or immunohistochemistry in virtually all parts of the brain, including the cerebral cortex, and spinal cord, in nerve endings abutting on the ventral horn motor cells, in the circumventricular structures, in the neurohypophysis, and in the pineal (for reviews, see Jackson and Reichlin[25] and Winokur and Utiger[26]). TRH has also been found in pancreatic islet cells and in various parts of the gastrointestinal tract. Although present in low concentrations in these areas, the aggregate in extrahypothalamic tissues exceeds the total amount in the hypothalamus. As the phylogenetic scale is descended, the concentration of TRH found in neural tissues outside the hypothalamus increases, so that in the frog, for example, the concentration in all extrahypothalamic brain is fully half that in the hypothalamus. In some species of frogs, TRH is found in the skin in concentrations higher than those found in the hypothalamus, an association presumed to be related to the embryological origin of skin cells in neuroectoderm. TRH has been detected in the most primitive vertebrate, the larval form of the lamprey; in the amphioxus, a provertebrate; and in snail nerve ganglia. Since the lamprey probably does not synthesize TSH, and amphioxus and snails lack a pituitary gland, it appears that the TRH molecule appeared in evolutionary development as a primitive neurosecretion prior to the development of TSH, and that the pituitary has "coopted" TRH as its regulatory hormone (for a review, see Jackson[27]). The same might be said for dopamine, which first appears in the nervous nets of the sponge, a primitive invertebrate.

The extensive extrahypothalamic distribution of TRH, its localization in nerve endings, and the presence of TRH receptors in brain tissue are strongly suggestive that it serves as a neurotransmitter or neuromodulator outside the hypothalamus (for reviews of its neurophysiological effects, see Barker[28] and Renaud *et al.*[29]).

When applied directly to a single neuron in the cortex, TRH suppresses spontaneous electrical activity, but appears to stimulate spinal motor neurons.

Neuropharmacological tests on experimental animals (even those hypophysectomized) indicate that TRH has a general stimulant activity[30] as shown by its reversal of barbituate sleeping time, enhancement of cerebral norepinephrine turnover, and enhancement of the excitatory action of dopamine in pargyline-pretreated mice. TRH also induces hyperthermia on central administration in the rat, suggesting a role in central thermoregulation. A number of authors have reported that TRH has a beneficial psychological effect in some depressed patients, but others have failed to confirm these findings.[30]

3.2.2. Gonadotropic-Hormone-Releasing Hormone [(GnRH), Luteinizing-Hormone-Releasing Hormone (LH-RH)]

It has been known for more than 20 years from the work of McCann and of Harris and their respective collaborators that extracts of hypothalamic tissue contained one or more biologically active substances capable of stimulating the release of gonadotropic hormones from the pituitary. This material was isolated in almost pure form from the hypothalami of stockyard animals by Guillemin and by Schally and their collaborators, and the structure was finally elucidated by Schally's group in 1971[31] (see Fig. 7).

Following intravenous injection, the naturally occuring LH-RH or its synthetic form brings about a prompt dose-related release of LH and FSH in man

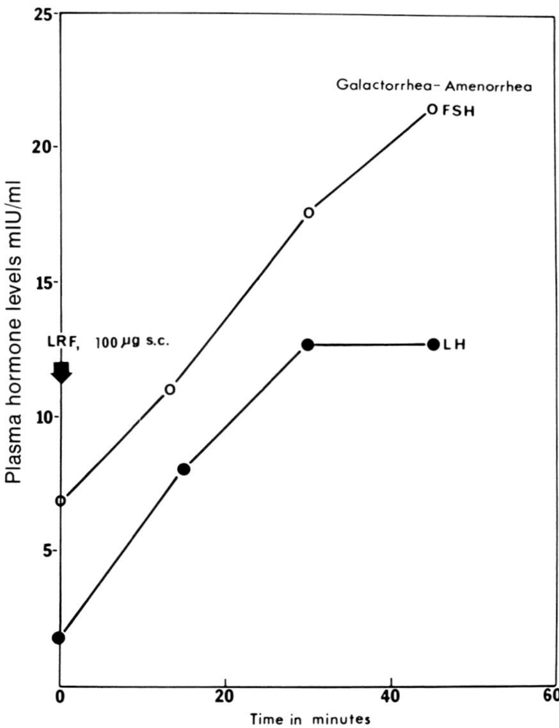

Fig. 9. Effect of LH-RH on release of gonadotropins in man.

(Fig. 9). The onset of effect on FSH release after a single bolus injection is somewhat delayed as compared with effects on LH secretion, the values peaking at 10–30 min after injection. The response to LH-RH is markedly influenced by the prior LH-RH secretory state, by the steroid milieu of the patient, by the time course of LH-RH injection, i.e., single dose, multiple pulses, or constant infusion, and perhaps by the patient's sex. Through secondary effects of pituitary activation, and under appropriately defined conditions, LH-RH can induce spermatogenesis and testosterone production in men with hypothalamic hypogonadotropic hypogonadism and ovulation in women with hypothalamic amenorrhea (for reviews, see Mortimer,[32] Frohman,[33] and Yen).[34]

Most reproductive neuroendocrinologists now believe that the LH-RH decapeptide is the only hypothalamic gonadotropin regulator and that observed dissociations of secretion are due to the interacting effects of prior hormone status, steroid pretreatment, and history of exposure to LH-RH, but some observations still cannot be explained by this unitary hypothesis.

Extrahypothalamic Distribution and Function of GnRH. Unlike TRH and somatostatin, almost all the GnRH in the brain is restricted to the hypothalamus and related neural structures. Small amounts are found in the circumventricular organs, including the pineal gland.[35,36] LH-RH (as in the case for TRH) has also been found in milk, suggesting that the breast, a dermal-derived structure with embryological origins analogous to the primitive neuroectoderm, which is the source of neuroendocrine cells generally, may have LH-RH-synthesizing capacity. The possibility that the breast concentrates LH-RH from the blood also has to be considered. On direct application to individual nerve cells, LH-RH from the blood also has to be considered. On direct application to individual nerve cells, LH-RH can enhance or depress certain populations of cells.[28,29] Even though this peptide is found in a very restricted area, responding cells are localized in many other areas of the brain. The most important neural effects of LH-RH appear to be those involved in regulation of mating behavior.[37] Direct injection of LH-RH into the hypothalamus has been reported to enhance female sexual responsivity even in animals lacking a pituitary and hence incapable of responding with gonadotropin–ovarian activation. The effects on sexual function in man are being investigated. There is evidence that LH-RH can stimulate sexual function in man unrelated to activation of pituitary function (cf. Moss *et al.*[37]).

3.2.3. Somatostatin

During the course of efforts to isolate GRF from hypothalamic extracts, Krulich and McCann discovered a fraction that inhibited GH release from pituitary incubates *in vitro*. They named the factor "growth-hormone-release-inhibitory factor" (GIF), and postulated that GH secretion was regulated by a dual control system, one stimulatory, the other inhibitory. Relatively little attention was paid to GIF when first discovered because it was thought by most workers to be a relatively nonspecific effect. Several years later, in 1973, Brazeau and a number of collaborators working in Guillemin's laboratory on the attempted isolation of GRF again identified the inhibitory factor, and with the background in methodology gained from earlier studies of TRH and LH-

RH were able in a relatively short time to isolate and identify a potent peptide from hypothalamic extracts that inhibited GH release in every assay system in which it was studied (for reviews, see Reichlin *et al.*[38] and Vale *et al.*[39]). The material, to which the name "somatostatin" was applied, is a 14-amino-acid peptide, lacking the amide and pyroglutamic acid termini that are characteristic of LH-RH and TRH, but containing an S–S cyclic bridge similar to that of vasopressin and oxytocin (see Fig. 7). That somatostatin is important as a physiological regulator of GH release is shown by studies in which the somatostatinergic pathways are damaged or endogenous somatostatin neutralized by treatment with antisomatostatin antibody.

Shortly after chemically synthesized somatostatin became available for study, it was found to inhibit the secretion of TSH, of glucagon, and of insulin (cf. Gerich and Lorenzi[40]). Subsequently, somatostatin has been shown to inhibit the secretion of many other secretory structures in the body (including virtually all the glands of the gastrointestinal tract) (cf. Arimura *et al.*[41]) (Table 2). Contemporary studies of somatostatin content of body tissues, carried out by radioimmunoassay and immunohistochemistry, showed that most tissues that respond to somatostatin contain this peptide in specialized neurosecretory cells. Thus, somatostatin, originally isolated from the hypothalamus, has been shown to be a widely distributed tissue component that in some settings acts as a paracrine secretion ("control of one cell by secretions of an adjacent tissue") and in others as a neuroendocrine secretion (as in the tuberohypophyseal neurons of the hypothalamus) (cf. Guillemin[42]).

Of the hypophysiotropic hormones thus far isolated, somatostatin has the highest extrahypothalamic concentration, both in other parts of the central nervous system and in extraneural structures, especially the gastrointestinal tract. In general, the major direct effect of somatostatin on nerve cells is to depress spontaneous activity.[28,29] In dorsal root ganglia, it probably modifies

TABLE 2. Glandular Secretions Inhibited by Somatostatin

Pituitary	GH TSH
Pancreas	Glucagon Insulin Vasoactive intestinal peptide (VIP)
Gastrointestinal tract	Gastrin Gastric acid VIP Cholecystokinin-pancreazymin Bombesin Motilin Secretin
Kidney	Renin
Thyroid	Calcitonin Thyroxine

centrally directed pain impulses by regulating substance P release in the dorsal root entry zone of the spinal cord. The physiological role of somatostatin in brain function remains to be elucidated.

3.2.4. Corticotropin-Releasing Factor (CRF)

Although CRF was the first of the releasing factors to be recognized and named by Saffran and Schally, its chemical nature is still unknown (for a review, see Krieger and Zimmerman[43]). A substance acting to release ACTH has been isolated from blood draining the primary portal plexus. Evidence has also been presented that CRF enters the general circulation and the cerebrospinal fluid. This material disappears after destruction of the "adrenotropic" region of the hypothalamus. Stress has also been shown to deplete the median eminence of CRF activity, and a few patients treated with purified hypothalamic fractions have responded with a rise in plasma corticoid levels, an effect thought to be due to induce ACTH release.

Vasopressin was initially thought by some to be CRF because it is secreted during stress and releases ACTH both *in vivo* and *in vitro* and because hypothalamic lesions that cause diabetes also block reflex ACTH discharge. However, several lines of evidence indicate that although vasopressin may under certain circumstances serve as *a* CRF, it is not *the* CRF.

3.2.5. Prolactin-Regulatory Factors (PIF, PRF)

In keeping with the observation that the hypothalamus exerts an *inhibitory* effect on prolactin secretion is the observation that hypothalamic extracts contain one or more substances inhibitory to prolactin release. This activity was termed "prolactin-inhibitory factor" (PIF) by Meites and collaborators. PIF had been identified in portal-vessel blood by Kamberi, Porter, and their collaborators, again satisfying the critical requirement of evidence for physiological significance of a hypophysiotropic hormone (for reviews, see Porter *et al.*,[12] Reichlin *et al.*,[38] and Vale *et al.*[39]).

Dopamine is the most important PIF. This biogenic amine, the secretory product of the tuberohypophyseal dopaminergic pathways, has recently been shown to be present in hypophyseal–portal vessel blood in sufficient concentration to inhibit prolactin release.[21] γ Aminobutyric acid (GABA), a constituent of hypothalamic extracts, is also an active PIF, but its presence in portal-vessel blood in appropriate concentrations has not yet been established. Several groups have also claimed that there is at least one additional PIF activity, distinct from the two that have already been mentioned. Dopamine alone can explain all the known prolactin-inhibitory functions of the hypothalamus, though not all the PIF activity of hypothalamic extracts.

Although the stalk section and transplantation experiments indicate that the predominant effect of the hypothalamus on prolactin secretion is inhibitory, the acute release of prolactin seen after suckling and acute stress have raised the possibility that there is a prolactin-releasing factor. Crude and partially purified extracts of hypothalamic tissue bring about the release of prolactin. Several well-characterized hypothalamic peptides also release prolactin on systematic injection. These include vasopressin, TRH, neurotensin, substance P, and β-endorphin (for reviews, see Müller *et al.*[24] and Boyd and Reichlin[44]). The effects of crude extracts have been shown to be independent of their content of ADH and TRH, but the other factors have not been excluded as the active substance. Further, the extent to which these factors are active by direct action on the pituitary, or by stimulation via the hypothalamus, is still not fully resolved.

4. Regulation of Secretion of the Tuberohypophyseal Neurons: Neuropharmacology of Hypothalamic Regulation

As outlined in previous sections, the tuberohypophyseal neurons form the "final common pathway" of neural control of the anterior pituitary and thereby serve as the ultimate neuroendocrine transducer. This group of neurons is acted on by the feedback effects of hormones secreted by target glands, such as the sex steroids, thyroid hormone, and cortisol, by pituitary peptide hormones (short-loop feedback control), by classic neurotransmitters (through which communication from the rest of the brain is mediated), and by neuropeptide modulators. This complex set of controls is integrated at the neuronal level for the regulation of anterior pituitary secretion (for reviews, see Hökfelt *et al.*,[6] Müller *et al.*,[24] and Weiner and Ganong[45]).

4.1. Neurotransmitter Regulation of Hypophysiotropic Neurons

The function of central bioaminergic neurotransmitters is of enormous importance for the understanding of psychiatric disease, of behavior, and of effect as well as control of the pituitary.

The structures of the important hypothalamic neurotransmitters are illustrated in Fig. 10.

4.1.1. Dopaminergic Pathways

An important group of bioaminergic neurons involved in anterior pituitary regulation arise mainly in the arcuate nucleus of the hypothalamus and are distributed to the median eminence (Fig. 11). This grouping, termed the "dopaminergic tuberohypophyseal system," is important mainly for its func-

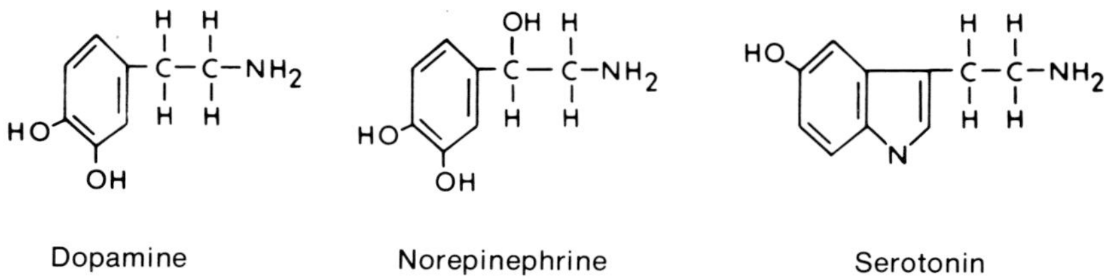

Fig. 10. Structure of principal monoaminergic neurotransmitters involved in hypophsiotropic hormone control.

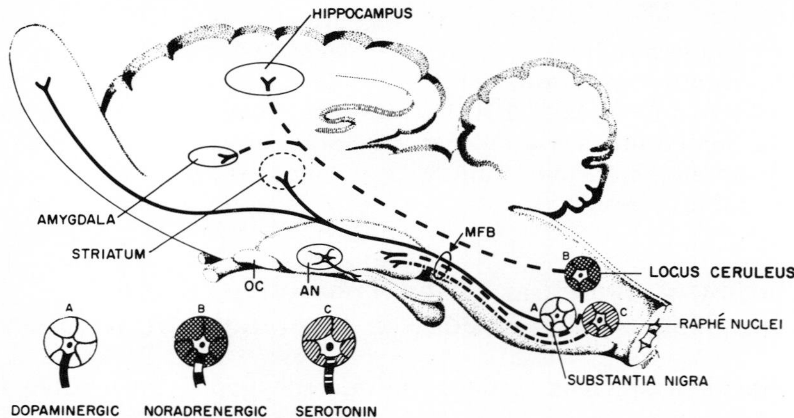

Fig. 11. Schematic outline of ascending monoaminergic pathways in the mammalian brain. The principal localization of the neurons containing norepinephrine, dopamine, and serotonin is in the mesencephalon and pons. Axons of these cells are distributed to widespread areas of the cortex, limbic system, and striatum. The dopaminergic system of the arcuate is an exception to the general system of distribution. (MFB) Medial forebrain bundle; (AN) arcuate nucleus; (OC) optic chiasm. From Martin *et al.*[5]; reproduced with permission of the F.A. Davis Company.

tion in direct control of anterior pituitary secretion. Two other relatively independent dopaminergic systems have also been identified. The best known, and the earliest to be recognized by neurologists, is that involved in extrapyramidal control, namely, the nigrostriatal pathways, which arise in the substantia nigra in the hindbrain, and are distributed to the caudate nucleus and other structures in the forebrain. Parkinson's disease is due to defects in this system. The third dopaminergic system arises in cells adjacent to the hypothalamus and projects to several hypothalamic regulatory areas. Dopaminergic neurotransmitters may be of importance by producing either direct effects on the pituitary or indirect effects on other tuberoinfundibular neurons (or both). This complexity of input underlines the problem of utilizing dopamine agonists and antagonists for analyzing the neuropharmacological coding of anterior pituitary regulation.

4.1.2. Noradrenergic Pathways[11]

All the cell bodies of origin of the noradrenergic pathways arise outside the hypothalamus in several nuclear groups in the hindbrain, the most conspicuous of which is the locus ceruleus, a cell grouping found in the floor of the fourth ventricle. From the locus ceruleus, noradrenergic fibers ascend to the hypothalamus and other midbrain and forebrain structures and descend into the spinal cord. The bulk of noradrenergic fibers involved in neuroendocrine control arise from areas adjacent to the locus ceruleus and also from cells anatomically close to the nucleus of the vagus nerve. These ascend in defined anatomical pathways and terminate on cell bodies of tuberohypophyseal neurons, neurohypophyseal neurons, and within the median eminence itself.

4.1.3. Serotonergic Pathways[11]

Most of the serotonergic neurons project to the hypothalamus from cell bodies located in the brainstem (raphe nuclei). They are extensively distributed to neurons, and to a lesser extent to the median eminence, and ependymal cells. Serotonin-containing nerve endings ramify over the ventricular surface of the brain. An intrinsic serotonin pathway within the hypothalamus analogous to the tuberohypophyseal dopamine pathway probably exists.

Dopamine, serontonin, and noradrenaline pathways are the principal control systems, but recent work has demonstrated the presence of adrenergic and histaminergic neural control systems. The cell bodies arise for the most part in hindbrain regions, but there are also smaller intrinsic bioaminergic systems self-contained in the hypothalamus.

4.1.4. Cholinergic Control

Tuberoinfundibular control is also exerted by cholinergic neurons.

Choline acetyltransferase, an enzyme marker of acetylcholine synthesis, is distributed in all defined nuclei in the hypothalamus, including the arcuate, and in the median eminence, two regions especially related to anterior pituitary control. Because only small changes have been noted in medial basal hypothalamic concentration of choline acetyltransferase after surgical isolation of this region of the brain, it has been proposed that there is "a cholinergic tuberoinfundibular pathway similar to the dopaminergic one, which may be responsible for the neuroendocrine effects of cholinergic agents."[23]

GABA has also been demonstrated in fairly high concentration in the hypothalamus and median eminence, and the presence of GABA-sensitive neurons has been demonstrated by microiontophoresis in the hypothalamic ventromedial nucleus as well as other sites in the "endocrine hypothalamus."

Neuropeptides with hypothalamic distribution of nerve endings are substance P, met-enkephalin (an endorphin), angiotensin II, neurotensin, gastrin, and cholecystokinin. The findings of met-enkephalin-containing cell bodies in the hypothalamus and a median eminence distribution supports the presence of an intrinsic control system for this peptide as well as a system with projections from other parts of the brain.

When called on to explain neural control of anterior pituitary secretion, the contemporary neuroendocrinologist suffers from an embarrassment of riches with regard to potential neurohumoral mediators. Summarized in Table 3 are the overall effects of the various classes of neurotransmitters and other hypothalamic regulators on anterior pituitary regulation. It should be borne in mind that a given effect of an agonist or antagonist may be due to direct or indirect effects on other regulatory systems and that many of the findings are not uniform in all studies in all animals and under all conditions.

4.2. Endocrine Significance of Neuropeptides

In addition to the enkephalins and the hypophysiotropic peptides, a number of other peptides have been demonstrated to occur in neurons distrib-

TABLE 3. Neurotransmitters and Anterior Pituitary Section[a]

Anterior pituitary secretion	Neurotransmitters[b]					
	NE	DA	5-HT	ACh	H	GABA
ACTH	↓→	↓→	↑	↑	↑	↓
TSH	↑	↓	↓	→	—	—
LH/FSH	↑	↑↓	↓→	↑	↑	↑
GH	↑	↑	↑	→	→	→↓
PRL	↑↓	↓	↑	↓↑	↑	↓↑

[a] Adapted from Müller *et al.*[49] and Weiner and Ganong.[45] Symbols: (↑) increase; (↓) decrease; (→) no change; (—) not known. The effects of various neurotransmitters is inferred from neuropharmacological studies using agonists, antagonists, and precursors. It must be *emphasized* that there are many inconsistencies and contradictions in the literature. These are due in part to species differences, prior functional status, lack of specificity of some drugs, and direct pituitary effects differing from hypothalamic effects.

[b] (NE) Norepinephrine (noradrenaline); (DA) dopamine; (5-HT) 5-hydroxytryptamine (serotonin); (ACh) acetylcholine; (H) histamine; (GABA) γ-amino-butyric acid.

uted in the hypothalamus and other brain regions (cf. Brownstein,[35] Brownstein *et al.*,[36] Reichlin *et al.*,[38] and Iversen *et al.*[46]). Almost all are represented in characteristic glandular cells of the gastrointestinal tract, believed to arise in embryological life from the primitive neuroectoderm.[10]

5. Interaction of the Hypothalamic–Pituitary Unit with Feedback Control by Target-Gland Secretions

Although the foregoing discussion has emphasized the close interaction of hypothalamus and pituitary, it must be emphasized that these interactions are but part of a larger control system in which hormones also play a regulatory role (cf. Martin *et al.*,[5] Reichlin,[47] and Labrie *et al.*[48]). TSH secretion is regulated by the negative-feedback effects of circulating thyroid hormone acting directly on the pituitary (pituitary–thyroid axis), and the positive stimulatory effect of TRH. Somatostatin also inhibits TSH secretion, as hypothalamic dopaminergic neurons. ACTH secretion is regulated by the negative-feedback effects of cortisol acting directly on the pituitary (pituitary–adrenal axis), interacting with the positive-drive effects of CRF. Cortisol may also exert negative-feedback influences on CRF secretion. The gonadotropic hormones are regulated by the gonadal secretions. In women, estrogens (the product of the ovary) have two kinds of effects. They may exert a negative-feedback effect, manifested by the rise in gonadotropin secretion that follows castration, and a positive-feedback effect, manifested by the surge in gonadotropin secretion observed at midcycle or following a pulse of estrogen stimulation. Estrogens act at both the hypothalamic and the pituitary level. In men, testosterone acts to tonically inhibit pituitary secretion of gonadotropins, both through the hypothalamus and, to a variable extent, on the pituitary directly. GH, which has no specific peripheral target organ, is believed to exert a "short-loop" feedback control on its own secretion, acting through a hypothalamic target. Prolactin, which like GH also lacks a specific target organ, also acts on the hypothalamus to inhibit the prolactin-regulatory hormones.

These interactions may account for the pathogenesis of some pituitary tumors (see Chapter 2), and they permit a wide variety of physiologically based tests of pituitary function, useful prior to surgery to evaluate the nature and extent of the disorder, and after surgery to evaluate the need for specific hormone replacement.

ACKNOWLEDGMENT. Studies from the author's laboratory alluded to in this article were supported by U.S.P.H.S. Grants #2R01 AM 16684 and #5T32 AM 07039.

References

1. D.M. Rioch, G.W. Wislocki, and J.L. O'Leary, A precis of preoptic, hypothalamic and hypophysial terminology with atlas, in: *The Hypothalamus* (Proceedings of the Association for Research in Nervous and Mental Disease), pp. 3–30, Hafner, New York, 1939.
2. P.M. Daniel, The anatomy of the hypothalamus and pituitary gland, in *Neuroendocrinology*, Vol. 1 (L. Martini and W.F. Ganong, eds.), pp. 15–80, Academic Press, New York, 1966.
3. H. Kobayashi and T. Matsui, Fine structure of the median eminence and its functional significance, in: *Frontiers in Neuroendocrinology* (W.F. Ganong and L. Martini, eds.), pp. 3–46, Oxford University Press, London, 1969.
4. W.E. Stumpf and L.D. Grant (eds.), *Anatomical Neuroendocrinology*, S. Karger, Basel, 1975.
5. J.B. Martin, S. Reichlin, and G.M. Brown, *Clinical Neuroendocrinology*, F.A. Davis, Philadelphia, 1977.
6. T. Hökfelt, R. Elde, K. Fuxe, O. Johansson, Ä. Ljungdahl, M. Goldstein, R. Luft, S. Efendic, G. Nilsson, L. Terenius, D. Ganten, S.L. Jeffcoate, J. Rehfeld, S. Said, M. Perez de la Mora, L. Possani, R. Tapia, L. Teran, and R. Palacios, Aminergic and peptidergic pathways in the nervous system with special reference to the hypothalamus, in: *The Hypothalamus* (S. Reichlin, R.J. Baldessarini, and J.B. Martin, eds.), pp. 60–135, Raven Press, New York, 1978.
7. S.A. Joseph and K.M. Knigge, The endocrine hypothalamus: Recent anatomical studies, in: *The Hypothalamus* (S. Reichlin, R.J. Baldessarini, and J.B. Martin, eds.), pp. 15–47, Raven Press, New York, 1978.
8. K.M. Knigge, S.A. Joseph, and G.E. Hoffman, Organization of LRH- and SRIF-neurons in the endocrine hypothalamus, in: *The Hypothalamus* (S. Reichlin, R.J. Baldessarini, and J.B. Martin, eds.), pp. 49–67, Raven Press, New York, 1978.
9. R. Defendini and E.A. Zimmerman, The magnocellular neurosecretory system of the mammalian hypothalamus, in: *The Hypothalamus* (S. Reichlin, R.J. Baldessarini, and J.B. Martin, eds.), pp. 137–152, Raven Press, New York, 1978.
10. A.G.E. Pearse and T. Takor Takor, Neuroendocrine embryology and the APUD concept, *Clin. Endocrinol. Suppl.* **5**:229–244, 1976.
11. K.G. Wingstrand, Microscopic anatomy, nerve supply and blood supply of the pars intermedia, in: *The Pituitary Gland*, Vol. 3 (G.W. Harris and B.T. Donovan, eds.), pp. 1–27, Butterworths, London, 1966.
12. J.C. Porter, R.L. Eskay, C. Oliver, N. Ben-Jonathan, J. Warberg, C.R. Parker, Jr., and A. Barnea, Release of hypothalamic hormones under *in vivo* and *in vitro* conditions, in: *Hypothalamic Peptide Hormones and Pituitary Regulation* (J.C. Porter, ed.), pp. 181–202, Plenum Press, New York, 1977.
13. S.J. Watson, C.W. Richard, III, and J.D. Barchas, Adrenocorticotropin in rat brain: Immunocytochemical localization in cells and axons, *Science* **200**:1180–1182, 1978.

14. G. Pelletier and R. Leclerc, Immunohistochemical localization of adrenocorticotropin in the rat brain, *Endocrinology* **104:**1426–1433, 1979.
15. J.N. Hayward, Functional and morphological aspects of hypothalamic neurons, *Physiol. Rev.* **57:**574–658, 1977.
16. D. Ganten, K. Fuxe, M.I. Phillips, J.F.E. Mann, and U. Ganten, The brain isorenin–angiotensin system: Biochemistry, localization and possible role in drinking and blood pressure regulation, in: *Frontiers in Neuroendocrinology,* Vol. 5 (W.F. Ganong and L. Martini, eds.), pp. 61–100, Raven Press, New York, 1978.
17. M. Rundgren and Fyhrquist Frej, Transient water diuresis and syndrome of inappropriate antidiuretic hormone secretion (SIADH) induced by forebrain lesions of different location, *Acta Physiol. Scand.* **103:**421–429, 1978.
18. S. Reichlin, Medical progress; Neuroendocrinology, *N. Engl. J. Med.* **269:**1246–1250 and 1296–1303, 1963.
19. G. Fink, The development of the releasing factor concept, *Clin. Endocrinol.* **5** (Suppl.):245s–260s, 1976.
20. R.M. Bergland and R.B. Page, Pituitary–brain vascular relations: A new paradigm, *Science* **204:**18–24, 1979.
21. D.M. Gibbs and J.D. Neill, Dopamine levels in hypophysial stalk blood in the rat are sufficient to inhibit prolactin secretion *in vivo, Endocrinology* **102:**1895–1900, 1978.
22. D.I. Krieger and E.M. Condon, Cyproheptadine treatment of Nelson's syndrome: Restoration of plasma ACTH circadian periodicity and reversal of response to TRF, *J. Clin. Endocrinol. Metab.* **46:**349–352, 1978.
23. E.E. Müller, G. Nistico, and U. Scapagnini, *Neurotransmitters and Anterior Pituitary Function,* Academic Press, New York, 1977.
24. E.E. Müller, D. Cocchi, V. Locatelli, E.A. Parati, and P. Mantegazza, Neurotransmitter control of growth hormone and prolactin secretion, in: *Central Regulation of the Endocrine System* (K. Fuxe, T. Hökfelt, and R. Luft, eds.), pp. 417–456, Plenum Press, New York, 1979.
25. I.M.D. Jackson and S. Reichlin, Distribution and biosynthesis of TRH in the nervous system, in: *Central Nervous System Effects of Hypothalamic Hormones and Other Peptides* (R. Collu, A. Barbeau, J.R. Ducharme, and J.-G. Rochefort, eds.), pp. 3–54, Raven Press, New York, 1979.
26. A. Winokur and R.D. Utiger, Thyrotropin-releasing hormone in the central nervous system: Distribution and degradation, in: *Central Nervous System Effects of Hypothalamic Hormones and Other Peptides* (R. Collu, A. Barbeau, J.R. Ducharme, and J.-G. Rochefort, eds.), pp. 55–73, Raven Press, New York, 1979.
27. I.M.D. Jackson, Phylogenetic distribution and function of the hypophysiotropic hormones of the hypothalamus, *Am. Zool.* **18:**385–399, 1978.
28. J.L. Barker, Physiological roles of peptides in the nervous system, in: *Peptides in Neurobiology* (H. Gainer, ed.), pp. 295–344, Plenum Press, New York, 1977.
29. L.P. Renaud, Q.J. Pittman, H.W. Blume, Y. Lamour, and E. Arnauld, Effects of peptides on central neuronal excitability, in: *Central Nervous System Effects of Hypothalamic Hormones and Other Peptides* (R. Collu, A. Barbeau, J.R. Ducharme, and J.-G. Rochefort, eds.), pp. 147–161, Raven Press, New York, 1979.
30. A.J. Prange, Jr., C.B. Nemeroff, P.T. Loosen, G. Bissette, A.J. Osbahr, III, I.C. Wilson, and M.A. Lipton, Behavioural effects of thyrotropin-releasing hormone in animals and man: A review, in: *Central Nervous System Effects of Hypothalamic Hormones and Other Peptides* (R. Collu, A. Barbeau, J.R. Ducharme, and J.-G. Rochefort, eds.), pp. 75–96, Raven Press, New York, 1979.
31. A.V. Schally, Aspects of hypothalamic regulation of the pituitary gland, *Science* **202:**18–28, 1978.
32. C.H. Mortimer, Gonadotropin-releasing hormone, in: *Clinical Neuroendocrinology* (L. Martini and G.M. Besser, eds.), pp. 213–236, Academic Press, New York, 1977.
33. L.A. Frohman, New understanding of human hypothalamic pituitary disease obtained through the use of synthetic hypothalamic hormones, in: *The Hypothalamus* (S. Reichlin, R.J. Baldessarini, and J.B. Martin, eds.), pp. 387–413, Raven Press, New York, 1978.
34. S.S.C. Yen, The human menstrual cycle (integrative function of the hypothalamic–pituitary–ovarian–endometrial axis), in: *Reproductive Endocrinology* (S.S.C. Yen and R.B. Jaffe, eds.), pp. 126–151, W.B. Saunders, Philadelphia, 1978.

35. M.J. Brownstein, Biologically active peptides in the mammalian central nervous system, in: *Peptides in Neurobiology* (H. Gainer, ed.), pp. 145–170, Plenum Press, New York, 1977.
36. M.J. Brownstein, M. Palkovits, J.M. Saavedra, and J.S. Kizer, Distribution of hypothalamic hormones and neurotransmitters within the diencephalon, in: *Frontiers in Neuroendocrinology*, Vol. 4 (L. Martini and W.F. Ganong, eds.), pp. 1–23, Raven Press, New York, 1976.
37. R.L. Moss, P. Riskand, and C. Dudley, The effects of LH-RH on sexual activities in animals and man, in: *Central Nervous System Effects of Hypothalamic Hormones and Other Peptides* (R. Collu, A. Barbeau, J. Ducharme, and J.-G. Rochefort, eds.), pp. 345–366, Raven Press, New York, 1979.
38. S. Reichlin, R. Saperstein, I.M.D. Jackson, A.E. Boyd, III, and Y. Patel, Hypothalamic hormones, *Annu. Rev. Physiol.* **38**:389–424, 1976.
39. W. Vale, C. Rivier, and M. Brown, Regulatory peptides of the hypothalamus, *Annu. Rev. Physiol.* **39**:473–527, 1977.
40. J.E. Gerich and M. Lorenzi, The role of the automatic nervous system and somatostatin in the control of insulin and glucagon secretion, in: *Frontiers in Neuroendocrinology*, Vol. 5 (W.F. Ganong and L. Martini, eds.), pp. 265–288, Raven Press, New York, 1978.
41. A. Arimura, D.H. Coy, M. Chihara, R. Fernandez-Durango, E. Samols, K. Chihara, C.A. Meyers, and A.V. Schally, Somatostatin, in: *Gut Hormones* (S.R. Bloom, ed.), pp. 437–445, Churchill Livingstone, Edinburgh, 1978.
42. R. Guillemin, Biochemical and physiological correlates of hypothalamic peptides: The new endocrinology of the neuron, in: *The Hypothalamus* (S. Reichlin, R.J. Baldessarini, and J.B. Martin, eds.), pp. 155–194, Raven Press, New York, 1978.
43. D.T. Krieger and E.A. Zimmerman, The nature of CRF and its relationship to vasopressin, in: *Clinical Neuroendocrinology* (L. Martini and G.M. Besser, eds.), pp. 364–392, Academic Press, New York, 1977.
44. A.E. Boyd, III, and S. Reichlin, Neural control of prolactin secretion in man, *Psychoneuroendocrinology* **3**:113–130, 1978.
45. R.I. Weiner and W.F. Ganong, Role of brain monoamines and histamine in regulation of anterior pituitary secretion, *Physiol. Rev.* **58**:905–976, 1978.
46. L.L. Iversen, R.A. Nicoll, and W.W. Vale, Neurobiology of peptides, *Neurosci. Res. Prog. Bull.* **16**(2):19, 1978.
47. S. Reichlin, Neuroendocrinology, in: *Textbook of Endocrinology* (R.H. Williams, ed.), pp. 774–831, W.B. Saunders, Philadelphia, 1974.
48. F. Labrie, J. Drouin, L. Lagace, L. Ferland, H. Beaulieu, V. Raymond, and J. Massicotte, Interactions between hypothalamic and peripheral hormones at the anterior pituitary level, in: *Central Regulation of the Endocrine System* (K. Fuxe, T. Hökfelt, and R. Luft, eds.), pp. 85–107, Plenum Press, New York, 1979.
49. E.E. Müller, G. Nistico, and U. Scapagnini, *Neurotransmitters and Anterior Pituitary Function*, Academic Press, New York, 1978.
50. V.L. Gay, The hypothalamus: Physiology and clinical use of releasing factors, *Fertil. Steril.* **23**:50, 1972.
51. W. Bargmann and E. Scharrer, The site of origin of the hormones of the posterior pituitary, *Am. Sci.* **39**:255–259, 1951.
52. S. Reichlin, Neural control of the pituitary gland: Normal physiology and pathophysiological implications, in: *Current Concepts*, pp. 1–59, Upjohn, Kalamazoo, Mich., 1978.

2

Etiology of Pituitary Adenomas

SEYMOUR REICHLIN

1. Introduction

Although pituitary adenomas have been found by routine autopsy study to be surprisingly common, their emergence as clinical problems is far less frequent. The factors that determine the incidence of adenoma and their growth are the subject of this chapter.

Systematic surveys of pituitaries of patients dying of various causes have shown an incidence as high as 22.6% (some with multiple tumors)[1] and as low as 8.8%.[2] Virtually all these tumors were unsuspected during life, although it must be emphasized that appropriate diagnostic studies were not carried out in these patients during life. The incidence increased with age. Using standard staining methods, Costello[1] classified the majority of the tumors as chromophobes (52.8%), the remaining being eosinophilic (7.5%), basophilic (27.2%), and mixed (12.4%). Adequate surveys of large series using specific antisera have not been published, but there is sufficient information from newer approaches to indicate that most of the chromophobe cells are in fact secretory.[2–4] In the studies of Conway *et al.*,[5] blood obtained from the tumor bed of a series of patients with chromophobe adenoma was rich in several anterior pituitary hormones, and more recently, Lipson *et al.*[6] have shown by tissue culture study that of 30 chromophobe adenomas, every one secreted at least one hormone, and one tumor had all six known anterior pituitary hormones. The high frequency of adenomas found at autopsy is in contrast to the relative low frequency presenting clinically. Pituitary adenomas make up about 10% of intracranial tumors, and brain tumors account for 1.7% of all cancer in the United States.[7] Of those coming to surgery in one clinic,[4] approximately 39% were prolactin (PRL)-secreting, 4% ACTH-secreting, 33% growth hormone (GH)-secreting, and 21% apparently nonsecretory. If one considers the incidence on the basis of clinical presentation, the overwhelm-

SEYMOUR REICHLIN • Tufts University School of Medicine; Division of Endocrinology, Department of Medicine, Tufts–New England Medical Center Hospital, Boston, Massachusetts 02111.

ing majority would be prolactinomas, with acromegaly relatively uncommon. In part, the relative infrequency of clinically apparent pituitary adenoma may be a function of available diagnostic tests. For example, the introduction of PRL radioimmunoassay by Friesen and his colleagues led to the recognition that many of the tumors that had previously been called chromophobic were in fact PRL-secreting, and that many cases of unexplained amenorrhea (even those unaccompanied by galactorrhea) were in fact due to PRL hypersecretion.[8]

It is still unknown whether the recent increase in diagnosed prolactinomas is due to improved diagnostic recognition or to some factor, such as the widespread use of contraceptive pills, that has increased the growth of tumor.[9]

In a recent unpublished survey from this clinic, Dr. Richard Goodman and his collaborators observed an incidence of 30% of abnormal pituitary sellas by polytomography in women systematically surveyed for the presence of galactorrhea without any evidence of pituitary disorder as determined by a battery of endocrine diagnostic tests. These findings can be interpreted to indicate that the incidence is the same as that previously shown in autopsy studies (cited above) or is an indication of lack of preciseness of currently available X-ray diagnostic procedures. Since many patients with microprolactinomas have been shown to have normal X rays at some time during the course of their disease (Chapter 4), it is likely that the incidence of the disorder is in fact underestimated.

2. Insights into the Pathogenesis of Adenoma Based on Embryological Considerations

Since the abnormal hyperplasia and growth of adenomas appear as an aberration of normal developmental sequences, one must first seek an etiological basis in embryogenesis. Since the time of Rathke, the adenohypophysis has been traditionally considered to be derived from an evagination of buccal ectoderm that takes up its place in close apposition to the down-growing neurohypophyseal process.[10] Studies in chick embryos[11] have more recently suggested that "far from being an ectodermal protrusion from the stomodeum, Rathke's pouch is a product of the ventral neural ridge." These workers also point out that the floor of the diencephalon arises from a more cranial part of the same neural ridge and that the two parts of the pituitary must therefore be regarded as having a common neuroectodermal origin.

This embryological coincidence thus places at least some of the anterior pituitary cells into the category of the amine content and Amine Precursor Uptake and Decarboxylation[11,12] (APUD) system, an acronym introduced by Pearse to describe their constant cytochemical properties.

Of known anterior pituitary cell types, it has been concluded on the basis of animal studies that adrenotropes and somatotropes are APUD cells and that PRL-secreting cells presumptively are.[11] The other pituitary cell types have not been shown conclusively to be part of this system, but it seems reasonable to assume that all the adenohypophyseal cells are neuroectoderm-derived. This inference is supported by the adenoma tissue culture studies of Lipson *et al.*[6] One tumor from an acromegalic patient secreted PRL, ACTH, thyroid-stimulating hormone (TSH), LH, and FSH; both ACTH-secreting tumors studied also contained PRL, and one each contained GH and LH; one PRL-secreting tumor released large amounts of all the other hormones, and there were many chromophobe adenomas that secreted various combinations of anterior pituitary hormones.

The presence of mixed somatotrophic and lactotrophic pituitary adenomas has been reported by Corenblum *et al.*,[13] and in the rat, estrogen administration induces the formation of pituitary tumor cell lines that secrete both PRL and GH. Although the classic requirement for demonstration of amine precursor uptake may not have been satisfied for all pituitary cell types, the occurrence of this wide variety of mixed cell types is good evidence for the existence of a single common cell type of origin for all pituitary cells; since some are proven to be of neuroectoderm origin, all must be.

These embryological considerations make more understandable the clinical association of polyglandular syndromes and the occurrence of ACTH- and GH-secreting tumors derived from organs other than pituitary. According to current widely held views, cells of the APUD system include a wide variety of bioamine- and peptide-secreting cells including virtually all the known endocrine glands; "paracrine" secretory cells in many viscera, especially the gastrointestinal tract; and a number of neural-crest-derived structures, the most important of which are the sympathetic ganglia, adrenal medulla, Schwann cells, pigment cells of the skin, and the C cell of the thyroid. It is noteworthy that all the cells of neural crest origin are capable of neoplastic transformation and that they may continue to secrete their characteristic hormone product, often in increased concentration. In the ectopic hormonal syndromes, ACTH hypersecretion may be the consequence of neoplastic transformation of a population of "clear cells" of the lung (oat-cell carcinoma), of carcinoid tumors of the intestine, of thymomas, and even of the adrenal medulla (pheochromocytoma).[12]

The factors that determine why a given neuroectodermal derivative may become neoplastic are still unknown. There is evidence that the specific milieu in which the neural-crest-derived cell grows may determine its differentiation. For example, the outgrowing sympathetic innervation of the adrenal does not develop characteristic catecholaminergic synthesizing enzymes unless in contact with the adrenal cortex.[14] Such responses are attributable to local organ-specific differentiating factors. In addition, some cells of the APUD series are responsive to nerve growth factor (NGF), a chemically characterized polypeptide originally isolated from mouse salivary gland, but now shown to be essential for the development of the sympathetic nervous system. NGF, a species-specific hormone, has been shown to promote local neurite development[15,16] not only in sympathetic ganglia cells, but also in neuroblastomas and pheochromocytoma. In addition, NGF has been reported to stimulate electrical excitability in a wide variety of APUDomas including neuroblastoma, pheochromocytoma, medullary thyroid carcinoma, bronchial carcinoid, oat-cell carcinoma, and pituitary adenoma (both human and rat tumor line), and in normal pancreatic islets and pituitary from mouse and frog, respectively.[16] The role of local differentiating factors and of circulating NGF in the appearance of adenoma is unknown. Tumors may arise due to excessive sensitivity to a normal local or circulating factor, in which case these conditioning elements may only be acting in a permissive fashion, or, due to mutational events, the growth may become independent of local regulatory factors (which tend to be differentiating and hence promoting an adult form). In a general sense, it must be recognized that tumor formation is widely believed to involve at least a two-stage process, including an initial inductive event (mutation, spontaneous, or viral- or radiation-induced) and a promoting factor that can be chemical or otherwise environmental. Unfortunately, these questions have not been well resolved in the case of neuroectodermal tumors in general or for the pituitary in particular.

Pituitary adenomas may occur in association with other endocrine hypersecretory states, the most common of which are hyperparathyroidism and pancreatic islet-cell tumors both benign and malignant (Werner's syndrome, multiple endocrine adenomatosis Type 1, multiple endocrine neoplasia Type 1).[17,18] Less common are tumors of adrenal cortex, thyroid, and rarely carcinoids, renal cortical tumors, and lipomas. In some pedigrees, as many as 65% have pituitary adenomas[18]; most are chromophobes, but acromegaly, and rarely prolactinomas, may occur.[19–21] The disease is inherited as an autosomal dominant. Although this condition is relatively rare, it is important to mention it because it emphasizes the role that genetic factors may play in pathogenesis of some tumors and links the pituitary cell to its embryological origin in common with other APUD cells (see above). Little is known about the course of development of this disorder or of the way in which the abnormal gene is expressed. If we can extrapolate from another polyglandular disorder, MEA type 2 (Sipple's syndrome), which does not involve the pituitary, but does involve parathyroid, thyroid C cells (medullary thyroid carcinoma), and adrenal medulla (pheochromocytoma), it is probable that adenomas pass through a stage of "hyperplasia" during the pretumorous phase.[22–25] In medullary thyroid carcinoma and pheochromocytoma, there is no evidence that the hyperplasia is a physiological response to excessive stimulation. Rather, the hyperplasia that is seen in the adrenal medulla and C cells of the thyroid occurs as a primary process in the setting of normal physiological stimulation.

In MEA type 1, the C cells become malignant while the pheochromocytoma cells rarely if ever become malignant. The reason for this difference in biological course (despite a common oncogenic gene) is unknown. Pituitary adenomas rarely become malignant in the true sense of the word. Local invasion is not uncommon, but metastasis is exceedingly rare, only 20 having been reported up to 1975.[26] These include extracranial metastases.

The bulk of adenomas encountered do not have a familial incidence.

3. Pituitary Adenomas Arising Due to Prolonged Hormonal Stimulation or Loss of Normal Negative-Feedback Control

3.1. Estrogen Effects

Extensive studies in the rodent, pioneered by Furth and collaborators,[27,29] have shown that prolonged administration of estrogens induces intense hyperplasia of the prolactinotrope cells, and the formation of pituitary tumors in genetically susceptible strains. In the rat, these tumors secrete PRL and GH from the same cell and have been called mammosomatotropic. They also secrete ACTH.[29] Such tumors have been used extensively for the study of regulation of pituitary secretion. It should be recognized that they are genetically heterogenous,[30] are malignant, and grow initially in estrogen-primed hosts, but later may show varying degrees of autonomy.

In the human, estrogen treatment sensitizes the pituitary to the stimulatory effects of thyrotropin-releasing hormone (TRH), increases the magnitude of GH responses to various stimuli, and stimulates the secretion of PRL. It is the effect of estrogen on PRL-secreting cells that is responsible for the worsening of preexistent prolactinomas during pregnancy and has been postulated to be a factor in the stimulation of clinically inapparent adenomas.[9] There is no clear evidence that estrogens alone can, in the human, induce tumor *de novo*. This may be a factor only of dose, since the effect of estrogens in the rodent is dose-dependent. The effects of estrogens on the pituitary are directly on these cells (not via the hypothalamus) and can be demonstrated in tissue culture. Estrogen receptors have been identified in pituitary cells.

3.2. Response to Loss of Negative-Feedback Control

In rodents, pituitary tumors have been shown to develop following thyroidectomy (TSH-secreting tumors). Such tumors can initially be transplanted only into thyroidectomized hosts (thyroxine-deficiency-dependent); after serial passages, they gain varying degrees of autonomy.[27] Soon after isolation, these tumors show normal responsivity to the usual controls; i.e., they are inhibited by thyroxine administration and stimulated by TRH. This has been demonstrated in the whole animals and also in tissue cultures.[31,32] Such tumors are commonly referred to as "Furth thyrotropic tumors" in recognition of the contributions of Jacob Furth to understanding this disorder. Analogous tumors arise rarely in the human who has suffered from longstanding hypothyroidism, usually due to Hashimoto's thyroiditis[33,34] (see Chapter 8). It is common to see enlargement of the pituitary fossa in chronic hypothyroidism, and in some patients, the tumor develops a degree of autonomy.

Another example of tumors secondary to long-standing target-gland deficiency is the rare occurrence of gonadotropin-secreting tumors[34,35] (see Chapter 8). Loss of negative-feedback control by glucocorticoids accounts for the progressive growth of a certain fraction of ACTH-secreting pituitary tumors, up to 20% [Nelson's syndrome (Chapter 7)], following adrenalectomy, but in such cases, the adenoma is present as a primary disorder arising initially in a setting of normal adrenal cortical function—glucocorticoid deficiency is a further conditioning factor.

It should be emphasized that primary TSH-secreting tumors also arise in otherwise normal individuals, as is the case for Cushing's disease. Also to be emphasized is that the secretion of most tumors is not restricted to a single hormone, although only one or at most two hormones dominate the clinical presentation. Detailed analysis of their secretion shows at least one or more other hormones.

X-ray exposure in rodents may induce ACTH-secreting tumors. An analogous disorder has not been observed in man. Large doses of X-irradiation in the human may cause hypopituitarism mainly through damage to hypothalamic function (see Chapter 21). Despite the theoretical importance of hormonal and deficient feedback in causing some tumors, only a few tumors in the human are apparently the response to such alterations in hormonal milieu. As in the case of genetically determined tumor, the defect appears to be intrinsic to the pituitary. Extrinsic hormonal factors in most cases are probably merely permissive to the neoplastic transformation.

4. Role of the Hypothalamus in Pathogenesis and Manifestations of Pituitary Adenomas

With the recognition that virtually all anterior pituitary functions depend on the hypothalamus (see Chapter 1), it has appeared reasonable to speculate that some adenomas may arise as a result of abnormal hypothalamic function and that some hypersecretory states may be due to hyperplasia. At the outset, it can be stated dogmatically that evidence definitively supporting this view has not been obtained to date.

The main approaches to this problem have been to determine the extent to which pituitary secretory responses in adenoma cases resemble the normal physiological response to test function, before and after removal of the adenoma, and to attempt to identify the presence of abnormal amounts of hypophysiotropic hormones in body fluids of patients with pituitary hypersecretion.

4.1. Physiological Responses in Patients with Pituitary Hypersecretion: Acromegaly

Many patients with acromegaly retain some residual of normal physiological responsivity.[36,37] For example, some show spontaneous surges in plasma GH level (Fig. 1),[38] partial suppression with glucose loading (Fig. 2),[39] and responses to hypoglycemia and arginine infusion (Fig. 3).[39]

However, there is also evidence that in acromegalics the GH control mechanism is qualitatively as well as quantitatively abnormal. Approximately 60% show "paradoxical" responses to glucose loading (that is, an increase, instead of a decrease, in blood GH levels), and sleep-induced GH release is not apparent. Unlike normal individuals, who show an increase in GH levels following the administration of L-dopa, acromegalics, almost without exception, show a decrease in GH levels following such treatment (Fig. 4).[40] In fact, the use of the potent dopamine agonist bromocriptine is a valuable aid for the suppression of GH in failed cases[41] (see Chapter 15). Since the inhibitory effect of L-dopa is blocked by carbidopa, an inhibitor of peripheral conversion of L-dopa to dopamine,[40] the tumor-cell membranes can be assumed to have dopamine receptors that are inhibitory to GH secretion. It is reasonable to postulate that under normal conditions, the effect of dopamine on the hypothalamus in stimulating the release of GH-RH predominates, so that the

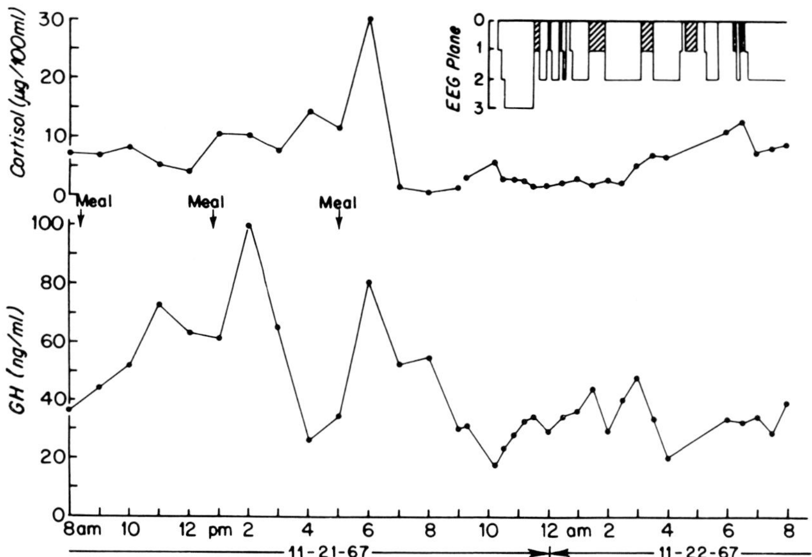

Fig. 1. Spontaneous fluctuations in blood GH levels in a patient with acromegaly. In contrast to the normal, blood GH levels were lower at night than in the day, and meals failed to suppress GH levels. Reprinted with permission of Cryer and Daughaday[38] and the *Journal of Clinical Endocrinology and Metabolism.*

direct inhibitory effects of dopamine are not manifested. Patients with acromegaly also show in more than half of the cases an increase in plasma GH following the injection of TRH,[40,43] a response that does not occur in normal individuals (Fig. 5). This effect has been attributed to the appearance of large numbers of TRH receptors on the abnormal adenoma. The finding of mixed

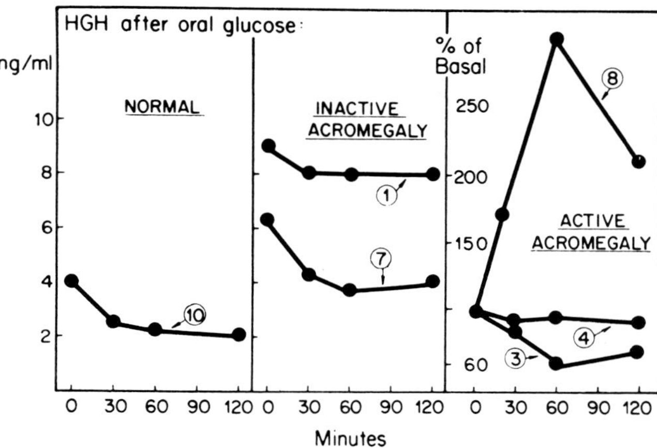

Fig. 2. Heterogenity of GH secretory responses to oral glucose administration in acromegalics. Some acromegalics behave like normals in displaying a fall in blood GH following glucose administration, whereas some show no change, or even paradoxical responses. Reprinted with permission from Lawrence *et al.*[39]

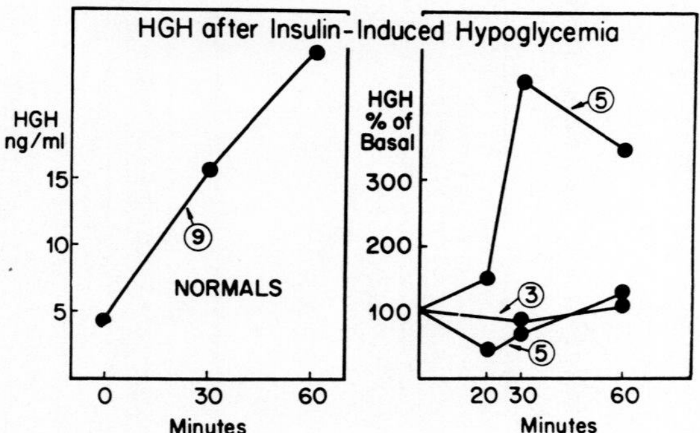

Fig. 3. Heterogenity of GH secretory responses to insulin-induced hypoglycemia in acromegalics. Five of 13 cases behaved like normals in showing an increase in plasma GH, but 3 others showed no change, and 5 showed a paradoxical lowering of plasma GH levels. These observations, as in Fig. 42, indicate a qualitative abnormality in GH regulation in some acromegalics. Reprinted with permission from Lawrence *et al.*[39]

cell populations (prolactinotropes, somatotropes) in the same tumor[14,44] favors an intrinsic pituitary abnormality.

Few cases of acromegaly have been studied in detail prior to, and after, apparent complete removal of a microadenoma. One case, reported by Hoyte and Martin,[45] showed return of normal responsiveness and loss of the paradoxical GH response to TRH and L-dopa. The extent to which this finding is typical of the disease is not known.

Efforts to identify excess secretion of GH-releasing factor (GH-RF) or decreased secretion of somatostatin have been made in acromegaly. From a theoretical point of view, excessive amounts of GH-releasing activity could bring about pituitary GH hypersecretion. For example, Saeed uz Zafar *et al.*[46] have reported the occurrence of acromegaly secondary to a bronchial carcinoid tumor and demonstrated that the tumor contained GH-RF activity and no GH and that the disease remitted following removal of the tumor. Similar cases of carcinoid had been reported previously, including one that apparently secreted GH, and GH-secreting adenomas may be associated with carcinoid.[46,47]

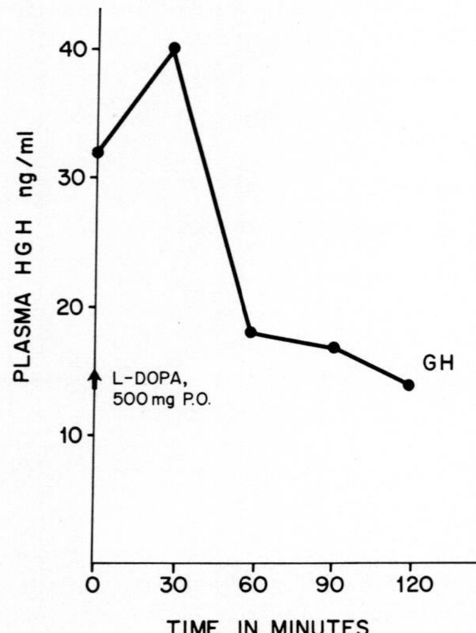

Fig. 4. Paradoxical suppressive effect of L-dopa on plasma GH in acromegalics.

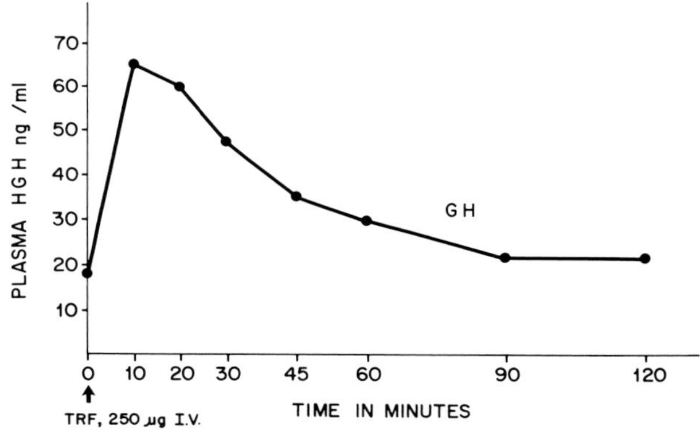

Fig. 5. Paradoxical release of GH after TRH administration in an acromegalic.

Proof of excessive secretion of GH-RF in acromegaly of the usual variety has been claimed by Hagen *et al.*,[48] who reported stimulation of release of GH from monkey pituitary *in vitro* following exposure to acromegalic plasma. Even if the finding were confirmed, it would still be only suggestive of hypothalamic GH-RF hypersecretion, since the specificity and tissue site of origin of the biological activity have not been established.

As to the possibility that acromegaly is due to somatostatin deficiency, measurements of cerebrospinal fluid somatostatin were made in acromegalic patients[49] (Urosa and Reichlin, unpublished), and all were within the normal range. Insofar as cerebrospinal fluid concentration can be taken as a reflection of somatostatin secretion rate (which is an unwarranted conclusion), these findings suggest that somatostatin deficiency is not a factor.

The critical problem in all studies of the role of the hypothalamus in the pathogenesis of acromegaly (as is true for the other pituitary hypersecretory disorders) is that definitive proof will require unambiguous methods for measurement of hypothalamic hormone secretion rate, preferably to include direct measurement of hypophyseal–portal blood concentrations.

The findings that some cases of acromegaly persist despite removal of all gland in contact with the base of the hypothalamus suggest a high degree of autonomy for the GH-secreting adenoma. In brief, a definitive answer cannot be given as to the role of hypothalamic hypersecretion in the pathogenesis of acromegaly. Further, there may be considerable heterogeneity in this disorder, some cases being due to well-localized adenomas (entirely due to intrinsic pituitary disease), while a smaller number may have mainly diffuse hyperplasia. It is this group that conceivably could be hypophysiotropogenic.

4.2. ACTH-Secreting Adenomas

Excessive secretion of glucocorticoids is most commonly secondary to ACTH hypersecretion, accounting for approximately 70% or more of cases of spontaneous Cushing's syndrome (Chapter 7). This group, characterized by bilateral hyperplasia of the adrenal cortex and an inappropriate elevation of ACTH (Cushing's disease), has been shown in various series to be accompanied by either radiological or histological evidence of adenoma of the pituitary in between 40 and 64%[50,51] (see Chapter 7). Recent series that have utilized arteriography and pleuridirectional tomography indicate an incidence of abnormality of 82% in Cushing's disease.[52] Exploration of the pituitary gland even in the absence of roentgen abnormalities revealed in the series of Tyrell *et al.*[53] 15 microadenomas in 20 patients, and in these and one other, removal of "suspicious" tissue resulted in a cure. In Hardy's series, all of ten patients with Cushing's disease were cured by microadenomectomy.[54] Thus, the majority of cases of this disorder appear to be due to ACTH-secreting adenomas; a few may be due to rather more diffuse hyperplasia of the adrenotrope cell or to minute tumors. Tests of function of the pituitary–adrenal axis have not succeeded in differentiating between these two types of cases. Following adrenalectomy, previously unrecognized tumors may become evident and established tumors become even larger (Nelson's syndrome). It is considered likely that such patients have had adenomas all along, but that intense growth is due to loss of normal feedback inhibition. Transient resistance to the feedback action of cortisol has also been observed in patients with primary Addison's disease.[55]

In attempts to determine whether the central nervous system may be involved in the pathogenesis of Cushing's disease, many studies have been carried out on the response of such patients to physiological stimuli and have become the basis of sophisticated and specific tests of the pituitary adrenal axis, but of themselves have not as yet established whether the disease is due to excessive secretion of a hypothalamic factor or whether the retention of some normal responses is due to residual CNS functions of the adenomatous tissue.

One hallmark of Cushing's disease is that the set point for feedback control of secretion of ACTH is established at a higher level. Much recent work reviewed by Jones[56] indicates that feedback effects of cortisol may be directed at the pituitary, and as well at the level of the hypothalamus or other central nervous system structures. Higher set point therefore cannot be taken as evidence for or against a pituitary abnormality as compared with brain hypersecretion of corticotropin-releasing factor (CRF).

More specific evidence of an intrinsic defect in the pituitary in Cushing's disease is the demonstration that some patients with this disorder show ACTH discharge following the administration of TRH,[57] a response never seen in normals; in some, the administration of dopamine agonists such as bromocriptine suppresses ACTH secretion, again a response not seen in the normal.[58] The latter observations (as in the analogous case of GH-secreting adenomas) are interpreted to indicate that the tumor has exposed the presence of TRH and dopamine receptors on adrenotrope cells, either through hypertrophy of receptors that have been there all along or through dedifferentiation. A direct effect of bromocriptine in experimental ACTH-secreting tumors *in vitro* has been demonstrated by MacLeod and Krieger.[59]

Cushing's disease patients characteristically lose normal circadian rhythms early in the disease, a finding that could be attributed to either pituitary or central nervous system abnormality. The finding that normal GH circadian rhythms are also lost in Cushing's disease and that this defect persists after clinical cure led Krieger[60] to propose that there is an intrinsic neural abnormality in such patients. However, it has been shown more recently that the abnormality gradually clears if sufficient time elapses.[61] In view of the finding that cortisol can produce a number of changes in brain function in man (including cerebral atrophy), it is equally likely that the changes are secondary to brain damage.

The use of neurotransmitter antagonists has recently been proposed by Krieger as a means of identifying a neural basis of Cushing's disease. The most interesting results have been obtained using the serotonin antagonist cyproheptadine, which is assumed to act on the serotonergic hypothalamic system regulating CRF secretion, although this conclusion is only inferential. Approximately 60% of cases are reported to respond, partially or completely, to this therapy, although it may take very high doses (up to 32 mg) or prolonged treatment (4–5 months) to see an effect.[62] Cyproheptadine also lowers ACTH in some cases of Nelson's syndrome[63] and restores circadian periodicity, and reverses paradoxical ACTH response to TRH.[57] Because of the undesirable side effects (drowsiness and obesity) and the superiority of the transsphenoidal adenomectomy approach, it is likely that responses to cryproheptadine may not prove to be of practical clinical value, but they do suggest that serotonin secretion may play a role in some patients. Krieger[60] suggests that "the existence of a subgroup of patients who do not respond to cyproheptadine raises the question that there may be at least two types of Cushing's disease, one dependent upon abnormal central nervous system drive (perhaps by a serotonergic mechanism), the other of primary pituitary origin, the latter perhaps representing those patients who respond to microadenomectomy." Until CRF secretion can be assessed directly or a specific CRF made available for direct testing of pituitary ACTH reserve, it will not be possible to determine whether serotonin antagonists are acting on the brain or on the pituitary in bringing about therapeutic responses.

A rare case of Cushing's disease apparently due to intrinsic hypothalamic disorder has been reported.[64]

The most convincing evidence that adrenotropic adenomas are not due to intrinsic brain disease is the study of ACTH regulatory responses in patients presumably cured by microadenomectomy. Several series have been published.[52,61,65,66] In general, these show a return to normal feedback regulatory control, and hence suggest that CRF secretion has been normal all along. Return to normal is associated with a transient period of hypoadrenalism. Most patients show a return to normal responsiveness to feedback inhibition by the "low-dose" dexamethasone test and normal responses to metyrapone.[52] In the patient of Lagerquist *et al.*,[61] circadian rhythms returned, as was true for the case of Bigos *et al.*[66] These authors provide a complete summary of the literature and also point out the association of galactorrhea, slight PRL excess secretion in Cushing's disease, and remission after surgery. Similar findings were reported by Schnall *et al.*[65]

Although these findings may not be uniform in all patients with Cushing's disease, the high incidence of microadenoma in this disease and complete cure following pituitary microadenomectomy is strong evidence that intrinsic pituitary disease underlies most instances of this disorder.

Efforts to demonstrate by direct study abnormalities in the secretion of CRF in patients with Cushing's disease have not been helpful. The chemical nature of CRF has not been established, and there are several substances with CRF activity, not all of which come from the hypothalamus and not all of which may be involved in pituitary regulation. Estimates of plasma or cerebrospinal fluid levels of bioassayable CRF activity (even if available) would likely not be specifically helpful because of the widespread distribution of CRF activity in both extrahypothalamic brain and in peripheral tissues.[67,68] It would be necessary to measure levels in portal-vessel blood to establish this point with certainty.

In the opinion of this author, the role of the brain in the pathogenesis of Cushing's disease has not been established. I believe that all the observations that have been made can be explained by the view that adenomas develop in the presence of a normal neural and steroid milieu. Abnormalities are intrinsic to the tumor. Normal regulatory influences are retained by the adenoma to a certain, somewhat variable degree.

4.3. Prolactin-Secreting Tumors

Many, but not all, cases of hyperprolactinemia can be shown to be due to adenomas (see Chapter 4). The precise frequency with which adenomas are present is still uncertain, and the role of the hypothalamus in the pathogenesis or maintenance of the disorder is still a subject of speculation.

Although no unique pattern characterizes PRL regulatory responses in patients with adenomas, it can be stated in general that such cases lose characteristic circadian rhythms and become less responsive to the stimulating effects of TRH and dopamine antagonists such as chlorpromazine and metoclopramide, but retain partial or complete responsivity to the inhibitory effects of dopamine agonists (see Chapter 4). The impaired responsiveness of the adenoma to secretagogues is not due to the fact that such patients already have high PRL levels because pregnant women, with similarly elevated PRL levels, show exuberant responses to TRH and metoclopramide.[69] The abnormality in the adenoma cases thus indicates either a defect in receptor mechanism or the presence of small, rapidly turning over pools of PRL.

Crucial to the question of whether there is an underlying nervous system abnormality is the extent to which normal PRL secretory responses return after removal of the microadenoma. This question has been addressed by Barbarino *et al.*,[69] who studied 7 women with PRL-secreting tumors before and after microadenomectomy. Prior to surgery, all had blunted or absent responses to metoclopramide and to TRH. After surgical cure (as indicated by return to menses and of PRL level to normal), responses to these physiological tests returned to normal in 6 of 7 cases (Fig. 6). In a series of 20 cases studied in our clinic,[70] 12 were cured and their secretory responses returned to normal. In the remainder, blood PRL levels remained elevated, and physiological responses were persistently abnormal. It is not clear whether these patients

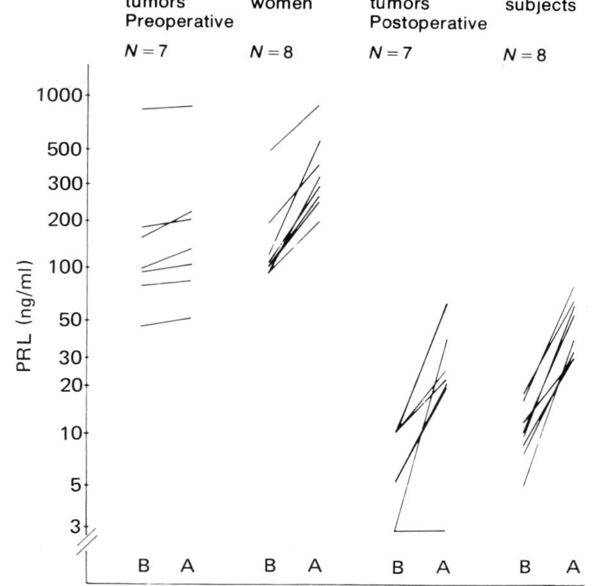

Fig. 6. Changes in PRL secretory response to TRH in pregnant women (with physiologically normally elevated plasma PRL levels), in patients with prolactinomas, and in prolactinoma patients following successful removal of an adenoma. Note that all pregnant women and all normals showed an increase in PRL after TRH administration, but that tumor cases showed blunted responses. In 6 of 7 cases, responses returned to normal following microadenomectomy, thus indicating that the remaining gland had been normal. These observations suggest that there is no underlying disturbance in pituitary–hypothalamic function in cases with microadenomas. Reprinted with permission from Barbarino *et al.*[69] and The Endocrine Society.

have an abnormality of CNS function or whether there is residual adenoma, despite the surgeon's perception that all tumor has been removed. In the series from our clinic, a study has been made of the pre- and postsurgical results of testing with L-dopa–carbidopa pretreatment. This approach, utilized by Fine and Frohman,[71] and also studied by Camanni *et al.*[42] in patients with acromegaly, is based on the fact that L-dopa is converted to dopamine in both the brain and the pituitary (and hence could theoretically act in either place), but that carbidopa (which blocks the enzymatic conversion step) acts only in regions outside the blood–brain barrier. Frohman and collaborators showed that L-dopa inhibition of PRL release in normals is not blocked by carbidopa, but is in tumors. The conclusion was drawn that in normals, the principal effect of L-dopa is at the level of the hypothalamus, while in adenoma patients, it is at the pituitary level. In 7 patients cured by microadenomectomy (Goodman *et al.*[70] and unpublished), all had abnormal responses to L-dopa–carbidopa, and all reverted to normal after microadenomectomy. We conclude that the microadenoma is an intrinsic abnormality in most patients.

These observations suggest at most a permissive role for the nervous system in the pathogenesis of prolactinoma. However, Van Loon[72] has provided data suggesting that there may be an underlying defect in peripheral catecholamine regulation in such patients. He found that normal individuals treated with bromocriptine showed a progressive decline in blood levels of dopamine, noradrenaline, and adrenaline, whereas those with prolactinoma showed increased levels. Although it is known from the animal studies of Fuxe *et al.*[73] that PRL stimulates dopamine turnover in the hypothalamus, the relevance of blood levels to hypothalamic levels is unknown. Van Loon demonstrated similar abnormalities in two other patients who had normal PRL levels following ablative surgery. The number of cases studied may be too small to generalize to all cases, and the time course of recovery of normal PRL-induced dopamine changes is not known. Nevertheless, the findings are provocative in suggesting an intrinsic disturbance of the autonomic nervous system in the prolactinoma syndrome.

An additional finding that suggests a hypothalamic abnormality in prolactinoma is the demonstration by Garthwaite and Hagen[74] of PRL-releasing activity in the plasma of patients with galactorrhea–amenorrhea, 8 of 13 of whom had demonstrable tumors. The forcefulness of this observation in providing convincing evidence of hypothalamic dysfunction in this disorder is conditioned by uncertainty as to the chemical nature of prolactin-releasing factor, of its site of secretion, and of the effect of microadenomectomy on its concentration. This interesting work will require further study.

ACKNOWLEDGMENT. Studies from the author's laboratory alluded to in this article were supported by U.S.P.H.S. Grants #2R01 AM 16684 and #5T32 AM 07039.

References

1. R.T. Costello, Subclinical adenomas of the pituitary gland, *Am. J. Pathol.* **12:**205, 1936.
2. W.F. McCormick and N.S. Halmi, Absence of chromophobe adenomas from a large series of pituitary tumors, *Arch. Pathol.* **92:**231, 1971.
3. A.M.T. Sirek, B. Corenblum, E. Horvath, B. Newcastle, C. Ezrin, and K. Kovacs, A new look at pituitary adenomas: Structure elucidating function, *Can. Med. Assoc. J.* **114:**225, 1976.
4. A.M. Landholt and H. Krayenbuhl, Progress in pituitary adenoma biology: Results of research and clinical applications, in: *Advances and Technical Standards in Neurosurgery*, Vol. 5, pp. 3–49, Springer-Verlag, Vienna and New York, 1971.
5. L.W. Conway, D.S. Schalch, R.D. Utiger, and S. Reichlin, Hormones in human pituitary sinusoid blood: Concentration of LH, GH and TSH, *J. Clin. Endocrinol. Metab.* **29:**446, 1969.
6. L.G. Lipson, I.Z. Beitins, P.D. Kornblith, J.W. McArthur, H.G. Friesen, B. Kliman, and R.N. Kjellberg, Tissue culture studies on human pituitary tumors: Radioimmunoassayable anterior pituitary hormones in the culture medium, *Acta Endocrinol.* **88:**239, 1978.
7. J.A. del Regato and H.J. Spjut, *Cancer*, C.V. Mosby, St. Louis, Missouri, 1977.
8. S. Reichlin, The prolactinoma problem (editorial), *N. Engl. J. Med.* **300:**313, 1979.
9. B.M. Sherman, J. Schlechte, N.S. Halmi, K.K. Chapler, C.E. Harris, T.M. Duello, J. VanGilder, and D.K. Granner, Pathogenesis of prolactin-secreting pituitary adenomas, *Lancet* **2:**1019–1021, 1978.
10. M. Banna, Terminology, embryology and anatomy, in: *Pituitary and Parapituitary Tumors* (J. Hankinson and M. Banna, eds.), pp. 1–12, W.B. Saunders, London, 1976.
11. T. Takor Takor and A.G.E. Pearse, Cytochemical identification of human and murine pituitary corticotrophs and somatotrophs as APUD cells, *Histochemie* **37:**207, 1973.
12. A.G.E. Pearse and T. Takor Takor, Neuroendocrine embryology and the APUD concept, *Clin. Endocrinol.* **5**(Suppl.):229, 1976.
13. B. Corenblum, A.M.T. Sirek, E. Horvath, K. Kovacs, and C. Ezrin, Human mixed somatotrophic and lactotrophic pituitary adenomas, *J. Clin. Endocrinol. Metab.* **42**(5):857, 1976.
14. G. Teitelman, H. Baker, T.H. Joh, and D.J. Reis, Appearance of catecholamine synthesizing enzymes during development of rat sympathetic nervous system: Possible role of tissue environment, *Proc. Natl. Acad. Sci. U.S.A.* **76**(1):509, 1979.
15. R.B. Campenot, Local control of neurite development by nerve growth factor, *Proc. Natl. Acad. Sci. U.S.A.* **74:**4516, 1977.
16. A.S. Tischler, M.A. Dichter, B. Biales, and L. Greene, Neuroendocrine neoplasms and their cells of origin, *N. Engl. J. Med.* **296:**919, 1977.

17. S.B. Baylin, The multiple endocrine neoplasia syndromes: Implications for the study of inherited tumors, *Semin. Oncol.* **5**:35, 1978.
18. R.A. DeLellis and H.J. Wolfe, Multiple endocrine adenomatosis syndromes: Origins and interrelationships, in: *Cancer Medicine*, 2nd ed. (J. Holland and E. Frei, eds.), Lea and Febiger, Philadelphia, 1979 (in press).
19. M. Vandeweghe, J. Schutyser, K. Braxel, and A. Vermuelen, A case of multiple endocrine adenomatosis with primary amenorrhea, *Postgrad. Med. J.* **54**:618, 1978.
20. H.E. Carlson, G.A. Levine, N.J. Goldberg, and J.M. Hershman, Hyperprolactinemia in multiple endocrine adenomatosis, Type I, *Arch. Intern. Med.* **138**:1807, 1978.
21. J.D. Veldhuis, J.E. Green III, E. Kovacs, T.J. Worgul, F.T. Murray, and J. M. Hammond, Prolactin-secreting pituitary adenomas. Association with multiple endocrine neoplasia, Type I, *Am. J. Med.* **67**:830–837, 1979.
22. H.J. Wolfe, K.E.W. Melvin, S.J. Cervi-Skinner, A.A. AlSaadi, J.F. Juliar, C.E. Jackson, and A.H. Tashjian, C-cell hyperplasia preceding medullary thyroid carcinoma, *N. Engl. J. Med.* **289**:437, 1973.
23. R.F. Gagel, K.E.W. Melvin, A.H. Tashjian, H.H. Miller, Z.T. Feldman, H.J. Wolfe, R.A. DeLellis, S. Cervi-Skinner, and S. Reichlin, Natural history of the familial medullary thyroid carcinoma–pheochromocytoma syndrome and the identification of preneoplastic stages by screening studies: A five year report, *Trans. Assoc. Am. Phys.* **88**:177, 1975.
24. K. Graze, I.J. Spiler, A.H. Tasjian, Jr., K.E.W. Melvin, S. Cervi-Skinner, R.F. Gagel, H.H. Miller, H.J. Wolfe, R.A. DeLellis, L. Leape, Z.T. Feldman, and S. Reichlin, Natural history of familial medullary thyroid carcinoma: Effect of a program for early diagnosis, *N. Engl. J. Med.* **299**:980, 1978.
25. R.A. DeLellis, H.J. Wolfe, R.F. Gagel, Z.T. Feldman, H.H. Miller, D.L. Gang, and S. Reichlin, Adrenal medullary hyperplasia: A morphometric analysis in patients with familial medullary thyroid carcinoma, *Am J. Pathol.* **83**:177, 1976.
26. A.M. Landolt, Ultrastructure of human sella tumors, *Acta Neurochir.*, Suppl. 22, 1975.
27. J. Furth and K.H. Clifton, Experimental pituitary tumours, in: *The Pituitary Gland* (G.W. Harris and B.T. Donovan, eds.), pp. 460–497, Butterworths, London, 1966.
28. A.B. Russfield, Tumors of endocrine glands and secondary sex organs, Public Health Service Publ. No. 1332, U.S. Government Printing Office, Washington, D.C., 1966.
29. G. Ueda, S. Takizawa, P. Moy, F. Marolla, and J. Furth, Characterization of four transplantable mammotropic pituitary tumor varients in the rat, *Cancer Res.* **10** and 28, 1963 and 1968.
30. C. Sonneschein, U.I. Richardson, and A.H. Tashjian, Jr., Chromosomal analysis, organ-specific function and appearance of six clonal strains of rat pituitary tumor cells, *Exp. Cell Res.* **61**:121, 1970.
31. L. Cacicedo, S.L. Pohl, and S. Reichlin, Biosynthesis of thyrotropin (TSH) by mouse thyrotropic tumor cells in primary culture: Inhibitory effect of triiodothyronine (T3) and thyroxine (T4), Program of the 58th Annual Meeting of the Endocrine Society, San Francisco, 1976 (abstract 259).
32. M.R. Blackman, M.C. Gershengorn, and B.D. Weintraub, Excess production of free alpha subunits by mouse pituitary thyrotropic tumor cells *in vitro*, *Endocrinology* **102**:499–508, 1978.
33. N.A. Samaan, B.M. Osborne, B. MacKay, M.E. Leavens, T.M. Duello, and N.S. Halmi, *J. Clin. Endocrinol. Metab.* **45**:903–911, 1977.
34. A.B. Russfield, Pituitary tumors, in: *Endocrine Pathology Decennial* (S.C. Sommers, ed.), pp. 41–79, Appleton-Century-Crofts, New York, 1975.
35. J.N. Friend, D.M. Judge, B.M. Sherman, and R.J. Santen, FSH secreting pituitary adenomas: Stimulation and suppression studies in two patients, *J. Clin. Endocrinol. Metab.* **43**:650–657, 1976.
36. W.H. Daughaday, P.E. Cryer, and L.S. Jacobs, The role of the hypothalamus in the pathogenesis of pituitary tumors, in: *Diagnosis and Treatment of Pituitary Tumors* (P.O. Kohler and G.T. Ross, eds.), pp. 26–34, Excerpta Medica, Amsterdam and New York, 1973.
37. W. Daughaday and P. Cryer, Growth hormone hypersecretion and acromegaly, *Hosp. Pract.* pp. 75–80, Aug. 1978.
38. P. Cryer and W. Daughaday, Regulation of growth hormone secretion in acromegaly, *J. Clin. Endocrinol. Metab.* **29**:386, 1969.
39. A.M. Lawrence, I.D. Goldfine, and L. Kirsteins, Growth hormone dynamics in acromegaly, *J. Clin Endocrinol. Metab.* **31**:239, 1970.

40. K. Janew, M. Aida, T. Tano, and K. Yoshinaga, Abnormal growth hormone responses to L-dopa and thyrotropin releasing hormone in patients with acromegaly, *Tohoku J. Exp. Med.* **121:**197, 1977.
41. G.M. Besser, J.A.H. Wass, and M.O. Thorner, Acromegaly—Results of long term treatment with bromocriptine, *Acta Endocrinol.* [*Suppl.*] (*Copenhagen*) **88**(216):187, 1978.
42. F. Camanni, G.B. Piccotti, F. Massara, G.M. Molinatti, P. Mantegazza, and E.E. Muller, Carbidopa inhibits the growth hormone and prolactin suppressive effect of L-dopa in acromegalic patients, *J. Clin. Endocrinol. Metab.* **47:**647, 1978.
43. K. Maeda, Critical review: Effects of thyrotropin releasing hormone on growth hormone release in normal subjects and in patients with depression, anorexia nervosa and acromegaly, *Kobe J. Med. Sci.* **22:**263, 1976.
44. E.A. Zimmerman, R. Defendini, and A.G. Frantz, Prolactin and growth hormone in patients with pituitary adenomas: A correlative study of hormone in tumor and plasma by immunoperoxidase technique and radioimmunoassay, *J. Clin. Endocrinol. Metab.* **38:**577, 1974.
45. K.M. Hoyte and J.B. Martin, Recovery from paradoxical growth hormone responses in acromegaly after transsphenoidal selective adenomectomy, *J. Clin. Endocrinol. Metab.* **41:**656, 1975.
46. M. Saeed uz Zafar. R.C. Mellinger, G. Fine, M. Szabo, and L.A. Frohman, Acromegaly associated with a bronchial carcinoid tumor: Evidence for ectopic production of growth hormone releasing activity, *J. Clin. Endocrinol. Metab.* **48:**66, 1979.
47. P.O. Sonkson, A.B. Ayres, M. Braimbridge, B. Corrin, D.R. Davies, G.M. Jeremiah, S.W. Oaten, C. Lowy, and T.E.T. West, Acromegaly caused by pulmonary carcinoid tumors, *Clin. Endocrinol* (*Oxford*), **5:**503, 1976.
48. T.C. Hagen, A.M. Lawrence, and L. Kirsteins, *In vitro* release of monkey pituitary growth hormone by acromegalic plasma, *J. Clin. Endocrinol.* **33:**448, 1978.
49. Y. Patel, K. Rao, and S. Reichlin, Somatostatin in human cerebrospinal fluid, *N. Engl. J. Med.* **296:**529, 1977.
50. C.M. Plotz, A.I. Knowlton, and C. Ragan, The natural history of Cushing's syndrome, *Am. J. Med.* **13:**597, 1952.
51. C.W. Burke and C.G. Beardwell, Cushing's syndrome, *Q. J. Med. N. Ser.* **42:**175, 1973.
52. R.M. Salassa, E.R. Laws, Jr., P.C. Carpenter, and R.C. Northcutt, Transsphenoidal removal of pituitary microadenoma in Cushing's disease, *Mayo Clin. Proc.* **53:**24, 1978.
53. J.B. Tyrell, R.M. Brooks, P.A. Fitzgerald, P. Coifaid, P.H. Forsham, and C. Wilson, Cushings disease: Selective transsphenoidal resection of pituitary mircoadenomas, *N. Engl. J. Med. 298:*753, 1978.
54. J. Hardy, Transsphenoidal surgery for hypersecreting adenomas, in: *Diagnosis and Treatment of Pituitary Tumors* (P.O. Kohler and G.T. Ross, eds.), pp. 179–198, American Elsevier, New York, 1973.
55. R. Clayton, V. Schriever, A.C. Burden, and R.D. Rosenthal, Secondary pituitary hyperplasia in Addison's disease, *Lancet,* Nov. 5, p. 954, 1977.
56. M.T. Jones, Control of corticotrophin (ACTH) secretion, in: *The Endocrine Hypothalamus* (S.L. Jeffcoate and J.S.M. Hutchinson, eds.), pp. 386–419, Academic Press, London, 1978.
57. D.T. Krieger and E.M. Condon, Cyproheptadine treatment of Nelson's syndrome: Restoration of plasma ACTH circadian periodicity and reversal of response to TRF, *J. Clin. Endocrinol. Metab.* **46:**349, 1978.
58. S.W.J. Lamberts and J.C. Birkenhagen, Bromocryptine in Cushing's disease, *J. Endocrinol.* **70:**315, 1976.
59. R.M. MacLeod and D.T. Krieger, Differential effect of ergotamine on ACTH and prolactin secretion, Program of the 58th Annual Meeting of the Endocrine Society, San Francisco, 1976 (abstract 317).
60. D.T. Krieger, The central nervous system and Cushing's disease, *Med. Clin. North Am.* **62:**261, 1978.
61. L.G. Lagerquist, A.W. Meikle, C.D. West, and F.H. Tyler, Cushing's disease with cure by resection of a pituitary adenoma: Evidence against a primary hypothalamic defect, *Am. J. Med.* **57:**826, 1974.
62. D.T. Krieger, L. Amorosa, and F. Linick, Cyproheptadine-induced remission of Cushing's disease, *N. Engl. J. Med.* **293:**893, 1975.
63. D.T. Krieger and M. Luria, Effectiveness of cyproheptadine in decreasing plasma ACTH concentration in Nelson's syndrome, *J. Clin. Endocrinol. Metab.* **43:**1179, 1976.

64. F.G. Berlinger, H.J. Ruder, and J.F. Wilber, Cushing's syndrome associated with galactorrhea, amenorrhea, and hypothyroidism: A primary hypothalamic disorder, *J. Clin. Endocrinol. Metab.* **45:**1205, 1977.
65. A.M. Schnall, J.S. Brodkey, B. Kaufman, and O.H. Pearson, Pituitary function after removal of pituitary microadenomas in Cushing's disease, *J. Clin. Endocrinol. Metab.* **47:**410, 1978.
66. S.T. Bigos, F. Robert, G. Pelletier, and J. Hardy, Cure of Cushing's disease by transsphenoidal removal of a microadenoma from a pituitary gland despite a radiographically normal sella turcica, *J. Clin. Endocrinol. Metab.* **45:**1251, 1977.
67. R.J. Witorsch and A. Brodish, Conditions for the reliable use of lesioned rats for the assay of CRF in tissue extracts, *Endocrinology* **90:**552, 1972.
68. N. Yasuda and M.A. Greer, Distribution of corticotropin releasing factor(s) activity in neural and extraneural tissues of the rat, *Endocrinology* **99:**944, 1976.
69. A. Barbarino, L. DeMarinis, G. Maira, E. Menini, and C. Anile, Serum prolactin response to thyrotropin-releasing hormone and metoclopramide in patients with prolactin-secreting tumors before and after transsphenoidal surgery, *J. Clin. Endocrinol. Metab.* **47:**1148, 1978.
70. R. Goodman, B. Biller, A.C. Mosses, M. Molitch, S. Feldman, and K. Post, Restoration of normal prolactin secretory dynamics after surgical cure of prolactinoma is evidence against underlying hypothalamic dysregulation, Program of the 61st Annual Meeting of the Endocrine Society, Anaheim, California, June 1979.
71. S.A. Fine and L.A. Frohman, Loss of central nervous system component of dopaminergic inhibition of prolactin secretion in patients with prolactin secreting pituitary tumors, *J. Clin. Invest.* **61:**973, 1978.
72. G.R. Van Loon, A defect in catecholamine neurons in patients with prolactin secreting pituitary adenoma, *Lancet* **2**(8095):868, 1978.
73. K. Fuxe, T. Hökfelt, A. Löfström, O. Johansson, L. Agnati, B. Everitt, M. Goldstein, S. Jeffcoate, N. White, P. Eneroth, J.A. Gustafsson, and P. Skett, On the role of neurotransmitters and hypothalamic hormones and their interactions in hypothalamic and extrahypothalamic control of pituitary function and sexual behaviour, in: *Subcellular Mechanisms in Reproductive Neuroendocrinology* (F. Naftolin, K.J. Ryan, and I.J. Davies, eds.), pp. 193–246, Elsevier, Amsterdam, 1976.
74. T.L. Garthwaite and T.C. Hagen, Plasma prolactin-releasing factor-like activity in the amenorrhea–galactorrhea syndrome, *J. Clin. Endocrinol. Metab.* **47:**885, 1978.

3

The Pathology of Pituitary Adenomas

LESTER S. ADELMAN

1. Traditional Concepts

Modern concepts of the biology of pituitary adenomas are dramatically different from those that were held from the time of Harvey Cushing [1] until only a few years ago. Application of techniques such as electron microscopy, immunofluorescence, and tissue culture to the study of pituitary adenomas, coupled with advances in the evaluation of the endocrinological state of patients with these tumors, has yielded information that required this revision of concepts. Because the traditional concepts dominated our thinking for so long, it is useful to review them.

These concepts are summarized by Kernohan and Sayre,[2] who classify pituitary adenomas into three types—eosinophilic, basophilic, and chromophobic. Eosinophilic adenomas are associated with increased growth hormone (GH) secretion and with acromegaly and gigantism. Basophilic adenomas secrete ACTH and are associated with Cushing's disease. Chromophobic adenomas are composed of cells that do not produce hormones and are therefore associated with hypopituitarism when they grow large enough to compress the normal gland.

As other pituitary hormones were discovered, additional differential stains have been developed to demonstrate the cells that produce them. At present, we can recognize by these methods two types of eosinophils, one that produces GH, and another that produces prolactin. Three varieties of basophils are recognized—the ACTH-producing cell, the thyroid-stimulating hormone (TSH)-producing cell, and a cell that produces both follicle-stimulating hormone (FSH) and luteninizing hormone (LH).[3]

Even this expanded classification, however, fails to produce the sort of correlation between histology and clinical hormonal state that one would expect. For example, one would expect that the amenorrhea–galactorrhea syn-

LESTER S. ADELMAN • Tufts University School of Medicine; Department of Pathology, Division of Neuropathology, Tufts–New England Medical Center Hospital, Boston, Massachusetts 02111.

drome of Forbes et al.[4] would be associated with prolactin-producing eosinophils; chromophobic tumors are found in many such patients.[5–7] Chromophobic tumors are found in close to half the patients with Cushing's disease[8] and acromegaly,[9] and have also been described in TSH-producing adenomas[10] and in tumors producing gonadotropins.[11] On the other hand, eosinophilic adenomas have been found in patients with hypopituitarism.[2,12]

Part of the explanation for these discrepancies between traditional expectations as to what the tumor type should be and what is actually found is the realization that the definition of a chromophobic cell is technologically determined. The idea that a large proportion of the cells in the normal pituitary gland are hormonally inactive stems from the inability to stain granules in them at the light-microscopic level. It is then postulated that tumors composed of similar cells will be hormonally inactive as well. In fact, at the electron-microscopic level, secretory granules can be found in virtually all cells in the normal gland and in most tumors. McCormick and Halmi[13] studied 145 adenomas found at autopsy, and 21 surgical specimens. Of the tumors from the autopsy series, 59% were acidophilic, 18% were basophilic, 16% were mixed, and only 6% were unclassified. Of the 21 surgical specimens, 19 were eosinophilic; the other 2 were too poorly preserved to classify. Granules were easily recognized by electron microscopy in tumors that appeared chromo-

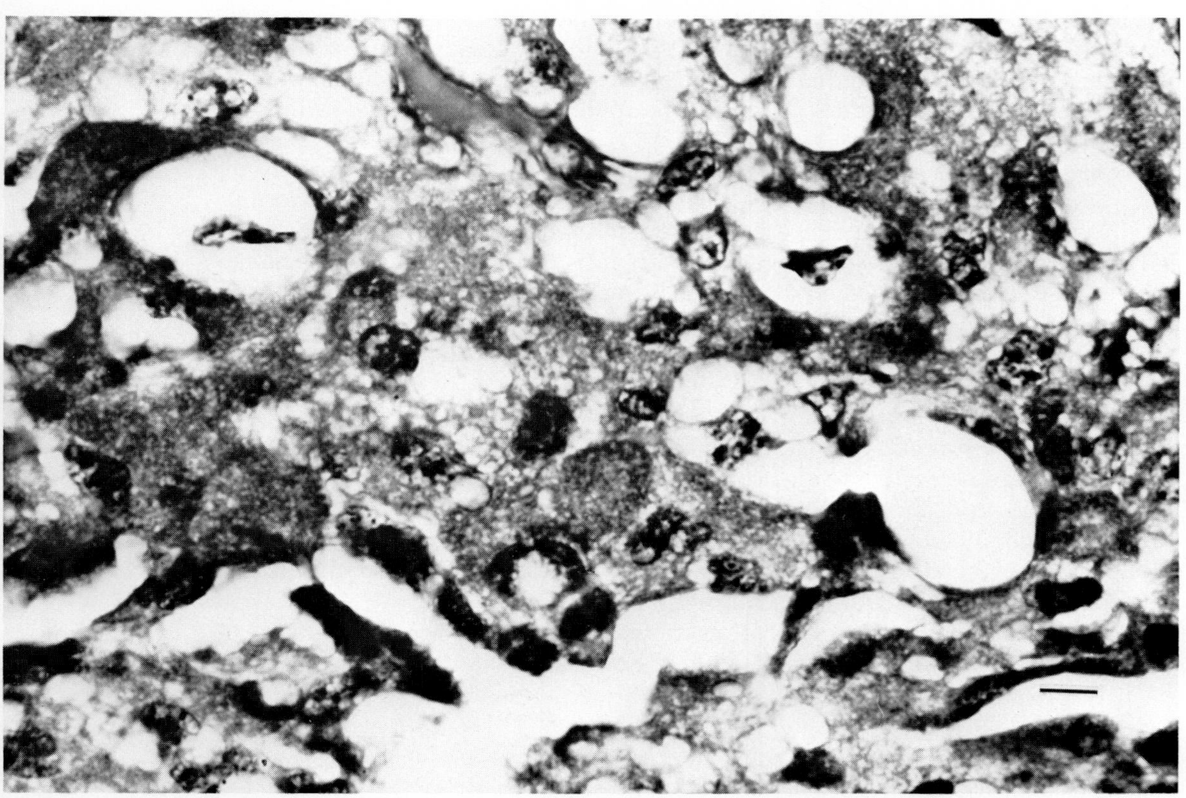

Fig. 1. Paraffin section of Bouin's-fixed specimen of pituitary adenoma from a patient with Nelson's syndrome. Granules are not apparent. Orange G–PAS–hematoxylin stain. Scale bar: 10 μm.

TABLE 1. Classification of Pituitary Adenomas

GH-producing (somatotropic) adenoma
Prolactin-producing adenoma (prolactinoma)
Acidophilic stem-cell adenoma
ACTH-producing (corticotropic) adenoma
TSH-producing (thyrotropic) adenoma
LH- and FSH-producing (gonadotropic) adenoma
Tumors producing more than one hormone (mixed adenomas)
Endocrinologically inactive tumors
  Oncocytic adenoma
  Nononcocytic adenoma

phobic in paraffin sections. Often, the granules can be seen in 1-μm sections of tissue fixed in glutaraldehyde and embedded in plastic as for electron microscopy, but examined in the light microscope. Figures 1 and 2 illustrate such a finding from a woman with Nelson's syndrome. Figure 1 shows an absence of stainable granules in Bouin's-fixed paraffin-embedded material; Fig. 2 shows abundant granules in glutaraldehyde-fixed material examined in the light microscope.

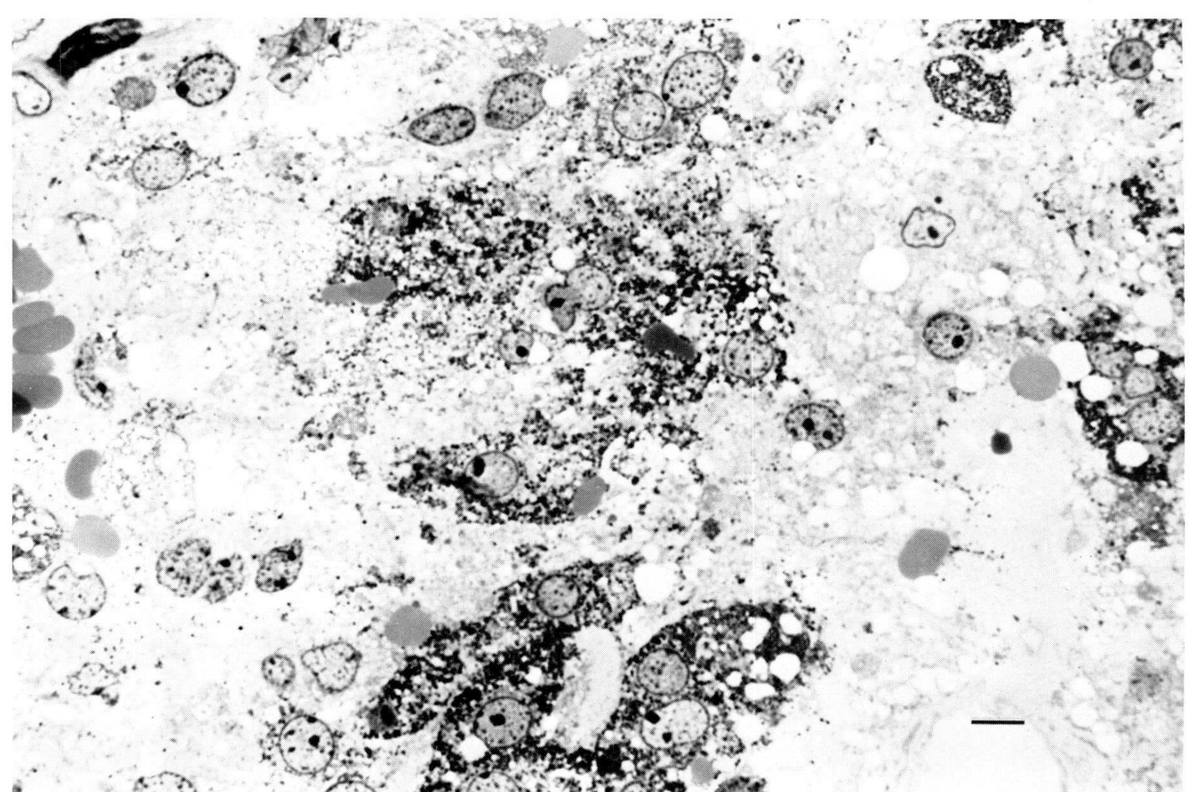

Fig. 2. Glutaraldehyde-fixed specimen from the same patient embedded in Araldite and sectioned at 1 μm. Granules are easily seen. Tolouidine blue stain. Scale bar: 10 μm.

Recent reviews of pituitary adenomas universally classify these tumors by the hormone or hormones produced, rather than by the functional properties of the cells.[14–18] The modern classification is summarized in Table 1.

2. Modern Techniques and Their Limitations

2.1. Electron Microscopy

The granules of the cells of the normal pituitary gland can be classified by their size and density, as seen in the electron microscope: Gray[19] found that the cells of the normal gland could be divided into six types, based on the size of granules in their cytoplasm. Cells with granules 100–160 nm in diameter were thought to contain TSH; those with granules 160–200 nm in diameter were thought to contain LH. Granules 200–270 nm in diameter were considered characteristic of FSH, and those 270–410 in diameter were correlated with ACTH. The granules of classic acidophils were larger: 410–500 nm for GH and 500–600 nm for prolactin. The identification of granules was not corroborated by parallel demonstration of hormones by immunological techniques. Furthermore, differences in granule sizes are most pronounced in resting cells. In actively secreting cells, granule size decreases and is not a reliable criterion by which to identify the hormone being produced.[20]

Some pituitary adenomas have granules that are easily recognized as GH[21] or prolactin.[6] But in many adenomas, granule size is not a reliable marker of the hormone being produced. In patients with acromegaly, Landolt and Rothenbühler[22] found granules between 160 and 342 nm, all of which were demonstrated to be GH by immunological stains. Granules of small size characteristic of basophils were found in acromegaly by Schecter[23] and in nonfunctioning tumors by Gray *et al.*[24] Small granules are characteristic of sparsely granulated adenomas,[22] and classification of these tumors must depend on features other than granule size. These features will be discussed below, but it is necessary to point out here that although some workers believe that classification of tumors by electron microscopy is easily accomplished,[15] others doubt that it can be done with reliability.[18]

Early studies suggested that patients with high serum hormone levels were more likely to have a sparsely granulated tumor than a densely granulated one.[25–26] Recent series show a poor correlation between granule size and serum hormone levels.[15,18,22] Although sparsely granulated tumors tend to be associated with ultrastructural signs of active synthesis such as prominence of the endoplasmic reticulum and Golgi apparatus, it is these signs of synthesis that are better correlates of high serum hormone levels, not the granule size. Furthermore, serum hormone levels depend on rate of release, as well as the rate of synthesis, and intracellular lysosomal digestion of formed hormone may keep the rate of release low even when synthesis is rapid.[27,28]

2.2. Immunological Staining

Isolation and purification of the pituitary hormones has permitted the development of antibodies directed against them. Cells containing a given hormone can be visualized by coupling the appropriate antibody with fluorescein and examining the specimen under a microscope with ultraviolet illumination. A second technique consists of reacting unlabeled antibody with the hormone antigen and then demonstrating the antigen–antibody complex with a fluorescein-label antibody directed against the globulins of the species in which the original antihormone antibody was made. For example, anti-human GH, made in the rabbit, can be visualized with fluorescein-labeled anti-rabbit globulin, made in the sheep. A third technique couples the sheep anti-rabbit globulin to peroxidase, rather than fluorescein. The peroxidase is then visualized by the 3,3′-diaminobenzidine reaction.[29] These techniques can be performed on formalin-fixed, paraffin-embedded material[30] (Fig. 3).

The peroxidase method has several advantages. The reaction product can be visualized at the light- and electron-microscopic levels.[31] Furthermore, the technique is more sensitive, even at the light-microscopic level. In somatotropic adenomas, the fluorescein technique stained only the heavily granulated cells, but the peroxidase technique stained sparsely granulated cells as well.[32]

Application of these methods to pituitary tumors has given further evidence that the traditional stains do not adequately reflect the hormone content of tumor cells. Prolactin was demonstrated by immunoperoxidase in 6 of 45 tumors that were chromophobic by histochemical techniques.[33] Of 28 tumors that were acidophilic on periodic acid–Schiff (PAS)–light green–Orange G stain, 8 were unstained by immunocytochemical techniques, 11 contained only prolactin, 3 contained only GH, and 6 contained both hormones.[34]

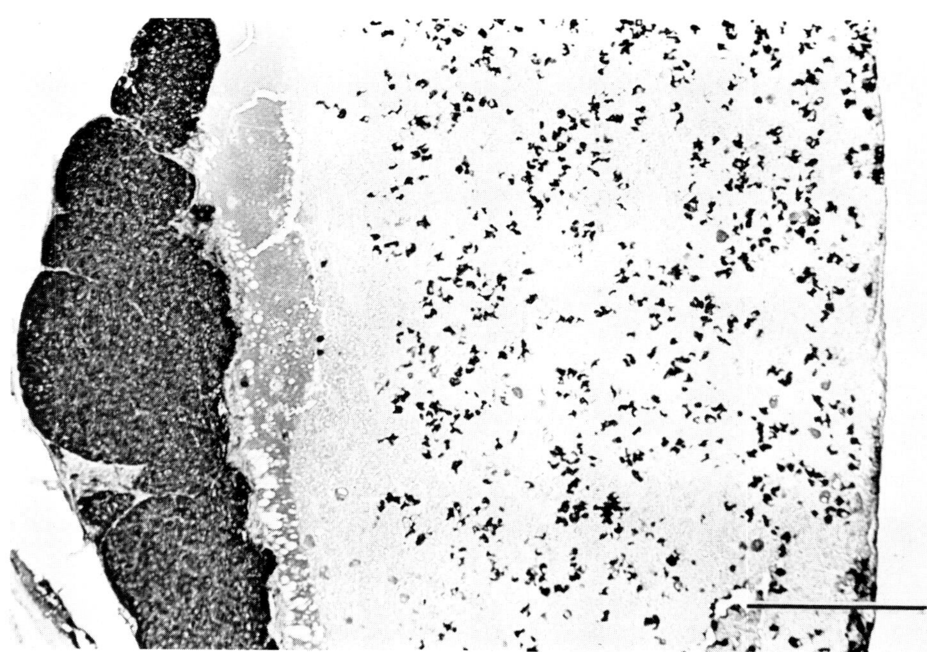

Fig. 3. ACTH-containing cells of the pituitary gland demonstrated by immunoperoxidase staining. The cells containing ACTH are black. Scale bar: 250 μm. Courtesy of Dr. Sean O'Briain, New England Medical Center.

Immunological staining is probably the most accurate method of determining which hormones are present in normal or neoplastic pituitary cells. Zimmerman *et al.*[35] found a good correlation between prolactin and GH levels in the serum of patients with pituitary adenomas and the demonstration of these hormones in their tumors by immunoperoxidase. Seven of eight patients with elevated serum GH showed GH in their tumors. Prolactin was seen in the tumor cells of 10 of 12 patients with elevated serum prolactin. Four patients had elevation of both GH and prolactin, and both hormones were stainable in each of the tumors removed from these patients. On the other hand, GH was found in the tumor of a patient with normal serum GH, and prolactin was found in a tumor from a patient with a normal serum prolactin level. In another study, two patients with pituitary adenomas thought to be secondary to hypothyroidism had tumors that did not stain with immunoperoxidase directed against TSH, although sparsely distributed granules measuring 120–200 nm were seen on electron microscopy.[36]

Immunoperoxidase, like electron microscopy, is limited to the demonstration of granules present at the moment of biopsy and does not measure rate of synthesis or release of hormones. Furthermore, a tumor may not make

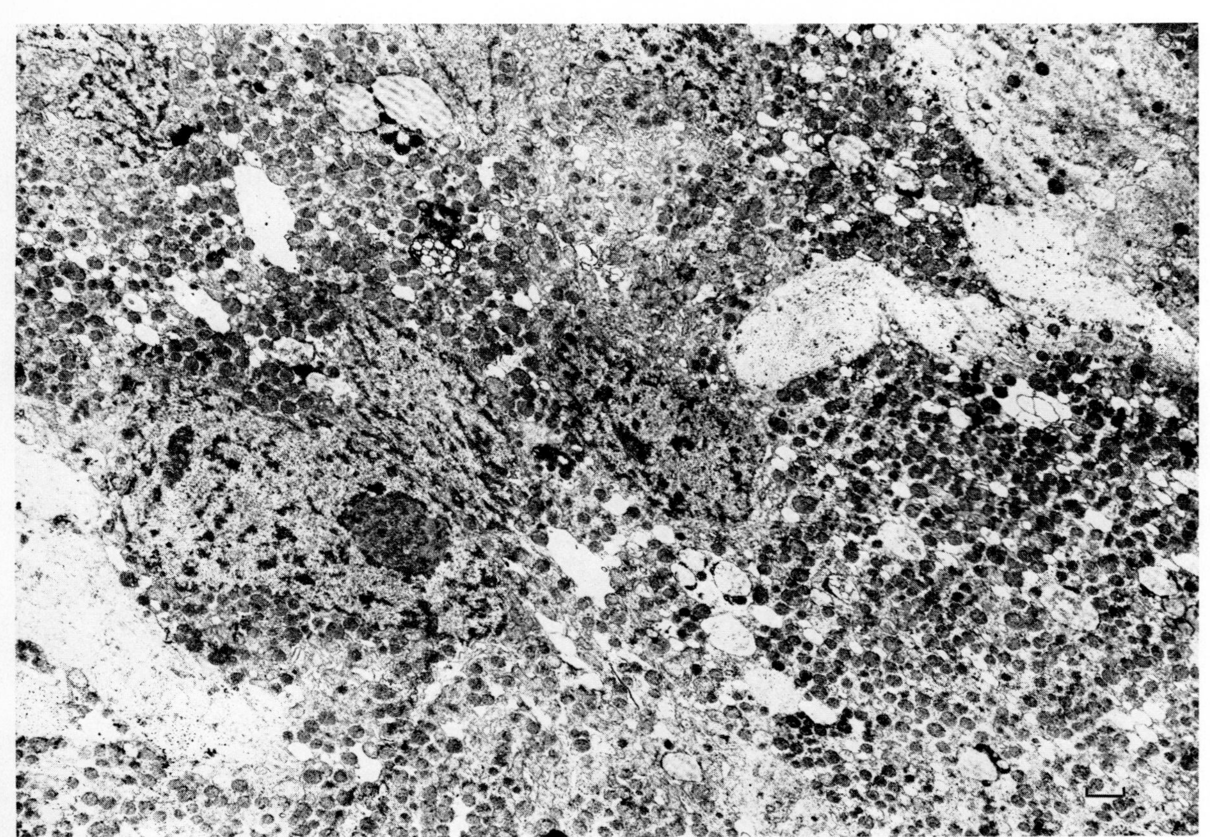

Fig. 4. Densely granulated somatotropic adenoma. This electron micrograph demonstrates numerous GH granules. Scale bar: 1 μm.

hormones identical to those made by normal cells, and the part of the molecule recognized by the antibody may not be the same as the part responsible for endocrinological activity.

3. Electron Microscopy of Pituitary Adenomas

3.1. Somatotropic (Growth-Hormone-Producing) Adenomas

Two varieties of this tumor are recognized: a densely granulated tumor and a sparsely granulated variant.[14,15] The two subtypes occur with equal frequency, so that about half the somatotropic tumors are densely granular and half are sparsely granular.[15,37] The electron-microscope appearance of the densely granulated tumors is similar to that of normal somatotropes.[14,15,21] The rough endoplasmic reticulum is prominent, as is the Golgi apparatus, and secretory granules are numerous, spherical, and electron-dense, and measure between 350 and 450 nm in diameter (Fig. 4).

The sparsely granulated variant shows much more cellular and nuclear pleiomorphism. The rough-surfaced endoplasmic reticulum and Golgi are again prominent, but the cells of these tumors also show marked proliferation of the smooth endoplasmic reticulum. Spherical aggregates of 12-nm filaments are characteristic of sparsely granulated somatotropic tumors.[38,39] Such masses have been found in 55% of GH-secreting tumors.[40] Centrioles and cilia are also found in these tumors and are often intermixed with the filamentous masses.[41] Tubular inclusions are found, not in the tumor cells, but in the endothelial cells of blood vessels.[42,43] They were found in 30% of adenomas from acromegalic patients, but in only 2% of adenomas without endocrine activity.[42] Granules are, by definition, more sparsely distributed in these tumors, but are found in almost every cell. They are smaller than those of the heavily granulated tumors, but could be demonstrated to contain GH by the immunoperoxidase technique.[22]

3.2. Prolactinomas

Again, a heavily granulated and a sparsely granulated variant are recognized.[44,45] In prolactinomas, the sparsely granulated variant is much more common than the densely granulated type, unlike the equal distribution of the subtypes in GH-secreting tumors.[15] The heavily granulated type is again composed of cells that are similar to their non neoplastic counterpart—the normal prolactin-producing cell in this case.[6] The rough endoplasmic reticulum and Golgi apparatus are prominent. The granules are of high electron density. They are the largest granules seen in pituitary adenomas, and are much larger than the GH granules, with an average size of 600 nm and a largest size of 1200 nm. Unlike GH granules, they are not always round; they are often oval or pleiomorphic.

Sparsely granulated adenomas, which are "chromophobic" by light microscopy, are the common prolactin-producing tumor.[12,15] They have even more prominent endoplasmic reticulum than the heavily granulated tumor; it often forms concentric whorls called "Nebenkerns." The Golgi is more prominent. The granules are much smaller than those of the heavily granulated variant; usually, they measure between 200 and 300 nm in diameter (Fig. 5). Extrusion of granules into the extracellular space distant from the capillaries is seen only in this tumor type and is called "misplaced exocytosis."[46] Dystrophic calcification, occurring in single necrotic cells undergoing fibrillary transformation, has been described only in prolactin-secreting tumors.[47]

3.3. Mixed Prolactin- and Growth-Hormone-Producing Tumors

These tumors have been found in patients who have acromegaly. In a series of six cases, five were also associated with elevated serum prolactin,[48] but since any pituitary tumor can produce hyperprolactinemia by interference with prolactin-inhibiting factor from the hypothalamus,[49,50] the tumor is defined by the anatomical demonstration of secretion of both hormones by tumor cells. Morphological evidence suggests that such tumors are composed of distinct populations of somatotropes and prolactin-secreting cells often ar-

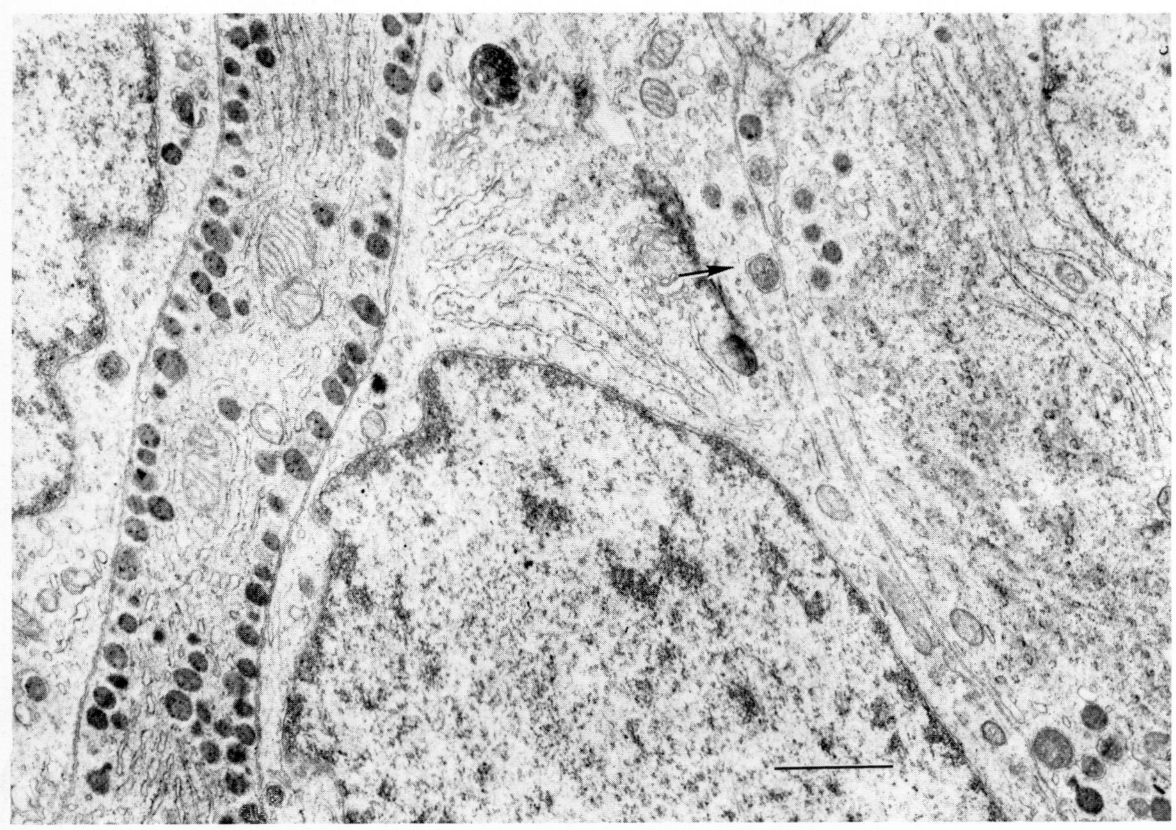

Fig. 5. Electron micrograph of a sparsely granulated prolactinoma. Note the abundant endoplasmic reticulin, variability of granule size, and the misplaced exocytosis (arrow). Scale bar: 1 μm.

ranged in groups,[48,51] but Landolt[18] has summarized theoretical evidence for production of both hormones by the same cell.

3.4. Corticotropic Adenomas

These adenomas show more ribosomes, both associated with the endoplasmic reticulum and free, than those previously described. Secretory granules, found in almost every cell, average 300–350 nm in size. The granules show considerable variation in electron density and tend to line up along the outer membranes of the cell[52,53] (Fig. 6).

Although a follicular arrangement of cells was present in a tumor from one patient with Cushing's disease,[54] this feature does not seem to be specific for any single type of pituitary cell.[55]

Perinuclear accumulations of 7-nm filaments occur in patients with Cushing's disease.[52,53] This is the electron-microscopic counterpart of Crooke's hyaline change.[56] Since this change correlates best with raised serum levels of adrenal cortical steroids,[57] it is not surprising that it is not seen in corticotropic adenomas from patients with Nelson's syndrome.[58,59]

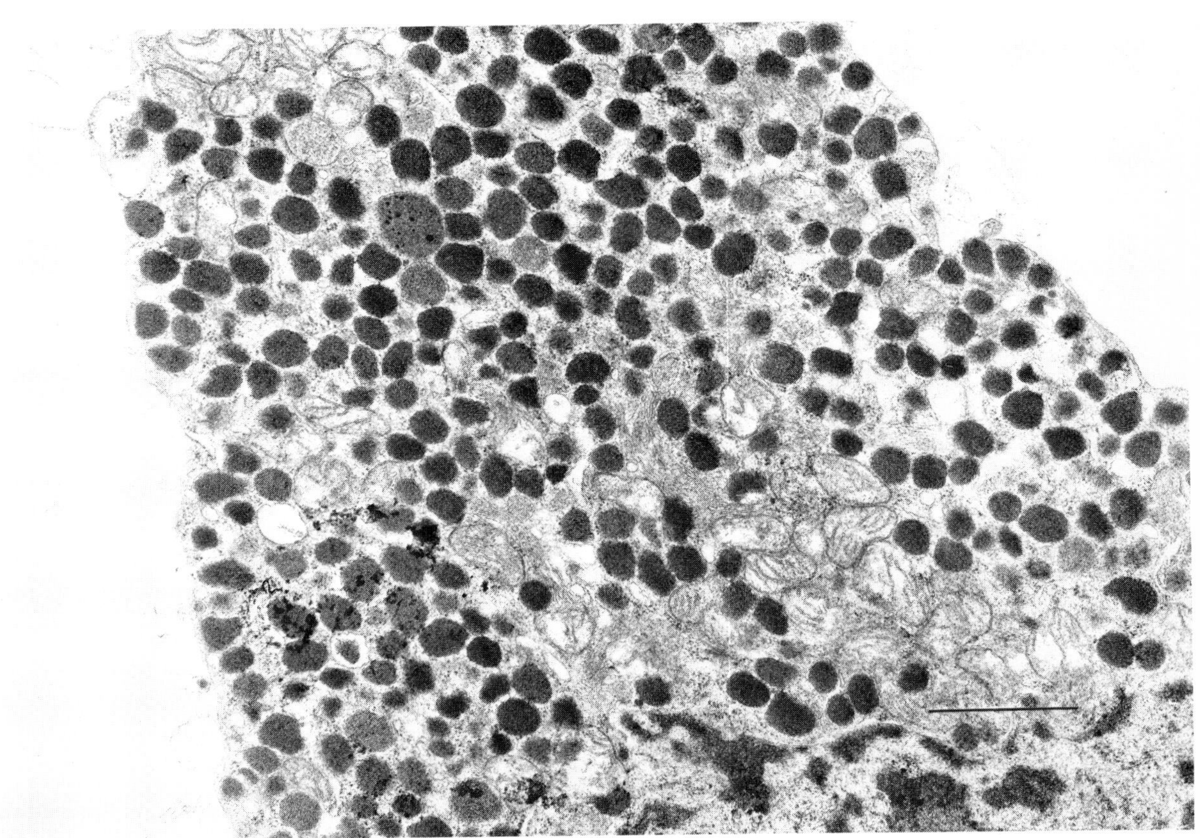

Fig. 6. Electron micrograph of a densely granulated corticotropic adenoma. Scale bar: 1 μm.

3.5. Thyrotropic Adenomas

Secretory granules 90–150 nm in diameter were found in adenomas from a patient with hypothyroidism[60] and a patient with hyperthyroidism.[61]

3.6. Gonadotropic Adenomas

The electron microscopy of these tumors has not been described.

3.7. Acidophilic Stem-Cell Adenomas[62]

Some patients with these tumors have moderate elevations of blood prolactin; others have normal levels. By light microscopy, they are ungranulated or have sparse eosinophilic granules. Immunoperoxidase reactions demonstrate both prolactin and GH in the cells. Ultrastructurally, they show features of both sparsely granulated prolactinomas (misplaced exocytosis) and sparsely granulated somatotropes (fibrous bodies and centrioles), often in the same cell.

3.8. Oncocytomas

Adenomas composed of oncocytes have cells larger than most other adenomas, but smaller than oncocytes in other organs. At the level of the light microscope, they appear either eosinophilic or chromophobic. The characteristic electron-microscopic feature is that the cytoplasm is packed with mitochondria, the cristae of which are deformed. Other organelles are scanty, but small numbers of secretory granules 100–150 nm may be found.[63,64] Small numbers of oncocytes were found in 3 normal glands examined for them and in 6 of 16 pituitary adenomas in which they were not the predominant cell.[65] Transitional forms among several types of granulated cells and oncocytes were seen, suggesting that they can arise from any cell type.[65] The features useful in distinguishing sparsely granulated tumors are summarized in Table 2.

4. Additional Features

4.1. Amyloid Production

Amyloid is occasionally found in pituitary adenomas. It is sometimes surrounded by histiocytes,[66] and it is composed of 7.5- to 9.5-nm filaments.[67]

TABLE 2. Features Useful in Distinguishing Sparsely Granulated Tumors from Each Other

Prolactinomas	Misplaced exocytosis, dystrophic calcification, Nebenkerns
Somatotropic tumors	Fibrous bodies (12 nm), centrioles, cilia
Corticotrope	Crooke's hyaline (7 nm)
Oncocytoma	Mitochondria

These features suggest that it is immunologically derived. On the other hand, it is found in adenoma cells as well as in the extracellular space,[68] and it does not contain tryptophan. This suggests that it is produced by the tumor cells and is similar to the nonimmunologically derived amyloid characteristic of other endocrine tumors of the APUD system of endocrine cells (see Chapter 2).

4.2. Hemorrhage and Infarction

Hemorrhage into pituitary adenomas was described by Cushing,[1] who called it "pituitary apoplexy." It is a cause of rapid neurological deterioration in such patients. Hemorrhage may occur in patients who do not show the clinical signs of pituitary apoplexy. In one series, 18 of 70 patients with pituitary adenoma had grossly visible hemorrhage at surgery.[69] Only 3 presented with clinical symptoms referable to the hemorrhage, and an additional 3 had a history compatible with previous bleeding. In the remainder, the hemorrhage was asymptomatic. Spontaneous infarction also occurs in pituitary adenomas, and may be clinically indistinguishable from hemorrhagic pituitary apoplexy.[70]

4.3. Carcinoma of the Pituitary Gland

Local invasion of adjacent tissues occurs occasionally in pituitary adenomas, and is not evidence of malignancy.[71] Seeding of the subarachnoid space and spread outside the cranium occur much more rarely, and are taken as biological evidence of malignancy. Although nuclear atypicism occurs in many otherwise innocent adenomas, most adenomas that behave in a malignant fashion have a higher mitotic index than their benign counterparts. Most reported cases have been associated with Cushing's syndrome[72–74]; only one case has been reported in a patient without this syndrome.[75]

5. Incidence of the Various Types of Pituitary Adenomas (Table 3)

In the series of Kovacs *et al.*[15] and of Landolt,[18] prolactin-producing adenomas are slightly more common than GH-producing tumors. In our own material, prolactin-producing tumors are by far the most common, but this probably reflects patterns of referral to our endocrinologists and neurosurgeons. Differences in referral patterns may also explain why ACTH-producing tumors constituted 14% of the material of Kovacs and co-workers, but only 4% of Landolt's.

It is clear that prolactinomas and somatotropic adenomas are far more common than tumors derived from basophils. Of the basophilic tumors, ACTH-producing adenomas are by far the most common; thyrotropic and gonadotropic tumors are rare. In the series of Kovacs and co-workers, almost all the prolactinomas, and half the somatotropic adenomas, were sparsely granular, but almost all the ACTH-producing tumors were heavily granulated.

TABLE 3. Relative Incidence of Various Types of Pituitary Adenomas

	Kovacs *et al.*[15]	Landolt[18]
Prolactinoma	25	39
GH	22	33
Mixed	5	—
Stem-cell	5	4
ACTH	14	4
TSH	1	—
Gonadotropic	0	—
(Undifferentiated)	26	24[a]

[a]Endocrine-inactive and oncocytoma.

Undifferentiated tumors are about as frequent as somatotropic tumors and prolactinomas.

If one adds the sparsely granulated tumors to the undifferentiated tumors in the series of Kovacs and co-workers, the total is about two thirds the cases. These are the traditional "chromophobes." Of these, abut a third were prolactinomas, a sixth were somatotropic, and half were hormonally inactive.

6. Frozen-Section Diagnosis of Pituitary Adenomas

The ability of surgeons to perform selective removal of small pituitary adenomas via the transphenoidal route, using the dissecting microscope, has made it important for the pathologist to be able to tell the surgeon whether a small fragment of tissue is adenoma or normal gland. In essence, the surgeon is asking the pathologist to define the margins of the tumor. Some adenomas are so poorly differentiated cytologically that distinguishing them from the normal gland can easily be done on conventionally stained sections. In more than half the cases, however, the tumor is well differentiated and special stains are required.

We have used an Orange G–hematoxylin stain to aid in making the distinction.[76] This takes advantage of the fact that the number of granules in adenoma cells tends to be about the same, from cell to cell. Thus, the cells of a tumor all have orangeophilic granules or are all unstained. Sections of normal gland usually contain eosinophils and therefore show both granulated and ungranulated cells. Orange G–PAS–hematoxylin stains were performed on the same pieces of tissue after Bouin's fixation and paraffin embedding. There was agreement in diagnosis between frozen sections and permanent sections in more than 90% of the sections examined. The intraoperative diagnosis of adenoma, in tissue thought to be grossly normal by the surgeon, has led to removal of additional tumor in several patients.[77] Another technique takes advantage of the relative paucity of reticulin in adenomas compared to normal gland and uses a rapid reticulin stain performed on frozen sections.[78]

References

1. H.C. Cushing, *The Pituitary Body and Its Disorders*, Lippincott, Philadelphia, 1912.
2. J.W. Kernohan and G.P. Sayre, *Tumors of the Pituitary Gland and Infundibulum*, Atlas of Tumor Pathology, Section X, Fascicle 36, Armed Forces Institute of Pathology, Washington, D.C. 1956.
3. M. Herlant and J.L. Pasteels, Histophysiology of human anterior pituitary, *Methods Achiev. Exp. Pathol.* **3:**250, 1967.
4. A.P. Forbes, P.H. Henneman, G.C. Griswald, and F. Albright, A syndrome characterized by galactorrhea, amenorrhea and low urinary FSH: Comparison with acromegaly and normal lactation, *J. Clin. Endocrinol.* **14:**265, 1954.
5. F. Robert and J. Hardy, Prolactin secreting adenomas, *Arch. Pathol.* **99:**625, 1975.
6. G.T. Peake, D.W. McKeel, L. Jarett, and W.H. Daughaday, Ultrastructural, histologic and hormonal characterization of a prolactin rich human pituitary tumor, *J. Clin. Endocrinol.* **29:**1383, 1969.
7. J. Trovillas, D. Pallo, and J. Tournaire, Les adénomes hypophysaires avec aménorhée–galactorhée isolée, *Lyon Med.* **236:**359, 1976.
8. R.L. Rovit and R. Berry, Cushing's syndrome and hypophysis, *J. Neurosurg.* **23:**270, 1965.
9. D.G. Young, R.C. Bahn, and R.V. Randall, Pituitary tumors associated with acromegaly, *J. Clin. Endocrinol. Metab.* **25:**249, 1965.
10. I. Jackson, Hyperthyroidism in a patient with a pituitary chromophobe adenoma, *J. Clin. Endocrinol. Metab.* **25:**491, 1965.
11. P.J. Snyder and F.H. Sterling, Hypersecretion of LH and FSH by a pituitary adenoma, *J. Clin. Endocrinol. Metab.* **42:**544, 1976.
12. P.D. Lewis and S. van Noorden, "Nonfunctioning" pituitary tumors, *Arch. Pathol.* **97:**178, 1974.
13. W.F. McCormick and N.S. Halmi, Absence of chromophobe adenomas from a large series of pituitary tumors, *Arch. Pathol.* **92:**231, 1971.
14. E. Horvath and K. Kovacs, Ultrastructural classification of pituitary adenomas, *Can. J. Neurol. Sci.* **3:**9, 1976.
15. K. Kovacs, E. Horvath, and C. Ezrin, Pituitary adenomas, in: *Pathology Annual 1977*, Part 2 (S.C. Sommers and P.P. Rosen, eds.), pp. 341–382, Appleton-Century-Crofts, New York, 1977.
16. A.M. Landolt, Ultrastructure of human sella tumors, *Acta Neurochir. Suppl.* **22:**1, 1975.
17. L. Olivier, E. Vila-Porcile, O. Racadot, F. Peillon, and J. Racadot, Ultrastructure of pituitary tumor cells: A critical study, in: *Ultrastructure in Biological Systems: The Anterior Pituitary* (A. Tixier-Vidal and M.G. Farquhar, eds.), pp. 231–276, Academic Press, New York, 1975.
18. A.M. Landolt, Progress in pituitary adenoma biology: Results of research and clinical applications, in: *Advances and Technical Standards in Neurosurgery* (H. Krayenbuhl, ed.), pp. 3–50, Springer-Verlag Vienna and New York, 1978.
19. A.B. Gray, Analysis of diameters of human pituitary hormone secretory granules, *Acta Endocrinol.* **85:**249, 1977.
20. M. Herlant, Introduction, in: *Ultrastructure in Biological Systems* (A. Tixier-Vidal and M.G. Farquhar, eds.), pp. 3–19, Academic Press, New York, 1975.
21. J. Schechter, Electron microscopic studies of human pituitary tumors. II. Acidophilic adenomas, *Am. J. Anat.* **138:**387, 1973.
22. A.M. Landolt and V. Rothenbühler, The size of growth hormone granules in pituitary adenomas producing acromegaly, *Acta Endocrinol.* **84:**461, 1977.
23. J. Schechter, Electron microscopic studies of human pituitary tumors. I. Chromophobic adenoma, *Am. J. Anat.* **138:**371, 1973.
24. A.B. Gray, I. Doniach, and P.N. Leigh, Correlation of diameters of secretory granules in clinically non-functioning chromophobe adenomas of the pituitary with those of normal thyrotrophs, *Acta Endocrinol.* **79:**417, 1975.
25. P.D. Lewis and S. van Noorden, Pituitary abnormalities in acromegaly, *Arch. Pathol.* **94:**119, 1972.
26. U. Schelin, Light and electron microscopical studies on pituitary adenomas in acromegaly, *Acta Pathol. Microbiol. Scand. Suppl.* **158:**1, 1962.
27. M.G. Farquhar, Processing of secretory products by cells of the anterior pituitary gland, in:

Subcellular Organization and Function in Endocrine Tissues (H. Heller and K. Lederis, eds.), pp. 79–124, Cambridge University Press, Cambridge, 1971.

28. M.G. Farquhar, E.H. Skutelsky and C.R. Hopkins, Structure and function of the anterior pituitary and dispersed pituitary cells: *In vitro studies*, in: *Ultrastructure in Biological Systems: The Anterior Pituitary* (A. Tixier-Vidal and M.G. Farquhar, eds.), pp. 83–135, Academic Press, New York, 1975.
29. P.K. Nakane, Application of peroxidase-labelled antibodies to the intracellular localization of hormones, *Acta Endocrinol. Suppl.* **153:**190, 1971.
30. A.C. Nieunenhuyzen Kruseman, G.T.A.M. Bots, and E. Lindeman, The immunohistochemical identification of hormone-producing cells in formalin-fixed, paraffin-embedded human pituitary tissue, *J. Pathol.* **117:**163, 1975.
31. P.K. Nakane and G.B. Pierce, Enzyme labelled antibodies for light and electron microscopic localization of tissue antigen, *J. Cell Biol.* **33:**307, 1967.
32. A.C. Nieunenhuyzen Kruseman, G.T.A.M. Bots, J. Lindeman, and A. Schaberg, Use of immunohistochemical and morphologic methods for the identification of human growth hormone–producing pituitary adenomas, *Cancer* **38:**1163, 1976.
33. K. Kovacs, B. Corenblum, A.M.T. Sirek, G. Penz, and C. Ezrin, Localization of prolactin in chromophobe pituitary adenomas: Study of human necropsy material by immunoperoxidase technique, *J. Clin. Pathol.* **29:**250, 1976.
34. N.S. Halmi and T. Duello, "Acidophilic" pituitary tumors: A reappraisal with differential staining and immunocytochemical techniques, *Arch. Pathol. Lab. Med.* **100:**346, 1976.
35. E.A. Zimmerman, R. Defendini, and A.G. Frantz, Prolactin and growth hormone in patients with pituitary adenomas: A correlative study of hormone in tumor and plasma by immunoperoxidase technique and radioimmunoassay, *J. Clin. Endocrinol. Metab.* **38:**577, 1974.
36. N.A. Samaan, B.M. Osborne, B. Mackay, M.E. Leavans, T.M. Duello, and N.S. Halmi, Endocrine and morphologic studies of pituitary adenomas secondary to primary hypothyroidism, *J. Clin. Endocrinol. Metab.* **45:**903, 1977.
37. F. Robert and J. Hardy, Prolactin-secreting adenomas: A light and electron microscopical study, *Arch. Pathol.* **99:**625, 1975.
38. R.R. Cardell and R.S. Knighton, The cytology of a human pituitary tumor: An electron microscopic study, *Trans. Am. Microsc. Soc.* **85:**58, 1966.
39. S.S. Schochet, Jr., W.F. McCormick, and N.S. Halmi, Acidophil adenomas with intracytoplasmic filamentous aggregates: A light and electron microscopic study, *Arch. Pathol.* **94:**16, 1972.
40. A.M. Landolt, Ultrastructure of human sella tumors, *Acta Neurochir. Suppl.* **22:**1, 1975.
41. E. Horvath, K. Kovacs, and C. Ezrin, Centrioles and cilia in non-tumorous anterior lobes and adenomas of the human pituitary, *Pathol. Eur.* **11:**81, 1976.
42. A.M. Landolt, H. Ryffel, H.U. Hosbach, and R. Wyler, Ultrastructure of tubular inclusions in endothelial cells of pituitary tumors associated with acromegaly, *Virchows Arch. Pathol. Anat. Histol.* **370:**129, 1976.
43. K. Kovacs, E. Horvath, K.P.H. Pritzker, and M.L. Schwartz, Pituitary growth hormone cell adenoma with cytoplasmic tubular aggregates in the capillary endothelium, *Acta Neuropathol.* **37:**77, 1977.
44. K. Kovacs, E. Horvath, B. Cornblum, A.M.T. Sirek, G. Penz, and C. Ezrin, Pituitary chromophobe adenomas consisting of prolactin cells: A histologic, immunocytological and electron microscopic study, *Virchows Arch. Pathol. Anat. Histol.* **366:**113, 1975.
45. K. Kovacs, Morphology of prolactin producing adenomas, *Clin. Endocrinol.* **6**(Suppl.):71s, 1977.
46. E. Horvath and K. Kovacs, Misplaced exocytosis: Distinct ultrastructural feature in some pituitary adenomas, *Arch. Pathol.* **97:**221, 1974.
47. A.M. Landolt and V. Rothenbühler, Pituitary adenoma calcification, *Arch. Pathol. Lab. Med.* **101:**22, 1977.
48. B. Corenblum, A.M.T. Sirek, E. Horvath, K. Kovacs, and C. Ezrin, Human mixed somatotrophic and lactotrophic pituitary adenomas, *J. Clin. Endocrinol. Metab.* **42:**857, 1976.
49. R.W. Turkington, L.E. Underwood, and J.J. Van Wyk, Elevated serum prolactin levels after pituitary-stalk section in man, *N. Engl. J. Med.* **295:**707, 1971.
50. M.T. Buckman and G.T. Peake, Prolactin in clinical practice, *J. Am. Med. Assoc.* **236:**871, 1976.

51. H. Guyda, F. Robert, E. Colle, and J. Hardy, Histologic, ultrastructural and hormonal characterization of a pituitary tumor secreting both hGH and prolactin, *J. Clin. Endocrinol. Metab.* **36:**531, 1973.
52. J. Racadot, F. Peillon, and E. Vila-Porcile, Les adénomes hypophysaires dans la maladie de Cushing: Étude de 21 cas, *Ann. Endocrinol.* **34:**753, 1973.
53. K. Kovacs and E. Horvath, Amphophil adenoma of the human pituitary gland with masses of cytoplasmic microfilaments, *Endokrinologie* **63:**402, 1974.
54. R.M. Bergland and R.M. Torack, An ultrastructural study of follicular cells in the human anterior pituitary, *Am. J. Pathol.* **57:**273, 1969.
55. E. Horvath, K. Kovacs, G. Penz, and C. Ezrin, Origin, possible function and fate of "follicular cells" in the anterior lobe of the human pituitary, *Am. J. Pathol.* **77:**199, 1974.
56. F.A. DeCicco, A. Dekker, and E.J. Unis, Fine structure of Crooke's hyaline change in the human pituitary gland, *Arch. Pathol.* **94:**65, 1972.
57. N.S. Halmi, W.F. McCormick, and D.A. Decker, Jr., The natural history of hyalinization of ACTH–MSH cells in man, *Arch. Pathol.* **91:**318, 1971.
58. K. Kovacs, E. Horvath, N.A. Kerenyi, and R.H. Sheppard, Light and electron microscopic features of a pituitary adenoma in Nelson's syndrome, *Am. J. Clin. Pathol.* **65:**337, 1976.
59. J.H. Garcia, H. Kalimo, and J.R. Givens, Human adenohypophysis in Nelson syndrome: Ultrastructural and clinical study, *Arch. Pathol. Lab. Med.* **100:**253, 1976.
60. R. Mornex, M. Tomasi, M. Caré, J. Farcot, J. Orgiazzi, and B. Rousset, Hyperthyroidie associée à un hypopituitarisme au cours de l'évolution d'une tumeur hypophysaire sécrétant TSH, *Ann. Endocrinol.* **33:**390, 1972.
61. A.S.Y. Leong, J.C. Chawla, and E.C. Teh, Pituitary thyrotropic tumor secondary to long-standing primary hypothyroidism, *Pathol. Eur.* **11:**49, 1976.
62. E. Horvath, K. Kovacs, W. Singer, C. Ezrin, and N.A. Kerenyi, Acidophil stem cell adenoma of the human pituitary, *Arch. Pathol. Lab. Med.* **101:**594, 1977.
63. K. Kovacs and E. Horvath, Pituitary "chromophobe" adenoma composed of oncocytes: A light and electron microscopic study, *Arch. Pathol.* **95:**235, 1973.
64. A.M. Landolt and U.W. Oswald, Histology and ultrastructure of an oncocytic adenoma of the human pituitary, *Cancer* **31:**1099, 1973.
65. K. Kovacs, E. Horvath, and J.M. Bilbao, Oncocytes in the anterior lobe of the human pituitary gland, *Acta Neuropathol.* **27:**43, 1974.
66. R. Schober and D. Nelson, Fine structure and origin of amyloid deposits in pituitary adenoma, *Arch. Pathol.* **99:**403, 1975.
67. J.M. Bilbao, K. Kovacs, E. Horvath, H.P. Higgins, and W.J. Horsey, Pituitary melanocorticotrophinoma with amyloid deposition, *Can. J. Neurol. Sci.* **2:**199, 1975.
68. J.M. Bilbao, E. Horvath, A.R. Hudson, and K. Kovacs, Pituitary adenoma producing amyloid-like substance, *Arch. Pathol.* **99:**411, 1975.
69. S. Mohanty, P.N. Tandon, A.K. Banerji, and B. Prakash, Hemorrhage into pituitary adenomas, *J. Neurol. Neurosurg. Psychiatr.* **40:**987, 1977.
70. J.P. Conomy, J.H. Ferguson, J.S. Brodkey, and H. Mitsumoto, Spontaneous infarction in pituitary tumors: Neurologic and therapeutic aspects, *Neurology* **25:**580, 1975.
71. P.O. Lundberg, B. Drettner, A. Hemmingsson, B. Stenkvist, and L. Wide, The invasive pituitary adenoma: A prolactin-producing tumor, *Arch. Neurol.* **34:**742, 1977.
72. H. Cohen and J.H. Dible, Pituitary basophilism associated with basophil carcinoma of the anterior lobe of the pituitary gland, *Brain* **59:**395, 1936.
73. W. Forbes, Carcinoma of the pituitary gland with metastases to the liver in a case of Cushing's syndrome, *J. Pathol. Bacteriol.* **59:**137, 1947.
74. R.M. Salassa, T.P. Kearns, J.W. Kernohan, R.G. Sprague, and C.S. McCarty, Pituitary tumors in patients with Cushing's syndrome, *J. Clin. Endocrinol. Metab.* **19:**1523, 1959.
75. V.St.E. D'Abrera, W.J. Burke, K.F. Bleasel, and L. Bader, Carcinoma of the pituitary gland, *J. Pathol.* **109:**335, 1973.
76. L.S. Adelman and K.D. Post, Intraoperative frozen section technique for pituitary adenomas, *Am. J. Surg. Pathol.* **3:**173, 1979.
77. K.D. Post, B.J. Biller, L.S. Adelman, M. Molitch, S.M. Wolpert, and S. Reichlin, Results of selective transsphenoidal adenomectomy in women with galactorrhea–amenorrhea, *J. Am. Med. Assoc.* **242:**158, 1979.
78. M.E. Velasco, S.D. Sindley, and U. Roessman, Reticulum stain for frozen-section diagnosis of pituitary adenomas, *J. Neurosurg.* **46:**548, 1977.

II

Clinical Features of Pituitary Tumors

4

Galactorrhea Syndromes

BRUCE J. BILLER, AUBREY BOYD III, MARK E. MOLITCH, KALMON D. POST, SAMUEL M. WOLPERT, and SEYMOUR REICHLIN

1. Introduction

With the advent of prolactin radioimmunoassay[1–4] and the development of sophisticated radiological techniques for visualization of the pituitary fossa,[5] it has become apparent that prolactin-producing pituitary adenomas are the most common pituitary disease seen in clinical practice.[6] Patients with prolactinomas often present with galactorrhea as the cardinal symptom,[7] and it has therefore become a major diagnostic dilemma to distinguish those patients who harbor adenomas from those with galactorrhea due to other causes. This chapter is designed to: (1) delineate and characterize the subgroup of galactorrhea patients with pituitary adenomas; (2) provide detailed, long-term follow-up of galactorrhea syndromes in order to define their natural history more precisely; (3) determine the influence of elevated prolactin levels on pituitary, adrenal, and ovarian function; and (4) study the etiological factors involved in galactorrhea. Results of initial study of 25 galactorrhea patients have recently been reported by our group.[8] We have now had the opportunity to extend the study in a more detailed fashion to an additional 45 patients. This larger sample of 70 galactorrhea patients provided a wider variety of clinical expression of this syndrome, led to revision of standards of prolactin

---

BRUCE J. BILLER, AUBREY BOYD III, MARK E. MOLITCH, and SEYMOUR REICHLIN • Tufts University School of Medicine; Department of Medicine, Division of Endocrinology, Tufts–New England Medical Center Hospital, Boston, Massachusetts 02111. *KALMON D. POST* • Tufts University School of Medicine; Department of Neurosurgery, Tufts–New England Medical Center Hospital, Boston, Massachusetts 02111. Dr. Biller's present address is: Department of Medicine, Massachusetts Institute of Technology, Cambridge, Massachusetts 02139. Dr. Boyd's present address is: Department of Internal Medicine, Division of Endocrinology and Metabolism, Baylor College of Medicine, Houston, Texas 77030. This chapter was presented in part at the 58th Annual Meeting, American College of Physicians, April 21, 1977, Dallas, Texas, and at the 29th Annual Meeting, Congress of Neurological Surgeons, October 13, 1977, San Francisco, California.

values associated with tumors, and modified our earlier interpretations of the significance of stimulation tests. These findings are analyzed and compared with studies of other investigators.[9–12]

2. Materials and Methods

2.1. Patients

Seventy women referred for evaluation of galactorrhea, with and without amenorrhea, were admitted to the Clincial Study Unit, New England Medical Center Hospital. Their clinical features and classification are outlined in Section 3.

2.2. Anatomical Evaluation of the Pituitary Fossa

All patients underwent sella polytomography at 1- to 2-mm intervals in the antero–posterior and lateral projections with the use of hypocycloidal-movement,[5] computerized tomography (CT scan) of the sella turcica, both with and without iodinated contrast material according to the technique described by Rozario *et al.*,[13] and complete ophthalmological evaluation, including visual-field testing by Goldmann perimetry. Most patients with abnormal sella polytomographs, CT scan or visual-field examinations underwent pneumoencephalography and selective carotid–vertebral angiography to further define the sella or parasellar region.

2.3. Endocrinological Evaluation of Galactorrhea Patients

Neuroendocrine regulation of prolactin (PRL) secretion was evaluated by measuring the response to (1) L-dopa (0.5 g by mouth),[14] (2) chlorpromazine (0.7 mg/kg intramuscularly up to a maximum of 50 mg),[15,16] (3) thyrotropin-releasing hormone (TRH) (500 μg intravenously),[17,18] and (4) insulin-induced hypoglycemia (0.15 U regular insulin/kg intravenously).[19,20] Responses in normal individuals for these and other tests of endocrine function are shown in Table 4. Serum levels of the other pituitary trophic hormones were also studied: Luteinizing hormone (LH) and follicle-stimulating hormone (FSH) were measured in the basal state and at 15, 30, 60, 90, and 120 min after administration of gonadotropin-releasing hormone (GnRH) (100 μg intravenously).[21,22] Growth hormone (GH) was measured in the fasting state and after insulin-induced hypoglycemia (0.15 U Regular insulin/kg intravenously)[20] and L-dopa (0.5 g by mouth).[23] Cortisol was measured at 08:00 hours and at 15, 30, 60, and 90 min after insulin-induced hypoglycemia (0.15 U Regular insulin/kg intravenously).[20] Estradiol-17β (E_2) was measured in the basal state at $t = 0$ during the GnRH test. Thyroid function was evaluated by measurement of serum thyroxine (T_4), triiodothyronine (T_3), and thyroid-stimulating hormone (TSH) in the basal state and at 15, 30, 60, 90, 120, and 150 min after administration of TRH (500 μg intravenously).[18] Posterior pituitary function was assessed by 14-hr dehydration testing according to the protocol described by Miller *et al.*[24] Normal controls were studied for comparison (see Table 3).

2.4. Assay Procedures

Pituitary hormones were measured by radioimmunoassay utilizing materials supplied by the National Pituitary Agency (NPA), National Institute for Arthritis, Metabolic Disease and Diabetes (NIAMDD). These include PRL,[2,4] GH,[25] thyrotropin (TSH), FSH, and LH. (The latter three hormones were assayed by methods supplied with NPA kits.) Results for LH and ESH were expressed in milli International Units per milliliter utilizing LER 907 as standard (biological potency 60 mIU/ng for LH and 20 mIU/ng for FSH). Human TSH standard A was provided by Dr. D.R. Bangham, International Laboratory for Biological Standards, Hampstead Laboratories, Holly Hill, London, and results are reported in microUnits per milliliter. T_3 was measured by radioimmunoassay by the method of Nejad *et al.*[26] and T_4 by the method of Bollinger and Reichlin (unpublished). E_2[27] and testosterone were measured by radioimmunoassay performed by Diamond Shamrock Medical Laboratory.

3. Results

3.1. Categories of Galactorrhea Patients

To ensure optimum therapy, differentiation of those patients with a PRL-secreting adenoma from those with more benign causes of galactorrhea is essential. Alterations in the sella turcica or abnormalities of visual fields are currently accepted as suggestive evidence for the existence of a pituitary tumor, but proof of a tumor usually requires surgical confirmation or gross evidence of a mass lesion by invasive neuroradiological studies. While the classic changes in sella architecture strongly suggesting a tumor are tilting of the sella floor to one side with erosion of the anterior wall,[28] sloping of the floor is a common anatomical variant[29] and when seen alone is not absolute evidence of an adenoma (see Chapter 13). Of the 70 women we evaluated for galactorrhea, 35 (50%) had abnormal sella polytomographs or visual-field examinations. A diagnosis of pituitary adenoma has been verified in 18 patients treated thus far by transsphenoidal adenomectomy and in 2 patients treated by proton-beam therapy (evidence of tumor provided by pneumoencephalography, arteriography, and cavernous sinography). These 20 patients constitute Group I, Verified Adenomas. The remaining 50 patients were classified into five separate groups on the basis of clinical, radiological, and hormonal features. These groups were further analyzed to determine whether patients with occult tumors could be detected among those with normal sella polytomographs on the basis of hormonal responses to neuroendocrine stimulation testing. The resulting characterization is summarized in Table 1. Group I, made up of the 20 established adenoma patients, all had galactorrhea, amenorrhea,[19] or oligomenorrhea,[1] low serum estradiol levels, elevated basal serum PRL levels, and abnormal sella polytomes or visual fields. Group II, Probable Adenomas, included 15 patients, all of whom had galactorrhea and

TABLE 1. Categories of Galactorrhea Patients

Findings	Group I	II	III	IV	V	VI
Galactorrhea	+	+	+	+	+	+
Oligomenorrhea/amenorrhea, low estradiol	+	±	+	+		
Elevated prolactin	+	±	+			+
Abnormal sella polytomography	+	+				

abnormal sella polytomes. Unlike those in Group I, 7 had normal basal PRL levels and 3 had normal menses and estradiol levels. While the abnormal polytomes were highly suggestive that prolactinomas were present, we do not have surgical verification of this diagnosis. Further testing, in fact, showed the empty sella syndrome in 3 of the patients[13] and occult primary hypothyroidism in 1.[30] Group III is identical to Group I in four features (galactorrhea, oligomenorrhea, low estradiol, and elevated PRL), but there were no radiographically evident tumors in any of the 15 patients. Group IV comprised 4 patients with galactorrhea, amenorrhea, and low estradiol, but with normal basal PRL and normal sella polytomographs. Group V comprised 15 patients who had galactorrhea unaccompanied by abnormalities of menstural function, estradiol, PRL, or sella polytomography. Group VI consisted of 1 patient with galactorrhea and elevated PRL, but normal menses and estradiol, and normal sella polytomographs.

3.2. Clinical Evaluation of Patients with Galactorrhea: Etiological Associations and Patient Complaints (Table 2)

Detailed historical surveys were performed in all patients to identify the association of childbirth, oral-contraceptive use, amenorrhea, drug use, or breast stimulation with the chief complaint of galactorrhea. In the patients taken as a whole, 18% had developed galactorrhea in the postpartum period, 24% had stopped birth-control pills immediately before the onset of galactorrhea, and 5% had primary amenorrhea. Secondary amenorrhea was found in 66%. Neurogenic causes of galactorrhea were found in 2 patients. One developed galactorrhea after laminectomy and X-ray therapy for a cervical ependymoma, while another practiced frequent manual breast-emptying to relieve painful postpartum engorgement. A drug-induced cause of galactorrhea was suspected in a single patient who developed galactorrhea during chlorpromazine therapy, but symptoms persisted after withdrawal of the drug, making a definite cause-and-effect relationship less likely. Half of all galactorrhea cases arose without obvious cause, including 10 with verified pituitary tumors. In patients with verified adenomas, galactorrhea appeared after pregnancy in 1 case, after contraceptive-pill use in 6, and in association with primary amenorrhea in 3 (Table 2). While amenorrhea occurred in all 20 established adenoma patients (Group I) and in 12 of 15 probable adenoma patients (Group II), half the patients with normal polytomographs (Groups III–VI) were also amenorrheic. Though 6 verified tumor patients and 3 "probable" tumor pa-

TABLE 2. Clinical Presentation of Women with Galactorrhea Syndromes

Categories	Total	Secondary amenorrhea	Primary amenorrhea	Spontaneous	Postpartum	Postpill
Established pituitary tumors (Group I: Verified adenomas)	20	17	3	10	1	6
Others with abnormal polytomes (Group II: Probable adenomas)	15	12	0	10	10	3
Normal polytomes (Groups III–VI)	35	17	2	15	15	8
TOTALS:	70	46 (66%)	5 (7%)	35 (50%)	26 (37%)	17 (24%)

tients had developed galactorrhea after discontinuing birth-control pills, 8 patients with normal sella polytomes also had postpill galactorrhea.

Patient complaints were systematically elicited and are summarized in Table 3. Headache (78%) and weight gain (40%) were common complaints among all patients with galactorrhea regardless of cause. Diminished libido and dyspareunia (28%), acne–seborrhea–hirsutism (22%), fatigue (21%), dry skin (17%), constipation (15%), and visual disturbances (diplopia, blurred vision, diminished acuity, impaired peripheral vision) (12%) occurred less frequently. While these complaints characterized the galactorrhea syndrome in general, there were no complaints sufficiently specific for established tumor patients that could aid in detecting occult adenomas among other groups. In particular, the symptom of headache was not specific to established tumor patients, occurring in 45% of those with normal sella polytomographs.

TABLE 3. Incidence of Clinical Complaints in Women with Galactorrhea Syndromes

Complaints	Total (%)	Established tumors (%)	All other patients	
			Abnormal polytomes (%)	Normal polytomes (%)
Headache	78	60	53	45
Weight gain	40	50	40	34
Decreased libido and dyspareunia	28	30	26	28
Acne/oily skin/hirsuitism	22	30	33	14
Fatigue	21	30	26	14
Dry skin	17	35	0	14
Constipation	15	35	6	8
Visual disturbances	12	15	13	11

3.3. Prolactin Secretion in Patients with Galactorrhea

Forty-two patients (60%) had hyperprolactinemia. However, basal PRL levels did not adequately differentiate among Group I, Verified Adenomas, and the five other patient groups. In our series, only basal PRL levels of greater than 260 ng/ml were invariably associated with radiologically and surgically verified pituitary tumors. An elevated basal serum PRL did not, by itself, constitute sufficient proof of a pituitary adenoma, since similar values were found in Groups III and VI, where no patient had radiographic or visual-field abnormalities (Fig. 1). Nonetheless, we have noted that 4 of the verified adenoma patients had made a transition from normal (Group III) to abnormal (Group I) sella polytomographs during 3 years of observation. Therefore, the normal polytomographs previously obtained in such patients did not, by themselves, totally exclude the presence of a small prolactinoma that might make its radiographic appearance only over a period of time. Last, a normal basal PRL level did not entirely exclude the existence of an adenoma: one verified adenoma case with initially elevated basal PRL levels (44 ng/ml) underwent asymptomatic, spontaneous, partial necrosis of the tumor (verified at surgery). She developed normal basal PRL values (19.8 and 17.9 ng/ml) preoperatively, values that overlapped with those in Groups II, IV, and V. In light of this occurrence, and the frequent finding of areas of hemorrhagic necrosis in other turmors, we cannot assign a lower limit of normal below which prolactinomas do not occur.

We next considered results of dynamic tests of PRL secretion. Of 12 established adenoma cases tested, 5 showed a blunted fall (33% decline from baseline) in PRL after oral L-dopa, a precursor of dopamine that stimulates receptors in pituitary PRL cells and in the hypothalamus[9] (Fig. 2 and Table 4). This pattern, indicative of attenuated dopamine responsiveness in 41% of

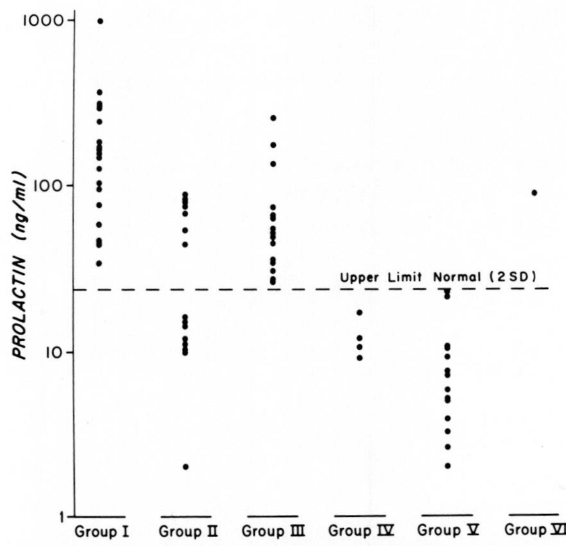

Fig. 1. Mean basal PRL levels in women with galactorrhea.

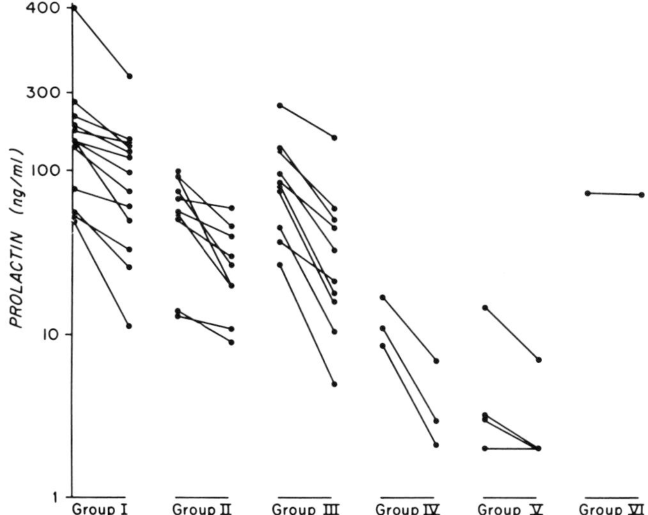

Fig. 2. PRL secretory response to L-dopa (0.5 g, p.o.) in women with galactorrhea.

TABLE 4. Incidence of Abnormal Responses to Neuroendocrine Stimulation Tests in Women with Galactorrhea Syndromes

	Agent								
	GnRH		L-Dopa	TRH		Chlorpromazine	Hypoglycemia		
Group	LH	FSH	PRL	PRL	TSH	PRL	PRL	hGH	Cortisol
I	3/16	1/15	5/12	16/16	7/16	14/14	9/10	4/18	2/17
II	0/8	0/7	3/9	7/12	2/11	6/8	3/5	2/11	1/13
III	0/9	0/9	0/10	9/9	0/10	9/9	7/7	3/11	0/13
IV	1/3	0/3	0/3	1/3	0/3	1/3	1/3	2/4	0/4
V	0/6	1/6	0/4	2/6	1/6	0/0	2/6	0/6	0/6
VI	0/1	0/1	1/1	1/1	0/1	0/0	1/1	0/1	0/1
TOTALS:	4/43 (9%)	2/41 (5%)	9/39 (23%)	36/47 (77%)	10/47 (21%)	30/34 (88%)	23/32 (72%)	11/51 (22%)	3/54 (6%)

Criteria for normal stimulation tests based (except where noted) on study of control group (number of cases shown in parentheses):
LH after GnRH: 3.75 times or more increase over baseline when E_2 levels are in early follicular range (11).
FSH after GnRH: 1.56 times or more increase over baseline when E_2 levels are in early follicular range (12).
PRL after L-dopa: 33.0% or greater fall from baseline level (5).
PRL after TRH: 2.33 times or more increase over baseline level (10).
TSH after TRH: 5.5 m IU/ml or more increase above baseline level (15).
PRL after chlorpromazine: 3.0 times or more increase above baseline level (6).
PRL after hypoglycemia: 28% or more increase above baseline level.[20]
hGH after hypoglycemia: 2.0 times or more increase above baseline level, with an increment of at least 8 ng/ml.[103]
Cortisol after hypoglycemia: 10 μg% or more increase above baseline and a value greater than 20 μg%.[103]

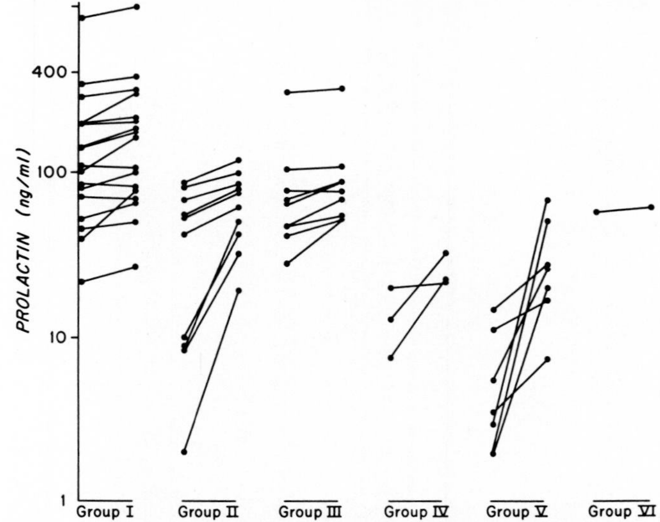

Fig. 3. PRL secretory response to TRH (500 μg, i.v.) in women with galactorrhea.

the verified adenoma cases tested, occurred in 33% of Group II patients, all of whom had abnormal sella X-rays. Blunted L-dopa responses were rare in other patients with galactorrhea (1 of 18), all of whom had normal X-rays. Thus, blunted responses to L-dopa suggest the existence of a PRL-secreting autonomous adenoma, but normal responses do not exclude tumor. PRL and TSH responses to TRH, a peptide known to directly stimulate pituitary release, were studied (Figs. 3 and 4 and Table 4). The PRL secretory response to

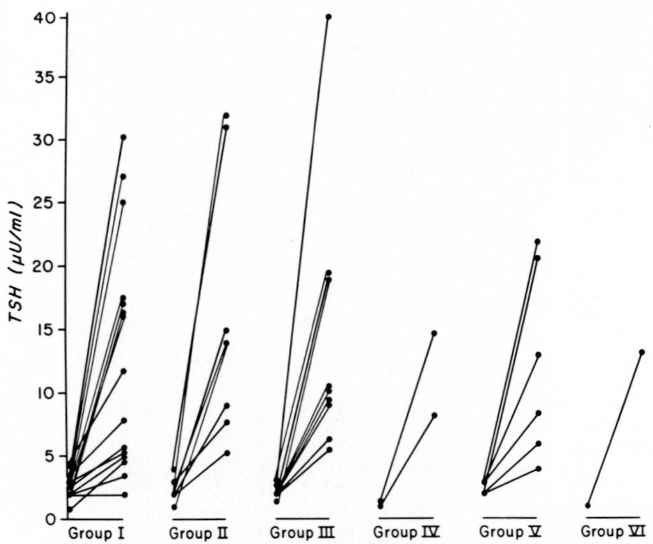

Fig. 4. TSH secretory response to TRH (500 μg, i.v.) in women with galactorrhea.

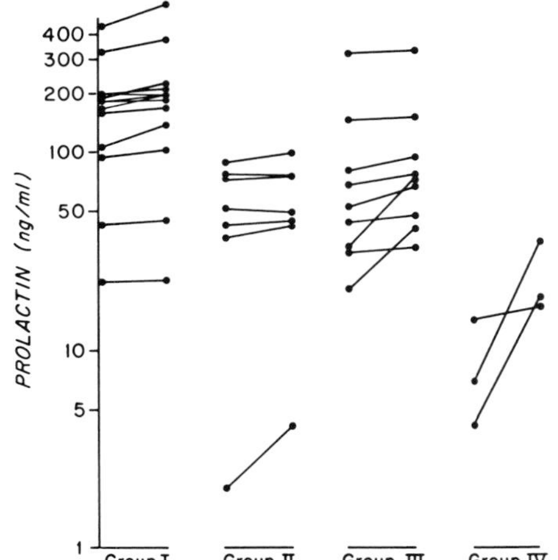

Fig. 5. PRL secretory response to chlorpromazine (0.7 mg/kg, i.m.) in women with galactorrhea.

TRH was blunted (less than 2.3 times baseline) in all cases of adenoma, and in 7 of 12 cases of probable adenoma (Group II). However, blunting was also observed in 13 of 19 other cases and hence does not discriminate among the various groups. Although a smaller proportion of established adenoma cases had a blunted TSH response to TRH (43%), only 3 of 31 cases in the other categories were abnormal. Therefore, low TSH reserve may be a helpful sign of tumor. Despite the high frequency of blunted TSH responses to TRH, all patients had normal serum T_4 and T_3 and were clinically euthyroid. Patients with adenomas tested with chlorpromazine and hypoglycemia, stimuli believed to act principally via the hypothalamus, showed responses that were indistinguishable from those of other galactorrhea patients (Figs. 5 and 6 and

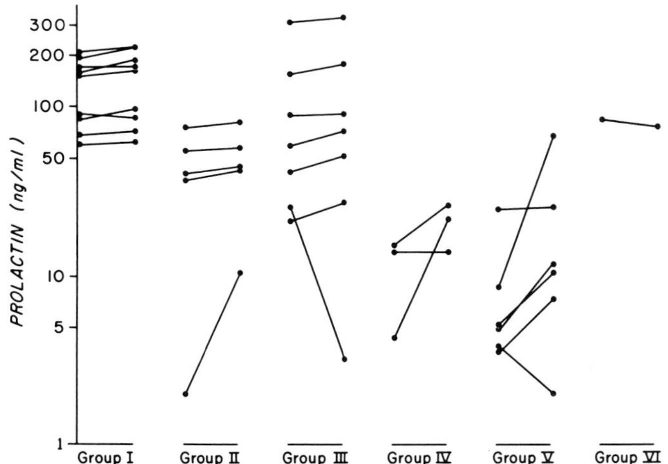

Fig. 6. PRL secretory response to insulin-induced (0.15 U/kg, i.v.) hypoglycemia in women with galactorrhea.

Table 4). Every one of the established adenoma patients had blunted PRL rise after chlorpromazine (less than 3 times baseline); after hypoglycemia, a blunted PRL rise (less than 28% above baseline) was seen in 90% of those tested. While such impaired responses may signify an alteration in hypothalamic function or pituitary responsivity to hypothalamic factors, the responses were not unique to any particular group and did not aid in differentiation between tumor and nontumor patients.

3.4. Gonadotropic Function in Patients with Galactorrhea

All verified adenoma cases (Group I) had amenorrhea or oligomenorrhea[47] and decreased serum estradiol levels (Fig. 7). Although decreased E_2 levels and menstural dysfunction were also noted in most of the Group II, Probable Adenoma, patients, these two features were also seen in all Group III and IV patients, none of whom had anatomical evidence of tumor. Virtually all patients with oligomenorrhea (Groups I–IV) had basal gonadotropin levels that were inappropriately low in the face of a chronic state of relative estrogen deficiency (Fig. 4 and Table 4). Nevertheless, only 3 established adenoma cases (Group I), 1 Group IV patient, and 1 Group V patient had blunted gonadotropin responses to GnRH (Figs. 8 and 9 and Table 4). Not only was gonadotropin response to GnRH normal in all other patients, but also there was no apparent difference in the response characteristics among groups. Thus, neither basal gonadotropins, basal estradiol, nor GnRH stimulation testing provided an endocrine profile of established adenomas that could separate occult tumors from the other galactorrhea patients.

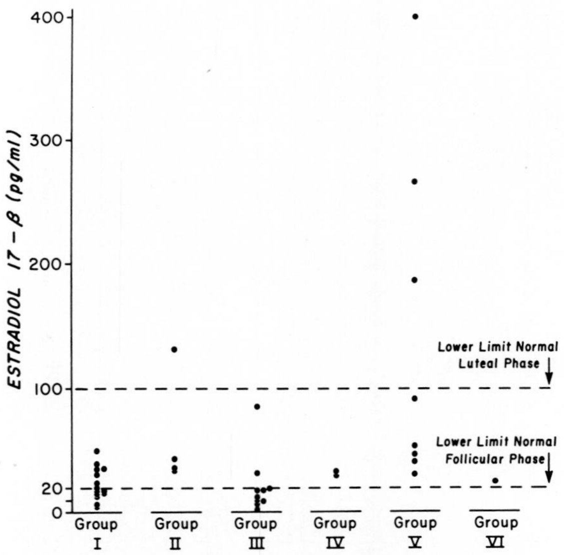

Fig. 7. E_2 levels in women with galactorrhea.

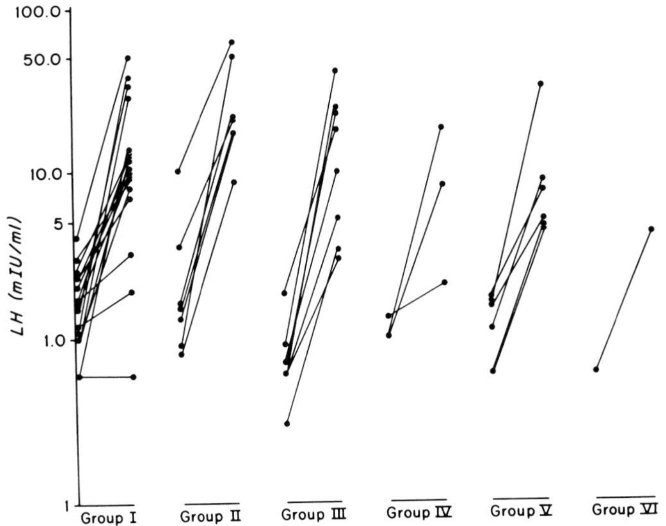

Fig. 8. LH secretory response to GnRH (100 μg, i.v.) in women with galactorrhea.

3.5. Growth Hormone, Adrenocorticotropin, and Antidiuretic Hormone Function in Patients with Galactorrhea

Two of the Group I, Verified Adenoma, patients had ACTH-reserve deficiency demonstrated by insulin-induced hypoglycemia and confirmed by overnight metyrapone testing[90] (Table 4), and four had GH-reserve deficiency

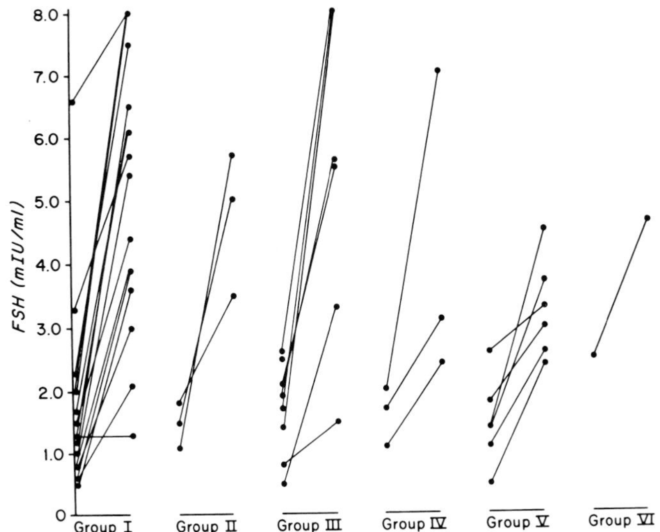

Fig. 9. FSH secretory response to GnRH (100 μg, i.v.) in women with galactorrhea.

on challenge with hypoglycemia and L-dopa.[23,103] ACTH-reserve deficiency was also documented in a single patient from Group II, while GH-reserve deficiency was discovered in two patients from Groups II and IV and three patients from Group III. Among the three cases in Group II, Probable Adenomas, one with GH-reserve deficiency was shown to have the empty sella syndrome on CT scan and pneumoencephalography.[13] Among all patients with galactorrhea, only one, a verified adenoma patient with suprasellar extension of the tumor, had abnormal antidiuretic hormone (ADH) function with a state of partial diabetes insipidus. Thus, stimulation testing of ACTH, GH, and ADH detected 14 patients with apparent hormone-reserve deficiencies, 7 of whom had established adenomas and 2 of whom had probable adenomas. However, the remaining 5 patients, all from Group III or IV, had no radiographic evidence of tumor, making the presence of such deficiencies only suggestive of an adenoma.

4. Discussion

Our study was designed to evaluate women presenting with galactorrhea. A number of investigators have sought to determine the incidence of galactorrhea in the general population. Friedman and Goldfien[31] found no breast secretion of any type in 114 nulliparous females. Vetter *et al.*[32] found galactorrhea in only 0.9% of nearly 5600 women examined. However, Jones and Gentile[33] studied 800 women, finding that 3.6% of anovulatory and 1.0% of ovulatory women had galactorrhea. Other studies, however, have found an appreciably higher incidence of galactorrhea, ranging from 12 to as high as 46%.[34–36] Such variability has been attributed by Buckman and Peake[37] to (1) breast examination technique, (2) different definition of galactorrhea, and (3) erroneous requirement for its presence in both breasts. In two separate studies, they report a 26% incidence among 50 normal women and a 22% incidence among 73 normal women, suggesting that the value of galactorrhea as a disease marker is, as yet, unknown, particularly among women with normal menses. However, the higher incidences were found in women who presented themselves for gynecological examination and may not be a true reflection of an entirely unselected population. We agree with Buckman and Peake[37] that proper breast-examination technique (gently, but firmly, milking the breast from all quadrants toward the nipple with the patient supine and leaning forward) is essential for detection of nonspontaneous galactorrhea. We emphasize that galactorrhea may be unilateral in 15–50% of cases,[34,35] may vary in the same individual from day to day, may manifest as only a single drop of breast secretion, and is frequently expressible only by direct pressure.[37] Moreover, we and others have found that neither the presence of occult or overt galactorrhea nor the amount of expressible milk correlates well with the serum PRL level.[12] Based on our own experience, and the data of other investigators, we view the presence of nonpuerperal lactation as an important marker of underlying pituitary–hypothalamic disease and a finding that demands further investigation.

While prolactinomas are now believed to represent approximately

33–70% of "chromophobe" adenomas,[6,38] their overall incidence is difficult to assess. In a study by Costello,[39] 265 (26.5%) of 1000 pituitary glands obtained during routine postmortem examination contained "subclinical adenomas," of which 52.8% were chromophobic, 27.2% basophilic, 7.5% eosinophilic, and 12.4% mixed. He noted the lack of historical or clinical indication of pituitary dysfunction in any case in which an adenoma was found, but the diligence with which such findings were sought can be questioned. These subclinical adenomas likely represent the base from which arise cases that attract our clinical attention because of galactorrhea and may reconcile the varied epidemiological studies on galactorrhea with our own results. We were able to verify the presence of adenoma in 29% of our patients overall and in 38% of those with both galactorrhea and menstrual dysfunction. Our high percentage of verified adenoma patients is biased by referral practices that tend to emphasize patients with already-documented radiographic abnormalities of the sella. Nonetheless, our findings are similar to those of Nader *et al.*,[7] who estimated a 48% incidence of tumor in 25 patients presenting with galactorrhea alone (prospective study) and a 58% incidence of tumors in 62 patients presenting with both galactorrhea and amenorrhea (retrospective study). Haesslein and Lamb[40] found that 53% of patients with galactorrhea and amenorrhea had adenomas, while Kase *et al.*[41] noted a 35% incidence among patients with galactorrhea. The data of Gomez *et al.*[10] and Canfield and Bates[42] also support an incidence of 37% in patients with galactorrhea. However, only a 15% incidence of tumors was detected by Tolis *et al.*[12] among 65 women with galactorrhea. This was paralleled by the recent report by Kleinberg *et al.*[11] showing an 18% tumor incidence among 42 women with galactorrhea alone and 34% among those with both galactorrhea and amenorrhea.

While all our patients presented with galactorrhea as their chief complaint, the literature also suggests that the absence of galactorrhea, either as a symptom or as a physical finding, in the face of irregular menses does not exclude underlying prolactinoma. Franks *et al.*[43] studied 106 women with secondary amenorrhea and found PRL elevations in 20% of those with so-called "functional amenorrhea" and in 12 of 13 with pituitary tumors, though only 3 patients in each group had galactorrhea. They emphasized that if galactorrhea had been taken as the index of excessive PRL secretion, at least two thirds of patients with hyperprolactinemia would not have been identified. This study supported earlier results reported by Frantz *et al.*[1] and Franks *et al.*,[44] and was reconfirmed in a subsequent investigation by Jacobs *et al.*,[45] who found a 22% incidence of hyperprolactinemia among 75 patients with amenorrhea alone, ranking it as the second most common cause of menstrual dysfunction in their series, a series in which only 30% of 35 women had galactorrhea. More recently, Franks *et al.*[46] reported a study of 60 patients with radiographic evidence of tumors and hyperprolactinemia, finding only a 28% incidence of galactorrhea. Last, Haesslein and Lamb[40] studied 144 women with secondary amenorrhea of greater than 6 month's duration, detecting 13 (9%) with evidence of pituitary tumor. Their analysis, however, indicated that if the amenorrhea was of 24 months' duration, 17% (12 of 71) had detectable tumors, and if the amenorrhea was longer than 5 years' duration, the likelihood of demonstrating tumor increased to 25%. Only one patient with amenorrhea of less than 24 months' duration had evidence of a pituitary tumor in their series.[40] Eight of our verified tumor patients, on the other hand, had oligo-/amenorrhea for less than 24 months, including two of less than 12 months' duration. We believe that the presence of galactorrhea alone demands further investigation of pituitary–hypothalamic function, since the likelihood of detecting a pituitary adenoma in this setting lies between 15 and 48%. When galactorrhea and amenorrhea occur together, the likelihood of detecting an adenoma rises to 34–59%. When amenorrhea occurs alone, 22% may have hyperprolactinemia, and the incidence of detectable adenomas will range between 9 and 34%.[7]

The historical data obtained from patients associating persistent lactation with the postpartum state, oral contraceptive use, primary amenorrhea, or other factors did not aid us in defining a subset more likely to harbor prolactinomas. Similar difficulties have been encountered by others and indicate that various eponyms commonly applied to galactorrhea syndromes do not have etiological or diagnostic value.[47–49] Kleinberg *et al.*[11] found that among 42 women with pituitary tumors, 15 (35%) noted galactorrhea postpartum, none had galactorrhea associated with birth-control pills, 5 (12%) had associated primary amenorrhea, and 22 (52%) developed spontaneously. On the other hand, Chang *et al.*[9] reported that in 34 women with galactorrhea or hyperprolactinemia and amenorrhea, 15 (75%) of 20 patients with proven adenomas had used oral contraceptives. Of 35 patients studies by Jacobs *et al.*,[50] 5 had associated primary amenorrhea. Haesslein and Lamb[40] found prolactinomas in 5 postpill and 2 postpartum patients and Gomez *et al.*[10] in 4 postpartum and 7 postpill patients. In the series of Tolis,[51] 34 of 65 women with galactorrhea–oligo-/amenorrhea developed the syndrome spontaneously or after the use of oral contraceptives. Because 4 of 11 with normal polytomes had adenomas found at surgery, Tolis considered the entire group of 34 patients to harbor microadenomas that were radiologically undetectable. We are not sure that the current evidence would support this assumption. Dr. Jules Hardy of Notre Dame Hospital, Montreal, reported that only 2 of 6 patients with normal sellas harbored adenomas (personal communication). We have demonstrated adenomas in 2 of 3 patients whose sella polytomographs were normal (unpublished). Dr. William Collins, Yale University, reported finding an adenoma in all 6 patients operated on with sella polytomographs read as normal, even retrospectively (personal communication).

Patient complaints, while characterizing the galactorrhea syndromes generally, did not assist in defining a group with occult tumors. Diminished libido and dyspareunia correlated well with hypoestrogenism, documented by us and others to be common among those with galactorrhea and amenorrhea.[11] Acne–seborrhea–mild hirsutism was seen in 22% of all patients. This complex of findings was mentioned in the original description of the Forbes–Albright syndrome,[49] by Lavric,[52] and is occasinally mentioned by others. There is some evidence that PRL exerts an action on the production of adrenal androgens,[53–55] and a recent study by Bassi *et al.*[56] found elevated plasma dehydroepiandrosterone sulfate (DHAS) and elevated free DHAS and urinary dehydroepiandrosterone (DHA) in 10 women with hyperprolactinemic amenorrhea. Lackelin *et al.*,[57] however, found normal levels of serum estrone, testosterone, androstenedione, and DHA in 18 prolactinoma patients. Serum testosterone levels in all our galactorrhea patients were within the normal range, making the etiology of this complaint still obscure. Headache, though a common symptom in established tumor patients, was seen in approximately equal frequency among other galactorrhea patients. Various authors emphasize the importance of headache in the diagnosis of sella and parasellar disease[58,59] and, more specifically, in the diagnosis of prolactinomas.[10] Our data do not support the differential value of this symptom. Weight gain in 40% of our patients corroborates observations made by Forbes *et al.*[49] and others.[38,57]

While Gomez *et al.*[10] felt that visual complaints were very suggestive of a pituitary tumor, only two patients in our series had confirmatory evidence of tumor on visual exam or visual-field testing, despite complaints in 12% of all patients of diplopia, blurred vision, and decreased peripheral vision. While we advocate such ophthalmological evaluation for all patients with galactorrhea to assist in planning therapy, the basis of such visual complaints is unknown in most cases. Thus, historical and clinical findings alone did not identify patients with occult tumors, and while they provide a basis for characterization of patients and stimulate investigation of the effect of PRL excess on other tissues, they rarely aided in defining the underlying pathology.

5. Roentgenographic Study

Hardy[60] contends that PRL-producing pituitary adenomas arise in the lateral wings of the pituitary gland, causing asymmetric enlargement of the sella. Large tumors are not a diagnostic problem and often cause abnormalities of the sella that appear on plain or coned-down views. Small prolactinomas, on the other hand, cause subtle changes that may be detected only with the use of polytomography.[10] Tomographic interpretation, however, must be done with great care, since minor changes may be seen in up to 30% of totally normal women.[61] The classic changes in sella architecture strongly suggesting a tumor are tilting of the sella floor to one side with erosion of the anterior wall.[28] However, sloping of the floor is a common anatomical variant, often associated with sphenoid sinus spetations, and when seen alone is not absolute evidence of an adenoma.[20] Some investigators have described the use of postero–anterior PA and lateral or coned-down views of the sella as the procedures of choice for screening patients with galactorrhea disorders,[10,43,45,59] reserving polytomography for those with abnormal plain films or elevated PRL levels. Other groups obtain both routine films and polytomographs on all patients.[7,9,50,51] We believe that there is sufficient clinical evidence to warrant the cost and radiation exposure of polytomographic examination in all patients with galactorrhea syndromes, and see little value in routine or coned-down views of the sella as a screening device: (1) Plain films and coned-down views of the sella were normal in 53% of our patients with abnormal polytomographs, an occurrence that has been mentioned by others.[17,63] (2) Polytomography maximizes the chance of detecting the earliest, subtle changes of a microadenoma in patients with previously normal radiographs and allows therapeutic intervention at a time when success is greatly enhanced. Correct diagnosis at this early stage avoids the use of costly, often ineffective therapies to induce menses. (3) Polytomography is the optimum study to guide the neurosurgical approach during selective tumor removal by providing the best data concerning localization. (4) Failure to find a tumor may increase the risk of visual deterioration during a medically induced pregnancy as reported by Gemzell[63] and others.[64–68]

6. Endocrine Evaluation in Differential Diagnosis

Analysis of basal PRL values indicated that a value of greater than 260 ng/ml was invariably associated with a pituitary adenoma. This supported the finding of Kleinberg *et al.*[11] that among 235 women with galactorrhea, PRL levels greater than 300 ng/ml were invariably associated with tumor, although it was somewhat higher than the 200 ng/ml limit suggested by Jacobs and Daughaday[69] and the 100 ng/ml limit of Gomez *et al.*[10] However, the number of our patients with established adenomas having a basal PRL level that was also found among other galactorrhea patients was high, representing an overlap of 86%, and prevented adequate discrimination on this basis alone. Other investigators have found similar results: Nader *et al.*[7] had overlap of basal PRL values of 48% of 25 women, Mroueh and Siler-Khodr[70] in 93% of 16 women, Tolis *et al.*[12] in 38% of 65 patients, Van Campenhout *et al.*[21] in 91% of 34 women, Friesen and Tolis[71] in 89% of 69 patients, and Kleinberg *et al.*[11] in 94% of 235 patients. While Jacobs *et al.*[50] demonstrated an overlap of basal PRL levels of only 7% in 27 untreated patients, the majority of studies support our contention that the level of PRL elevation does not distinguish tumor from nontumor unless a level of greater than 260 ng/ml is achieved. Even then, case reports of patients with empty sella syndrome, idiopathic galactorrhea and amenorrhea, and primary hypothyroidism with galactorrhea having basal PRL levels considerably above 300 ng/ml appear in the literature,[7,70,72] so that for a given patient, assignment to the tumor or nontumor group on the basis of basal PRL alone is not possible. Last, because one of our verified adenoma patients developed a normal PRL level following the spontaneous, partial necrosis of tumor with retention of galactorrhea–amenorrhea, we were unable to assign a lower limit of basal PRL below which one could be certain that no tumor was present. Several authors have also reported normal PRL levels in patients with verified tumors.[4,7,10,11,73] Thus, while elevated basal PRL is most typical of prolactinomas, it is not possible to definitely exclude a tumor among galactorrhea patients when PRL is normal. However, Lindstedt and Cullberg[74] raise the intriguing issue of what a "normal" PRL concentration should be in amenorrheic patients. They argue that estrogens in normal cycling women stimulate PRL synthesis and release, resulting in higher PRL levels for fertile compared with postmenopausal women. Since women with galactorrhea–amenorrhea are chronically hypoestrogenemic, PRL levels in the normal range for fertile women are inappropriately elevated for them. Although this is a cogent argument, more data on patients with normal PRL and the presence of prolactinomas will be needed to clarify this point.

Our finding of inappropriately low basal gonadotropin levels in the face of chronic hypoestrogenism among all patients with combined galactorrhea and oligo-/amenorrhea corresponds to the findings of most other authors.[9,12,43,50,75] On the other hand, Gomez *et al.*[10] and Van Campenhout *et al.*[21] found that FSH and LH levels often are in the range of the normal follicular phase. Although the values may be in the range of normal, what is important to emphasize is that they are usually inappropriately low for the degree of ovarian failure that is manifested.

The mechanism of gonadrotropin inhibition in the galactorrheic state has received much study. That the disorder is due to deranged hypothalamic function is suggested by the finding that gonadotropin secretory responses to injection of luteinizing-hormone-releasing hormone (LH-RH) in our series was normal in all but 5 cases, a result paralleling numerous other studies.[10,50,62,75–81] Nonetheless, in our series, and in certain of the reports cited above, there were some patients with blunted[21,50,57,81,82] or exaggerated[9,21,50,57,75] gonadotropin responses to LH-RH. Thus, we concur with the statement of Van Campenhout *et al.*[21] that variable responses to LH-RH injection can be seen in patients with prolactinomas, as well as in patients with more benign causes of galactorrhea–amenorrhea, and that this test is of no aid in differential diagnosis. Further evidence for a hypothalamic origin of the disordered gonadotropin secretion is the finding that pulsatile LH secretion is diminished in the absence of normal pituitary responsiveness to LH-RH.[83] Most workers believe, as Tolis and collaborators have proposed,[84] that the defect represents an effect of PRL excess, since normal gonadotropin secretion is usually restored by removal of the adenoma. However, four of our patients manifested amenorrhea, low estradiol levels, and inappropriately low gonadotropins despite normal PRL levels. It is possible that they have transient spikes of PRL secretion that were missed, or that their hypothalamic–pituitary axis is hypersensitive to the effects of normal PRL levels. Further evidence of derangement of hypothalamic or pituitary function is the finding that patients with galactorrhea–amenorrhea syndrome fail to show normal estrogen-induced sensitization response to LH-RH.[85] In addition to an effect of PRL at the level of the hypothalamus or pituitary, McNattey *et al.*[86] showed that PRL directly impaired progesterone secretion from cultures of granulosa cells, and Seppala *et al.*[87] found impaired corpus luteum function in two women with hyperprolactinemia.

The occurrence of blunted responses to orally administered L-dopa was suggestive of the presence of a PRL-producing tumor, occurring in 41% of Group 1, Verified Adenomas, and 33% of Group II, Probable Adenomas, all of whom had abnormal sella polytomes. Only 1 of 18 other galactorrhea patients demonstrated a blunted fall in PRL after this agent. L'Hermite *et al.*[88] detected blunted L-dopa responses in half their tumor patients, while Kleinberg *et al.*[11] found blunting in 44% of tumor patients, but in only 13% of those with other causes of galactorrhea. Wiebe *et al.*[62] showed similar nonsuppressibility in 50% of patients with definite prolactionomas, one of whom had no radiographic evidence of tumor. However, Healy *et al.*[89] described blunted responses to L-dopa in all 18 women with hyperprolactinemia, only 2 of whom had surgically confirmed prolactinomas. In one series, Tollis *et al.*[90] also found that the mean percentage decrease after L-dopa was blunted in tumor patients compared to normals, but in another series, Tolis *et al.*[12] reported no diagnostic discrimination using this test, with only 1 of 6 tumor patients and 6 of 12 other galactorrhea patients showing a blunted response. In our earlier study reported by Boyd *et al.*,[8] 3 of 4 adenoma patients had blunted PRL responses after L-dopa, a result seen in only 1 of 10 other galactorrhea patients. Thus, the bulk of evidence suggests that an attenuated fall in PRL after L-dopa administration is suggestive of a prolactinoma, but a normal response does not exclude a tumor.

We found impaired PRL response to intravenous TRH in every one of the verified tumor patients, but also in 76% of all other groups with galactorrhea. The surprisingly high incidence of such impaired responses might imply that attenuation is characteristic of all galactorrhea syndromes. Alternatively, it might signify, as Tolis[51] suggests, that subclinical adenomas are present in the patients with normal polytomes who evidence blunted response patterns. The prognostic significance of this finding is unclear at present and must await prolonged follow-up of these patients to see whether tumors subsequently develop. Review of the literature indicates that similar response patterns appear frequently in patients with PRL secretory disorders. Healy *et al.*[89] tested 18 women with hyperprolactinemia–amenorrhea and found all to be unresponsive to TRH, including 2 with pituitary tumors. Jacobs *et al.*[50] found subnormal increases of PRL after TRH in all 35 patients with hyperprolactinemia–amenorrhea, of whom 12 had defined tumors. Kleinberg *et al.*[11] showed marked blunting in 15 of 16 tumor patients and 7 of 24 other galactorrhea patients, a higher percentage of abnormality among tumor vs. nontumor patients than with any other provocative test in their hands. Snyder *et al.*[18] detected abnormal stimulation after TRH in 14 of 17 patients with abnormal sella radiographs and hyperprolactinemia. Results similar to these have been recorded by other authors.[69,77,81,82,88] On the other hand, consistently normal PRL rises after TRH have been found by Tolis *et al.*[51,90] and Tyson[81] in patients both with and without known tumors. Recently, Lamberts *et al.*[17] studied 24 patients with verified prolactinomas: in 9, an increase of greater than 100% of basal occurred, while in 4, there was a rise of between 5 and 100% and in 11 an increase of less than 50%. These responses were noted to be independent of the presence or absence of suprasellar extension of tumor. Nonetheless, Lamberts *et al.*[17] concluded that while responses varied, an absent rise might always indicate a pituitary tumor. Many theories have been advanced to account for such impaired responses to TRH, including (a) autonomy of adenomatous cells by loss or alteration of cell-surface receptors; (2) an ultra-short-loop feedback system whereby excessive PRL release by microadenoma tissue inhibits PRL production by contralateral normal lactotropes; (3) tumor cells already secreting at maximal capacity, unable to produce further increments when stimulated; and (4) release of prolactin-inhibitory factor (PIF) activity during TRH administration.

While only 2 of 7 tumor patients had blunted TSH responses to TRH in our initial study,[8] 7 of 16 tumor patients demonstrated blunting in the current expanded study. The presence of blunted TSH responses to TRH in 43% of verified adenomas and only 9% of other galactorrhea groups, despite normal concentrations of thyroid hormones and clinical euthyroidism, remains unexplained. To our knowledge, only Snyder *et al.*[18] reported similar findings in 7 of 19 patients with prolactinomas. Since estrogens are known to modulate TSH secretion from the human pituitary,[91] a possible explanation might be the degree of chronic hypoestrogenism among verified tumor patients. However, equally low levels of estradiol were seen in Group II and Group III patients, but only two patients from these groups demonstrated a blunted TSH response after TRH. Other theoretical explanations include loss or alteration of pituitary TRH receptors or a direct inhibitory effect of elevated serum PRL on TSH release. PIF activity may be increased in an attempt to exert control over semiautonomous lactotropes, and simultaneously act to impair TSH release. Supporting this theory is the report that L-dopa (a precursor of dopamine, the putative PIF) lowered TSH levels in idiopathic galactorrhea,[92] in primary myxedema,[93,94] and in galactorrhea–amenorrhea associated with primary hypothyroidism.[30] Although the precise cause of impaired TSH response to TRH is unknown, we feel that its presence may be taken as suggestive of a prolactinoma.

Chlorpromazine and hypoglycemia were used to assess the hypothalamic component of pituitary PRL regulation, although recent evidence suggests that chlorpromazine may also act directly on the pituitary.[95] We found blunted responses to chlorpromazine in every one of the verified adenoma patients and blunted responses to hypoglycemia in 90%. However, differentiation between tumor and nontumor patients was difficult, since the overall incidence of blunted responses among the other galactorrhea patients was 88% for chlorpromazine and 71% for hypoglycemia. Chlorpromazine has been utilized by others in evaluating galactorrhea patients. Boyd *et al.*[8] found blunted PRL responses to chlorpromazine in 4 of 6 adenomas and in 4 of 12 other galactorrhea patients. Tolis *et al.*[90] described blunted PRL responses to this agent in 10 patients with pituitary tumors, only 2 of whom had hyperprolactinemia. Kleinberg *et al.*[11] found blunted chlorpromazine rises in all 9 patients with verified prolactinomas and in 19 of 36 patients with other forms of galactorrhea. They concluded that lack of effective modulation by PIF was common in all forms of galactorrhea, but it was not known whether the defect resided in abnormal hypothalamic regulation of PIF or in a defective pituitary response to PIF, or both.[11] Furthermore, they suggested that a normal chlorpromazine response provided evidence against a tumor, a fact that appears to be supported by our present data, although longer follow-up is necessary among the normal responders to assess its certainty. However, Zarate *et al.*[82] demonstrated normal responses to chlorpromazine in 8 of 16 patients with galactorrhea and amenorrhea, including 2 of 5 with pituitary tumors. Malarkey[96] studied five women who would fit into our Group III, and all had absent chlorpromazine responses, as did six patients who would fit into our Group II, Probable Adenomas. Del Pozo *et al.*[77] found blunted responses in four patients and Pearson *et al.*[97] found an impaired response in most, but not all, pituitary tumor patients. Thus, the bulk of evidence suggests that a blunted response of PRL to chlorpromazine is highly suggestive of a prolactinoma, but it may be seen in its absence. Moreover, a normal response can occur in the face of a known tumor, so that for a given patient, the use of the chlorpromazine test to determine the presence or absence of an occult pituitary tumor is quite limited. As mentioned for the PRL response to TRH, one could suggest that if the majority of patients with galactorrhea disorders had radiographically undetectable adenomas, the blunted responses would be characteristic of occult tumors. Indeed, Jacobs *et al.*[50] have speculated that in most patients, with or without X-ray abnormalities, in whom no other cause of hyperprolactinemia can be found, microadenomas exist.

Our analysis of pituitary reserves of ACTH, GH, and ADH detected 7 instances of dysfunction among the 20 verified adenoma patients and 7 among the 50 other patients with galactorrhea. While this finding had no descriminating value in detecting hidden adenomas, documentation of ACTH-reserve deficiency in any patient carries with it therapeutic implications for steroid coverage during intercurrent stressful illnesses or during stressful diagnostic procedures to avoid the precipitation of partial or complete adrenal insufficiency. Some clinicians would even argue that all such patients should be placed on daily maintenance corticosteroids once an ACTH-reserve deficiency is adequately documented to protect them from the hazards and morbidity of reserve-deficiency progression. The frequency of GH-reserve deficiency and ACTH-reserve deficiency in patients with pituitary tumors in general has been assessed by others. Weisberg *et al.*[38] studied 100 patients with enlarged sella turcicas, of whom 27 had a primary intrasellar tumor. Among this group, 12 of 14 had GH-reserve deficiency and 10 of 24 had ACTH-reserve deficiency. Rabkin and Frantz[98] reported a high incidence of GH-reserve deficiency and a 50% incidence of ACTH-reserve deficiency among pituitary tumor patients. The data on prolactinoma patients alone are less uniform. Gomez *et al.*[10] found normal GH and ACTH reserve in 15 patients with galactorrhea, while Wiebe *et al.*[62] found normal ACTH reserve in 4 galactorrhea patients and normal GH reserve in 3. However, Kase *et al.*[41] found marginal or subnormal GH reserve in 17 patients with galactorrhea disorders, and Boyar *et al.*[99] found abnormal GH secretion in 3 of 7 patients with hyperprolactinemia. This degree of dysfunction was not supported by Tolis *et al.*,[12] who documented only 2 of 10 tumor patients with GH-reserve deficiency, only 1 of 10 with ACTH-reserve deficiency, and normal function in the other 55 galactorrhea patients. Chang *et al.*[9] likewise found 6 of 33 tumor patients with GH-reserve deficiency and 3 of 29 with ACTH-reserve deficiency. The low frequency of ACTH and GH deficiency is probably due to the relatively early stage at which prolactinomas are detected. Although infrequent, deficiencies of potential clinical significance do exist, and justify adequate assessment of ACTH reserve by insulin-induced hypoglycemia or metyrapone testing, or both. Prolonged follow-up will be required to determine whether women with GH- and ACTH-reserve deficiencies will untimately prove to have harbored tumors.

7. Natural History of Adenomas

Our analysis of clinical, hormonal, and radiographic data allows us to construct a hypothetical schema for women with galactorrhea syndromes that suggests possible pathophysiological relationships (Fig. 10). Other authors

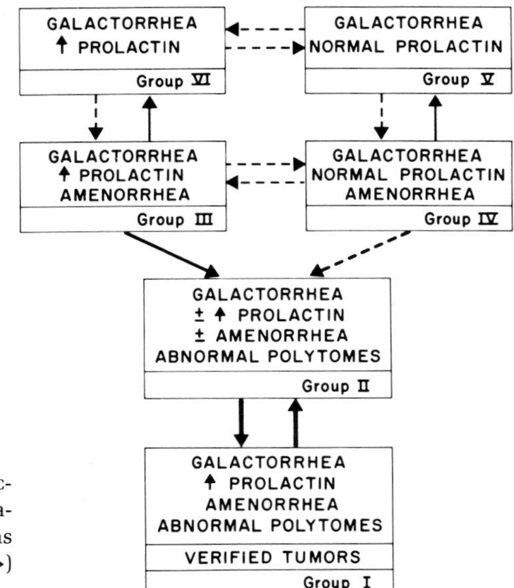

Fig. 10. Proposed schema for women with galactorrhea illustrating interrelationships among patient groups. (→) Intergroup transition patterns that have been observed among 70 patients; (- - -→) hypothetical transitions.

have observed patients to make transitions from one type of galactorrhea disorder to another,[8,10,42,100,101] and our experience also suggests that this is not uncommon. Five patients have been observed to make a transition from Group III to Groups I/II by developing abnormal polytomographs over 1–3 years. Moreover, six Group V patients recalled, in the distant past, spontaneous resolution of associated oliogo-/amenorrheic states that had been present from 6 to 12 months. Likewise, three of our original Group III patients have had spontaneous resolution of amenorrhea while under our observation, thus making a transition to Group VI. Finally, one verified adenoma patient had spontaneous restoration of ovulatory menses just prior to transsphenoidal selective adenomectomy. Therefore, we believe that the occurrence of amenorrhea is of little value in distinguishing among groups of patients with galactorrhea. Transitions from one group to another occur frequently, with galactorrhea being retained. This evolution of symptoms may represent a continuum of the same pituitary–hypothalamic disorder, one in which we believe that many patients with galactorrhea will ultimately be shown to harbor pituitary adenomas. Our inability to detect very early PRL microadenomas stems both from the limits of current radiological technology and from the pervasive biochemical disturbances seen in all galactorrhea syndromes that render differential endocrine testing so difficult.

8. Conclusions

Our data indicate that no test or combination of tests of prolactin, gonadotropins, thyrotropin, or estradiol could definitively distinguish which patients with normal sella polytomes harbored occult prolactinomas. However, the finding of a blunted PRL response to L-dopa, a blunted TSH response to TRH, or a mean basal PRL of greater than 260 ng/ml was very suggestive of the presence of an adenoma. While attenuated PRL responses to TRH and chlorpromazine were characteristic of prolactinomas, their high frequency among all other galactorrhea patients limits their diagnostic use at present. As more well-studied patients with currently normal polytomographs make a transition to abnormal radiographs, these stimulation tests may assume predictive importance in the early diagnosis of prolactinomas. Despite the current lack of specificity, we do feel that complete hormonal profiles of galactorrhea patients are clinically useful. Though ACTH-reserve deficiency was infrequent (5% incidence overall), its presence carries therapeutic implications. A complete evaluation also ensures the exclusion of occult disease that may mimic a prolactinoma: the demonstration by CT scan and pneumoencephalography[13] of the empty sella syndrome in three patients and the detection of subclinical primary hypothyroidism[30] by TRH testing in one patient in Group II, Probable Adenomas, emphasizes this point. Thorough hormonal and radiographic evaluation also uncovered a patient in Group IV with a variant of the empty sella syndrome associated with gonadotropin and GH deficiencies.[102] Clearly, the therapeutic decisions for these patients are much different than for prolactinoma patients or for those with galactorrhea of unknown etiology. Ultimately, however, the essential feature for the definitive preoperative diagnosis of PRL-producing pituitary tumors remains anatomical evidence by sella polytomography or visual-field examination. On the basis of our experience with these 70 patients, we feel that women who present with the symptom of galactorrhea should have the following initial evaluation: (1) determination of mean basal serum PRL; (2) measurement of T_4 and TSH; (3) sella polytomography; (4) CT scan of sella; (5) Goldmann visual-field testing; and (6) assessment of ACTH reserve. In patients with initially negative studies, these tests should be repeated at 1- to 2-year intervals to detect the earliest appearance of previously occult tumors. We do not recommend routine LH-RH or chlorpromazine testing at present. On the other hand, our findings do suggest that the occurrence of a mean basal PRL greater than 260 ng/ml, blunted TSH response to TRH, or blunted PRL response to L-dopa indicates a high probability that an adenoma is present, and these dynamic tests can be useful in diagnostic assessment of galactorrhea patients.

ACKNOWLEDGMENTS. This study was supported in part by General Clinical Research Center Grant No. FR0054, by NIAMDD Grants AM16684 and AM07039, and by a Grant in Aid from Sandoz, Inc.

References

1. A.G. Frantz, D.L. Kleinberg, and G.L. Noel, Studies on prolactin in man, *Recent Prog. Horm. Res.* **28:**527, 1972.
2. P. Hwang, H. Guyda, and H. Friesen, A radioimmunoassay for human prolactin, *Proc. Natl. Acad. Sci. U.S.A.* **68:**1902, 1971.
3. L.S. Jacobs, I.K. Mariz, and W.H. Daughaday, A mixed heterologous radioimmunoassay for human prolactin, *J. Clin. Endocrinol. Metab.* **34:**484, 1972.

4. Y.N. Sinha, F.W. Selby, U.J. Lewis, and W.P. Vanderlaan, A homologous radioimmunoassay for prolactin, *J. Clin. Endocrinol. Metab.* **36:**509, 1973.
5. J.L. Vezina and T.J. Sutton, Prolactin secreting pituitary microadenomas, *Am. J. Roentgenol. Radium Ther. Nucl. Med.* **120:**46, 1974.
6. S. Franks, H.S. Jacobs, and J.D.N. Nabarro, Studies of prolactin in pituitary disease, *J. Endocrinol.* **67:**55, 1975.
7. S. Nader, K. Mashiter, F.H. Doyle, and G.F. Joplin, Galactorrhea, hyperprolactinemia and pituitary tumors in the female, *Clin. Endocrinol.* **5:**245, 1976.
8. A.E. Boyd, III, S. Reichlin, and R.N. Turksoy, Galactorrhea–amenorrhea syndrome: Diagnosis and therapy, *Ann. Intern. Med.* **87:**165, 1977.
9. R.J. Chang, W.R. Keye, J.R. Young, C.B. Wilson, and R.B. Jaffe, Detection, evaluation and treatment of pituitary microadenomas in patients with galactorrhea and amenorrhea, *Am. J. Obstet. Gynecol.* **128:**357, 1977.
10. F. Gomez, F. Reyes, and C. Faiman, Nonpuerperal galactorrhea and hyperprolactinemia, *Am. J. Med.* **62:**648, 1977.
11. D.L. Kleinberg, G.L. Noel, and A.G. Frantz, Galactorrhea: A study of 235 cases, including 48 with pituitary tumors, *N. Engl. J. Med* **296:**589, 1977.
12. G. Tolis, M. Somma, J. Van Campenhout, and H. Friesen, Prolactin secretion in sixty-five patients with galactorrhea, *Am. J. Obstet. Gynecol.* **118:**91, 1974.
13. R. Rozario, S.B. Hammerschlag, K.D. Post, S.M. Wolpert, and I.M. Jackson, Diagnosis of empty sella with C-T scan, *Neuroradiology* **13:**85, 1977.
14. M. Buckman, M. Kaminsky, M. Conway, and G.T. Peake, Utility of L-dopa and water loading in evaluation of hyperprolactinemia, *J. Clin. Endocrinol. Metab.* **36:**911, 1973.
15. H. Friesen, H. Guyda, R. Hwang, J.E. Tyson, and A. Barbeau, Functional evaluation of prolactin secretion: A guide to therapy, *J. Clin. Invest.* **51:**706, 1972.
16. D.L. Kleinberg, G.L. Noel, and A.G. Frantz, Chlorpromazine stimulation and L-dopa suppression of plasma prolactin in man, *J. Clin. Endocrinol. Metab.* **33:**873, 1971.
17. S.W.J. Lamberts, J.C. Birkenhager, and H.G. Kwa, Basal and TRH stimulated prolactin in patients with pituitary tumors, *Clin. Endocrinol.* **5:**709, 1976.
18. P.J. Snyder, L.S. Jacobs, M.M. Robello, F.S.H. Sterling, R.N. Shore, R.D. Utiger, and W.H. Daughaday, Diagnostic value of thyrotrophin-releasing hormone in pituitary and hypothalamic disease, *Ann. Intern. Med.* **81:**751, 1974.
19. G. Copinschi and M. L'Hermite, Effects of glucocorticoids on pituitary hormonal responses to hypoglycemia: Inhibition of prolactin release, *J. Clin. Endocrinol. Metab.* **40:**442, 1975.
20. P.D. Woolf, L.A. Lee, W. Leebaw, D. Thompson, U. Lilavivathana, R. Brodows, and R. Campbell, Intracellular glucopenia causes prolactin release in man, *J. Clin. Endocrinol. Metab.* **45:**377–382, 1977.
21. J. Van Campenhout, S. Papas, P. Blanchet, H. Wyman, and M. Somma, Pituitary responses to synthetic luteinizing hormone–releasing hormone in thirty-four cases of amenorrhea or oligo-amenorrhea associated with galactorrhea, *Am. J. Obstet. Gynecol.* **127:**723, 1977.
22. S.S.C. Yen, R. Rebar, G. Vandenberg, F. Naftolin, Y. Ehara, S. Engblom, K.J. Ryan, K. Benirschke, J. Rivier, M. Amoss, and R. Guillemin, Synthetic lutenizing hormone–releasing factor: A potent stimulator of gonadotropin release in man, *J. Clin. Endocrinol. Metab.* **34:**1108, 1972.
23. V.V. Weldon, S.K. Gupta, M.W. Haymond, A.S. Pagliara, L.S. Jacobs, and W.H. Daughaday, The use of L-dopa in the diagnosis of hyposomatotropism in children, *J. Clin. Endocrinol. Metab.* **36:**42, 1973.
24. M. Miller, A.M. Moses, and D.H. Streeten, Recognition of partial defects in antidiuretic hormone secretion, *Ann. Intern. Med.* **73:**721, 1970.
25. D.S. Schalch and M.L. Parker, A sensitive double antibody immunoassay for human growth hormone in plasma, *Nature (London)* **203:**1141, 1964.
26. I. Nejad, J. Bollinger, M.A. Mitnick, P. Sullivan, and S. Reichlin, Measurement of plasma and tissue triiodothyronine concentration in the rat by radioimmunoassay, *Endocrinology* **96:**773, 1975.
27. G. Orczyk, B.V. Caldwell, and H. Behrman, Estrogens, estradiol, estrone, estriol, in: *Methods of Hormone Radioimmunoassay* (B. Jaffe and H. Behrman, eds.), pp. 333–345, Academic Press, New York, 1974.

28. G. Guiot and B. Thibaut, L'extirpation des adenomes hypophysaires par voie transsphenoidale, *Neurochirurgia (Stuttgart)* **1**:133, 1959.
29. C. Radberg, Some aspects of the asymmetrical enlargement of the sella turcica, *Acta Radiol. Diagn. (Stockholm)* **1**:152, 1963.
30. W.R. Keye, Jr., B. Hoyuen, R.F. Knopf, and R.B. Jaffe, Amenorrhea, hyperprolactinemia and pituitary enlargement secondary to primary hypothyroidism, *Obstet. Gynecol.* **48**:697, 1976.
31. S. Friedman and A. Goldfien, Breast secretion in normal women, *Am. J. Obstet. Gynecol.* **104**:846, 1969.
32. L. Vetter, F. Knauer, and H. Wyss, Galactorrhea, *Arch. Gynaekol.* **216**:81, 1974.
33. J.R. Jones and G.P. Gentile, Incidence of galactorrhea in ovulatory and anovulatory females, *Obstet. Gynecol.* **45**:13, 1975.
34. M.V. Lavric, Breast secretion in nulligravid women, *Am. J. Obstet. Gynecol.* **112**:1139, 1972.
35. A.B. Shevach and W.N. Spellacy, Galactorrhea and contraceptive practices, *Obstet. Gynecol.* **38**:286, 1971.
36. R. Wenner, Physiologisch und pathologische Lactation, *Arch. Gynaekol.* **204**:171, 1976.
37. M.T. Buckman and G.T. Peake, Incidence of galactorrhea (letter to the editor), *J. Am Med. Assoc.* **236**:2747, 1976.
38. L. Weisberg, E.A. Zimmerman, and A.G. Frantz, Diagnosis and evaluation of patients with an enlarged sella turcica, *Am. J. Med.* **61**:590, 1976.
39. R. Costello, Subclinical adenoma of the pituitary gland, *Am. J. Pathol.* **12**:205, 1936.
40. H.C. Haesslein and E.J. Lamb, Pituitary tumors in patients with secondary amenorrhea, *Am. J. Obstet, Gynecol.* **125**:759, 1956.
41. N. Kase, J. Androle, and L. Sobrinho, Endocrine diagnosis of pituitary tumor in galactorrhea syndromes, *Am. J. Obstet. Gynecol.* **114**:321, 1972.
42. C.J. Canfield and R.W. Bates, Nonpuerperal galactorrhea, *N. Engl. J. Med.* **273**:897, 1965.
43. S. Franks, M.A.F. Murray, A.M. Jequier, S.J. Steele, J.D.N. Nabarro, and H.S. Jacobs, Incidence and significance of hyperprolactinemia in women with amenorrhea, *Clin. Endocrinol.* **4**:597, 1975.
44. S. Franks, D.N.L. Ralphs, V. Seagroatt, and H.S. Jacobs, Prolactin concentrations in patients with breast cancer, *Br. Med. J.* **4**:320, 1974.
45. H.S. Jacobs, M.G.R. Hull, M.A.F. Murray, and S. Franks, Therapy-oriented diagnosis of secondary amenorrhea, *Horm. Res.* **6**:268, 1975.
46. S. Franks, J.D.N. Nabarro, and H.S. Jacobs, Prevalence and presentation of hyperprolactinemia in patients with "functionless" pituitary tumors, *Lancet* **1**:778, 1977.
47. J. Agronz and E.B. Del Castillo, A syndrome characterized by estrogenic insufficiency, galactorrhea and decreased urinary gonadotrophins, *J. Clin. Endocrinol. Metab.* **13**:79, 1953.
48. J. Chiari, Bericht über die in den Jahren 1848 bis inclusive 1851 an der gynaekologischen Abtheilung in Wein beobachteten Frauenkrankheiten im engern Sinne des Wortes, in: *Klinik der Geburtshilfe und Gynaekologie* (J. Chiarl, C. Brown, J. Spaeth, and Erlagen, eds.). pp. 363–415, Verlag von Ferdinand Enke, 1855.
49. A.P. Forbes, P.H. Henneman, G.C. Griwold, and F. Albright, Syndrome characterized by galactorrhea, amenorrhea and low urinary FSH, comparison with acromegaly and normal lactation, *J. Clin. Endocrinol. Metab.* **14**:265, 1954.
50. H.S. Jacobs, S. Franks, M.A.F. Murray, M.G.R. Hull, S.J. Steele, and J.D.N. Nabarro, Clinical and endocrine features of hyperprolactinemia amenorrhea, *Clin. Endocrinol.* **5**:439, 1976.
51. G. Tolis, Galactorrhea–amenorrhea and hyperprolactinemia: Pathophysiological aspects and diagnostic tests, *Clin. Endocrinol.* **6**(Suppl.):81s, 1977.
52. M.V. Lavric, Galactorrhea and amenorrhea with polycystic ovaries, *Am. J. Obstet. Gynecol.* **104**:814, 1969.
53. M. Lis, C. Gilordeau, and M. Chretien, Effect of prolactin on corticosterone production by rat adrenals, *Clin. Res.* **21**:1027, 1974.
54. M. Seppala and E. Hirvonen, Raised serum prolactin levels associated with hirsutism and amenorrhea, *Br. Med. J.* **4**:144, 1975.
55. A.O. Thorner, A.S. McNeilly, C. Hogan, and G.M. Besser, Long-term treatment of galactorrhea and hypogonadism with bromocriptine, *Br. Med. J.* **2**:419, 1974.
56. F. Bassi, G. Guisti, L. Borsi, S. Cattaneo, P. Gianotti, G. Forti, M. Pazzagli, C. Vigiani, and M.

Serio, Plasma androgens in women with hyperprolactinemic amenorrhea, *Clin. Endocrinol.* **5**:61, 1977.

57. G.C.L. Lackelin, S. Abu-Fadil, and S.S.C. Yen, Functional delineation of hyperprolactinemic amenorrhea, *J. Clin. Endocrinol. Metab.* **44**:1163, 1977.
58. H. Krieger, Sella and juxtasellar disease: A neurologic viewpoint, *Hosp. Pract.* **95**:95–103, 1975.
59. J.E. Kurnick, C.R. Hartman, E.G. Lufkin, and F.D. Hofeldt, Abnormal sella turcica, *Arch. Intern. Med.* **137**:111, 1977.
60. J. Hardy, Transsphenoidal surgery of hypersecreting pituitary tumors, in: *Diagnosis and Treatment of Pituitary Tumors* (P.O. Kohler and G.T. Ross, eds.), pp. 179–194, Excerpta Medica, Amsterdam, 1973.
61. H.A. Swanson and G. DuBoulay, Borderline variants of the normal pituitary fossa, *Br. J. Radiol.* **48**:366, 1975.
62. R.H. Wiebe, C.B. Hammond, and L.G. Borchert, Diagnosis of prolactin-secreting pituitary microadenoma, *Am. J. Obstet. Gynecol.* **126**:993, 1976.
63. C. Gemzell, Induction of ovulation in infertile women with pituitary tumors, *Am. J. Obstet. Gynecol.* **121**:311, 1975.
64. D.F. Child, H. Gordon, K. Mashiter, and G.F. Joplin, Pregnancy, prolactin and pituitary tumors, *Br. Med. J.* **4**:87, 1975.
65. T. Kajtar and G.H. Tomkin, Emergency hypophysectomy in pregnancy after induction of ovulation, *Br. Med. J.* **4**:88, 1971.
66. S.W.J. Lamberts, H.J. Seldenrath, H.G. Kwa, and J.C. Birkenhager, Transient bitemporal hemianopsia during pregnancy after treatment of galactorrhea–amenorrhea syndrome with bromocriptine, *J. Clin. Endocrinol. Metab.* **44**:180, 1977.
67. G.I.M. Swyer, V. Little, and B.J. Harries, Visual disturbance in pregnancy after induction of ovulation, *Br. Med. J.* **4**:90, 1971.
68. A.O. Thorner, G.M. Besser, A. Jones, J. Dacie, and A.E. Jones, Bromocriptine treatment of female infertility: Report of 13 pregnancies, *Br. Med. J.* **4**:694, 1975.
69. L.S. Jacobs and W.H. Daughaday, Pathophysiology and control of prolactin secretion in patients with pituitary and hypothalamic disease, in: *Human Prolactin* (J.L. Pasteels and C. Rolyn, eds.), p. 189, Excerpta Medica, Amsterdam, 1973.
70. A.M. Mroueh and T.M. Siler-Khodr, Bromerocriptine therapy in cases of amenorrhea–galactorrhea, *Am. J. Obstet. Gynecol.* **127**:291, 1977.
71. H.G. Friesen and G. Tolis, The use of bromocriptine in the galactorrhea–amenorrhea syndromes: The Canadian Cooperative Study, *Clin. Endocrinol.* **9**(Suppl.)91s, 1977.
72. T. Hsu, J.R. Shapiro, J.E. Tyson, A.L. Leddy, and A.T. Paz-Guevara, Hyperprolactinemia associated with the empty sella syndrome, *J. Am. Med. Assoc.* **235**:2002, 1976.
73. W.B. Malarkey and J.C. Johnson, Pituitary tumors and hyperprolactinemia, *Arch. Intern. Med.* **136**:40, 1976.
74. G. Lindstedt and G. Cullberg, What is a "normal" prolactin concentration in amenorrhea? (letter to the editor), *Lancet* **1**:757, 1977.
75. D.F. Archer, J.W. Sprong, H.R. Nankin, and J.B. Josimovich, Pituitary and gonadotrophin response in women with idiopathic hyperprolactinemia, *Fertil. Steril.* **27**:1158, 1976.
76. T. Aono, A. Myake, T. Shiroji, T. Kinugasa, T. Onishi, and K. Kurachi, Impaired LH release following exogenous estrogen administration in patients with amenorrhea–galactorrhea syndrome, *J. Clin. Endocrinol. Metab.* **42**:696, 1976.
77. E. Del Pozo, L. Varga, H. Wyss, G. Tolis, H. Friesen, R. Wenner, L. Vetter, and A. Uettwiler, Clinical and hormonal responses to bromocriptine (CB 154) in the galactorrhea syndromes, *J. Clin. Endocrinol. Metab.* **39**:18, 1974.
78. P. Fossati, M. Asfour, M. L'Hermite, J. Buvat, J.P. Gosnault, and M. Hedouin-Quipuempois, Étude de la fonction gonadotrope dans 12 cas de galactorrhea avec hypogonadisme, microdeformation de la sella turcique et hyperprolactinemie, *Ann. Endocrinol. (Paris)* **36**:329, 1975.

78a. P.O. Lundberg, Clinical evaluation of the luteinzing hormone–releasing hormone (LH-RH) test in cases with anatomically verified disorders of the hypothalamo–pituitary region. *Acta Neurol. Scand.* **49**:461, 1973.

79. C.H. Mortimer, G.H. Besser, A.D. McNeilly, J.C. Marshall, P. Harsoulis, W.M.G. Turnbridge,

A. Gomez-Pan, and A. Hall, Luteninizing hormone and follicle stimulating hormone releasing hormone test in patients with hypothalamic–pituitary–gonadal dysfunction, *Br. Med. J.* **4:**73, 1973.

80. R.F. Spark, J. Pallotta, F. Naftolin, and R. Clemens, Galactorrhea–amenorrhea syndromes: Etiology and treatment, *Ann. Intern. Med.* **84:**532, 1976.
81. J.E. Tyson, B. Andreasson, J. Huth, B. Smith, and H. Zacur, Neuroendocrine dysfunction in galactorrhea–amenorrhea after oral contraceptive use, *Obstet. Gynecol.* **46:**1, 1975.
82. A. Zarate, L.S. Jacobs, and E.S. Canales, Functional evaluation of pituitary reserve in patients with the amenorrhea–galactorrhea syndrome utilizing luteinizing releasing hormone (LH-RH), L-dopa and chlorpromazine, *J. Clin. Endocrinol. Metab.* **37:**855, 1973.
83. H.G. Bohnet, H.G. Dahlen, W. Wuitke, and H.R.G. Schneider, Hyperprolactinemic anovulatory syndrome, *J. Clin. Endocrinol. Metab.* **39:**18, 1976.
84. G. Tolis and H.G. Friesen, Prolactin and human reproduction, *Can. Med. Assoc. J.* **115:**709, 1976.
85. M.R. Glass, R.W. Shaw, W.R. Butt, R. Logan-Edwards, and D.R. London, An abnormality of estrogen feedback in amenorrhea–galactorrhea, *Br. Med. J.* **3:**204, 1975.
86. K.P. McNattey, R.S. Sawyers, and A.S. McNeilly, A possible role for prolactin in the control of steroid secretion by the human graffian follicle, *Nature (London)* **250:**653, 1974.
87. M. Seppala, E. Hirvoen, and T. Ranta, Hyperprolactinemia and luteal insufficiency, *Lancet* **1:**229, 1976.
88. M. L'Hermite, M. Degueldre, and A. Caufriez, Prolactin secretion: The impact of dynamic studies, *Pathol. Biol. (Paris)* **23:**769, 1975.
89. D.L. Healy, R.J. Pepperell, J. Stackdale, W.J. Bremmer, and H.G. Burger, Pituitary autonomy in hyperprolactinemic secondary amenorrhea; Results of hypothalamic pituitary testing, *J. Clin. Endocrinol. Metab.* **44:**809, 1977.
90. G. Tolis, M. Goldstein, and H. Friesen, Functional evaluation of prolactin secretion in patients with hypothalamic–pituitary disorders, *J. Clin. Invest.* **52:**783, 1973.
91. F. Sanchez-Franco, M.D. Garcia, L. Cacicedo, A. Marten-Zuno, and F. Escobar de Rey, Influence of sex phase of the menstrual cycle on thyrotropin (TSH) response to thyrotropin-releasing hormone (TRH), *J. Clin. Endocrinol. Metab.* **37:**736, 1973.
92. R.B. Jaffe, B. Hoyuen, and W.R. Keye, Jr., Physiologic and pathologic profiles of circulating human prolactin, *Am. J. Obstet. Gynecol.* **117:**757, 1973.
93. B. Rapoport, S. Refetoff, V.S. Fang, and H.G. Friesen, Suppression of serum thyrotrophin (TSH), by L-dopa in chronic hypothyroidism: Interrelationships in the regulation of TSH and prolactin secretion, *J. Clin. Endocrinol. Metab.* **36:**256, 1973.
94. S. Refetoff, V.S. Fang, B. Rapoport, and H.G. Friesen, Interrelationships in the regulation of TSH and PRL secretion in man: Effects of L-dopa, TRH, and thyroid hormone in various combinations, *J. Clin. Endocrinol. Metab.* **38:**450, 1974.
95. D.L. Kleinberg, G.L. Noel, and A.G. Frantz, Implications of circulating prolactin (letter), *N. Engl. J. Med.* **297:**55, 1977.
96. W.B. Malarkey, Nonpuerperal lactation and normal prolactin regulation, *J. Clin. Endocrinol. Metab.* **40:**198, 1975.
97. O.H. Pearson, J.S. Brodkey, and B. Kaufman, Endocrine evaluation and indications for surgery of functional pituitary adenomas, *Clin. Neurosurg.* **21:**26, 1974.
98. M.T. Rabkin and A.G. Frantz, Hypopituitarism: A study of growth hormone and other endocrine functions, *Ann. Intern. Med.* **64:**1197, 1966.
99. R.M. Boyar, S. Kapen, J.W. Finklestein, M. Perlow, J.F. Sassin, D.K. Fukushima, E.D. Weitzman, and L. Hellman, Hypothalamic–pituitary function in diverse hyperprolactinemic states, *J. Clin. Invest.* **53:**1588, 1974.
100. W.H. Daughaday, The adenohypophysis, in: *Textbook of Endocrinology* (R.H. Williams, ed.), p. 31, W.B. Saunders, Philadelphia, 1974.
101. J.M. Maas, Amenorrhea–galactorrhea syndrome: Before, during and after pregnancy, *Fertil. Steril.* **18:**857, 1967.
102. M. Farber, R. Facog, R.N. Turksoy, and J. Rogers, The primary empty sella syndrome, *Obstet. Gynecol.* **49**(Suppl.):2s–5s, 1977.
103. F.C. Greenwood, J. Landon, and T.C.B. Stamp, The plasma sugar, free fatty acid, cortisol and growth hormone response to insulin I: In control subjects. *J. Clin. Invest.* **45:**429, 1966.

5

Prolactin-Secreting Adenomas in the Male

RICHARD H. GOODMAN, MARK E. MOLITCH, KALMON D. POST, and IVOR M.D. JACKSON

1. Introduction

Prolactin-secreting tumors are the most common hormone-secreting pituitary tumors in women and may be the most common hormone-secreting tumors in men as well. It is only within the last five years, with the advent of sensitive radioimmunoassays for prolactin, that the often subtle and varied clinical presentations of these tumors have become apparent. Women with prolactin-secreting tumors (also called prolactinomas) usually present with amenorrhea or galactorrhea, or both, in association with a modestly elevated serum prolactin level in the 50–200 ng/ml range. Plain skull X-rays are often normal, and abnormalities such as focal erosion or enlargement of the sella turcica are detectable only with pleuridirectional tomography. In women with galactorrhea and amenorrhea, the incidence of verified pituitary adenomas has been reported to be as high as 30–50%[1,2] (Chapter 4).

In comparison with the situation in women, prolactin-secreting tumors in men are usually considerably larger at the time of presentation, and abnormalities are readily seen even on plain skull films. The symptoms of hyperprolactinemia in men—impotence, decreased libido, and perhaps infertility—are frequently not ascribed to a pituitary adenoma, and the diagnosis is often not made until the late development of tumor-mass effects, including visual-field defects, headaches, CSF rhinorrhea, and even hypothalamic function disturbances from suprasellar extension. In this regard, these tumors present similarly to nonfunctioning adenomas.

We have had the opportunity to evaluate ten men with prolactin-secret-

---

RICHARD H. GOODMAN, MARK E. MOLITCH, and IVOR M.D. JACKSON • Tufts University School of Medicine; Department of Medicine, Division of Endocrinology, Tufts–New England Medical Center Hospital, Boston, Massachusetts 02111. *KALMON D. POST* • Tufts University School of Medicine; Department of Neurosurgery, Tufts–New England Medical Center Hospital, Boston, Massachusetts 02111.

ing tumors. Their clinical presentation, laboratory and radiographic evaluation, and clinical course are described below. These patients are compared to ten men with nonsecreting adenomas and to women with prolactinomas, who are described in detail in Chapter 4.

2. Results

2.1. Males with Prolactin-Secreting Tumors

Ten men with hyperprolactinemia and pituitary tumors were evaluated in the Clinical Study Unit of Tufts–New England Medical Center Hospital. Details of their presenting symptoms, laboratory data, and clinical courses are outlined in Table 1. Patients ranged in age from 32 to 62 years (mean 46 years). Nine of the patients complained of impaired sexual function, either decreased libido, impotence, or both. In two patients (cases 1 and 2) with diabetes mellitus, the relationship of impotence to the pituitary tumor was unclear. Low testosterone and gonadotropin levels in these two patients suggest that the pituitary lesion was responsible for their sexual dysfunction. In a third patient with diabetes mellitus (case 7), impotence antedated the development of diabetes by several years. Three patients developed gynecomastia and one developed galactorrhea during their course. Three patients were morbidly obese (case 2, 130 kg; case 7, 131 kg; case 8, 235 kg), and only four of the ten were of normal weight. The mean weight of the patients was 108 kg. Two patients manifested severe psychological disturbances, consisting mainly of sociopathic behavior.

Headache was a presenting complaint of four patients. One patient presented with a third, fifth, and sixth cranial nerve palsy, and one patient presented with CSF rhinorrhea due to extension of tumor into the sphenoid sinus. Enlargement of the sella turcica on X-ray was detected as an incidental finding in one patient (case 2).

The mean basal prolactin level was 1378 ng/ml, with values ranging from 188 to 4480 ng/ml. The results of dynamic studies of prolactin regulation are shown in Fig. 1. In the six patients who were tested with L-dopa (500 mg orally), the average suppression of serum prolactin was 44±7%. In two patients, L-dopa was administered after pretreatment with carbidopa (50 mg p.o. q6h), a peripheral inhibitor of dopa decarboxylation. Suppression of serum prolactin levels in these two patients was only 7.5±0.5%, significantly less than after L-dopa alone ($p<0.05$), suggesting defective hypothalamic regulation of prolactin secretion.[3] Prolactin responses to insulin-induced hypoglycemia ($n=2$) or thyrotropin-releasing hormone (TRH) (500 μg i.v.) ($n=4$) were blunted (7.5±2.5% and 43±30% increase from baseline, respectively). Testosterone and gonadotropin values were low except in the single patient (case 5) whose sexual function was normal. In this patient, serum testosterone was in the low normal range (281 ng/dl) despite a serum prolactin level of 2100 ng/ml. Deficiencies in either growth hormone (GH), ACTH, or thyroid-stimulating hormone (TSH) reserve were noted in five patients, but only one patient presented with panhypopituitarism, and one was panhypopituitary following previous pituitary surgery.

TABLE 1. Males with Prolactin-Secreting Tumors

Case no.	Presenting symptoms	Laboratory[a]	Radiographic	Therapy[b]	Course
1	Lethargy Impotence Decreased libido Diabetes mellitus	Prolactin: 1960 ng/ml L-Dopa: 39% suppression Carbidopa: 7% suppression Testosterone: 52 ng/dl LH: 1.2 mIU/ml FSH: 1.3 mIU/ml ACTH: low (metyrapone) GH: low (L-dopa) TSH: normal (TRH)	+SSE	RTX	
2	Obesity Impotence Diabetes mellitus	Prolactin: 188 ng/ml L-Dopa: 35% suppression TRH: No response Testosterone: 30 ng/dl LH: 0.6 mIU/ml FSH: 0.7 mIU/ml ACTH: normal (metyrapone) TSH: normal (TRH)	−SSE	RTX	Prolactin 263 ng/ml following RTX
3	Impotence Decreased libido Visual-field defect Gynecomastia Hypothyroidism	Prolactin: 358 ng/ml L-Dopa: 48% suppression TRH: 130% rise Testosterone: 55 ng/ml LH: 0.6 mIU/ml FSH: 0.7 mIU/ml ACTH: normal GH: normal (L-dopa) TSH: normal (TRH) 1° hypothyroidism	+SSE	TA RTX	Prolactin 49 ng/ml following TA Panhypopituitary Potency improved on testosterone
4	Headaches Impotence Decreased libido Visual-field defect Gynecomastia	Prolactin: 2546 ng/ml ACTH: normal (hypoglycemia) GH: low (L-dopa) TSH: normal	+SSE	TA RTX	Prolactin 1629 ng/ml following TA Panhypopituitary Prolactin decreased to 18 ng/ml on bromocriptine Potency poor on bromocriptine, testosterone
5	CSF rhinorrhea Normal sexual function	Prolactin: 2100 ng/ml L-Dopa: 20% suppression Carbidopa: 8% suppression Hypoglycemia: 5% increase TRH: No response Testosterone: 281 ng/dl ACTH: normal (hypoglycemia) GH: low (L-dopa, hypoglycemia) TSH: normal (TRH)	+SSE	TA RTX	Prolactin 1256 ng/ml following TA

(continued)

TABLE 1. (*continued*)

Case no.	Presenting symptoms	Laboratory	Radiographic	Therapy	Course
6	Headaches Impotence Decreased libido Cranial-nerve defects Visual-field defects	Prolactin: 705 ng/ml Testosterone: 19 ng/dl LH: 0.4 mIU/ml FSH: 2 mIU/ml ACTH: normal TSH: normal	−SSE	TA RTX	Prolactin 288 ng/ml following TA Potency improved on testosterone
7	Headache Lethargy Impotence Decreased libido Visual-field defect	No laboratory evaluation available	−SSE	Frontal craniotomy RTX Repeat craniotomy	Prolactin 240 ng/ml following surgery Obesity Panhypopituitary Galactorrhea Diabetes mellitus Prolactin increased to 1370 ng/ml Impotent on testosterone Begun on bromocriptine
8	Impotence Decreased libido Obesity	Prolactin: 370 ng/ml L-Dopa: 71% suppression Testosterone: 20 ng/dl LH: 0.6 mIU/ml FSH: 0.8 mIU/ml ACTH: normal GH: normal (arginine) TSH: normal (TRH)	−SSE	Proton beam	Prolactin 70 ng/ml following proton beam Prolactin increased to 324 ng/ml TSH: low (TRH) GH: low (L-dopa, arginine) Impotent on testosterone Begun on bromocriptine
9	Impotence Decreased libido Panhypopituitary	No prolactin available Testosterone 10 ng/dl LH 3.1 mIU/ml FSH 3.1 mIU/ml ACTH low TSH low	+SSE	TA RTX	Prolactin 834 ng/ml following TA Persistent diabetes insipidus Panhypopituitary Gynecomastia Impotent on testosterone
10	Status post removal of chromophobe adenoma and RTX 20 yr previously: Headaches Impotence Decreased libido Panhypopituitary Visual-field defect	Prolactin: 4480 ng/ml L-Dopa: 49% suppression TRH: 40% increase Hypoglycemia: 10% increase LH, FSH: low (LRF)	+SSE	TA RTX Transethmoidal surgery Frontal craniotomy	Recurrent visual defects Persistent elevation in prolactin (1000–3000 ng/ml) Potency improved on testosterone Prolactin 12 ng/ml on bromocriptine

[a] Stimulatory tests of endocrine function are given in parentheses.
[b] (TA) Transsphenoidal adenomectomy; (RTX) radiotherapy, (SSE) suprasellar extension.

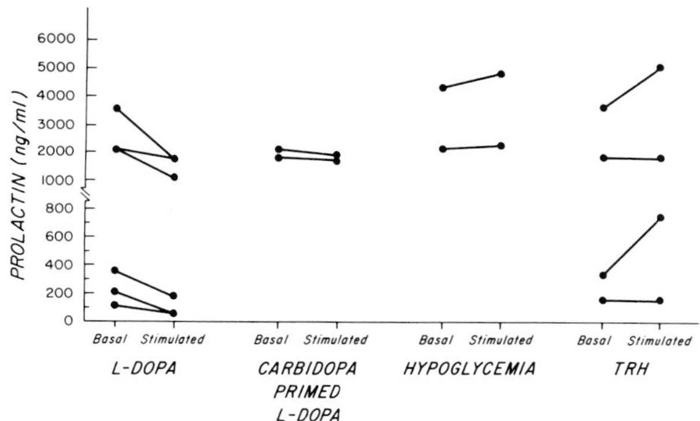

Fig. 1. Prolactin responses to L-dopa, carbidopa-primed L-dopa, hypoglycemia, and TRH in males with prolactin-secreting adenomas. In normal men, prolactin increases 1.4–8.4 times over baseline after hypoglycemia[65] and 3.8 times over baseline after TRH.[66]

Abnormalities of the sella turcica were seen on plain skull X-rays in all patients and variously consisted of gross sella enlargement, a double appearance of the floor with erosion, and backward displacement of the dorsum. Sella pleuridirectional tomography was useful in demonstrating focal areas of erosion and sphenoid sinus invasion. Computerized axial tomographic (CT) scanning or pneumoencephalography revealed suprasellar extension of tumor in six patients. Five of these six patients had defects on Goldmann visual-field testing. The overall incidence of visual-field defects was 50%.

Patients were treated with either transsphenoidal adenomectomy or frontal craniotomy and radiotherapy (7 patients), radiotherapy (5000 rads) alone (2 patients), or proton-beam (1 patient) depending on their clinical circumstances. No patients were cured by these procedures; all remained hyperprolactinemic. Two patients (cases 7 and 10) have required repeated surgical procedures for recurrent visual impairment. Case 10 remains hyperprolactinemic despite four surgical procedures and a course of radiotherapy.

Following treatment, the relationship among serum prolactin levels, testosterone levels, and sexual function was variable (Table 1). Three patients regained normal sexual function after treatment with supplemental testosterone despite persistent hyperprolactinemia. Our experience with bromocryptine in this group of patients has been limited. Although serum prolactin levels have fallen (in one instance to within the normal range) in the four patients treated with this agent, potency has not been markedly improved.

2.2. Males with Nonsecreting Tumors

Males with nonsecreting chromophobe adenomas are considered in Table 2. Presenting symptoms in patients in this group were often very similar to those seen in men with prolactin-secreting tumors (Table 3). The average age at presentation was 55 years. Impotence or decreased libido was noted in nine patients. One patient (case 16) presented with a third cranial nerve palsy and

TABLE 2. Males with Nonsecreting Tumors

Case no.	Presenting symptoms	Laboratory	Radiographic	Therapy	Course
11	Lethargy Hypothyroidism Impotence Decreased libido Visual-field defect	Prolactin: 18.3 ng/ml L-Dopa: 71% suppression TRH: 48% increase Testosterone: 142 ng/dl LH: 0.8 mIU/ml FSH: 3.8 mIU/ml GH: low (L-dopa) TSH: low (TRH)	+SSE	TA	Prolactin 9 ng/ml following TA Potency improved on testosterone
12	Visual-field defect Normal sexual function	Prolactin: 8.2 ng/ml Testosterone: 630 ng/dl TSH: normal	+SSE	TA RTX Frontal craniotomy	Recurrent visual-field defects Impotent Hypothyroid
13	Decreased libido Impotence Lethargy	Prolactin: 13.6 ng/ml TRH: 180% increase Hypoglycemia: 7% increase Testosterone: 80 ng/dl LH: 1.2 mIU/ml FSH: 1.4 mIU/ml ACTH: low (hypoglycemia) GH: low (hypoglycemia) TSH: normal (TRH) Partial diabetes insipidus	+SSE	TA RTX	Prolactin 7.6 following TA Potency improved on testosterone
14	Decreased libido Impotence Panhypopituitary Visual-field defect	Prolactin: 4 ng/ml	+SSE	Frontal craniotomy TA RTX	Recurrent visual-field defects Panhypopituitary Potency poor on testosterone
15	Hypothyroid Decreased libido Visual-field defect	Prolactin: 10.4 ng/ml L-Dopa: 71% suppression TRH: 43% increase Chlorpromazine: 25% increase Testosterone: 440 ng/dl TSH: low GH: low (L-dopa) ACTH: low (hypoglycemia)	−SSE	TA	
16	Impotence Headaches Cranial-nerve defect Gynecomastia	Prolactin: 7 ng/ml L-Dopa: 30% suppression TRH: 33% increase Testosterone: 250 ng/dl LH: 0.7 mIU/ml FSH: 2.0 mIU/ml GH: low (L-dopa) TSH: low (TRH) ACTH: low	+SSE	TA RTX	Prolactin 10.5 ng/ml following TA Potency improved on testosterone Gynecomastia resolved

(continued)

gynecomastia. No patients had galactorrhea, and none was morbidly obese. The mean weight of the patients with nonsecreting chromophobe adenomas was 89 kg. None of the patients with nonsecreting tumors had diabetes mellitus.

The average basal prolactin level in the patients with nonsecreting chromophobe adenomas was 10.6±1.3 ng/ml. Testosterone values were low in seven patients. In all but one of these patients with low testosterone levels, the gonadotropin levels were also low.

Seven patients (70%) with nonsecreting tumors had evidence of TSH-reserve deficiency in preoperative testing, either hypothyroidism in association with low TSH levels or subnormal TSH responses to TRH administration.[4] Of the male patients with prolactin-secreting tumors, only 13% had a deficiency in TSH reserve preoperatively. ACTH-reserve deficiency, documented by stimulation with hypoglycemia or metyrapone, was detected in five patients (50%) with nonsecreting tumors. By contrast, the incidence of ACTH-reserve deficiency in males with prolactin-secreting tumors was 25%.

Dynamic testing of prolactin secretion blunted responses to TRH administration in all six patients tested preoperatively (Fig. 2). Prolactin levels also failed to rise normally in two patients tested with insulin-induced hypo-

TABLE 2. (*continued*)

Case no.	Presenting symptoms	Laboratory[a]	Radiographic	Therapy[b]	Course
17	Decreased libido Impotence Headaches	Prolactin: 7.6 ng/ml L-Dopa: 76% suppression TRH: 102% increase Testosterone: 440 ng/dl TSH: normal (TRH) GH: low (L-dopa) ACTH: normal (metyrapone)	+SSE	TA RTX	Prolactin 5 ng/ml following TA, no response to TRH Potency poor despite normal testosterone
18	Decreased libido Impotence Panhypopituitary	Prolactin: 12.3 ng/ml	−SSE	RTX	Potency improved on testosterone Motor disturbance possibly 2° to RTX
19	Decreased libido Impotence Hypothyroid	Prolactin: 9.8 ng/ml TRH: 55% increase Testosterone: 20 ng/dl LH: 0.6 mIU/ml FSH: 0.6 mIU/ml TSH: low ACTH: normal (hypoglycemia) GH: low (L-dopa)	−SSE	TA	Prolactin 6.4 ng/ml following TA Potency poor on testosterone
20	Headaches Decreased libido Impotence Visual-field defect	Prolactin: 15 ng/ml Testosterone: 10 ng/ml FSH: 47 mIU/ml TSH: low GH: low (arginine)	+SSE	TA RTX	Prolactin 5 ng/ml following TA Potency improved on testosterone

TABLE 3. Comparison of Men with Prolactinomas and Nonsecreting Tumors and Women with Prolactinomas (All Surgically Verified Tumors)

	Males		Females
	Prolactin secreting	Non-secreting	prolactin-secreting
Total number	10	10	30
Age at presentation (years)	46	55	27
Gonadal dysfunction			
Amenorrhea	—	—	94%
Impotence/decreased libido	90%	90%	—
Headaches	40%	30%	60%
Visual-field defect	50%	50%	15%
Morbid obesity	30%	0%	0%
Diabetes	30%	0%	0%
Galactorrhea	10%	0%	100%
Gynecomastia	30%	10%	—
Abnormal plain skull X-rays	100%	100%	—
Suprasellar extension	60%	70%	20%
Prolactin	1378 ng/ml	10.6 ng/ml	168 ng/ml
Partial hypopituitarism[a]			
Gonadotropin deficiency	86%	60%	100%
TSH-reserve deficiency	13%	70%	26%
ACTH-reserve deficiency	25%	50%	7%
GH-reserve deficiency	67%	100%	10%
Panhypopituitarism[a]	11%	30%	0%

[a]Patients with prior pituitary surgery excluded.

glycemia or chlorpromazine. This blunting of prolactin response is similar to that seen in males with prolactin-secreting tumors (see Fig. 1). The blunted prolactin responses in patients with nonsecreting chromophobe adenomas may be related to the high incidence of panhypopituitarism. Either replacement of pituitary tissue by tumor or secondary effects of hypopituitarism could be responsible for the failure of prolactin to respond appropriately to stimulation. In this regard, however, it is noteworthy that two patients with nonsecreting tumors (cases 13 and 17) had blunted prolactin responses to TRH administration despite normal TSH responses, and one of these (case 17) additionally had normal testosterone levels and ACTH reserve. The high incidence of abnormal prolactin responses to TRH in patients with either prolactin-secreting or nonsecreting tumors makes this test of little use in the diagnosis of a prolactinoma.

GH responses to hypoglycemia, arginine, or L-dopa (500 mg p.o.) administration were typically depressed in patients with either prolactin-secreting (67% of patients) or nonsecreting (100% of patients) tumors. In four patients with nonsecreting tumors who underwent L-dopa tests, prolactin levels fell by an average of 62±11% from baseline, similar to the suppression seen in normals and in patients with prolactin-secreting tumors.

Similar to those found in all men with prolactin-secreting tumors, plain

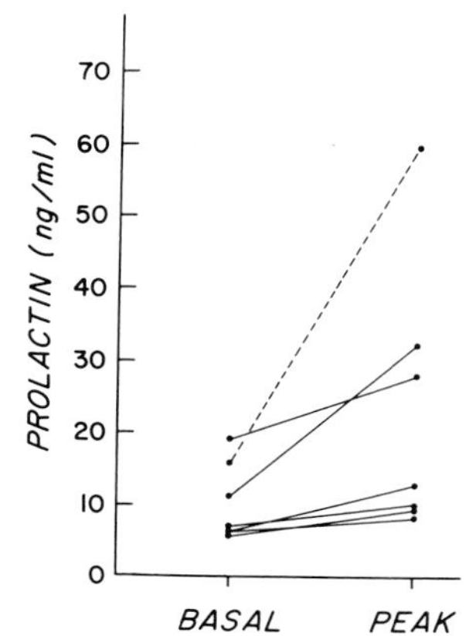

Fig. 2. Prolactin responses to TRH administration in men with nonsecreting pituitary tumors. (----) Normal response.[66]

skull X-rays were abnormal in all men with nonsecreting adenomas. CT scan and pneumoencephalography showed a 70% incidence of suprasellar extension of tumor. Goldmann visual-field testing revealed defects in five patients (50%).

All but one patient with a nonsecreting tumor was operated on, eight by the transsphenoidal route and one by a subfrontal approach. All ten received irradiation. It is difficult to compare the postoperative course of patients with nonsecreting tumors to the course of those with prolactinomas. First, there is no easily identifiable tumor marker in patients with nonsecreting tumors. Second, several of the patients with nonsecreting adenomas were panhypopituitary prior to surgery. Two patients with nonsecreting tumors have required repeated surgery for recurrent visual-field deficits. Another patient (case 18) developed choreiform movements possibly secondary to radiation toxicity. Gynecomastia resolved postoperatively in case 16, even though prolactin and testosterone values were unchanged from the preoperative levels.

3. Discussion

In our series, males with prolactin-secreting tumors appear to have larger, more aggressive tumors than do women. Impotence, decreased libido, and visual-field abnormalities were common presenting features in men with either prolactin-secreting or nonsecreting adenomas. The response to ablative therapy was far inferior to that seen in women, even in women with comparable-size prolactinomas.[5] Whether the marked differences in clinical manifestations of prolactin-secreting tumors in men and women are due to the delayed detection of these tumors in men or to some innate biological difference in the adenomas is uncertain. Although basal prolactin levels were considerably higher in males with prolactin-secreting tumors than in females, stimulatory tests of prolactin secretion were not noticeably different.

The incidence of diminished sexual function and visual-field abnormalities in men with nonsecreting adenomas was similar to that in men with prolactin-secreting tumors (Table 3). The incidence of morbid obesity was greater in men with prolactin-secreting tumors (30 vs. 0%), as was the incidence of gynecomastia (30 vs. 10%) and galactorrhea (10 vs. 0%). It is unknown whether the greater frequency of diabetes mellitus in males with prolactin-secreting tumors (30 vs. 0%) reflects a diabetogenic effect of prolactin[6] or whether this is secondary to the higher incidence of obesity. An increased frequency of diabetes mellitus has not been noted in most series of women with prolactin-secreting tumors, including our own (Chapter 4). Panhypopituitarism appears to be more common in patients with nonsecreting than in those with prolactin-secreting tumors (30 vs. 11%). The postoperative course appears to be more benign in men with nonsecreting adenomas, but this is difficult to determine in the absence of an easily identifiable tumor marker.

Several reports of men with prolactin-secreting tumors have appeared in the literature (Table 4).[7–30] In some early cases,[7,8,10] the diagnosis of a prolactin-secreting tumor has been suspected because of the occurrence of gynecomastia or galactorrhea in a male with a chromophobe adenoma. Since one of our patients with a nonsecreting adenoma also developed gynecomastia, we feel that documented hyperprolactinemia is necessary to confirm the diagnosis of a prolactinoma.

The average age of patients in Table 4 at the time of presentation was 35 years, slightly younger than the patients in our series, and patients as young as 12 years old have been described.[21] Disturbances in sexual function, either decreased libido or impotence, were noted in over 90% of patients in some studies[27,29]; other studies have found men with prolactin-secreting tumors to be "endocrinologically normal."[26] In our patients, the presence of sexual dysfunction did not discriminate between males with nonsecreting and those with prolactin-secreting tumors.

Several of the patients listed in Table 4 were markedly obese. Franks *et al.*[28] attributed the obesity in their patients with prolactin-secreting tumors to associated hypogonadism. In our series, patients with prolactin-secreting tumors had a clearly higher incidence of hypogonadism, indicating that other factors may also be important. These factors might include the degree of hypothalamic involvement, the influence of other hormonal deficiencies, or perhaps an effect of prolactin itself. In support of the latter possibility, prolactin has been shown to have a stimulatory effect on eating behavior in several animal species.[31]

Although earlier studies suggested that the frequency of gynecomastia and galactorrhea in males with prolactinomas may exceed 50–60% (Table 4), more recent studies have found the incidence to be much lower.[17,27–29,32] In our patients, 30% had gynecomastia and 10% had galactorrhea. Although this incidence of gynecomastia was slightly greater than that seen in men with non-secreting adenomas, the association between hyperprolactinemia and gynecomastia is unclear. Several studies have suggested that patients with gynecomastia have normal serum prolactin levels,[9,12,33] but in other studies, hyperprolactinemia has been seen in 19–25% of patients with gynecomastia.[34,35] Buckman and Peake[35] have provided evidence suggesting that prolactin-secretory dynamics, as determined by phenothiazine ingestion or water-loading, are abnormal in patients with gynecomastia. Twenty-four-hour

TABLE 4. Males with Prolactin-Secreting Tumors[a]

Reference	Age	Gyn.[b]	Gal.[b]	Prolactin	Sexual function	Visual fields
Moehlig[7]	52	+	?	?	Impotent	Normal
McCullagh *et al.*[8]	26	+	+	?	Impotent	Normal
Forsyth *et al.*[9]	25	+	+	5000 ng/ml	Impotent	—
Racodot *et al.*[10]	38	+	+	?	—	Normal
	31	+	−	?	—	Abnormal
Finn and Mount[11]	18	−	+	?	Normal	Normal
	32	+	+	Elevated	Normal	Abnormal
Volpe *et al.*[12]	24	+	+	60 ng/ml	Impotent	Normal
Besser *et al.*[13]	25	+	+	1000 ng/ml	Impotent	Normal
	36	+	+	1500 ng/ml	Impotent	Normal
Boyar and Hellman[14]	38	+	−	500 ng/ml	Impotent	Normal
Thorner *et al.*[15]	20–36			30–1572 ng/ml	Impotent	—
4 cases	(28)	?	(100%)	(644 ng/ml)	(100%)	—
Rogal and Rosen[16]	32	?	+	3000 ng/ml	—	—
Zimmerman *et al.*[17]	17–60	?	?	37–3000 ng/ml	—	—
6 cases	(40)			(1544 ng/ml)	—	—
Child *et al.*[18]	55	?	?	30 ng/ml	Impotent	—
Malarkey and Johnson[19]	18	−	−	4800 ng/ml	Impotent	—
	44	−	−	292 ng/ml	Impotent	—
Schroffner[20]	13	−	−	5527 ng/ml	Normal	Normal
Van Meter *et al.*[21]	12	+	+	41 ng/ml	—	Normal
Koenig *et al.*[22]	18	−	+	58–246 ng/ml	Impotent	Normal
Antunes *et al.*[23]	16–73			21–10,000 ng/ml	—	—
16 cases	(40)	?	(13%)	(1507 ng/ml)	—	—
McKenna *et al.*[24]	38	+	+	65 ng/ml	Impotent	Normal
Carlson *et al.*[25]	26–49	−	−	30–800 ng/ml		Abnormal
3 cases	(35)			(298 ng/ml)		(33%)
Osamura *et al.*[26]	24–45	−	−	103–8240 ng/ml	Normal	Abnormal
11 cases	(32)			(1961 ng/ml)	(100%)	(100%)
Nagulesparen *et al.*[27]		−	−	Elevated	Impotent	Abnormal
22 cases	—			—	(94%)	—
Franks *et al.*[28]	16–61			14–5300 ng/ml	Impotent	—
21 cases	(39)	(14%)	−	(1085 ng/ml)	(81%)	—
Carter *et al.*[29]	20–65			76–22,000 ng/ml	Impotent	Abnormal
22 cases	(38)	(14%)		(880 ng/ml)	(91%)	(41%)
McGregor *et al.*[30]	24	−	−	8000 ng/ml	Impotent	Abnormal

[a] Mean values are given in parentheses where applicable.
[b] (Gyn.) Gynecomastia; (Gal.) galactorrhea.

prolactin-secretory rates may be a more sensitive measure of subtle hyperprolactinemia, but these studies have not as yet been performed.

Another approach to studying the role of prolactin in the development of gynecomastia has been to manipulate prolactin levels with bromocryptine. There are several examples of gynecomastia resolving after bromocriptine therapy in patients with prolactin-secreting tumors.[13,36] Since bromocriptine may cause an elevation in circulating testosterone levels in men with prolactinomas,[28,29] resolution of gynecomastia in these patients may simply be due to correction of the low androgen levels. There are, however, examples of men with prolactin-secreting tumors whose gynecomastia resolved after bromocriptine therapy despite persistently low testosterone levels,[13] implying that hyperprolactinemia *per se* may cause breast enlargement in men. Further confusing the issue is the report by Jaffiol *et al.*[37] describing men with idiopathic gynecomastia, normal sexual function, and normal prolactin levels in whom gynecomastia resolved following treatment with bromocriptine. Larger studies comparing men with prolactin-secreting tumors to those with nonsecreting tumors may be helpful in establishing the role of hyperprolactinemia in the development of gynecomastia.

The incidence of galactorrhea in our male patients with prolactinomas was similar to that described in other recent studies.[23,27–29] Although uncommon, the occurrence of galactorrhea in a male has an extraordinarily high likelihood of being due to a prolactin-secreting tumor. Kleinberg *et al.*[2] found that 6 of 13 men with galactorrhea had pituitary tumors. If drug-induced causes of galactorrhea are excluded, the incidence of documented pituitary tumors in men with galactorrhea in their study approaches 70%. This figure would probably be even higher if patients bearing adenomas with normal X-rays were included. Cases of histologically documented prolactin-secreting tumors in men with normal sella tomography have recently been reported.[24] The relatively infrequent occurrence of galactorrhea in men with prolactinomas as compared to women may be due to prior estrogen priming of the female breast.[38]

Prolactin-secreting tumors in men are typically larger than those in women[23] and more likely to be associated with visual-field defects.[32] Our study confirms these findings (see Table 3). The incidence of visual-field abnormalities has varied from 20 to 100% in several large series.[17,26,27,29,32] In our series, half the patients had visual-field defects. Whether this high incidence of visual-field impairment reflects the inability to detect early clinical manifestations of prolactinomas in men or increased aggressiveness of these tumors is unknown. The later age of presentation and occasional detection of prolactinomas as an incidental finding in men[32] suggests that these tumors are not diagnosed until a later stage in their development. In our series, prolactin-secreting and nonsecreting tumors in men were not distinguishable radiographically.

Prolactin levels in men with tumors are far higher than those in women; in our series, as in others,[26,28] the average basal prolactin exceeded 1000 ng/ml. Serum testosterone values have been reported to be generally low, and gonadotropin levels are usually low[27,29] or not elevated appropriately[28] in relation to the level of testosterone. Our findings were similar. Despite the large size of these prolactin-secreting tumors, panhypopituitarism is surprisingly infrequent.

Detailed comparisons of prolactin-secretory dynamics in men and women with prolactinomas have not been performed in prior studies. Franks *et al.*[28] did report blunted prolactin responses to TRH administration in seven male patients with prolactin-secreting tumors, however. The TSH responses to TRH in these patients were normal. The prolactin response to TRH stimulation was blunted in most of our male patients with prolactin-secreting adenomas, similar to our findings in women (Chapter 4). The finding that prolactin responses to TRH were blunted in all six patients with nonsecreting adenomas tested indicates that this test may not be useful for diagnosing a prolactin-secreting tumor. In our male patients with prolactinomas, the reduction in prolactin in response to L-dopa of 44±7% was comparable to the usual response in normal individuals[3] and in women with microadenomas.[39] Similar reductions in prolactin levels following L-dopa administration in males have been described in case reports by others.[12,20,21] It thus appears that males with large tumors and markedly elevated prolactin levels, females with microadenomas and moderately elevated prolactin levels, and normal individuals are equally sensitive to dopaminergic inhibition despite differences in estrogen levels. The diminished suppression of prolactin after L-dopa with carbidopa pretreatment in our two men so tested is similar to the findings in women with prolactinomas[3,39] and suggests defective hypothalamic regulation of prolactin secretion in both sexes when an adenoma is present.

The relationship between hyperprolactinemia and hypogonadism has been studied by the use of stimulatory tests of gonadotropin and testosterone secretion, but interpretation of results obtained in several published series is difficult because many of the patients studied had been operated on previously or had received radiotherapy. Following administration of lutenizing-hormone-releasing hormone (LH-RH), both blunted[27] and normal[28,29] gonadotropin-secretory responses have been reported. Administration of human chorionic gonadotropin (hCG) has also given inconsistent results. Franks *et al.*[28] and Carter *et al.*[29] reported normal testosterone elevations following hCG administration in their male patients with prolactin-secreting tumors, but Thorner *et al.*[40] and Ambrosi *et al.*[41] found blunted responses to hCG in hyperprolactinemic males. When the hyperprolactinemia was corrected by surgery or bromocriptine therapy, testosterone responses to hCG increased toward normal. Stimulatory tests of gonadotropin and testosterone secretion were not performed in our patients.

The role of prolactin in modulating male sexual function remains controversial. In animal models, there is evidence for both a stimulatory[42–48] and an inhibitory[49–51] effect of prolactin on sexual function. There is also evidence in humans that prolactin might participate in testosterone regulation. Rubin *et al.*[52] have noted that the nocturnal rise in testosterone is preceded by an increase in prolactin levels. The elevation in serum prolactin seen following administration of haloperidol or TRH is also associated with an increase in testosterone secretions.[53–55] Treatment with sulpiride, a dopaminergic antagonist, has been reported to cause hyperprolactinemia and an exaggeration of the testosterone response to hCG.[56] In other studies, however, Magrini *et al.*[57] found that sulpiride administration had no effect on the testosterone response to hCG. As mentioned above, the testosterone response to hCG was also variable in hyperprolactinemic men with prolactin-secreting tumors. Varma *et al.*[58] have shown that administration of ovine prolactin to normal men has no effect on androgen production. Decreasing serum prolactin levels with methysergide, a serotonin antagonist, does not appear to affect testosterone levels.[59]

Although gonadal unresponsiveness to gonadotropins may contribute to the sexual impairment found in men with prolactin-secreting tumors, the frequent ineffectiveness of supplemental testosterone therapy[27,29] in restoring potency in hyperprolactinemic patients remains unexplained, and suggests a direct suppressive effect of prolactin. In support of this possibility, Magrini *et al.*[57] have shown that hyperprolactinemia may interfere with testosterone metabolism. These workers administered hCG to healthy men after inducing hyperprolactinemia with sulpiride. Despite normal testosterone responses to hCG, the rise in dihydrotestosterone was blunted, suggesting the possibility of interference with the enzyme 5α-reductase, which converts testosterone to dihydrotestosterone. Similar responses were noted when hyperprolactinemia was the result of pituitary-stalk section. In both instances, bromocriptine restored dihydrostestosterone responses to normal.

In several studies, bromocriptine therapy has led to normalization of serum prolactin levels and in some instances[28,29] to elevation in the serum testosterone. Other studies have shown no improvement in testosterone levels following bromocriptine therapy.[27] It is of interest that sexual function may improve after bromocriptine therapy despite persistently low testosterone levels[27] or before testosterone levels have risen appreciably,[28] again suggesting a direct suppressive effect of prolactin. The observations of Carter *et al.*[29] that elevations in serum LH often do not precede the increases in testosterone levels during bromocriptine therapy support the hypothesis that hyperprolactinemia may cause gonadal unresponsiveness to gonadotropins. The relationship among prolactin, testosterone, and sexual function in our patients was variable.

Unlike the experience in women,[5,60] surgical removal of prolactinomas in men is usually unsuccessful in restoring sexual function and returning prolactin levels to normal.[27–29] None of our patients was cured by surgery and irradiation or irradiation alone. Nonetheless, surgery or irradiation or both are still indicated in most patients to relieve the mass effects of the adenoma and to prevent further tumor growth. Surgery or radiotherapy appears to be curative in only a few reported cases.[11,21,24]

Histological studies have not revealed differences between prolactin-secreting tumors occurring in men and women. Immunoperoxidase staining has demonstrated that tumors in men, like those in women, are rich in prolactin compared to adjacent pituitary tissue.[17,26] These observations are consistent with the hypothesis that prolactin-secreting tumors can arise spontaneously in the pituitary, rather than developing as a result of abnormal hypothalamic influences.[39]

4. Conclusion

Comparisons between prolactin-secreting tumors in men and women are limited by the delay in the diagnosis in men. Further studies of the interaction between prolactin and male gonadal function may allow earlier recognition and decreased morbidity. Several reports have suggested that infertile males have slightly elevated prolactin levels[16,62] and that male fertility is improved in these mildly hyperprolactinemic patients following bromocryptine therapy.[63,64] Although these patients did not have radiographic evidence of pituitary tumors, the possibility of small microadenomata cannot be excluded. Long-term follow-up of infertile males may result in the definition of a subgroup of patients, like women with galactorrhea and amenorrhea, with a high incidence of pituitary tumors.

In summary, males with prolactin-secreting adenomas appear to present differently from females with prolactinomas. In general, men have macro-adenomas that often result in considerable suprasellar extension and visual-field defects. These tumors are frequently associated with decreased libido, impotence, and perhaps infertility, but these symptoms are either misdiagnosed by the physician or ignored by the patient. It is unclear whether the large size of the tumors is due to their prolonged period of growth because these symptoms are ignored or because there is an innate biological difference in the growth characteristics of these tumors compared to those occurring in women. Unfortunately, these large tumors in men respond poorly to surgery or irradiation, or both, so that every effort should be made to diagnose these tumors early. The recognition that prolactin-secreting tumors may make up a significant percentage of the causes of male hypogonadism, impotence, and infertility may lead to the earlier diagnosis of these tumors with consequent improvement in their prognosis.

References

1. S. Nader, K. Mashiter, F.H. Doyle, and F.G. Joplin, Galactorrhea, hyperprolactinemia, and pituitary tumors in the female, *Clin. Endocrinol.* **5:**245, 1976.
2. D.L. Kleinberg, G.L. Noel, and A.G. Frantz, Galactorrhea: A study of 235 cases, including 48 with pituitary tumors, *N. Engl. J. Med.* **296:**589, 1977.
3. S.A. Fine and L.A. Frohman, Loss of central nervous system component of dopaminergic inhibition of prolactin secretion in patients with prolactin-secreting pituitary tumors, *J. Clin. Invest.* **61:**973, 1978.
4. P.J. Snyder, L.S. Jacobs, M.M. Robello, F.S.H. Sterling, R.N. Shore, R.D. Utiger, and W.H. Daughaday, Diagnostic value of thyrotropin-releasing hormone in pituitary and hypothalamic disease, *Ann. Intern. Med.* **81:**751, 1974.
5. K.D. Post, B.J. Biller, L.S. Adelman, M.E. Molitch, S.M. Wolpert, and S. Reichlin, Results of transsphenoidal adenomectomy in women with galactorrhea–amenorrhea, *J. Am. Med. Assoc.* **242:**158, 1979.
6. R. Landgraf, A. Weissmann, R. Horl, and M.M.C. Landgraf-Leurs, Is prolactin a diabetogenic hormone?, *Diabetologia* **11:**357, 1975.
7. R.C. Moehlig, Pituitary tumor associated with gynecomastia, *Endocrinology* **15:**529, 1929.
8. E.P. McCullagh, J.G. Alivisatos, and C.A. Schaffenburg, Pituitary tumor with gynecomastia and lactation—a case report, *J. Clin. Endocrinol. Metab.* **16:**397, 1956.
9. I.A. Forsyth, G.M. Besser, C.R.W. Edwards, L. Francis, and R.P. Myres, Plasma prolactin activity in inappropriate lactation, *Br. Med. J.* **3:**225, 1971.
10. J. Racodot, E. Vila-Porcile, and F. Peillon, Adénomes hypophysaires a cellules a prolactine: Etude structurale et ultrastructurale; corrélations anatomocliniques, *Ann. Endocrinol. (Paris)* **32:**298, 1971.
11. J.E. Finn and L.A. Mount, Galactorrhea in males with tumors in the region of the pituitary gland, *J. Neurosurg.* **35:**723, 1971.
12. R. Volpe, D. Killinger, C. Bird, A.F. Clark, and H. Friesen, Idiopathic galactorrhea and mild hypogonadism in a young adult male, *J. Clin. Endocrinol. Metab.* **35:**684, 1972.
13. G.M. Besser, L. Parke, C.R.W. Edwards, I.A. Forsyth, and A.S. McNeilly, Galactorrhea: Successful treatment with reduction of plasma prolactin levels by brom-ergocryptine, *Br. Med. J.* **3:**669, 1972.
14. R.M. Boyar and L. Hellman, Syndrome of benign nodular adrenal hyperplasia associated with feminization and hyperprolactinemia, *Ann. Intern. Med.* **80:**389, 1974.

15. M.O. Thorner, A.S. McNeilly, C. Hagan, and G.M. Besser, Long-term treatment of galactorrhea and hypogonadism with bromocriptine, *Br. Med. J.* **2:**419, 1974.
16. A.D. Rogal and S.W. Rosen, Prolactin of apparent large molecular size: The major immunoactive prolactin component in plasma of a patient with a pituitary tumor, *J. Clin. Endocrinol. Metab.* **38:**714, 1974.
17. E.A. Zimmerman, R. Defendini, and A.G. Frantz, Prolactin and growth hormone in patients with pituitary adenomas; a correlative study of hormone in tumor and plasma by immunoperoxidase technique and radioimmunoassay, *J. Clin. Endocrinol. Metab.* **38:**577, 1974.
18. D.F. Child, S. Nades, K. Mashifer, M. Kjeld, L. Banks, and T.R. Fraser, Prolactin studies in "functionless" pituitary tumors, *Br. Med. J.* **1:**604, 1975.
19. W.B. Malarkey and J.C. Johnson, Pituitary tumors and hyperprolactinemia, *Arch. Intern. Med.* **136:**40, 1976.
20. W.G. Schroffner, Prolactin-secreting pituitary tumor in early adolescence, *Arch. Intern. Med.* **136:**1164, 1976.
21. Q.L. Van Meter, F.J. Garcia, J.W. Hayes, and C.B. Wilson, Galactorrhea in a 12 year old boy with a chromophobe adenoma, *J. Pediatr.* **90:**756, 1977.
22. M.P. Koenig, K. Zuppinger, and B. Liechti, Hyperprolactinemia as a cause of delayed puberty: Successful treatment with bromocriptine, *J. Clin. Endocrinol. Metab.* **45:**825, 1977.
23. J.L. Antunes, E.M. Housepian, A.G. Frantz, D.A. Holub, R.M. Hui, P.W. Carmel, and D.O. Quest, Prolactin-secreting pituitary tumors, *Ann. Neurol.* **2:**148, 1977.
24. T.J. McKenna, A.D. Glick, C.A. Cobb, and L.S. Jacobs, Galactorrhea and hypogonadism associated with a radiologically-inapparent prolactin-secreting pituitary tumor, *Acta. Endocrinol.* **87:**225, 1978.
25. H.E. Carlson, G.A. Levine, N.J. Goldberg, and J.M. Hershman, Hyperprolactinemia in multiple endocrine adenomatosis, type I, *Arch. Intern. Med.* **138:**1807, 1978.
26. R.Y. Osamura, K. Watanabe, A. Teramoto, K. Hirakawa, N. Kawano, and S. Morii, Male prolactin secreting pituitary adenomas in humans studies by peroxidase-labelled antibody method, *Acta. Endocrinol.* **88:**643, 1978.
27. M. Nagulesparen, V. Ang, and J.S. Jenkins, Bromocriptine treatment of males with pituitary tumours, hyperprolactinemia, and hypogonadism, *Clin. Endocrinol.* **9:**73, 1978.
28. S. Franks, H.S. Jacobs, N. Martin, and J.D.N. Nabarro, Hyperprolactinemia and impotence, *Clin. Endocrinol.* **8:**277, 1978.
29. J.N. Carter, J.E. Tyson, G. Tolis, S. Van Vliet, C. Faiman, and H.G. Friesen, Prolactin-secreting tumors and hypogonadism in 22 men, *N. Engl. J. Med.* **299:**847, 1978.
30. A.M. McGregor, M.F. Scanlon, K. Hall, D.B. Cook, and R. Hall, Reduction in size of a pituitary tumor by bromocriptine therapy, *N. Engl. J. Med.* **300:**291, 1979.
31. C.S. Nicoll, Physiological actions of prolactin, in: *Handbook of Physiology,* Section 7: Endocrinology, Vol. IV (R.O. Greep and E.B. Astwood, eds.), pp. 253–292, American Physiological Society, Washington, D.C. 1974.
32. S. Franks, J.D.N. Nabarro, and H.S. Jacobs, Prevalence and presentation of hyperprolactinemia in patients with "functionless" pituitary tumors, *Lancet* **1:**778, 1977.
33. R.W. Turkington, Serum prolactin levels in patients with gynecomastia, *J. Clin. Endocrinol.* **34:**62, 1972.
34. A.G. Frantz, D.L. Kleinberg, and G.L. Noel, Studies on prolactin in man, *Recent Prog. Horm. Res.* **28:**527, 1972.
35. M.T. Buckman and G.T. Peake, Abnormal regulation of prolactin secretion in patients with gynecomastia, *Clin. Res.* **22:**162A, 1974.
36. P. Fossati, G. Strauch, and J. Tourniare, Etude de l'activité de la bromocriptine dans les états d'hyperprolactinemie, *Nouv. Presse Med.* **5:**1687, 1976.
37. C. Jaffiol, M. Rubin, A. Orsetti, and J. Mirouze, Le. hormones gonadotropes de la prolactine au cours des gynecomasties, *Ann. Endocrinol.* (*Paris*) **37:**469, 1976.
38. A.G. Frantz, Prolactin, *N. Engl. J. Med.* **298:**201, 1978.
39. R. Goodman, B. Biller, A.C. Moses, M. Molitch, Z. Feldman, and K. Post, Restoration of normal prolactin secretory dynamics after surgical cure of prolactinoma is evidence against underlying hypothalamic dysregulation, Abstracts of The Endocrine Society, 61st Annual Meeting, June 13–15, 1979, p. 159.
40. M.O. Thorner, G.M. Besser, C. Hagen, and A.S. McNeilly, The relationship between prolactin

and gonadotrophins: Effects of clomiphene administration in normal men, *J. Endocrinol.* **63:**43, 1974.

41. B. Ambrosi, R. Elli, M. Gaggini, M. Rondena, and G. Faglia, Prolactin-secreting tumors and hypogonadism in men, *N. Engl. J. Med.* **300:**563, 1979.
42. A. Bartke, Effects of prolactin on spermatogenesis in hypophysectomized mice, *J. Endocrinol.* **49:**311, 1971.
43. A. Bartke, Effects of prolactin and luteinizing hormone on the cholesterol stores in the mouse testes, *J. Endocrinol.* **49:**317, 1971.
44. N. Musto, A.A. Hafiez, and A. Bartke, Prolactin increases 17β-hydroxysteroid dehydrogenase activity in the testes, *Endocrinology* **91:**1106, 1972.
45. A.A. Hafiez, C.W. Lloyd, and A. Bartke, The role of prolactin in the regulation of testis function: The effects of prolactin and luteinizing hormone on the plasma levels of testosterone and androstenedione in hypophysectomized rats, *J. Endocrinol.* **52:**327, 1972.
46. C. Aragona and H.G. Friesen, Specific prolactin binding sites in the prostate and testes of cats, *Endocrinology* **97:**677, 1975.
47. F.J. Bex and A. Bartke, Testicular LH binding in the hamster: Modification by photoperiod and prolactin, *Endocrinology* **100:**1223, 1977.
48. C. Aragona, H.G. Bohnet, and H.G. Friesen, Localization of prolactin binding in prostate and testis: The role of serum prolactin concentration on the testicular LH receptor, *Acta Endocrinol.* **84:**402, 1977.
49. V.S. Fang, S. Refetoff, and R.L. Rosenfield, Hypogonadism induced by a transplantable, prolactin-producing tumor in male rats: Hormonal and morphological studies, *Endocrinology* **95:**991, 1974.
50. A. Bartke, M.S. Smith, S.D. Michael, F.G. Peron, and S. Dalterio, Effects of experimentally-induced chronic hyperprolactinemia on testosterone and gonadotropin levels in male rats and mice, *Endocrinology* **100:**182, 1977.
51. S.J. Winters and D.L. Loriaux, Suppression of plasma luteinizing hormone by prolactin in the male rat, *Endocrinology* **102:**864, 1978.
52. R.T. Rubin, P.R. Gouin, A. Lubin, R.E. Poland, and K.M. Pirke, Nocturnal increase of plasma testosterone in men: Relation to gonadotropins and prolactin, *J. Clin. Endocrinol. Metab.* **40:**1027, 1975.
53. R.T. Rubin, R.E. Poland, and B.B. Tower, Prolactin-related testosterone secretion in normal adult men, *J. Clin. Endocrinol. Metab. 42:*112, 1976.
54. R.T. Rubin, R.E. Poland, J.R. Sowers, and J.M. Hershman, Influence of methyl-TRH-induced prolactin increase on serum testosterone levels in normal adult men, *J. Clin. Endocrinol. Metab.* **46:**830, 1978.
55. R.T. Rubin, R.E. Poland, I. Sobel, B.B. Tower, and W.D. Odell, Effects of prolactin and prolactin plus luteinizing hormone on plasma testosterone levels in normal adult men, *J. Clin. Endocrinol. Metab.* **47:**447, 1978.
56. B. Ambrosi, P. Travaglini, P. Beck-Peccoz, R. Bara, R. Elli, A. Paracchi, and G. Faglia, Effect of sulpiride-induced hyperprolactinemia on serum testosterone response to HCG in normal men, *J. Clin. Endocrinol. Metab.* **43:**700, 1976.
57. G. Magrini, J.R. Ebiner, P. Burekhardt, and J.P. Felber, Study on the relationship between plasma prolactin levels and androgen metabolism in man, *J. Clin. Endocrinol. Metab.* **43:**944, 1976.
58. M.M. Varma, C.A. Huseman, and J. Johanson, Effect of prolactin on adrenocortical and gonadal function in normal men, *J. Clin. Endocrinol. Metab.* **44:**760, 1977.
59. L.S. Jacobs, W.B. Mendelson, R.T. Rubin, and J.E. Bauman, Failure of nocturnal prolactin suppression by methylsergide to entrain changes in testosterone in normal men, *J. Clin. Endocrinol. Metab.* **46:**561, 1978.
60. J. Hardy, H. Beauregard, and F. Robert, Prolactin-secreting pituitary adenomas: Transsphenoidal microsurgical treatment, in: *Progress in Prolactin Physiology and Pathology* (C. Robyn and M. Harter, eds.), pp. 361–370, Elsevier/North Holland, Amsterdam, 1978.
61. R. Roulier, A. Mattei, A. Reuter, and P. Franchimont, Etude de la prolactine dans les stérilités et les hypogonadismes masculins, *Ann. Endocrinol. (Paris)* **37:**285, 1976.
62. P. Falaschi, G. Frajese, A. Rocco, G.M. Besser, and L.H. Rees, Prolactin and idiopathic oligospermia, *Lancet* **1:**667, 1979.

63. K. Saidi, R.V. Wenn, and F. Sharif, Bromocriptine for male infertility, *Lancet* **1:**250, 1977.
64. S. Segal, W.Z. Polishuk, and M. Ben-David, Hyperprolactinemic male infertility, *Fertil. Steril.* **27:**1425, 1976.
65. G. Copinschi, M. L'Hermite, R. Leclercq, J. Goldstein, L. Vanhaelst, E. Viragoro, and C. Robyn, Effects of glucocorticoids on pituitary hormonal responses to hypoglycemia: Inhibition of prolactin release, *J. Clin. Endocrinol. Metab.* **40:**442, 1975.
66. G. Schwinn, A. von zur Muhlen, J. Kubberling, E. Halves, K.W. Wenzel, and H. Meinhold, Plasma prolactin levels after TRH and chlorpromazine in normal subjects and patients with impaired pituitary function, *Acta Endocrinol.* **79:**663, 1975.

6

Growth-Hormone-Secreting Pituitary Adenomas

IVOR M.D. JACKSON

1. Introduction

Acromegaly is a rare endocrinopathy that is estimated to occur with a frequency of one in 5000–15,000 patients.[1] The term, derived from the Greek *akron* (extremity) and *megale* (great), was first used by Marie[2] in 1886 to describe two patients with a syndrome in which hypertrophy of the extremities was the most striking clinical feature. His clinical description delineated the classic features of this condition, viz., marked enlargement of the hands and feet, prognathism, macroglossia, thickened skin associated with headache, joint pain, and lethargy. Although a relationship to the pituitary was postulated, Marie interpreted autopsy findings of a pituitary tumor in acromegaly as evidence of adenohypophyseal insufficiency (for a historical review, see Lawrence *et al.*[3]). It was Harvey Cushing[4] who in 1909 first used the term "hyperpituitarism" in relation to acromegaly, and his concept was provided with a firm scientific basis following the demonstration by Evans and Long that gigantism could be produced in rats by injection of a pituitary gland extract.

So gradual may be the development of acromegaly that gross distortion of appearance can occur before the patient seeks medical help. However, variability in the course of the disease is common,[5] and acromegaly of short duration, so called "fugitive acromegaly," occasionally occurs, as first reported by Bailey and Cushing.[6] This entity was used by these authors to describe features suggestive of acromegaly, which had apparently shown no progression, in patients with pituitary tumors. It is probably a form of "burned-out acromegaly" that results from infarction of the tumor ("pituitary apoplexy") or failure of the tissues to show further growth despite continued growth hor-

IVOR M.D. JACKSON • Tufts University School of Medicine; Department of Medicine, Division of Endocrinology, Tufts–New England Medical Center Hospital, Boston, Massachusetts 02111.

mone (GH) hypersecretion. Plateauing of growth has been observed in the rat despite continued treatment with exogenous GH.[5]

Acromegaly is an insidious disorder that most commonly presents between the third and fifth decades with growth of the acral parts. Such patients will often give a history of increase in shoe or glove size, coarsening of facial features, tightening of a ring, or the necessity for frequent changes in their dental prostheses. If a GH-secreting pituitary adenoma develops in the teens, or earlier, before the epiphyses of the long bones have closed, gigantism occurs. Should the GH hypersecretion persist after the epiphyseal plates have fused, so called acromegalic gigantism is present. Pituitary gigantism is exceptionally rare, and the victims of this condition have been local celebrities or circus curiosities or both.[7] Whereas acromegaly is slightly more common in women than in men, gigantism has been reported almost invariably in males only.

It is apparent that in the past decade, a marked alteration in the type of patient with acromegaly presenting for treatment has taken place, consequent on the ready availability of assays for serum GH. An increasing number of patients are being diagnosed in whom only minor acromegalic changes have occurred and in whom appropriate treatment may produce almost complete reversal of the soft-tissue abnormalities.

2. Pathogenesis of Acromegaly

The pathophysiological disturbance in the development of pituitary adenomas is reviewed in Chapter 2. Two major theories have been put forward: (1) One proposes that a primary pituitary somatotropic adenoma secretes GH autonomously (adenohypophyseal hypothesis). (2) The other proposes that a primary defect in the hypothalamus produces a marked increase in the putative growth-hormone-releasing factor (GH-RF) relative to growth-hormone-release-inhibiting hormone (somatostatin); the result is somatotrope proliferation and GH hypersecretion (hypothalamic hypothesis). The concepts are not mutually exclusive, for chronic hyperstimulation of the somatotropes may well lead to neoplasia. For further discussion, see Chapter 2 and Daughaday and Cryer.[8]

3. Pathology of Acromegaly

Although conventionally associated with eosinophil adenomas, the tumors are frequently chromophobe or mixed eosinophil–chromophobe. However, immunohistochemical staining demonstrates a high degree of correlation between GH hypersecretion as determined by immunoreactive GH levels in the circulation and staining of GH in the tumor, regardless of the hematoxylin and eosin (H and E) tinctorial qualities.[9]

4. Clinical Features of Acromegaly

The symptoms and signs of acromegaly reflect the effects of GH on soft-tissue growth and on intermediary metabolism, the associated impaired secretion of other pituitary hormones, and the effects of the pituitary adenoma as an intracranial-space-occupying lesion.

4.1. Acral Changes

The alterations in bones and soft tissues are especially marked in the hands, feet, and face. The thickening of the skin and subcutaneous tissue appears to reflect connective-tissue overgrowth accompanied by an increase in interstitial fluid (evidence supporting this view is derived from the marked reduction in acral size that often occurs within 24 hr of the surgical treatment of the pituitary tumor). In the patients reported by Lawrence *et al.*,[3] acral changes had been present for over 7 years at the time of initial presentation, and coarsening of the facial features was evident in almost all, though nearly 25% had not noted such changes for themselves.

Skin-fold thickness may be helpful diagnostically in the evaluation of acromegaly. Wright and Joplin[10] found that skin-fold measurements from the dorsum of the hand were abnormally thick in 71% of patients with definite acromegaly. The thickness of the heel pad is usually much increased in acromegaly. Radiological measurements have shown that heel-pad thickness greater than 25 mm is characteristic of acromegaly, while a value less than 18 mm is normal, with levels in the 18- to 25-mm range being equivocal.

The hands appear "spadelike," and X-ray examination shows cortical thickening with "tufting" of the terminal phalanges. Although osteophytes at the level of the epiphyses of the long bones are common, the bony changes in the skull are the most striking. The increase in length and thickness of the mandible produces a "lantern jaw" with a marked degree of prognathism. The coarsening of the facial soft tissues is compounded by overgrowth of the frontal, malar, and nasal bones. The sinuses are often much enlarged. Occasionally, there is excessive growth of a jaw, nose, or orbital ridge with sparing of the other bones of the face.[5]

Over 80% of acromegalics complain of hyperhidrosis and an oiliness of the skin that leads to an unpleasant odor. This occurs particularly in the early "active" stage of the disease and is associated with an increase in the basal metabolic rate (BMR).

4.2. Headaches

Headaches are frequently encountered, being present in 50–75% of all patients.[3,11] The headaches are of different varieties and may be located in the fronto-orbital, fronto-temporal, retro-orbital, occipito-cervical, or at the vertex. The pain is usually dull and annoying in type, but occasionally a stabbing pain, reminiscent of trigeminal neuralgia, occurs.

The cause of the headaches is unknown, but has been thought to reflect stretching of the diaphragma sellae or torsion of blood vessels with stimulation of nerve endings. In the patients studied by Pickett *et al.*,[12] five of six patients with suprasellar extension of a pituitary adenoma had headaches, but so did six of nine in whom the tumor was confined to the sella. In this series, headaches did not correlate with size of the pituitary fossa, thickening of the calvarium, or displacement of the vessels on arteriography. A purely frontal or occipital headache was noted in five of the patients with suprasellar extension, and in three of them it was exacerbated by coughing.

Visual-field disturbances usually reflect suprasellar extension of the pituitary adenoma (see Chapter 13). The characteristic deficit is bitemporal hemianopia with an upper quadrantic hemianopia being the earliest sign. However, other visual abnormalities occur, including homonomous and unilateral hemianopias, that may reflect prefixation or postfixation of the optic chiasma, or possibly eccentric expansion of the tumor.

4.3. Neuromuscular Changes

The recognition of an association of acromegaly with lethargy and weakness is as old as the description of acromegaly itself. Marie's original two cases had weakness and wasting of the proximal muscles of the limbs. More recent studies with electromyography have demonstrated the existence of a proximal myopathy in about half of all acromegalic subjects,[13] though serum enzymes and muscle biopsy are usually normal.[12]

Acroparesthesias and numbness are early symptoms of acromegaly, and the most common cause is the carpal-tunnel syndrome. Not infrequently, patients presenting with acromegaly may have had surgical correction of the carpal-tunnel syndrome within the previous year without the acromegaly itself being recognized. Factors contributing to the development of the carpal-tunnel syndrome in acromegaly are multiple and include encroachment by bone and soft tissues on the carpal tunnel, involvement of the median nerve by a "hypertrophic" neuropathy, altered fluid balance in the carpal tunnel, and possible changes in nerve metabolism. However, the rapid improvement and early decrease in hand volume after pituitary surgery suggest that sodium and water retention caused by GH[14] increases the volume of the soft tissues in the carpal tunnel and produces nerve compression.[12] Less commonly, generalized peripheral neuropathy occurs that is characterized by paresthesias in the hands and feet, numbness and absent reflexes in the lower limbs, associated with muscle weakness and atrophy. The peripheral nerves may be palpably thickened ("hypertrophic neuritis") due to perineural and/or endoneural fibrous proliferation.[15] Other causes of neuropathy in acromegaly include nerve entrapment, the possible metabolic effects of GH itself on neural tissue, and complications such as diabetes mellitus and hypothyroidism.

In the series of patients reported by Pickett *et al.*,[12] the presence of myopathy or the carpal-tunnel syndrome could not be correlated with the magnitude of GH elevation of any secondary endocrine derangement, but myopathy was associated with a longer duration of the acromegaly. Although the carpal-tunnel syndrome shows early improvement after hypophysectomy, myopathy reverses much more slowly and may indeed persist.

4.4. Skeletal and Bony Changes

Bony overgrowth leads to abnormal joint mechanisms and gives rise to arthralgias. However, some of the articular symptoms are probably due to thickening of the joint capsule and ligaments. In the initial phases of the disease, articular cartilage proliferates, but later erodes with the production of a severe arthritis that cannot be readily distinguished from osteoarthritis.[16]

Although it has been postulated that acromegaly is associated with osteoporosis, several recent roentgenographic and densitometric studies have failed to disclose evidence of osteoporosis (for a review, see Aloia *et al.*[17]). There is some evidence, however, that differential bone remodeling with an increase in cortical bone accompanied by a reduced trabecular bone mass occurs in untreated acromegaly. When reduction of the GH level is achieved with treatment, cortical apposition may decrease. Since the increased cortical bone mass may aid the prevention of vertebral fractures, lowering the GH level as well as hypogonadism consequent on pituitary ablative procedures may impose on the treated acromegalic patient an increased susceptibility to fractures.[17]

4.5. Other Organs

Generalized enlargement of various organs of the body occurs. Cardiomegaly is common and is associated with hypertension, atherosclerosis, and frequently the development of congestive cardiac failure in the fifth and sixth decades. It is felt by many that there is a true cardiomyopathy in acromegaly, but this view remains controversial.

Hepatomegaly often occurs, and kidney hypertrophy may result in a substantial increase in the creatinine clearance above normal. Enlarged salivary glands can usually be appreciated on physical examination. Penile enlargement also occurs.

5. Effects of Acromegaly on Other Endocrine Functions

The pituitary tumor may compress normal pituitary tissue and thus give rise to anterior pituitary failure with hypothyroidism, hypocortisolism, and hypogonadism, though such panhypopituitarism tends to occur only late in the disease.[18] Galactorrhea is common in females and may reflect either concomitant hyperprolactinemia or the height of the GH level, since GH itself is lactogenic in bioassays for prolactin. There is one report of a patient with acromegaly and galactorrhea–amenorrhea with two pituitary adenomas, one of which secreted GH and the other prolactin.[19]

Although the frequent presence of a goiter and excess sweating suggests the possibility of thyrotoxicosis accompanying acromegaly, in most instances direct measurement of thyroid hormones (T_4 and T_3) and thyroid-stimulating hormone (TSH) by radioimmunoassay have given levels within the normal range, so that many workers have concluded that the hypermetabolism of acromegaly is an effect of GH excess. Nevertheless, there have been a small number of reports linking acromegaly with pituitary-TSH-induced thyrotoxicosis (for a review, see Cooper *et al.*[20]). Thyroid nodularity with "hot" and "cold" areas on scanning is often present, and thyrotoxicosis due to a hyperfunctioning nodule (Plummer's disease) could occur on this basis.

Adrenocortical function is usually normal, though the reserve may be diminished. Early in the disease, metyrapone testing frequently leads to an exuberant response of the urine 17-ketosteroids that may reflect hyperplasia of the adrenal cortex. Likewise, adrenal hyperplasia with secretion of a mineralocorticoid, not yet characterized, has been suggested as a possible etiological factor in the genesis of the hypertension associated with this disorder. Gonadotropic secretion is reduced in many subjects and frequently leads to impotence in males and menstrual irregularities in females. The frequently associated hyperprolactinemia in acromegaly may play a role in the gonadal insufficiency.

Unless there is an associated parathyroid adenoma (see Section 8), parathyroid function is not increased and the serum calcium is normal. The serum inorganic phosphate is often increased due to the effect of GH on renal tubular secretion. Hypercalciuria is, however, frequently present.

Diabetes mellitus may be present in 25% of all acromegalics with as many as 50% having impaired glucose tolerance. There is now much evidence that the insulin resistance of acromegaly is due to abnormalities in the insulin receptor that may be caused by the increased circulating levels of GH.[21] This leads secondarily to hyperinsulinism. It is possible that some acromegalics with frank diabetes mellitus are those who are genetically predisposed to the diabetes for which there may be an increased prevalence in acromegaly. Diabetic retinopathy is not infrequently observed, but Kimmelstiel–Wilson kidney disease is rare. Following pituitary surgery, glucose tolerance usually improves due to the fall in the GH levels. Occasionally, however, severe hyperglycemia occurs in the immediate postoperative period, necessitating insulin administration, a requirement that may persist.[22]

6. Diagnosis of Acromegaly

The laboratory tests utilized in the diagnosis and evaluation of acromegaly are outlined in Chapter 11. In brief, the serum GH level in acromegaly is characterized by: (1) lack of suppression and sometimes a paradoxical rise following glucose administration; (2) marked instability during the day, in some cases with a rise associated with lack of sleep; (3) variable responses to insulin hypoglycemia, arginine infusion, mixed meals, and exercise, with occasionally a paradoxical decrease following these stimuli; (4) a rise in GH in about 50% of cases following intravenous thyrotropin-releasing hormone (TRH) and luteinizing-hormone-releasing hormone (LH-RH) injection; and (5) a paradoxical reduction following administration of dopaminergic drugs,

L-dopa, apomorphine, and bromocriptine (see also Faglia *et al.*[23]). There is a high correlation between the GH response to TRH administration and its suppression with dopaminergic agents.

Radiological tests utilized in the diagnosis of the pituitary adenoma are outlined in Chapter 14.

7. Treatment of Acromegaly

Therapy in acromegaly is directed toward removal of the pituitary tumor and reduction of the GH levels—ideally with preservation of other modalities of pituitary function. The adenoma may be treated by surgery (Chapters 16 and 18); heavy-particle irradiation, e.g., proton-beam (Chapter 22); or cobalt-beam radiotherapy (conventional X-irradiation) (Chapter 21). Various pharmacological agents have been used to treat acromegaly, but with the possible exception of bromocriptine, there is no definite effect on tumor growth. (See Chapter 15 for further details on the role of drugs in the treatment of acromegaly.)

Therapy for deficits of other anterior pituitary hormones, diabetes mellitus, and cardiovascular complications such as hypertension may be required.

8. Associated Tumors

Pituitary adenomas in acromegaly may be part of the multiple endocrine adenomatosis syndrome (MEA Type I), and as such may be accompanied by adenomas of the parathyroid, islets of Langerhans, and adrenal cortex. Although it has been suggested that the incidence of cancer might be increased in acromegaly, evidence in support of this view is equivocal.[24] There have, however, been seven reports of acromegaly coexisting with an intracranial meningioma.[25]

9. Causes of Acromegaly Other Than a Pituitary Adenoma

Carcinoid tumors of the lung are occasionally associated with acromegaly as part of the pluriglandular syndrome (MEA Type I). There have also been a number of reports describing cure of acromegaly following removal of the lung tumor.[26] In some instances, it appears that the carcinoid contained large quantities of immunoreactive GH, and in others, GH-RF activity has been identified.[27] Cure of acromegaly by operative removal of an islet-cell tumor of the pancreas has also been described.[28] Substantial amounts of immunoreactive-hGH-like activity were detected in the tumor tissue extract.

10. Differential Diagnosis

Cerebral gigantism (Sotos' syndrome) may be confused clinically with gigantism due to a pituitary adenoma secreting GH. The former condition is characterized by excessive growth in early childhood, acromegalic features, and advanced osseous maturation.[29] GH-secretory dynamics are usually normal, and no evidence of a pituitary tumor is present. The pathogenesis of the disorder is unknown.[30]

Pachydermoperiostosis (Touraine-Solenti-Golé syndrome), or idiopathic hypertrophic osteoarthropathy, is a familial condition characterized by thickening of the skin, finger-clubbing, and coarsening of the acral features. GH levels are normal in this syndrome.

11. Prognosis in Acromegaly

Patients with pituitary adenomas secreting GH may be particularly susceptible to pituitary apoplexy, giving rise to an "empty sella" syndrome that in some[31] but not all[32] instances may result in complete remission of the acromegaly. Antecedent estrogen therapy that may stimulate the growth of tumor tissue may be a causal factor in some cases.

Apart from the morbidity in acromegaly, there is an increased mortality.[24] In acromegalic patients in the fifth and sixth decades, there is an increased number of deaths due to cardiovascular and respiratory disease in male patients, and to cerebrovascular and respiratory disease in female patients. Total deaths due to malignant neoplasms were no more than expected, but an excess of these occurred in female patients aged 65–74 years. Increased mortality was associated with hypertension and clinical diabetes, but not with chemical diabetes. Optic chiasmal compression and sex of the patient did not correlate statistically with increased mortality. There is some evidence of a reduced mortality rate in those acromegalics who had received treatment directed at their pituitary tumors.

12. Summary

Gigantism and acromegaly are uncommon disorders that result from excess GH secretion, usually from a pituitary adenoma. The underlying disorder of hypothalamic–pituitary function is not known with certainty, but the condition gives rise to considerable morbidity as a result of the facial disfiguration, acral growth, headaches, neuromuscular and visual disturbances, arthritis, hypermetabolism, diabetes mellitus, and hypogonadism consequent on GH hypersecretion and/or effects of the pituitary tumor itself. There is an increased mortality due to cardiovascular complications (hypertension, atherosclerosis) and diabetes mellitus, so that early treatment is an important goal. The ready availability of radioimmunoassays for GH permits this condition to be diagnosed at an early stage, and newer surgical, radiotherapeutic, and pharmacological approaches allow the acromegaly to be more readily cured or controlled with preservation of, or less damage to, normal anterior pituitary functions.

References

1. N.P. Christy, Acromegaly, in: *Cecil–Loeb Textbook of Medicine* (P.B. Beeson and W. McDermott, eds.), Vol. 2, 12th ed., p. 1277, W.B. Saunders, Philadelphia, 1967.
2. P. Marie, Sur deux cas d'acromégalie; hypertrophie singulière, non congénitale, des extrémités superieures, inférieurs et céphalique, *Rev. Med. (Paris)* **6**:297, 1886.
3. J.H. Lawrence, C.A. Tobias, J.A. Linfoot, J.L. Born, J.T. Lyman, C.Y. Chong, E. Manougi an, and W.C. Wei, Successful treatment of acromegaly: Metabolic and clinical studies in 145 patients, *J. Clin. Endocrinol. Metab.* **31**:180, 1970.
4. H. Cushing, Partial hypophysectomy for acromegaly with remarks on the function of the hypophysis, *Ann. Surg.* **50**:1002, 1909.
5. W.H. Daughaday, The adenohypophysis, in: *Textbook of Endocrinology*, 5th ed. (R.H. Williams, ed.), pp. 31–77, W.B. Saunders, Philadelphia, 1974.
6. P. Bailey and H. Cushing, Studies in acromegaly. VIII. The microscopical structure of the adenomas in acromegalic dyspituitarism (fugitive acromegaly), *Am. J. Pathol.* **4**:545, 1928.
7. F. Drimmer, There were giants in the earth, in: *Very Special People*, pp. 269–322, Amjon Publishers, New York, 1973.
8. W.H. Daughaday and P.E. Cryer, Growth hormone hypersection and acromegaly, *Hosp. Pract.* **13**:75, 1978.
9. E.A. Zimmerman, R. Defendini, and A.G. Frantz, Prolactin and growth hormone in patients with pituitary adenomas: A correlative study of hormone in tumor and plasma by immunoperoxidase technique and radioimmunoassay, *J. Clin. Endocrinol. Metab.* **38**:577, 1974.
10. A.D. Wright and G.F. Joplin, Skin-fold thickness in normal subjects and in patients with acromegaly and Cushing's syndrome, *Acta Endocrinol.* **60**:705, 1969.
11. P.C. Eskildsen, P.A. Svendsen, L. Vang, and J. Nerup, Long term treatment of acromegaly with bromocriptine, *Acta Endocrinol.* **87**:687, 1978.
12. J.B.E. Pickett, R.B. Layzer, S.R. Levin, *et al.*, Neuromuscular complications of acromegaly, *Neurology* **25**:638, 1975.
13. F.L. Mastaglia, D.D. Barwick, and R. Hall, Myopathy in acromegaly, *Lancet* **2**:907, 1970.
14. E.G. Biglieri, C.D. Waltington, and P.H. Forsham, Sodium retention with human growth hormone and its subfractions, *J. Clin. Endocrinol. Metab.* **21**:361, 1961.
15. P.A. Low, J.G. McCleod, J.R. Turtle, *et al.*, Peripheral neuropathy in acromegaly, *Brain* **97**:139, 1974.
16. J.H. Kellgren, J. Ball, and G.K. Tutton, The articular and other limb changes in acromegaly: Clinical and pathological study of 25 cases, *Q. J. Med.* **21**:405, 1952.
17. J.F. Aloia, Z. Petrak, K. Ellis, and S.H. Cohn, Body composition and skeletal metabolism following pituitary irradiation in acromegaly, *Am. J. Med.* **61**:59, 1976.
18. A.L. Plummer, R.V. Randall, and B.L. Riggs, Active acromegaly with anterior pituitary failure, *Metabolism* **18**:469, 1969.
19. G. Tolis, G. Bertrand, S. Carpenter, and J.M. McKenzie, Acromegaly and galactorrhea–amenorrhea with two pituitary adenomas secreting growth hormone or prolactin, a case report, *Ann. Int. Med.* **89**:345, 1978.
20. D.S. Cooper, E.C. Ridgway, and F. Maloof, Unusual types of hyperthyroidism, *Clin. Endocrinol. Metab.* **7**:199, 1978.
21. M. Muggeo, R.S. Bar, Roth, J., *et al.*, Two abnormalities in insulin binding to its receptor in the insulin resistance of acromegaly, *Clin. Res.* **26**:310a, 1978.
22. E.M. Bunick, H. Schnidek, R.L. Lavine, *et al.*, Insulin-dependent diabetes mellitus: Sudden onset following hypophysectomy in an acromegalic patient, *J. Am. Med. Assoc.* **238**:1047, 1977.
23. G. Faglia, A. Paracchi, C. Ferrari, and P. Beck-Peccoz, Evaluation of the results of transsphenoidal surgery in acromegaly by assessment of the growth hormone response to thyrotrophin-releasing hormone, *Clin. Endocrinol.* **8**:373, 1978.
24. A.D. Wright, D.M. Hill, C. Lowy, and T.R. Fraser, Mortality in acromegaly, *Q. J. Med.* **39**:1, 1970.
25. E.M. Bunick, L.C. Mills, and L.I. Rose, Association of acromegaly and meningiomas, *J. Am. Med. Assoc.* **240**:1267, 1978.

26. P.H. Sonksen, A.B. Ayren, M. Brainbridge, *et al.*, Acromegaly caused by pulmonary carcinoid tumours, *Clin. Endocrinol.* **5**:503, 1976.
27. L.A. Frohman, M. Szabo, M.E. Stachura, S. Zafar, R.C. Mellinger, and G. Fine, Growth hormone–releasing activity in an extract of a bronchial carcinoid associated with acromegaly, *Clin. Res.* **26**:702A, 1978.
28. R.H. Caplan, L. Koob, R.M. Abellera, *et al.*, Cure of acromegaly by operative removal of an islet cell tumor of the pancreas, *Am. J. Med.* **64**:874, 1978.
29. J.F. Sotos, P.R. Dodge, D. Muirhead, *et al.*, Cerebral gigantism in childhood: A syndrome of excessively rapid growth with acromegalic features and a non-progressive neurologic disorder, *N. Engl. J. Med.* **271**:109, 1964.
30. J.F. Sotos, E.A. Cutler, and P. Dodge, Cerebral gigantism, *Am. J. Dis. Child.* **131**:625, 1977.
31. I. Login and R.J. Santen, Empty sella syndrome: Sequela of the spontaneous remission of acromegaly, *Arch. Intern. Med.* **135**:1519, 1975.
32. M.E. Molitch, G.B. Hieshima, S. Marcovitz, I.M.D. Jackson, and S. Wolpert, Co-existing primary empty sella syndrome and acromegaly, *Clin. Endocrinol.* **7**:261, 1977.

7

ACTH-Secreting Adenomas

MARK E. MOLITCH

1. Introduction

Cushing's *syndrome* refers to the clinical and biochemical manifestations due to hypercortisolism of any cause. Hypercortisolism may be due to (1) pharmacological administration of glucocorticoids or adrenocorticotropic hormone (ACTH); (2) excessive, autonomous secretion by an adrenal adenoma or carcinoma; (3) excessive adrenal secretion secondary to increased pituitary secretion of ACTH; or (4) excessive adrenal secretion secondary to the ectopic secretion of ACTH or possibly corticotropin-releasing factor (CRF) by a neoplasm. Cushing's *disease* specifically refers to the entity of excess ACTH secretion by the pituitary with resultant bilateral adrenal hyperplasia and hypercortisolism. Because therapeutic modalities for these entities are different, careful endocrinological and radiological evaluations are needed to differentiate between them.

The recent discoveries of the opiate receptor and the endogenous opiate-like peptides have provided exciting new information regarding the neuroendocrine regulation of ACTH secretion and have provided new diagnostic measures that will be helpful in the diagnosis of Cushing's disease. Furthermore, research into the bioaminergic regulation of ACTH secretion has not only provided new insights into the pathogenesis of Cushing's disease, but has also resulted in pharmacological agents that are clinically valuable in the treatment of many patients.

2. Regulation of ACTH Secretion

ACTH secretion is controlled by the hypothalamus, mediated by CRF interacting with negative feedback by glucocorticoids (Fig. 1). Although CRF

MARK E. MOLITCH • Tufts University School of Medicine; Department of Medicine, Division of Endocrinology, Tufts–New England Medical Center Hospital, Boston, Massachusetts 02111.

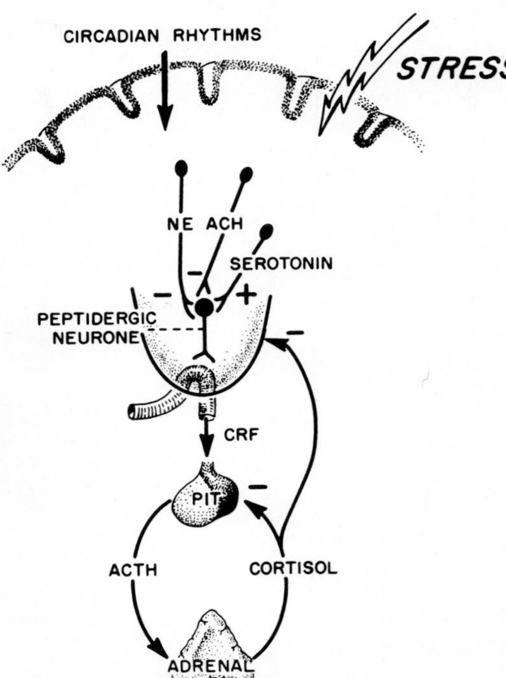

Fig. 1. Diagram of the regulation of ACTH secretion. For details, see the text. (NE) Norepinephrine; (ACH) acetylcholine; (CRF) corticotropin-releasing factor; (PIT) pituitary; (ACTH) adrenocorticotropic hormone. From Martin *et al.*,[2] p. 180, with permission.

was the first releasing factor identified in hypothalamic extracts, its structure remains to be elucidated. The highest concentrations of CRF are found in the median eminence and the arcuate, dorso-medial, ventro-medial, and periventricular nuclei,[1] and this corresponds to physiological data in animals showing the medial basal hypothalamus to be important in the excitatory control of ACTH release.[2]

The glucocorticoids, released by ACTH stimulation, exert negative feedback at both the hypothalamic and pituitary levels (the long feedback loop).[2] Additionally, ACTH may exert negative feedback at the hypothalamic level on its own secretion in what has been termed "short-loop" feedback.[3] In this short-loop feedback, the ACTH probably reaches the hypothalamus via retrograde flow in the portal vessels,[4–6] but perhaps via the systemic circulation. Recently, ACTH has been found to be widely distributed in the brain, but it is uncertain whether this is due to (1) retrograde flow up the portal vessels from the pituitary, (2) leakage into the cisternae, or (3) *de novo in situ* synthesis.[7,8] Immunocytochemical studies have shown that both ACTH and lipotropin (LPH) are similarly distributed both in cell bodies and in a beaded fashion along axons, suggesting that these substances may even have a neurotransmitter or neuromodulator function,[9] perhaps as part of the widespread peptidergic neurotransmitter system.

The interaction of the short-loop and long-loop feedback systems and CRF determines the physiological "set point" controlling cortisol levels in blood. ACTH and cortisol are both secreted episodically, cortisol secretion occurring 5–10 min following an ACTH rise.[10] ACTH and cortisol secretion follow a diurnal pattern, the highest levels of ACTH and cortisol occurring between 6 and 7 A.M. in most individuals and the lowest occurring in the late evening.[10] In virtually all forms of Cushing's syndrome, depression, and various brain disorders (hypothalamic diseases, syphilis, Wernicke's encephalopathy, and lesions associated with impaired consciousness), diurnal variation is lost.[2] As is discussed in Chapter 11, this loss of diurnal variation may be useful in establishing a diagnosis of Cushing's syndrome.

The bioaminergic regulation of CRF and ACTH secretion is poorly understood. Serotonin has been shown to be both stimulatory[11] and inhibitory[12] to ACTH secretion. However, cyproheptadine, a drug with antiserotonin and anti-histamine properties, has been shown to reduce ACTH and cortisol levels in some patients with Cushing's disease[13] (see Chapter 15). There appear to be both excitatory and inhibitory catecholamine pathways, and alpha-adrenergic stimulation promotes ACTH release while beta stimulation inhibits ACTH release.[2] Cholinergic pathways appear to be stimulatory also.[2] In addition to bioamines, prostaglandins may also be important in the hypothalamic regulation of CRF release.[14]

3. Relationship of ACTH to β-Lipotropin and the Endorphins

In the past few years, peptides that appear to be the endogenous substances that interact with the opiate receptors in the brain have been identified and characterized (for reviews, see Guillemin[15] and Uhl *et al.*[16] Purification and sequencing of these substances have revealed them to be fragments of the hormone β-lipotropin (β-LPH); for example, the opioid peptide met-enkephalin has the sequence 61–65 of β-LPH and β-endorphin has the sequence 61–91. Of great interest is the finding that melanocyte-stimulating hormone (β-MSH), long held to be responsible for the abnormal pigmentation in Cushing's disease, is also a fragment of β-LPH and is essentially an artifact of extraction procedures.[17]

Radioimmunoassays of ACTH, β-LPH, and β-endorphin have shown serum levels of these substances to parallel each other in a wide variety of circumstances, including Addison's disease, Cushing's disease, insulin-induced hypoglycemic stimulation, and steroid suppression.[18,19] Furthermore, immunohistochemical studies have shown β-LPH and ACTH to be present in the same secretory granules of the same cells of the pituitary.[20] Most recently, evidence has been obtained showing that in the corticotroph cells of the pituitary, the initial molecule that is synthesized is a 31,000-dalton protein (known as 31K or proopiocortin) that is the common precursor for both β-LPH and ACTH,[21–23] as shown in Fig. 2. Finally, the finding of calcitonin in similar cells of the pituitary by immunohistochemical techniques suggests that it may be homologous with a portion of the 31K precursor.[24]

The concomitant secretion of the endogenous opiate ligands and ACTH raises important questions as to the function of these substances. It has been proposed that just as the ACTH secretion in times of stress readies the body to handle that stress, so will the release of the various fragments of β-LPH ready

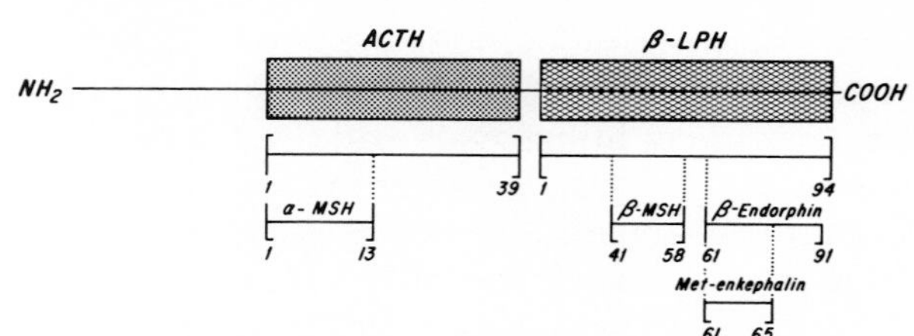

Fig. 2. Hypothetical structure of "proopiocortin" or "31K," the putative precursor to LPH and ACTH. (ACTH) Adrenocorticotropic hormone; (β-LPH) β-lipotropic hormone; (NH_2) amino-terminal end; (COOH) carboxy-terminal end; (MSH) melanocyte-stimulating hormone. Modified from Roberts and Herbert.[22]

the mind to handle that stress via either neurotropic or psychotropic pathways.[19] As will be discussed later, it is possible that the increased secretion of β-LPH and its fragments in patients with Cushing's disease may be responsible for some of the psychopathology seen in that disorder. Measurements of β-LPH and some of its fragments may also be helpful diagnostically in differentiating among the different varieties of Cushing's syndrome.

4. Clinical Features of Cushing's Syndrome

Most of the clinical features of Cushing's syndrome are due to excessive secretion of glucocorticoids, but there are variations due to differing patterns of hormone secretion and to the underlying cause. Excluding iatrogenic steroid and ACTH administration, Cushing's syndrome is quite uncommon, only three to five cases presenting to large centers per year. Of those manifesting the classic findings of Cushing's syndrome, about 10% will have adrenal adenomas, 10% will have adrenal carcinoma, and the rest will have pituitary-dependent ACTH hypersecretion.[25]

Truncal obesity with increased dorsal, ventral, supraclavicular, and mediastinal fat deposition accompanied by thin arms and legs is one of the most common symptoms (Fig. 3). The skin is usually thinned and fragile with the subcutaneours vasculature showing through stretched areas, resulting in purplish striae. Bruising is due to both skin and blood-vessel fragility. Infections and poor wound healing occur in 40% of cases. Facial plethora is common and is due to steroid-induced erythema as well as to the thinning of the skin. Oligo-/amenorrhea or impotence occur in 70–80% of patients. A proximal myopathy occurs in 80%, and low back pain from osteoporosis occurs in about 50%. Hirsutism and acne occur in 50–75% due to excess androgen secretion.[25–27] Although hypertension occurs in about 85%, the mechanism is still unclear; in the majority of patients studied, plasma renin activity and concentration have been elevated, plasma renin substrate has been normal or increased, and the hypertension has decreased in response to the infusion of saralasin, a competitive antagonist of angiotensin II,[28,29] indicating that the hypertension is mediated through the renin–angiotensin system and is not due to excessive mineralocorticoid activity. Finally, about 90% of patients have glucose intolerance, but only 20–25% develop significant fasting hyperglycemia, polyuria, and polydipsia.[27]

Mental symptoms occur frequently in all forms of Cushing's syndrome. The clinical picture ranges from mild anxiety to severe depression, with acute, psychiatric confusional states occurring occasionally.[30] Although depression tends to be the dominant psychopathology with endogenous Cushing's syndrome, euphoria is the most common finding in patients made Cushingoid with exogenous steroids.[31] It is of great importance to distinguish between the depression of Cushing's syndrome and the elevated cortisol levels seen in many psychiatrically depressed patients (see Section 5). The hypercortisolism of depression does not appear to be sufficient to cause the metabolic and tissue effects usually associated with Cushing's syndrome, however.

In children, many of these clinical features of Cushing's syndrome may be absent; however, the one finding that is almost always present is growth retardation,[32,33] although obesity is also often present.[34,35] Although it is rare for a patient with Cushing's syndrome to become pregnant, neonatal adrenal insufficiency due to excessive steroid crossing the placenta has been reported[36]; careful monitoring of such newborns is therefore mandatory.

Special features of the various types of Cushing's syndrome deserve emphasis. Adrenal carcinomas are usually so inefficient in producing steroids that by the time Cushingoid features become manifest, the tumor is usually quite large and often palpable. These tumors often behave as though the 11-hydroxylation step is blocked, leading to relatively high 11-deoxycortisol (Compound "S") levels compared to cortisol levels. Urinary 17-ketosteroids are often elevated out of proportion to the 17-hydroxycorticosteroids, resulting in a greater incidence of hirsutism and virilization in women compared to

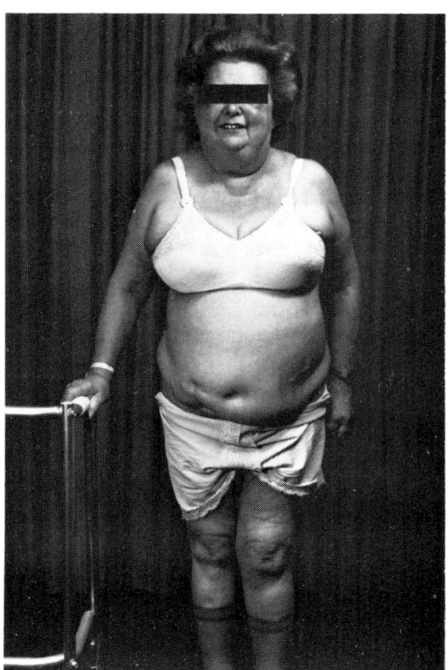

Fig. 3. A 62-year-old patient with Cushing's disease. Note the centripetal fat distribution, facial plethora, and rounded facies.

TABLE 1. Tumors Associated with the Ectopic ACTH Syndrome[a]

Type	Percentage
Carcinoma of lung	50
Thymomas	10
Pancreatic carcinoma	10
Bronchial adenomas and carcinoid	5
Neural crest (e.g., pheochromocytoma)	5
Medullary carcinoma of thyroid	5
Miscellaneous (e.g., ovary, colon, prostate, breast, liver, thyroid, kidney, stomach)	15

[a] Data from Liddle *et al.*,[39] Odell and Wolfsen,[40] and Rosenberg *et al.*[41]

other types of Cushing's syndrome.[27,37] Feminization also occasionally occurs in men with adrenal carcinoma.[38]

The clinical presentation of patients with ectopic ACTH syndrome is usually different than the presentations of the other types of Cushing's syndrome. In these patients, ACTH and cortisol levels are very high, and pigmentation, hypokalemia, hypertension, glucose intolerance, and marked weakness are the most striking findings. The usual changes in skin, bones, and fat tissue that are due to long-standing hypercortisolism are usually not found in the ectopic ACTH syndrome, since the course is often too short for these findings to develop owing to the underlying malignancy.[39,40] However, in cases in which the neoplasm is very slow-growing, e.g., bronchial adenomas, all the features of Cushing's syndrome may be present. The most common types of tumors associated with the ectopic ACTH syndrome are given in Table 1. A particularly interesting example of full-blown Cushing's syndrome occurring due to a neoplasm is the ectopic production of ACTH in association with calcitonin secretion in some cases of medullary carcinoma of the thyroid.[41] Because of the recent finding that calcitonin may be present along with the 31K prohormone for ACTH and LPH in pituitary,[24] it is not surprising that these two hormones should be found together in cases of medullary carcinoma of the thyroid. To date, no one has reported calcitonin measurements in patients with Cushing's disease.

Although most carcinomas appear to secrete ACTH,[42–44] the ectopic ACTH syndrome does not occur in all these patients. Most of this ACTH is present in a higher-molecular-weight precursor form (20,000 daltons) referred to as "big" ACTH, or "pro" ACTH, from which ACTH can be liberated by tryptic digestion. The "expression of the clinically apparent ectopic ACTH syndrome appears to be related to enzymatic ability of the tumor to convert pro ACTH to bioactive ACTH."[40] Since LPH appears to be made by the same tumors at the same time as big ACTH,[44] it is tempting to speculate that the original substance made by all these tumors is the same 31K or "proopiocortin" made by the pituitary.

Although some patients with the ectopic ACTH syndrome have been found to have material present in extracts of the tumors that appears to have corticotropin-releasing properties,[45–46] such estimates were based on bioassays. Confirmation of this work will depend on the final structural identification of CRF and the demonstration of idential material in tumor extracts.

5. Laboratory Diagnosis of Cushing's Disease

As discussed in Chapter 11, the first step in the diagnosis of a patient with Cushing's disease is to establish the presence of Cushing's syndrome (hypercortisolism) itself. Although elevated basal urinary 17-hydroxycorticosteroids and plasma cortisol levels and loss of diurnal variation in steroid levels usually accompany Cushing's syndrome, these findings are neither uniform nor specific,[47] and it is necessary to establish that there is some degree of adrenal nonsuppressibility by exogenous steroids. The overnight dexamethasone suppression test (1 mg at midnight) is the simplest screening test, and patients with Cushing's syndrome do not have cortisol values the next morning below 6 μg/dl as normals should.[47–49] An elevated 24-hr urinary free cortisol measurement has similar diagnostic sensitivity.[47] Therefore, a normal overnight dexamethasone test (8 A.M. cortisol less than 6 μg/dl) or a normal 24-hr urinary free cortisol effectively excludes Cushing syndrome, and no other tests need be performed. Exceptions are exceedingly rare. Abnormal results necessitate further evaluation.

Once nonsuppressibility by the overnight dexamethasone suppression test or an elevated 24-hr urinary free cortisol is found, then a full 2-day low-dose dexamethasone suppression test (0.5 mg every 6 hr for 48 hr) should be carried out as outlined in Chapter 11 to confirm the diagnosis of Cushing's syndrome. In the low-dose test, a 24-hr excretion of 17-hydroxycorticosteroids in excess of 2–5 mg is indicative of Cushing's syndrome.[50,51] A number of tests may then be performed to differentiate among the different types of Cushing's syndrome. High-dose dexamethasone suppression (2 mg every 6 hr for 48 hr) results in suppression of plasma or urinary glucocorticoids by 50% or more in patients with Cushing's disease, but not in patients with the other varieties of Cushing's syndrome.[25,50,51] Rarely, higher doses of dexamethasone are needed to suppress glucocorticoid production in Cushing's disease. In addition to suppression testing, stimulation of the hypothalamic–pituitary–adrenal axis by metyrapone (see Chapter 11) is also helpful. In Cushing's disease, there is an exaggerated rise after 750 mg metyrapone every 4 hr for 6 doses to a level over 36 mg/day of urinary 17-hydroxycorticosteroids that is not seen in the other varieties of Cushing's syndrome.[25]

In recent years, the radioimmunoassay for ACTH has become more widespread and is now readily available from commercial laboratories. ACTH levels are easily detectable and are usually elevated in Cushing's disease and in the ectopic ACTH syndrome, but they are suppressed in adrenal adenomas and carcinomas.[25] ACTH levels should also be drawn along with the plasma and urinary steroids during dexamethasone testing and metyrapone testing; in Cushing's disease, ACTH and cortisol levels will usually decrease with high-dose dexamethasone and may rise with metyrapone, but in the ectopic ACTH syndrome, there will be no alteration in either ACTH or steroid levels.

Recently, serum β-LPH measurements have been used together with ACTH measurements in evaluating patients with Cushing's disease[52]; although varying ratios of LPH to ACTH have been suggested to be helpful in differentiating pituitary adenomas from pituitary hyperplasia[53] and pituitary from ectopic ACTH production,[54] it is too early to reach firm conclusions in this regard.

Although it was initially proposed that stimulation tests with exogenous ACTH would help to differentiate among the various types of Cushing's syndrome, it has been found that this test is quite nonspecific, adrenal adenomas and even carcinomas occasionally responding to ACTH.[25] Furthermore, ACTH administration to patients with Cushing's disease has been associated with adrenal hemorrhage.[55–56] For these reasons, ACTH stimulation tests should be performed with caution.

Although the tests as outlined above are reasonably straightforward, certain situations arise that require special care for proper interpretation of test results. One potential source of confusion in interpreting overnight dexamethasone suppression tests is the presence of elevated cortisol levels due to an increase in cortisol binding globulin, an effect of concurrent estrogen administration. This effect is dose-dependent, small doses of estrogens (0.625 and 1.25 mg of conjugated estrogens) having no effect,[57] but larger doses of estrogens causing higher cortisol levels.[48] Dexamethasone suppression testing in individuals taking phenytoin (Dilantin®) may be inaccurate,[58–59] because the dexamethasone is metabolized more quickly due to phenytoin-induced hepatic enzymes.

In obese patients, urinary 17-hydroxycorticosteroid excretion may be elevated, but the value can be corrected by expressing the results in relation to creatinine exretion as milligrams per gram creatinine, normal values being 2.0–6.5 mg/g creatinine.[60] Urinary free cortisol measurements are normal in obesity, however.[47,60] The plasma cortisol level after an overnight dexamethasone test may also be elevated in obesity,[47] but full 48-hr low- and high-dose dexamethasone suppression tests suppress 17-hydroxycorticosteroid excretion to less than 4 mg/24 hr, as in normals. Urinary free cortisol responses are also suppressed to normal.[47]

Severe, unipolar, endogenous depression is associated with a marked disruption of the normal hypothamic–pituitary axis, giving rise to a biochemical profile that may be quite similar to that of Cushing's disease. Depressed patients may show high absolute blood levels of cortisol with a lack of diurnal variation,[61] high urinary 17-hydroxycorticosteroids and free cortisol,[62] high ACTH levels, and resistance to dexamethasone suppression.[25] The most difficult problem arises in the differential diagnosis between severe depression due to Cushing's disease vs. hypercortisolism secondary to depression. Besser and Edwards[25] regard the cortisol response to hypoglycemia as being helpful in distinguishing between these two entities, rising normally in depressed patients but not in patients with Cushing's disease. However, we and others[63] have found that some patients with Cushing's disease do respond to hypoglycemia with a rise in ACTH and cortisol, so that we feel that this test is not particularly helpful in this regard. In some patients, a decisive conclusion regarding which disease is primary may occur only following successful ther-

TABLE 2. Dexamethasone Suppression Test in a Patient with Cushing's Disease and Severe Depression

Dexamethasone dose (mg)	Plasma cortisol (μg/dl)	Urinary free cortisol (μg/24 hr)
2	33.8	435
8	30.2	148
16	8.8	62
32	5.3	46

apy of the primary disease process. In one patient that we have seen with severe depression requiring electroconculsive therapy, and only mild clinical changes suggestive of Cushing's disease, cure of the hypercortisolism of his Cushing's disease by bilateral adrenalectomy resulted in a complete resolution of his depression within 48 hr.

Another common condition in which a diagnosis of Cushing's syndrome may be made erroneously is alcoholism. Several patients have now been described who were alcoholics and who had Cushingoid appearances, high plasma and urinary corticosteroid levels with a lack of diurnal variation, and resistance to suppression with the overnight dexamethasone suppression test. After several days in the hospital off alcohol, all these values returned to normal.[64] The mechanisms for these findings are unknown.

Occasionally, patients who have Cushing's syndrome do not respond in the appropriate fashion to the various stimulation and suppression tests. Some patients with Cushing's disease do not show suppression of glucocorticoid secretion when given 8 mg dexamethasone/day, but will with even higher doses; an example of this phenomenon is illustrated in Table 2, which shows good suppression only at 16 mg/day in the patient with Cushing's disease and severe depression described above. On the other hand, an adrenocortical carcinoma responsive to ACTH stimulation and dexamethasone suppression has been described.[65] Some ectopic ACTH-secretory tumors, especially bronchial adenomas, may be partially suppressible by dexamethasone and stimulatable by metyrapone.[66] Some cases of Cushing's disesae are characterized by only periodic hypersecretion at regular intervals separated by periods of normal ACTH secretion.[67] In such patients, suppression and stimulation testing will vary markedly depending on whether the patient was in a hypersecreting or a normal-secreting phase. These fluctuating levels probably account for the so-called "paradoxical" increase in cortisol secretion after dexamethasone.

6. Pathogenesis of Cushing's Disease

There has been considerable controversy in recent years as to whether Cushing's disease begins as hypothalamic derangement in which there is an oversecretion of CRF leading to an excess secretion of ACTH by the pituitary or whether it is a primary pituitary disease due to an adenoma. Because CRF has not been identified and cannot be assayed accurately, the evidence on each side of this controversy remains indirect.

Evidence that the primary site of dysfunction is in the hypothalamus comes largely from the work of Krieger and colleagues. Studies of patients with Cushing's disease that was active or in remission (after irradiation) showed absent growth hormone (GH) responses to hypoglycemia, pyrogen, and sleep, reflecting abnormal hypothalamic function.[68] Similarly, the nocturnal rise in prolactin has not been found in patients with Cushing's disease, implying hypothalamic dysfunction.[69] Additionally, Krieger and colleagues have demonstrated complete normalization of ACTH and cortisol levels in three patients with Cushing's disease by the administration of large doses of cyproheptadine, an antiserotonin drug that presumably works at the hypothalamic level to reduce CRF secretion.[13]

On the other hand, there are now several reports of normal hypothalamic–pituitary function including detailed testing of the hypothalamic–pituitary–adrenal axis following removal of ACTH-secreting microadenomas from patients with Cushing's disease.[70–73] These studies imply that the primary disease resided in the pituitary adenoma and that hypothalamic function was normal.

Prior to the past five or ten years, most radiological evaluations of the pituitary in Cushing's disease were confined to standard skull films or "coned" views of the sella, and these studies revealed "tumors" to be present in 10–15% of patients.[74,75] The development of newer tomographic techniques with hypocycloidal or triaxial spiral movement (see Chapter 14) has dramatically altered the percentage of patients showing abnormal studies. Of 33 consecutive patients seen at the Mayo Clinic from 1974 to 1977 with Cushing's disease, only 1 patient had an abnormal sella on plain skull films, but of the other 31 in whom triaxial spiral tomograms were done, 12 showed evidence of a microadenoma that was later confirmed by surgical exploration.[75] Furthermore, in 6 patients who had normal sella tomograms, carotid angiography suggested the presence of a microadenoma, but this was verified by surgery in only 5, no tumor being found in the sixth patient. Thus, in this series,[75] tumors were found at surgery in 17 of 32 patients (53%) who had normal plain skull films. Late postoperative testing in 10 patients revealed normal diurnal variation in 7 of 8, dexamethasone suppression testing in 6 of 6 tested, and metyrapone testing in 5 of 5 tested.

Tyrell *et al.*[76] have gone one step further in that they performed surgical exploration of the sella on 20 consecutive patients with Cushing's disease diagnosed only by endocrinological biochemical criteria, including 8 with normal sella polytomography and 12 with abnormal polytomography suggestive of a microadenoma. Of these 20 patients, 18 were able to undergo adequate sellar exploration (in 2, a large venous sinus prevented access to the sella), and definite, pathologically confirmed tumors were found in 15. In the other 3 patients, selective removal of abnormal-appearing tissue that was insufficient in quantity for adequate pathological examination resulted in cure of the Cushing's disease. In the 6 patients in whom late (over 1 year) postoperative evaluations were performed, normal hypothalamic–pituitary–adrenal function was demonstrable, including normal suppressibility and diurnal variation.

It thus appears that pituitary tumors are present in the overwhelming majority of patients with Cushing's disease. The fact that hypothalamic–pituitary–adrenal function appears to be entirely normal once the effects of prolonged high amounts of ACTH and cortisol have worn off in all patients tested following selective adenoma resection argues against a primary hypothalamic dysfunction with secondary pituitary disease. One case has also been reported of failure of pituitary stalk section in the treatment of Cushing's disease.[67] The suggestion that a tumor is the primary site of the disease is not incompatible with observed findings of Krieger and others. As Lagerquist *et al.*[70] conclude, the site of steroid feedback in Cushing's disease is most likely the pituitary. It is quite possible that the hypothalamus exerts some influence over these pituitary tumors and that they are not completely autonomous, thus explaining the observed effects of antiserotonin agents. Such incomplete autonomy has been well described in both GH-secreting[77] and prolactin-secreting (see Chapter 4) pituitary tumors as well as many other endocrine adenomas. The altered prolactin and GH responses found in Krieger's patients may be related to the presence of an ACTH-secreting tumor or irradiation or both, since such abnormalities revert to normal following microadenomectomy in the few patients studied.[73,76] There is evidence against the abnormal GH dynamics being related to the tumor only, however, in that Tyrrell *et al.*[71] found that GH dynamics were normal in nine patients who had had bilateral adrenalectomy and who had no radiologic evidence of pituitary tumors. However, we now know, from the later work of this group,[76] that most of those patients probably have tumors that are too small to see radiologically. Interestingly, patients with radiological evidence of progressive tumor growth following adrenalectomy (Nelson's syndrome) have abnormal GH-secretory dynamics despite the normalization of plasma cortisol.[71] The evidence now available therefore favors a primarily pituitary origin of Cushing's disease due to ACTH-secretory adenomas that are not completely autonomous. It is still possible that some cases will be due to hypothalamic dysfunction, but these would be uncommon.

7. Therapy of Cushing's Disease

When considering the various types of therapy that have been used in treating Cushing's disease, one should keep in mind the four characteristics of the ideal therapy as outline by Orth and Liddle[78]: (1) to correct the hypercortisolism; (2) to eradicate any tumor that itself may threaten health; (3) to avoid varying degrees of endocrine deficiency; and (4) to avoid permanent dependency on hormone-replacement therapy. As will be discussed, selective transsphenoidal adenomectomy appears to come closest to these ideals.

Therapy in Cushing's disease may be aimed at the hypothalamus, the pituitary, the adrenals, or the target organs affected by the hypercortisolism. The medical therapy of Cushing's disease is dealt with in detail in Chapter 15. Medical therapy should in general be regarded as adjunctive or interim therapy; it often causes enough of a reduction in hypercortisolism to enable the patient to tolerate surgery better or to obtain rapid clinical improvement while awaiting the results of irradiation.

The results of Salassa *et al.*[75] and Tyrrell *et al.*[76] as outlined in the previous section are striking arguments for the use of transsphenoidal selective adenomectomy in the therapy of Cushing's disease. Similar results have been achieved by Hardy and Vezina[79] (see Table 3). Transsphenoidal surgery in general has very low mortality and low morbidity (see Chapter 18), and the results of the three large series mentioned above show remarkably little morbidity, most patients retaining normal pituitary function. Such low morbidity reflects the fact that these patients almost all had microadenomas and that the neurosurgery was performed in experienced centers.

About 10–15% of cases present with tumors large enough to be visible on plain skull films. Such tumors are much more prone to be locally invasive than other pituitary tumors.[80] In the series of Welbourn *et al.*,[80] of seven patients with abnormal plain skull X-rays, four of the pituitary tumors were found to be locally invasive at surgery or autopsy. Furthermore, these tumors are also more prone to have distant metastases than other types of pituitary tumors, albeit such behavior is quite rare even for Cushing's disease.[81] Because of their experience, Welbourn *et al.*[80] have recommended that some form of radiotherapy be administered following surgery if the tumors appear at all invasive. Our own approach has been to perform as close to a total hypophysectomy as possible when there is evidence of invasion and follow this with irradiation if the neurosurgeon feels that not all tissue could be removed or if ACTH levels remain elevated. The undesirability of panhypopituitarism appears to be clearly outweighed by the morbidity and mortality of progressive local invasion.

Irradiation of the pituitary has been used as primary therapy in Cushing's disease by several groups. It has usually been used in milder cases because of the lag period of 1–12 months before clinical remissions may be seen. In the

TABLE 3. Comparison of Radiotherapy to Transsphenoidal Surgery in the Treatment of Cushing's Disease

Therapy	Series	Year	Total number of patients	Cured	Improved	No change
Transethmoidal hypophysectomy	Fletcher *et al.*[86]	1971	10	6	3	1
Transsphenoidal adenomectomy	Hardy and Vezina[79]	1976	20	14	3	3
	Salassa *et al.*[75]	1978	18	16	—	2
	Tyrrell *et al.*[76]	1978	20	17	—	3
Radiotherapy	Heuschele and Lampe[83]	1967	16	10	—	6
	Orth and Liddle[78]	1971	44	10	13	21
	Edmonds *et al.*[82]	1972	15	9	1	5
	Jennings *et al.*[84,a]	1977	15	12	—	3
^{198}Au or ^{90}Y implants	Burke *et al.*[85]	1973	55	27	6	22

[a] Children only.

past, 4000–5000 rads were usually given over 4–5 weeks (see Chapter 21). In the largest series, reported by Orth and Liddle,[78] only 10 of 44 patients achieved a cure and 13 of 44 were improved, while 21 of 44 were unchanged and required other therapy (usually bilateral adrenalectomy). Better results were found by Edmonds *et al.*,[82] who reported that 9 of 15 patients achieved cures, 1 was improved, and 5 of 15 remained unchanged, and by Heuschele and Lampe,[83] who reported cures in 10 of 16 patients. Recently, it has been found that children with Cushing's disease are much more responsive to irradiation than adults, cures being obtained in 12 of 15 such patients.[84] In these children, growth and sexual development resumed normally following normalization of cortisol levels. In all series of patients undergoing conventional irradiation, the side effects of the irradiation have been negligible; hypopituitarism has not been a problem. Yttrium-90 and other radioactive needle implantations into the pituitary have not been employed frequently in this country. However, Burke *et al.*[85] have had considerable success, with 27 of 55 patients said to be cured and 6 of 55 improved. Arguments against the use of radioactive implants center around the fact that if the sella is to be entered surgically anyway, why not just perform an adenomectomy?

The surest and fastest method of curing Cushing's disease is to perform a bilateral total adrenalectomy, although rarely ectopic adrenal tissue can continue to hypersecrete.[87–89] Such surgery renders the patient completely dependent on exogenous therapy with glucocorticoid and mineralocorticoid replacement. The operative mortality for such a procedure is 3–4% in experienced hands, but postoperative wound infections and bleeding can also be a problem.[90] In the past, this method of therapy had been reserved for patients who did not respond to pituitary irradiation or who had evidence of severe hypercortisolism as manifested by severe depression, hypertension unresponsive to antihypertensive medications, severe myopathy, or severe osteoporosis, and therefore required urgent relief of the hypercortisolism.

One of the most problematic of the long-term complications of bilateral adrenalectomy for Cushing's disease is the development of Nelson's syndrome (Fig. 4). In 1958, Nelson *et al.*[91] reported the development of hyperpigmentation associated with an enlarging, ACTH-secreting pituitary tumor 3 years following bilateral adrenalectomy in a patient with Cushing's disease whose sella had not been enlarged on plain skull films at the time of the adrenalectomy. The definition of Nelson's syndrome in the literature has been variable, meaning sellar enlargement alone, hyperpigmentation alone, or both together, in different series. If one adheres to the definition of Nelson's syndrome as the development of sellar enlargement and hyperpigmentation following bilateral adrenalectomy in patients with initially normal sellas on plain skull films, the incidence ranges from 3 to 38%, the largest series showing incidences of 5–10%.[34,74,80,90,92,93] In children, as many as 25% have been found to develop Nelson's syndrome.[94] The time course of development of these tumors ranges from 1 to 16 years, and these tumors prove to be locally invasive 10–25% of the time. Although it has been suggested that pituitary irradiation may prevent the development of Nelson's syndrome,[67] this has been disputed.[92] The recent findings of microadenomas in most patients with Cushing's disease make it highly likely that patients with Nelson's syndrome

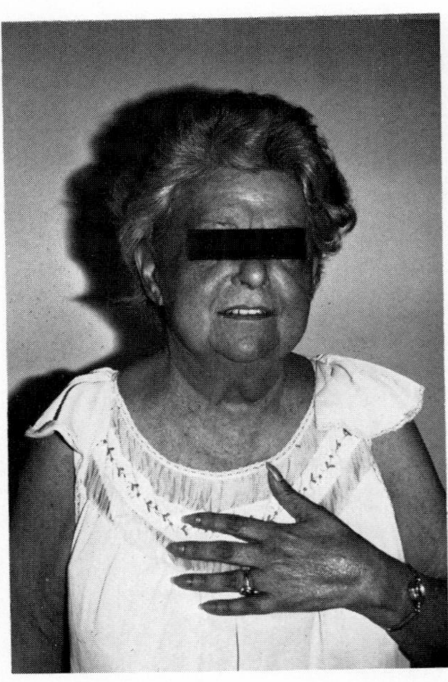

Fig. 4. Same patient as in Fig. 3 who had bilateral adrenalectomy in the time between these two photographs. Note the development of marked hyperpigmentation as well as the partial resolution of Cushingoid features.

had tumors present prior to adrenalectomy that become larger only following adrenalectomy. Clearly, these tumors are partially responsive to circulating glucocorticoid levels (as demonstrable by dexamethasone suppression testing); lowering of the high circulating cortisol levels by adrenalectomy removes the partial inhibition of ACTH release by cortisol, so that ACTH levels go even higher and tumor growth occurs. It is not clear why only some patients develop Nelson's syndrome, but it may be due to the degree of inhibition exerted by the circulating cortisol levels. Some have advocated treating all patients who undergo bilateral adrenalectomy as the first procedure, with prophylactic pituitary irradiation. We believe that all patients subjected to bilateral adrenalectomy as the initial therapy should have yearly determinations of ACTH levels, visual fields, and possibly sella polytomography performed to detect the development of Nelson's syndrome at an early stage; since it is unlikely that tomograms will detect an enlarging tumor before ACTH levels rise, it is probably sufficient to monitor ACTH levels every 6–12 months. The finding that these tumors are sometimes invasive warrants this close surveillance.

The overall treatment plan for each patient must be individualized. On the basis of the most recent evidence cited above, transsphenoidal selective adenomectomy would appear to be the treatment of choice if an experienced neurosurgeon is available along with suitable support facilities and personnel and if the patient is able to tolerate surgery. Preoperative preparation with metyrapone or aminoglutethimide (see Chapter 15) can often be helpful in this regard. In children, it would appear that irradiation probably has similar success. When the degree of hypercortisolism is severe, then transsphenoidal surgery will correct this quickly, but if this is not available, then bilateral adrenalectomy would be the next best choice. With large pituitary tumors, total hypophysectomy plus postoperative irradiation would seem appropriate. Finally, very mild cases of Cushing's disease may be treated with irradiation alone, but consideration should also be given to transsphenoidal surgery because of its lack of morbidity and speed of achieving a cure. If future neurosurgical series continue to duplicate the results of Salassa *et al.*[75] and Tyrrell *et al.*,[76] transsphenoidal surgery may well be considered as the treatment of choice for Cushing's disease even in the absence of sella abnormalities.

8. Management of Patients Undergoing Ablative Therapy

All patients who are going to have specific therapy for their Cushing's disease should have a full evaluation of their pituitary function (aside from ACTH) prior to therapy (for details of testing, see Chapter 11). Because of pressure effects of a tumor or because of the effect of hypercortisolism, a variable percentage will be found to have defects of one or more pituitary hormones. It is important to document these so as to be able to evaluate the results of therapy when retesting is performed later. It is even more important to detect the presence of hypothyroidism due to TSH deficiency (although this is rare) so that thyroid-hormone replacement may be completed before subjecting the patient to surgery, since there are some risks to operating on patients who are hypothyroid (for a discussion of these risks, see Molitch[95]).

Successful transsphenoidal adenomectomy results in a period of hypocortisolism lasting from 3 to 24 months,[75,76] due to the prior suppression of the normal hypothalamic–pituitary–adrenal axis by the high cortisol levels. This period of recovery is as long as that for patients receiving exogenous steroids,[96] even though the adrenals are hyperresponsive. Evidently the disordered feedback system requires a long time for resetting no matter where the system is perturbed. During this period of hypocortisolism, the patient will need steroid therapy.

Since normal individuals secrete 200–300 mg/24 hr of cortisol in the face of severe stress,[27] we recommend giving 300 mg/day of hydrocortisone on the day of pituitary surgery (and also in other operations or in the face of severe stress for up to 1 year following pituitary surgery). Specifically, 100 mg hydrocortisone sodium succinate is given intramuscularly on call to the operating room, and 100 mg is given as an intravenous drip during the procedure. Then the dexamethasone that is given in high doses for most neurosurgical procedures will be sufficient for any steroid needs. The dexamethasone is usually tapered over the next 4–6 days, and the patient should be sent home on twice maintenance dose of hydrocortisone (i.e., 40–60 mg daily) for about 2–4 weeks to help the body to come down to physiological cortisol levels gradually.[27] This dose should then be gradually tapered down to 20 mg in the morning and 10 mg hydrocortisone in the afternoon for about 2 months. Then the evening dose should be dropped for about 2–3 months and the dose of hydrocortisone in the morning can be tapered by 2.5 mg/day every 1–2 weeks to 10 mg.[97] When the patient has been taking 10 mg daily for several weeks, the 8 A.M. cortisol is checked prior to the morning dose monthly, and when this level reaches 10 μg/dl, some degree of restoration of function can be assumed and exogenous steroids can be discontinued.[97] Once steroids have been totally withdrawn, it is prudent to check the response of the hypothalamic–pituitary–adrenal axis through pyrogen or insulin-induced hypoglycemic stimulation when such testing is practical. Patients withdrawn in such a manner are still considered to be at risk for developing adrenal insufficiency at surgery or due to other major stresses for over 1 year following pituitary surgery, and steroid "coverage" during such stresses is necessary (see Table 4). At 4–6 weeks following pituitary surgery, patients should also receive testing of the other pituitary hormones (see Chapters 11 and 20) to assess their status and the need for other hormonal replacement.

Patients undergoing bilateral adrenalectomy should also receive 50–100 mg hydrocortisone the night before surgery. On the day of surgery, 100 mg should be given intramuscularly on call to the operating room, 100 mg should be infused intravenously during the procedure, and 100 mg should be given intramuscularly that evening. The steroid dosage can then be tapered as shown in Table 4. When the total dose of hydrocortisone per day is less than 75–100 mg, fludrocortisone (Florinef®) should be given in doses of 0.05–0.1 mg daily orally to provide mineralocorticold. These patients should also be placed on twice maintenance dose of glucocorticoids for 2–4 weeks to help the patient readjust before going to normal maintenance doses of hydrocortisone 20 mg in the morning and 10 mg in the afternoon or prednisone 2.5–5 mg in the morning and 2.5 mg in the afternoon. Such patients will obviously need to have their steroid dosage increased in times of stress (see Table 4).

After radiation therapy, patients with still-active Cushing's disease and patients in remission often do not demonstrate normal increments in cortisol after pyrogen or hypoglycemic stimulation.[68] Because of this, these patients will also need steroid coverage following irradiation for periods of stress (see Table 4). During radiation therapy, patients should be maintained on twice the maintenance dose because of the stress of the irradiation.

TABLE 4. Glucocorticoid Therapy for Major Surgery and Stress

1. Hydrocortisone 100 mg i.m. the night prior to surgery
2. Hydrocortisone 100 mg i.m. in A.M. on call to O.R.
3. Hydrocortisone 100 mg i.v. over course of surgery
4. Hydrocortisone 100 mg i.m. or i.v. evening of surgery
5. Postoperative day (POD) 1: Hydrocortisone 50–100 mg[a] i.m. or i.v. q 8 hr
6. POD 2: Hydrocortisone 25 mg i.m. or i.v. q 8 hr
7. POD 3: Hydrocortisone 25 mg i.m., i.v., or p.o. q 12 hr
   Fludrocortisone (Florinef) 0.1 mg p.o. daily[b]
8. POD 4: Hydrocortisone 20 mg in A.M., 10 mg in P.M.
   Fludrocortisone 0.05–0.1 mg daily

[a] For major procedures, unstable course, or supervening infection, the higher figures should be used with slower tapering.

[b] Fludrocortisone is necessary only in patients who have undergone bilateral adrenalectomy.

9. Conclusions

The recent demonstration that microadenomas are present in most patients who have radiologically normal sellas has shifted the focus of attention away from the hypothalamus and back toward the pituitary as originally proposed by Harvey Cushing. The initiating event in this ACTH-secreting adenoma formation remains unknown, but the lack of abnormal ACTH regulation once the adenoma is removed suggests that there is no basic hypothalamic dysfunction in most cases. It is intriguing that ACTH-secreting tumors, like many other endocrine tumors, do not have complete autonomy. These tumors remain variably responsive to a variety of modulating factors.

The other major new findings in the understanding of Cushing's disease relate to the interrelationship between ACTH and LPH. The information that these hormones are probably initially synthesized as a single large protein and that β-MSH is a part of LPH explains the relationship between ACTH and MSH that has been observed over the years. The measurement of LPH may turn out to be easier than the measurement of ACTH, which has some technical problems, so that this new information may be of direct clinical benefit.

Thus, the most basic of molecular research may contribute directly to the earlier diagnosis of Cushing's disease, and it is precisely these early-diagnosed patients, with their microadenomas, who may benefit from the recent clinical data about the feasibility of transsphenoidal adenomectomy. The next few years should show the fruits of this blending of basic and clinical research in the form of better patient care.

References

1. D.T. Krieger and E.A. Zimmerman, The nature of CRF and its relationship to vasopressin, in: *Clinical Neuroendocrinology* (L. Martini and G.M. Besser, eds.), pp. 363–391, Academic Press, New York, 1977.
2. J.B. Martin, S. Reichlin, and G.M. Brown, *Clinical Neuroendocrinology*, F.A. Davis, Philadelphia, 1977.
3. M. Motta, F. Piva, and L. Martini, The role of "short" feedback mechanisms in the regulation of adrenocorticotropin secretion, *Prog. Brain Res.* **32:**25, 1970.
4. B. Török, Structure of the vascular connections of the hypothalamo–hypophysial region, *Acta Anat.* **59:**84, 1964.
5. R.M. Bergland, S.L. Davis, and R.B. Page, Pituitary secretes to brain: Experiments in sheep, *Lancet* **2:**276, 1977.
6. C. Oliver, R.S. Mical, and J.C. Porter, Hypothalamic–pituitary vasculature: Evidence for retrograde blood flow in the pituitary stalk, *Endocrinology* **101:**598, 1977.
7. D.T. Krieger, A. Liotta, and M.J. Brownstein, Presence of corticotropin in brain of normal and hypophysectomized rats, *Proc. Natl. Acad. Sci. U.S.A.* **74:**648, 1977.
8. R. Moldow and R.S. Yalow, Extrahypophysial distribution of corticotropin as a function of brain size, *Proc. Natl. Acad. Sci. U.S.A.* **75:**994, 1978.
9. S.J. Watson, C.W. Richard III, and J.D. Barchas, Adrenocorticotropin in rat brain: Immunocytochemical localization in cells and axons, *Science* **200:**1180, 1978.
10. E.D. Weitzman, D. Fukushima, C. Nogeire, H. Roffwarg, T.F. Gallagher, and L. Hellman, Twenty-four hour pattern of the episodic secretion of cortisol in normal subjects, *J. Clin. Endocrinol. Metab.* **33:**14, 1971.
11. D.T. Krieger, Serotonin regulation of ACTH secretion, *Ann. N.Y. Acad. Sci.* **297:**527, 1977.

12. J. Vernikos-Danellis, K.J. Kellar, D. Kent, C. Gonzales, P.A. Berger, and D. Barchas, Serotonin involvement in pituitary–adrenal function, *Ann. N.Y. Acad. Sci.* **297:**518, 1977.
13. D.T. Krieger, L. Amorosa, and F. Linick, Cyproheptadine-induced remission of Cushing's disease, *N. Engl. J. Med.* **293:**893, 1975.
14. S.M. McCann, S.R. Ojeda, P.G. Harms, J.E. Wheaton, D.K. Sundberg, and C.P. Fawcett, Control of adenohypophyseal hormone secretion by prostaglandins, in: *Subcellular Mechanisms in Reproductive Neuroendocrinology* (F. Naftolin, K.J. Ryan, and J. Davies, eds.), pp. 407–422, Elsevier, Amsterdam, 1976.
15. R. Guillemin, Endocrinology of the neuron, in: *The Hypothalamus* (S. Reichlin, R.J. Baldessarini, and J.B. Martin, eds.), pp. 155–194, Raven Press, New York, 1978.
16. G.R. Uhl, S.R. Childers, and S.H. Snyder, Opioid peptides and the opiate receptor, in: *Frontiers in Neuroendocrinology*, Vol. 5 (W.F. Ganong and L. Martini, eds.), pp. 289–378, Raven Press, New York, 1978.
17. I. Bachelot, A.R. Wolfsen, and W.D. Odell, Pituitary and plasma lipotropins: Demonstration of the artifactual nature of β-MSH, *J. Clin. Endocrinol. Metab.* **44:**939, 1977.
18. L.S. Rees, Human adrenocorticotropin and lipotropin (MSH) in health and disease, in: *Clinical Neuroendocrinology* (L. Martini and G.M. Besser, eds.), pp. 401–441, Academic Press, New York, 1977.
19. R. Guillemin, T. Vargo, J. Rossier, S. Minick, N. Ling, C. Rivier, W. Vale, and F. Bloom, β-Endorphin and adrenocorticotropin are secreted concomitantly by the pituitary gland, *Science* **197:**1367, 1977.
20. G. Pelletier, R. LeClerc, F. Labrie, J. Cote, M. Chretien, and M. Lis, Immunohistochemical localization of β-lipotropic hormone in the pituitary gland, *Endocrinology* **100:**770, 1977.
21. R.E. Mains, B.A. Eipper, and N. Ling, Common precursor to corticotropins and endorphins, *Proc. Natl. Acad. Sci. U.S.A.* **74:**3014, 1977.
22. J.L. Roberts and E. Herbert, Characterization of a common precursor to corticotropin and β-lipotropin: Identification of β-lipotropin peptides and their arrangement relative to corticotropin in the precursor synthesized in a cell-free system, *Proc. Natl. Acad. Sci. U.S.A.* **74:**5300, 1977.
23. M. Rubinstein, S. Stein, and S. Udenfriend, Characterization of pro-opiocortin, a precursor to opioid peptides and corticotropin, *Proc. Natl. Acad. Sci. U.S.A.* **75:**669, 1978.
24. L.J. Deftos, D. Burton, B.D. Catherwood, H.B. Bone, J.G. Parthemore, R. Guillemin, W.B. Watkins, and R.Y. Moore, Demonstration by immunoperoxidase histochemistry of calcitonin in the anterior lobe of the rat pituitary, *J. Clin. Endocrinol. Metab.* **47:**457, 1978.
25. G.M. Besser and C.R.W. Edwards, Cushing's syndrome, *Clin. Endocrinol. Metab.* **1:**451, 1972.
26. C.M. Plotz, A.I. Knowlton, and C. Ragan, The natural history of Cushing's syndrome, *Am. J. Med.* **13:**597, 1952.
27. G.W. Liddle, The adrenal cortex in: *Textbook of Endocrinology* (R.H. Williams, ed.), pp. 233–283, W.B. Saunders, Philadelphia, 1974.
28. L. Krakoff, G. Nicolis, and B. Amsel, Pathogenesis of hypertension in Cushing's syndrome, *Am. J. Med.* **58:**216, 1975.
29. T.G. Dalakos, A.N. Elias, G.H. Anderson Jr., D.H.P. Streeten, and E.T. Schroeder, Evidence for an angiotensinogenic mechanism of the hypertension of Cushing's syndrome, *J. Clin. Endocrinol. Metab.* **46:**114, 1978.
30. Q.R. Regestein, L.I. Rose, and G.H. Williams, Psychopathology in Cushing's syndrome, *Arch. Intern. Med.* **130:**114, 1972.
31. C.K. Smith, J. Barish, J. Correa, and R.H. Williams, Psychiatric disturbance in endocrine disease, *Psychosom. Med.* **34:**69, 1972.
32. P.A. Lee, V.V. Weldon, and C.J. Migeon, Short stature as the only clinical sign of Cushing's syndrome, *J. Pediatr.* **86:**89, 1975.
33. I.L. Solomon and E.J. Schoen, Juvenile Cushing syndrome manifested primarily by growth failure, *Am. J. Dis. Child.* **130:**200, 1976.
34. R.G. McArthur, M.D. Cloutier, A.B. Hayles, and R.G. Sprague, Cushing's disease in children: Findings in 13 cases, *Mayo Clin. Proc.* **47:**318, 1972.
35. D.H.P. Streeten, F.H. Faas, M.J. Elders, T.G. Dalakos, and M. Voorhess, Hypercortisolism in childhood: Shortcomings of conventional diagnostic criteria, *Pediatrics* **56:**797, 1975.

36. K. Kreines and W.D. DeVanx, Neonatal adrenal insufficiency associated with maternal Cushing's syndrome, *Pediatrics* **47:**516, 1971.
37. A.M. Hutter, and D.E. Kayhoe, Adrenal cortical carcinoma: Clinical features of 138 patients, *Am. J. Med* **41:**580, 1966.
38. W.K. Stewart, L.W. Fleming, and H.H. Wotiz, The feminizing syndrome in male subjects with adrenocortical neoplasms, *Am. J. Med.* **37:**455, 1964.
39. G.W. Liddle, W.E. Nicholson, D.P. Island, D.N. Orth, K. Abe, and S.C. Lowder, Clinical and laboratory studies of ectopic humoral syndromes, *Recent Prog. Horm. Res.* **25:**283, 1969.
40. W.D. Odell and A.R. Wolfsen, Humoral syndromes associated with cancer, *Annu. Rev. Med.* **29:**379, 1978.
41. E.M. Rosenberg, T.J. Hahn, D.N. Orth, L.J. Deftos, and K. Tanaka, ACTH-secreting medullary carcinoma of the thyroid presenting as severe idiopathic osteoporosis and senile purpura: Report of a case and review of the literature, *J. Clin. Endocrinol. Metab.* **47:**255, 1978.
42. G. Gewirtz and R.S. Yalow, Ectopic ACTH production in carcinoma of the lung, *J. Clin. Invest.* **53:**1022, 1974.
43. W.D. Odell, A. Wolfsen, Y. Yoshimoto, R. Weitzman, and D. Fisher, Ectopic peptide synthesis: A universal concomitant of neoplasia, *Clin. Res.* **25:**149A, 1977.
44. A. Wolfsen and W. Odell, Big-ACTH and β-lipotropin: Production by colon and lung cancer, *Clin. Res.* **25:**107A, 1977.
45. G.V. Upton and T.T. Amatruda Jr., Evidence for the presence of tumor peptides with corticotropin-releasing factor–like activity in the ectopic ACTH syndrome, *N. Engl. J. Med.* **285:**419, 1971.
46. T. Suda, H. Demura, R. Demura, I. Wakabayashi, K. Nomura, E. Odagiri, and K. Shizume, Corticotropin-releasing factor–like activity in ACTH producing tumors, *J. Clin. Endocrinol. Metab.* **44:**440, 1977.
47. R.L. Eddy, A.L. Jones, P.F. Gilliland, J.D. Ibarra Jr., J.Q. Thompson, and J.F. McMurry Jr., Cushing's syndrome: A prospective study of diagnostic methods, *Am. J. Med.* **55:**621, 1973.
48. C.A. Nugent, T. Nichols, and F.H. Tyler, Diagnosis of Cushing's syndrome: Single dose suppression test, *Arch. Intern. Med.* **116:**172, 1965.
49. C.T. Sawin, G.A. Bray, and B.A. Idelson, Overnight suppression test with dexamethasone in Cushing's syndrome, *J. Clin. Endocrinol. Metab.* **28:**422, 1968.
50. G.W. Liddle, Tests of pituitary–adrenal suppressibility in the diagnosis of Cushing's syndrome, *J. Clin. Endocrinol. Metab.* **12:**1539, 1960.
51. T. Nichols, C.A. Nugent, and F.H. Tyler, Steroid laboratory tests in the dignosis of Cushing's syndrome, *Am. J. Med.* **45:**116, 1968.
52. T. Suda, A. Liotta, and D.T. Krieger, Plasma lipotropin (LPH) and ACTH secretion in normal subjects and patients with pituitary–adrenal disease, Program of the 60th Annual Meeting of the Endocrine Society, p. 224, 1978.
53. E. Wiedemann, T. Saito, and J.A. Linfoot, Elevated plasma β-lipotropin in Cushing's disease due to pituitary adenoma, Program of the 60th Annual Meeting of the Endocrine Society, p. 227, 1978.
54. J.J.H. Gilkes, L.H. Rees, and G.M. Besser, Plasma immunoreactive corticotrophin and lipotrophin in Cushing's syndrome and Addison's disease, *Br. Med. J.* **1:**996, 1977.
55. J.H. Pratt, C.T. Sawin, and J.C. Melby, Remission of Cushing's disease after administration of adrenocorticotropin, *Am. J. Med.* **57:**949, 1974.
56. J.F. Redman and F.H. Faas, Acute unilateral adrenal hemorrhage following ACTH administration in a patient with Cushing's syndrome, *Am. J. Med.* **61:**533, 1976.
57. G.L. Treece, D.J. Magelssen, and B.L. Fariss, Conjugated estrogens and the overnight dexamethasone suppression test, *Obstet. Gynecol.* **50:**407, 1977.
58. E.E. Werk Jr., Y. Choi, L. Sholiton, C. Olinger, and N. Hague, Interference in the effect of dexamethasone by diphenylhydantoin, *N. Engl. J. Med.* **281:**32, 1969.
59. N. Hague, K. Thrasher, E.E. Werk Jr., H.C. Knowles Jr., and L.J. Sholiton, Studies on dexamethasone metabolism in man; effect of diphenylhydantoin, *J. Clin. Endocrinol. Metab.* *34:*44, 1972.
60. D.H.P. Streeten, C.T. Stevenson, T.G. Dalakos, J.J. Nicholas, L.G. Dennick, and H. Fellerman, The diagnosis of hypercortisolism: Biochemical criteria differentiating patient from lean and

obese normal subjects and from females on oral contraceptives, *J. Clin. Endocrinol. Metab.* **29:**1191, 1969.

61. E.J. Sachar, L. Hellman, H.P. Roffwarg, F.S. Halpern, T.K. Fukushima, and T.F. Gallagher, Disrupted 24 hour patterns of cortisol secretion in psychotic depression, *Arch. Gen. Psychiatry* **28:**19, 1973.
62. P.G. Ettigi and G.M. Brown, Psychoneuroendocrinology of affective disorder; an overview, *Am. J. Psychiatry* **134:**493, 1977.
63. R. Demura, H. Demura, T. Nunokawa, H. Baba, and K. Miura, Responses of plasma ACTH, GH, LH and 11-hydroxycorticosteroids to various stimuli in patients with Cushing's syndrome, *J. Clin. Endocrinol. Metab.* **34:**852, 1972.
64. L.H. Rees, G.M. Besser, W.J. Jeffcoate, D.J. Goldie, and V. Marks, Alcohol induced pseudo–Cushing's syndrome, *Lancet* **1:**726, 1977.
65. E.J. Rayfield, L.I. Rose, J.P. Cain, R.G. Dluhy, and G.H. Williams, ACTH-responsive, dexamethasone-suppressible adrenocortical carcinoma, *N. Engl. J. Med.* **284:**591, 1971.
66. A.M.S. Mason, J.G. Ratcliffe, R.M. Buckle, and A.S. Mason, ACTH secretion by bronchial carcinoid tumours, *Clin. Endocrinol.* **1:**3, 1972.
67. G.W. Liddle, Cushing's syndrome, *Ann. N.Y. Acad. Sci.* **297:**594, 1977.
68. D.T. Krieger and S.M. Glick, Growth hormone and cortisol responsiveness in Cushing's syndrome, *Am. J. Med.* **52:**25, 1972.
69. D.T. Krieger, P.J. Howanitz, and A.G. Frantz, Absence of nocturnal elevation of plasma prolactin concentrations in Cushing's disease, *J. Clin. Endocrinol. Metab.* **42:**260, 1976.
70. L.G. Lagerquist, A.W. Meikle, C.D. West, and F.H. Tyler, Cushing's disease with cure by resection of a pituitary adenoma: Evidence against a primary hypothalamic defect, *Am. J. Med.* **57:**826, 1974.
71. J.B. Tyrrell, J. Wiener-Kronish, M. Lorenzi, R.M. Brooks, and P.H. Forsham, Cushing's disease; growth hormone response to hypoglycemia after correction of hypercortisolism, *J. Clin. Endocrinol. Metab.* **44:**218, 1977.
72. S.T. Bigos, F. Robert, G. Pelletier, and J. Hardy, Cure of Cushing's disease by transsphenoidal removal of a microadenoma from a pituitary gland despite a radiographically normal sella turcica, *J. Clin. Endocrinol. Metab.* **45:**1251, 1977.
73. A.M. Schnall, J.S. Brodkey, B. Kaufman, and O.H. Pearson, Pituitary function after removal of pituitary microadenomas in Cushing's disease, *J. Clin. Endocrinol. Metab.* **47:**410, 1978.
74. R.M. Salassa, T.P. Kearns, J.W. Kernohan, R.G. Sprague, and C.S. MacCarty, Pituitary tumors in patients with Cushing's syndrome, *J. Clin. Endocrinol. Metab.* **19:**1523, 1959.
75. R.M. Salassa, E.R. Laws Jr., P.C. Carpenter, and R.C. Northcutt, Transsphenoidal removal of pituitary microadenoma in Cushing's disease, *Mayo Clin. Proc.* **53:**24, 1978.
76. J.B. Tyrrell, R.M. Brooks, P.A. Fitzgerald, P.B. Cofoid, P.H. Forsham, and C.B. Wilson, Cushing's disease; selective transsphenoidal resection of pituitary microadenomas, *N. Engl. J. Med.* **298:**753, 1978.
77. A.M. Lawrence, I.D. Goldfine, and L. Kirsteins, Growth hormone dynamics in acromegaly, *J. Clin. Endocrinol. Metab.* **31:**239, 1970.
78. D.N. Orth and G.W. Liddle, Results of treatment in 108 patients with Cushing's syndrome, *N. Engl. J. Med.* **285:**243, 1971.
79. J. Hardy and J.L. Vezina, Transsphenoidal neurosurgery of intracranial neoplasm, *Adv. Neurol.* **15:**261, 1976.
80. R.B. Welbourn, D.A.D. Montgomery, and T.L. Kennedy, The natural history of treated Cushing's syndrome, *Br. J. Surg.* **58:**1, 1971.
81. L. des Quieroz, N.O. Facure, J.J. Facure, N.P. Modesto, and J.L. deFaria, Pituitary carcinoma with liver metastases and Cushing syndrome, *Arch. Pathol.* **99:**32, 1975.
82. M.W. Edmonds, W.J.K. Simpson, and J.W. Meakin, External irradiation of the hypophysis for Cushing's disease, *Can. Med. Assoc. J.* **107:**860, 1972.
83. R. Heuschele and I. Lampe, Pituitary irradiation for Cushing's syndrome, *Radiol. Clin. Biol.* **36:**27, 1967.
84. A.S. Jennings, G.W. Liddle, and D.N. Orth, Results of treating childhood Cushing's disease with pituitary irradiation, *N. Engl. J. Med.* **297:**957, 1977.
85. C.W. Burke, F.H. Doyle, G.F. Joplin, R.N. Arnot, D.P. Macerlean, and T.R. Fraser, Cushing's disease: Treatment by pituitary implantation of radioactive gold or yttrium seeds, *Q. J. Med.* **42:**693, 1973.

86. R. Fletcher, G.A. Dalton, M.H.B. Carmalt, and W.T. Smith, The treatment of Cushing's syndrome by transethmoidal hypophysectomy, *Acta. Endocrinal.* **67:**(Suppl. 155):163, 1971.
87. D.E. Schteingart, J.W. Conn, L.M. Lieberman, and W.H. Beierwaltes, Persistent or recurrent Cushing's syndrome after "total" adrenalectomy, *Arch. Intern. Med.* **130:**384, 1972.
88. G.O. Strauch and L. Vinnick, Persistent Cushing's syndrome apparently cured by ectopic adrenalectomy, *J. Am. Med. Assoc.* **222:**183, 1972.
89. P.D. Papapetrou and I. Jackson, Cortisol secretion in Nelson syndrome: Persistence after "total" adrenalectomy for Cushing syndrome, *J. Am. Med. Assoc.* **234:**847, 1974.
90. H.W. Scott Jr., G.W. Liddle, J.L. Mulherin Jr., T.J. McKenna, S.L. Stroup, and R.K. Rhamy, Surgical experience with Cushing's disease, *Ann. Surg.* **185:**524, 1977.
91. D.H. Nelson, J.W. Meakin, J.B. Dealy Jr., D.D. Matson, K. Emerson Jr., and G.W. Thron, ACTH producing tumor of the pituitary gland, *N. Engl. J. Med.* **259:**161, 1958.
92. T.J. Moore, R.G. Dluhy, G.H. Williams, and J.P. Cain, Nelson's syndrome; frequency, prognosis, and effect of prior pituitary irradiation, *Ann. Intern. Med.* **85:**731, 1976.
93. K.L. Cohen, R.H. Noth, and T. Pechinski, Incidence of pituitary tumors following adrenalectomy. A long term follow-up study of patients treated for Cushing's disease, *Arch. Intern. Med.* **138:**575, 1978.
94. N.J. Hopwood and F.M. Kenny, Incidence of Nelson's syndrome after adrenalectomy for Cushing's disease in children, *Am. J. Dis. Child.* **131:**1353, 1977.
95. M.E. Molitch, Endocrinology, in: *Management of Medical Problems in Surgical Patients* (M.E. Molitch, ed.), F.A. Davis, Philadelphia, 1980 (in press).
96. A.L. Graber, R.L. Ney, W.E. Nicholson, D.P. Island, and G.W. Liddle, Natural history of pituitary–adrenal recovery following long term suppression with corticosteroids, *J. Clin. Endocrinol. Metab.* **25:**11, 1965.
97. R.L. Byyny, Withdrawal from glucocorticoid therapy, *N. Engl. J. Med.* **295:**30, 1976.

8

Thyrotropin- and Gonadotropin-Secreting Pituitary Adenomas

IVOR M.D. JACKSON

1. Introduction

Pituitary tumors that secrete growth hormone (GH), ACTH, and prolactin have been well characterized and result in distinct clinical syndromes. In contast, pituitary adenomas that secrete thyroid-stimulating hormone (TSH) or gonadotropins[follicle-stimulating hormone (FSH) and luteinizing hormone (LH)] are infrequent in clinical practice and consequently less well appreciated by clinicians managing patients with pituitary disorders. Caughey[1] drew attention to the fact that prolonged deprivation of the negative-feedback hormone secreted by the target organ can lead to hyperplasia and subsequently adenomatous transformation of the appropriate tropic-hormone-secreting adenohypophyseal cell. More recently, it has been recognized that primary tumors of the pituitary occur that secrete TSH or gonadotropins without prior thyroidal or gonadal failure. Further, it appears that pituitary adenomas may, on occasion, secrete peptides similar to, but not identical with, the authentic hormone, for although immunoreactivity is recognized by radioimmunoassay, the molecular species is not biologically active. Such circumstances may apply to all pituitary tumors including those that produce TSH and gonadotropins.

2. TSH-Secreting Pituitary Adenomas

Increased adenohypophyseal TSH secretion most commonly occurs in response to primary thyroid failure. However, recent reports suggest that pituitary tumors that secrete TSH may be less rare than was once thought. In this

IVOR M.D. JACKSON • Tufts University School of Medicine; Department of Medicine, Division of Endocrinology, Tufts–New England Medical Center Hospital, Boston, Massachusetts 02111.

section, the syndromes of inappropriate, or excess, TSH secretion will be reviewed, with particular emphasis on those resulting from pituitary adenomas.

2.1. Primary Hypothyroidism

The effects of long-standing thyroid insufficiency on the pituitary gland in man have been known for over a century. In 1851, long before there was any understanding of a pituitary–thyroid axis, Niépce[2] reported the presence of an enlarged pituitary in a series of goitrous cretins at autopsy. Recently, in a group of 26 patients with primary hypothyroidism, Yamada *et al.*[3] reported that 81% had an abnormal enlargement of the sella turcica. The magnitude of increase in sella turcica volume showed a positive correlation with the serum TSH and was inversely related to the levels of serum thyroxine (T_4) and triiodothyronine (T_3). Similar findings were also reported by Bigos *et al.*,[4] who found that sella volume determined by polytomography was significantly greater than normal in the more severe cases of hypothyroidism, in whom GH and ACTH reserve were significantly diminished.

A pituitary tumor is especially likely to occur when the hypothyroidism is prolonged,[5] analagous to the thyrotropic tumor that occurs in the mouse following thyroid ablation.[6] Vagenakis *et al.*[7] reviewed the association of primary hypothyroidism and pituitary tumor and described two cases of their own. In a total of 14 adult patients who had been carefully studied, visual fields were normal in 12, and suprasellar extension, demonstrated by pneumoencephalography, was reported in 2 cases. In most patients, pituitary function was otherwise normal; panhypopituitarism was present in both cases reported by Vagenakis and co-workers. Thyroid autoantibodies were found in many subjects, indicating Hashimoto's thyroiditis as the probable etiology of their hypothyroidism. The serum TSH was markedly elevated, but suppressed fully in all patients following physiological thyroid-hormone replacement. The return of the serum TSH to normal was associated with a reduction in pituitary tumor size as evidenced by improvement in visual fields. This syndrome has also been described in children with juvenile hypothyroidism associated with premature pubertal development and galactorrhea.[8] Within 8 months of starting thyroid medication, there was regression of the sexual precocity, cessation of the galactorrhea, and reduction in sella turcica volume on skull X-ray. Although normalization of pituitary fossa size suggests that hyperplasia of the pituitary thyrotropes was present in these cases, neoplastic change, exquisitely sensitive to thyroid-hormone suppression, as may occur with mouse thyrotropic tumors,[6] is not excluded. The etiology of the premature sexual development and galactorrhea in children with primary hypothyroidism is unknown. The possibilities include hypothalamic dysfunction due to "myxedema of the hypothalamus," which might block the inhibitory CNS effects on the onset of puberty and impair the secretion of prolactin-inhibitory factor (PIF). Enchanced responsivity of the pituitary lactotropes to hypothalamic thyrotropin-releasing hormone (TRH), without necessarily invoking increased TRH secretion, is an alternate and/or additional consideration. It is also possible that the increase in TSH itself directly stimulates the gonad, for high-affinity TSH receptors are present in the mammalian testis.[9,10] Prolactin itself may directly affect the hormonal secretion of gonadal and adrenal glands, since receptors for this peptide are present in such sex-steroid-producing tissues.

2.2. Primary Hypothalamic–Pituitary Disease

Some patients with established primary hypothalamic and/or pituitary disease who are hypothyroid are found to have paradoxically elevated immunoreactive (IR) TSH levels with exaggerated TSH response to TRH stimulation.[11,12] This elevation may represent the concomitant association of a primary thyroid disorder with hypothalamic–pituitary disease. The possibility that TSH with impaired biological activity is being secreted must also be considered, for there have been reports of patients with pituitary tumors who have elevated TSH levels by radioimmunoassay but normal levels by cytochemical assay,[13] a method sensitive to biological action. Primary hypothyroidism in these cases is unlikely in view of their normal thyroidal-radioiodine-uptake response to exogenous TSH. A third possibility to be conjectured is an altered "set point" for pituitary TSH secretion, consequent on impaired hypothalamic secretion of somatostatin, for Arimura and Schally[14] have shown that passive immunization with antisomatostatin antiserum in the rat causes a marked elevation in basal TSH levels as well as an enhanced TSH response to TRH stimulation. However, for hypothyroidism to occur in the context of somatostatin deficiency, some impairment of secretion of TRH or TSH or both would also have to be postulated.

2.3. Pituitary Hyperthyroidism ("TSH Toxicosis")

In contrast to the usual finding of suppressed TSH unresponsive to TRH in thyrotoxicosis,[17] there have been reports of 19 patients to this year with clinical and chemical evidence of hyperthyroidism associated with inappropriately elevated TSH levels (for reviews, see Cooper *et al.*[15] and Tolis *et al.*[16]). Of the 19 cases, 14 had tumors of the pituitary. These were associated in a few instances with GH or prolactin hypersecretion, though most demonstrated no other endocrine abnormality. There were no reports of infiltrative exophthalmopathy, though 1 patient developed Graves' disease following craniotomy. The other 5 subjects had no clinical or radiological evidence of a pituitary tumor. In the patient described by Tolis *et al.*,[16] frank symptoms of thyrotoxicosis including nervousness, flushing, and palpitations were present; clinical evaluation revealed a diffuse goiter and bitemporal hemianopsia. Radiological investigation showed suprasellar extension of the pituitary tumor. The α-subunit in the blood was also elevated (see also Chapter 11), a finding noted in most cases of TSH-secreting pituitary adenomas.[18] Neither TSH nor the α-subunit showed a rise in response to TRH stimulation. Lack of suppression of ^{131}I uptake in the thyroid gland by exogenous thyroid hormone is the usual finding in tumor patients. Although the patient reported by Horn *et al.*[19] showed a fall in serum TSH with both L-dopa and bromocriptine, no change in serum TSH following L-dopa was found by Tolis *et al.*[16]

The patient of Tolis *et al.*[16] underwent transsphenoidal removal of her pituitary adenoma with preservation of normal pituitary tissue. Immunohistochemical staining revealed heavily granulated thyrotropes in the tumor tissue. One year following *pituitary* surgery, the patient was euthyroid and no longer had a goiter. Similarly, radiation or surgical therapy applied to the pituitary gland has resulted in remission of thyrotoxicosis in other tumor cases.

Since the association of a pituitary chromophobe adenoma and hyperthyroidism may occur by chance,[20,21] Tolis *et al.*[16] have proposed that the following criteria should be fulfilled for the diagnosis of a thyrotropin-secreting pituitary tumor causing thyrotoxicosis:

1. Measurement of a supranormal serum TSH despite increased concentration of thyroid hormones.
2. Presence of a pituitary tumor.
3. Identification of thyrotopes in the tumor.
4. Disappearance of hyperthyroidism after removal of the pituitary tumor.

The *non*tumor patients reported with "TSH toxicosis" had all received prior treatment with ^{131}I or partial thyroidectomy for their hyperthyroidism, and in most instances the thyrotoxicosis had been difficult to control.[15] Unlike the case with the tumor patients, the α-subunit in these patients was normal and, along with the TSH, rose appropriately on TRH stimulation.[18] Partial suppression of TSH and ^{131}I uptake following T_3 administration occurs in this group.[22] The nature of the underlying pathophysiology in this group of patients is unknown. Whether these subjects harbor a microadenoma and might go on to develop frank evidence of a pituitary tumor later requires further follow-up. It seems likely that an altered set point for thyroid hormone–TSH interaction exists, and may reflect a state of resistance of the pituitary thyrotrope to feedback thyroid-hormone regulation.[22]

Unlike the group of patients described above who have clinical evidence of thyrotoxicosis and appear to have selective resistance at the pituitary level to thyroid hormone, patients have been described with a generalized tissue resistance to thyroid hormone, who, in spite of elevated circulating levels of thyroid hormone and inappropriately raised TSH concentrations, are clinically euthyroid or even mildly hypothyroid.[23,24] These patients demonstrate no evidence of a pituitary tumor.

2.4. Summary

The various disorders that give rise to elevated TSH levels are summarized in Table 1. Pituitary adenomas that secrete TSH are uncommon. Nevertheless, recognition of the various syndromes produced is important from the standpoint of patient management. The presence of an elevated TSH in a patient with an enlarge sella turcica and hypothyroidism may result from a primary disorder of the thyroid *per se* due to prolonged loss of negative feedback; these patients usually respond satisfactorily to thyroid-hormone suppression alone. In some patients with primary hypothalamic–pituitary disease, the raised serum TSH reflects concomitant primary thyroid failure, and in others the secretion of an IR-TRH with impaired biological activity. Some

TABLE 1. Conditions that Cause Elevated Serum TSH Levels

1. Primary hypothyroidism
   a. Thyrotrope hyperplasia (physiological)
   b. Adenomatous or neoplastic change of the thyrotrope
2. Primary hypothalamic–pituitary disease with hypothyroidism
   a. Concomitant primary thyroid disease
   b. Serum TSH is immuno- but not bioactive
   c. ??Hypothalamic disorder (?complete somatostatin deficiency with partial TRH deficiency)
3. Pituitary-TSH-induced hyperthyroidism ("TSH toxicosis")
   a. Pituitary adenoma (primary)
   b. "Nontumor" (?selective resistance of the thyrotrope to thyroid hormone; ??pituitary microadenoma)
4. Generalized tissue resistance to thyroid hormone (Refetoff's syndrome)

patients with pituitary adenomas secreting TSH develop thyrotoxicosis and need to be separated from a nontumorous variety wherein the pathophysiology appears to be a partial resistance at the pituitary level to thyroid-hormone suppression. A more generalized abnormality of tissue thyroid-hormone receptors also occurs, but these patients do not have symptoms or signs of thyrotoxicosis and are clinically euthyroid or slightly hypothyroid.

3. FSH- and LH-Secreting Pituitary Adenomas

Pituitary tumors that secrete gonadotropins have been reported rarely. This may be because they are uncommon or are poorly recognized. In this section, I will review the clinical and diagnostic features of these adenomas. Their importance lies in the fact that recognition provides a "tumor marker" that may be of much help in refining the efficacy of treatment and possibly aid in diagnosis.

3.1. Adenomas Associated with Chronic Hypogonadism

There is evidence that gonadectomy in certain strains of rodents leads to hyperplasia and later to neoplasia of pituitary gonadotropes,[25] in a manner analogous to the development of pituitary tumors that secrete TSH in experimental animals subjected to thyroidectomy. Similarly, in humans, long-standing hypogonadism has been reported to lead to pituitary adenoma formation.[1] Such pituitary tumors have been reported in both Klinefelter's syndrome[26] and Turne's syndrome.[27] In states of chronic hypogonadism, the diagnosis of a gonadotropin-secreting adenoma is difficult to establish, particularly early in its development, since elevation in serum gonadotropins is a physiological response to the abolition of the negative-feedback suppression from the gonad. Although an enlarged sella turcica in a patient with hypogonadism and elevated serum levels of FSH or LH or both suggests that a tumor of the gonadotropes has developed,[28,29] proof that the excess gonadotropin originated from the tumor, and not the nonadenomatous adjacent pituitary tissue, requires immunocytology of gonadotropic hormones in the tumor cell cytoplasm and/or demonstration of FSH and/or LH release by tumor cells in culture.[30,31]

Cunningham and Huckins[32] described a hypogonadal patient with a chromophobe adenoma of the pituitary who had normal-sized testes and elevated plasma levels of FSH and prolactin, but reduced LH and testosterone. Plasma FSH and LH increased following luteinizing-hormone-releasing hormone (LH-RH) administration, but FSH was not suppressed by exogenous testosterone. The patient described by Woolf and Schenk[31] was a 28-year-old man with a pituitary adenoma associated with an elevated serum FSH, reduced LH, and a slightly low testosterone of 235 ng/dl (normal: 300–1000 ng/dl). His testes were normal in size, and his sperm count was normal. The clinical findings in these two reports are somewhat reminiscent of the "fertile eunuch" syndrome,[33] a condition characterized by eunuchoidism with spermatogenesis and usually normal FSH levels, but low LH and testosterone. Indeed, the testicular biopsy in one of these cases showed a similar histology.[32] It remains possible that disordered testicular feedback in the "fertile eunuch" syndrome may occasionally lead to an FSH-secreting pituitary adenoma. Some patients with gonadotropin-secreting pituitary adenomas, apparently following prolonged hypogonadism, could have had a primary pituitary disorder in which there was secretion of an abnormal gonadotropin similar to that described for TSH. Although no definite example of such a tumor has been reported to date, a hypogonadal male, the product of a consanguineous mating, has been described with an elevated serum IR-LH that was biologically inactive.[34]

3.2. Primary Pituitary Adenomas That Secrete Gonadotropins

Recently, there have been a number of reports of gonadotropin-secreting tumors developing in males in whom there was no evidence of hypogonadism either preceding or at the time of presentation.[30] The ages of these patients have usually ranged from 45 to 65 years, and FSH has been the dominant gonadotropin secreted in most subjects.[35,30]

Snyder and Sterling[36] reported a patient (51-year-old male) with a pituitary adenoma that appeared to be hypersecreting both FSH and LH. Although serum concentrations of testosterone, free testosterone, and dihydrotestosterone were above normal, the patient had diminished libido possibly related to concomitant hyperprolactinemia. Serum LH and FSH increased in response to both LH-RH *and* TRH administration. In another case of an FSH- and LH-secreting pituitary adenoma in a 50-year-old male, libido and potency were well maintained and were associated with a normal sperm count and serum testosterone.[37] LH-RH administration in this case did not stimulate an increase in serum FSH or LH, although partial suppression to exogenous testosterone was demonstrated.[37]

Those conditions that give rise to excess circulating gonadotropins are summarized in Table 2. Fewer than ten patients in all have been described in

TABLE 2. Conditions that Cause Elevated Serum Gonadotropin Levels

1. Primary hypogonadism
   a. Gonadotrope hyperplasia (physiological)
   b. Adenomatous or neoplastic change of the gonadotrope
2. Primary pituitary adenoma
   a. FSH-secreting
   b. FSH- *and* LH-secreting[a]
3. Secretion of an abnormal gonadotropin that is immunoreactive but not bioactive[b]

[a] A gonadotropin-producing adenoma secreting solely LH has not been described to date.
[b] This syndrome might account for some cases of gonadotropin-secreting pituitary adenomas secondary to hypogonadism.

whom pituitary tumors have been clearly proven to secrete gonadotropin(s). These adenomas are difficult to diagnose primarily because they produce no easily recognizable clinical syndrome that readily separates them from nonfunctioning pituitary tumors. Most, if not all, patients with a gonadotropin-secreting tumor have presented late and usually because of visual-field defects.[38] Excluding those tumors associated with chronic primary hypogonadism, the presence of normal-size testes in a subject with an apparent nonfunctioning pituitary tumor should alert the physician to the possibility of a gonadotropin-secreting tumor. Many of these patients have diminished libido, and in these circumstances, the tumor is predominantly FSH-secreting,[31,32,35] In some cases, the etiology of the pituitary adenoma may be related to antecedent testosterone deficiency (?a form of the "fertile eunuch" syndrome), but in other cases, the FSH-secreting adenoma is clearly primary. One of the cases described by Kovacs *et al.*[30] presented with impotence, high serum FSH, and low serum testosterone; following resection of the pituitary tumor, the serum testosterone level rose to normal and sexual potency returned. Those patients in whom the tumor secreted both FSH and LH demonstrated either normal[37,38] or diminished[36] libido and potency. Increased testosterone levels[36] did not ensure normal sexual function. No cases of heightened sexual activity associated with gonadotropin-secreting pituitary adenomas have been reported.

The degree of autonomy of these tumors varies. Following LH-RH stimulation, serum FSH and LH have shown an enhanced,[30,36] blunted,[35] or absent response. Partial suppression of one or both of the gonadotropins occurred with exogenous testosterone.[35,37]

3.3. Summary

Pituitary adenomas that secrete gonadotropins are very rare. Such tumors have been reported in cases of long-standing hypogonadism. It is assumed that the prolonged hyperplasia of the gonadotropes subsequently results in adenomatous change. Primary tumors of the pituitary that secrete gonadotropins, usually FSH alone but occasionally accompanied by LH, have been described in older males in whom there is no antecedent hypogonadism. The clinical syndrome is similar to that found in nonfunctioning tumors.

Libido and sexual function are frequently diminished, occasionally preserved, but never enhanced. Recognition of the nature of these adenomas will provide a tumor marker.

References

1. J.E. Caughey, The aetiology of pituitary tumours: The role of hypogonadism, *Australas. Ann. Med.* **6:**93, 1957.
2. B. Niépce, Traite due goitre et du crétinisme, suivi de la statistique des goitreux et des crétins dans le basin del'Isere en Savoie, dans les departements de l'Isere, des Hautes-Alpes et de Basses-Alpes, Balliere, Paris, 1851.
3. T. Yamada, T. Tsukui, K. Ikejiri, Y. Yukimura, and M. Kotani, Volume of sella turcica in normal subjects and in patients with primary hypothyroidism and hyperthyroidism, *J. Clin. Endocrinol. Metab.* **42:**817, 1976.
4. S.T. Bigos, E.C. Ridgway, I.A. Kourides, and F. Maloof, Spectrum of pituitary alterations with mild and severe thyroid impairment, *J. Clin. Endocrinol. Metab.* **46:**317, 1978.
5. I.M.D. Jackson, Pituitary enlargment resulting from primary thyroid disease, *Proc. R. Soc. Med.* **63:**578, 1970.
6. J. Furth, J.N. Dent, W.T. Burnett, and E.L. Gadsden, The mechanism of induction and the characteristics of pituitary tumors induced by thyroidectomy, *J. Clin. Endocrinol. Metab.* **15:**81, 1955.
7. A.G. Vagenakis, K. Dole, and L.E. Braverman, Pituitary enlargement, pituitary failure and primary hypothyroidism, *Ann. Intern. Med.* **85:**195, 1976.
8. J.J. Van Wyck and M.M. Grumbach, Syndrome of precocious menstruation and galactorrhea in juvenile hypothyroidism: An example of hormonal overlap in pituitary feedback, *J. Pediatr.* **57:**416, 1960.
9. T.F. Davies, B.R. Smith, and R. Hall, Binding of thyroid stimulators to guinea pig testis and thyroid, *Endocrinology* **103:**6, 1978.
10. S.M. Amir, R.C. Sullivan, and S.H. Ingbar, Binding of bovine thyrotropin to receptors in rat testis and its interaction with gonadotropins, *Endocrinology* **103:**111, 1978.
11. G. Faglia, P. Beck-Peccoz, C. Gerrari, B. Ambrosi, A. Spada, P. Travaglini, and S. Paracchi, Plasma thyrotropin response to thyrotropin-releasing hormone in patients with pituitary and hypothalamic disorders, *J. Clin. Endocrinol. Metab.* **37:**595, 1973.
12. Y.C. Patel and H.G. Burger, Serum thyrotropin (TSH) in pituitary and/or hypothalamic hypothyroidism: Normal or elevated levels and paradoxical response to thyrotropin-releasing hormone, *J. Clin. Endocrinol. Metab.* **37:**190, 1973.
13. V.B. Peterson, A.M. McGregor, P.E. Belchetz, R.S. Elkeles, and R. Hall, The secretion of thyrotrophin with impaired biological activity in patients with hypothalamic–pituitary disease, *Clin. Endocrinol.* **8:**397, 1978.
14. A. Arimura and A.V. Schally, Increase in basal and thyrotropin-releasing hormone (TRH)–stimulated secretion of thyrotropin (TSH) by passive immunization with antiserum to somatostatin in rats, *Endocrinology* **98:**1069, 1976.
15. D.S. Cooper, E.C. Ridgway, and F. Maloof, Unusual types of hyperthyroidism, *Clin. Endocrinol. Metab.* **7:**199, 1978.
16. G. Tolis, C. Bird, G. Bertrand, J.M. McKenzie, and C. Ezrin, Pituitary hyperthyroidism—case report and review of the literature, *Am. J. Med.* **64:**177, 1978.
17. M.M. Kaplan and R.D. Utiger, Diagnosis of hyperthyroidism, *Clin. Endocrinol. Metab.* **7:**97, 1978.
18. I.A. Kourides, E.C. Ridgway, B.D. Weintraub, S.T. Bigos, M.C. Gershengorn, and F. Maloof, Thyrotropin induced hyperthyroidism: Use of alpha and beta subunit levels to identify patients with pituitary tumors, *J. Clin. Endocrinol. Metab.* **45:**534, 1977.
19. K. Horn, F. Erhardt, R. Fahlbusch, C.R. Pickhardt, K. von Werder, and P.C. Scriba, Recurrent

goiter, hyperthyroidism, galactorrhea and amenorrhea due to thyrotropin and prolactin-producing pituitary tumor, *J. Clin. Endocrinol. Metab.* **43:**137, 1976.

20. L. Carneiro, K.J. Dorrington, and D.S. Munro, Relation between long-acting thyroid stimulator and thyroid function in thyrotoxicosis, *Lancet* **2:**878, 1966.
21. G. Burke, Hyperthyrodism and demonstration of circulating long-acting thyroid stimulator following hypophysectomy for chromophobe adenoma, *J. Clin. Endocrinol. Metab.* **27:**1161, 1967.
22. M.C. Gershengorn and B.D. Weintraub, Thyrotropin-induced hyperthyroidism caused by selective pituitary resistance to thyroid hormone: A new syndrome of "inappropriate secretion of TSH," *J. Clin. Invest.* **56:**633, 1975.
23. S. Refetoff, L.T. DeWing, and L.S. DeGroot, Familial syndrome combining deaf-mutism, stippled epiphyses, goiter and abnormally high PBI: Possible target organ refractoriness to thyroid hormone, *J. Clin. Endocrinol. Metab.* **27:**279, 1967.
24. B.-A. Lamberg, Congenital euthyroid goitre and partial peripheral resistance to thyroid hormones, *Lancet* **1:**854, 1973.
25. W.E. Griesbach and H.D. Purves, Basophil adenomata in the rat hypophysis after gonadectomy, *Br. J. Cancer* **14:**49, 1960.
26. A.S. Burt, L. Reiner, R.B. Cohen, and R.C. Sniffen, Klinefelter's syndrome: Report of an autopsy, with particular reference to the histology and histochemistry of the endocrine glands, *J. Clin. Endocrinol. Metab.* **14:**719, 1954.
27. L.W. Kelly, Jr., Ovarian dwarfism with pituitary tumor, *J. Clin. Endocrinol. Metab.* **23:**50, 1963.
28. S.J. Gordon and A.M. Moses, Multiple endocrine organ refractories to trophic hormone stimulation: A patient with an enlarged sella turcica and increased FSH secretion, *Ann. Intern. Med.* **63:**313, 1965.
29. B.F. Bower, Pituitary enlargement secondary to untreated primary hypogonadism, *Ann. Intern. Med.* **69:**107, 1968.
30. K. Kovacs, E. Horvath, G.R. VanLoon, N.B. Newcastle, C. Ezrin, and A.A. Rosenbloom, Pituitary adenomas associated with elevated blood follicle–stimulating hormone levels: A histologic, immunocytologic and electron microscopic study of two cases, *Fertil. Steril.* **29:**622, 1978.
31. P.D. Woolf and E.A. Schenk, An FSH-producing pituitary tumor in a patient with hypogonadism, *J. Clin. Endocrinol. Metab.* **38:**561, 1974.
32. G.R. Cunningham and C. Huckins, An FSH and prolactin-secreting pituitary tumor: Pituitary dynamics and testicular histology, *J. Clin. Endocrinol. Metab.* **44:**248–253, 1977.
33. E.P. McCullagh, J.C. Beck, and C.A. Schaffenburg, A syndrome of eunuchoidism with spermatogenesis, normal urinary FSH and low or normal ICSH: "Fertile eunuchs," *J. Clin. Endocrinol. Metab.* **13:**489, 1953.
34. L. Axelrod, R.M. Neer, and B. Kliman, Hypogonadism in a male with immunologically active, biologically inactive luteinizing hormone: An exception to a venerable rule, *Clin. Res.* **26:**610A, 1978.
35. J.N. Friend, D.M. Judge, B.M. Sherman, and R.J. Santen, FSH-secreting pituitary adenomas: Stimulation and suppression studies in two patients, *J. Clin. Endocrinol. Metab.* **43:**650, 1976.
36. P.J. Snyder and F.H. Sterling, Hypersecretion of LH and FSH by a pituitary adenoma, *J. Clin. Endocrinol. Metab.* **42:**544, 1976.
37. R. Demura, O. Kubo, H. Demura, and K. Shizume, FSH and LH secreting pituitary adenoma, *J. Clin. Endocrinol. Metab.* **45:**653, 1977.
38. R. Luboshitzky and D. Barzilai, Suprasellar extension of tumour associated with increased cerebrospinal fluid activity of LH and FSH, *Acta Endocrinol. (Copenhagen)* **87:**673, 1978.

9

Nonsecreting Adenomas

MARK E. MOLITCH

1. Introduction

Pituitary adenomas that are not hormone-secreting are probably the most common pituitary tumors and may be present in as much as 10–25% of the population. Although the vast majority of such tumors are completely asymptomatic, some patients with large tumors present with visual-field disturbances, headaches, or hypopituitarism. The introduction of the newer radiographic techniques of tomography of the sella at 1 to 2-mm cuts using hypocycloidal movement has brought forth the information that we may now be able to diagnose nonfunctioning microadenomas in patients.

2. Prevalence

In 1936, Costello[1] reported a remarkable study of autopsy examinations of the pituitary from the Mayo Clinic. This series consisted of 1000 pituitaries obtained in the course of routine postmortem examination; none of the patients was known to have clinically significant pituitary disease (as far as was known in 1936). In these 1000 pituitaries, Costello found adenomas in 225 with a prevalence of up to 35–40% in the 50 to 60-year-old age group. There was no sex difference in the frequency of tumors. Although specific information on size was not provided, Costello stated that the "majority of adenomas were found to be 1.5 mm or larger in diameter." The only other series comparable in size in the literature is the study of the pituitaries in 1600 consecutive autopsies at the University of Iowa by McCormick and Halmi.[2] Adenomas were found in 145 of these 1600 pituitaries, and of these, 3 patients were known to have had acromegaly and 2 patients were known to have had Cushing's disease. Therefore, 140 of the 1600 pituitaries (8.8%) were thought to

MARK E. MOLITCH • Tufts University School of Medicine; Department of Medicine, Division of Endocrinology, Tufts–New England Medical Center Hospital, Boston, Massachusetts 02111.

contain nonfunctioning tumors. In this series, tumors varied "from a fraction of a millimeter to 10 mm in diameter." Another study of only 50 pituitaries examined at autopsy revealed 8 (16%) to have microadenomas, mostly less than 1 mm in diameter.[3]

It is apparent from these studies, therefore, that 9–25% of pituitaries may harbor adenomas that are usually microadenomas (10 mm). These studies all predate the availability of the prolactin radioimmunoassay, and it is not clear how many of these tumors were functional, secreting prolactin. Recently, studies of 98 patients with abnormal sellas by polytomography have shown that 72 (74%) had hyperprolactinemia.[4,5] However, most of these patients presented because of galactorrhea, amenorrhea, or impotence, so that these series are biased toward finding patients with hyperprolactinemia. Undoubtedly, most nonfunctioning small adenomas go unrecognized.

In our own ongoing series of patients presenting with galactorrhea (for details of the studies performed on the first 70 patients in this series, see Chapter 4), we have found abnormal sella polytomograms in a substantial portion of women with normal prolactin blood levels. In Fig. 1, the number of patients with normal and abnormal polytomograms is shown with regard to prolactin levels. Of the 63 patients presenting with galactorrhea and prolactin levels under 20 ng/ml, 30% had abnormal sella turcicas by tomography. The findings on these tomograms were predominantly those of focal erosion or bulging, or both, and were comparable to those seen in our hyperprolactinemic patients who had had surgical removal of tumors found at similar sites of tomographic abnormalities. It is unclear at present what the true nature of these tomographic abnormalities is in our normoprolactinemic patients with galactorrhea (the majority of whom had normal menses). The fact that these abnormalities are the same as in those patients with surgically verified prolactin-secreting adenomas would suggest that they indeed repre-

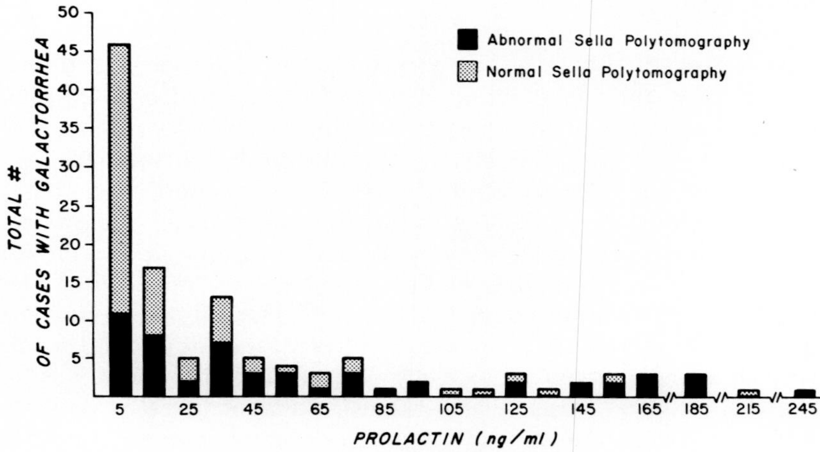

Fig. 1. Frequency of abnormal sella polytomograms occurring in patients with galactorrhea according to serum prolactin levels. The upper limit of normal of prolactin in this assay is 25 ng/ml. From R. Goodman, B. Biller, M. Molitch, Z. Feldman, K. Post, S. Wolpert, and S. Reichlin (unpublished data).

sent adenomas most of the time. However, it is unclear whether they are (1) nonsecreting microadenomas found incidentally in the evaluation of patients with galactorrhea or (2) microadenomas secreting prolactin in low amounts. The large percentage of women in our series who may have nonsecreting microadenomas is compatible with the autopsy studies of Costello[1] mentioned above. Only surgical exploration of these women would provide adequate proof for the suggestion that all these women with tomographic abnormalities harbor nonsecreting microadenomas, but we have not felt that surgical exploration or other ablative therapy was justified in these women. Recently, Geehr *et al.*[6] studied a group of 15 normoprolactinemic patients with galactorrhea or amenorrhea or both and only minimal tomographic abnormalities; surgical exploration in 6 cases revealed microadenomas in all,[6] lending support to our own findings.

3. Presentation

Nonsecreting pituitary adenomas are diagnosed only because of the mass effects of the adenomas, and these mass effects can be symptomatic or asymptomatic. The symptomatic mass effects are due to pressure effects on adjacent structures giving rise to visual-field defects from optic-nerve impingement, ophthalmoplegias from cavernous sinus compression and cranial nerve damage, varying degrees of hypopituitarism from either pressure on the adjacent normal pituitary or interference with blood flow in the portal vessels of the stalk, and headache. Clearly, all these effects can occur in hormone-secreting tumors as well. Often, the clinical manifestations of the hormone oversecretion of these tumors (i.e., acromegaly, Cushing's disease, and galactorrhea–amenorrhea–impotence) bring the patient to a physician's attention before the tumors grow large and therefore only in the early stages of the mass effects. Patients of both sexes with growth hormone (GH)- and ACTH-secreting tumors and women with prolactinomas often have small tumors that may be visible only on detailed polytomography. Non-hormone-secreting tumors, however, are usually large enough to be easily visualized on plain skull films by the time they produce visual-field defects, ophthalmoplegia, headaches, or hypopituitarism. The nonsecreting "microadenomas" are usually asymptomatic, as noted above, although they may present in association with galactorrhea in some patients.

Frequently, patients will have only mild headaches or be completely asymptomatic, and an enlarged sella is found incidentally on skull films taken for some nonrelated reason. In the series of 100 patients with enlarged sellas evaluated by Weissberg *et al.*,[7] 18 patients were completely asymptomatic; 27 of these 100 patients had adenomas that were not secreting GH or ACTH, and 4 of these were completely asymptomatic. Overall, about 10–15% of patients with nonsecreting adenomas big enough to cause sella abnormalities on routine skull films have been found to be asymptomatic, 50–60% to have visual-field defects, 10–15% to have extraocular muscle palsy, and 20–50% to have varying degrees of hypopituitarism (more precise figures are hard to obtain because most of the patients in each series were studied prior to the introduction of the prolactin radioimmunoassay, and therefore the "hypogonadism" said to be present could have been due to hyperprolactinemia in some cases).[7–9]

4. Differential Diagnosis

The differential diagnosis of the causes of an enlarged sella in patients without hormonal oversecretion (with or without other symptoms) is extensive (see Chapter 10). In the series of Weissberg *et al.*,[7] of the 65 patients who did not have visual abnormalities, acromegaly, or Cushing's disease and in whom diagnoses were obtained, 27 had primary intrasellar tumors, 25 had the empty sella syndrome, and 13 had primary extrasellar conditions (craniopharyngioma, 2; chordoma, 2; sarcoidosis, 2; hydrocephalus, 2; metastases to sella, 1; eosinophilic granuloma, 1; atypical pinealoma, 1; parasellar meningioma, 1; and pseudotumor cerebri, 1). Other rare causes of an enlarged sella include astrocytoma, glioma, ganglioneuroma, sarcoma, choroid plexus papilloma of the 4th ventricle, ophthalmic artery aneurysm,[8] aneurysm of the internal carotid artery,[10] Rathke's cleft cyst,[11] pituitary abscess,[12] and primary arachnoid cyst of the sella.[13]

The most common and therefore the most important entities that can cause confusion in the diagnosis of nonsecreting adenomas are craniopharyngiomas and the empty sella syndrome. In the series of Kurnick *et al.*,[8] craniopharyngiomas were one third as common as pituitary tumors, but in the series of Weissberg *et al.*,[7] they were only one thirteenth as common. In addition to causing erosion and enlargement of the sella, craniopharyngiomas cause visual-field abnormalities in 70–80%, extraocular muscle palsy in 10–20%, varying degrees of hypopituitarism in 40–50%, and headaches in 70–80% of cases, figures similar to those given for nonsecreting adenomas[8,14,15] (see Chapter 10).

The empty sella syndrome has been found to be as common as pituitary adenomas by Weissberg *et al.*[7] In this syndrome, the sella is partially filled with CSF, which can be demonstrated as air filling this "empty" space on pneumoencephalography. The empty sella syndrome is believed to develop either as a result of the spontaneous infarction of either normal or tumorous pituitary or as a result of the transmission of CSF pressure through a defective sellar diaphragm.[16] In this syndrome, the sella is usually symmetrically enlarged without focal erosions, but many cases will have irregularly enlarged sellas with areas of erosion,[16] thus mimicking adenomas. In patients with this syndrome, visual-field defects are uncommon but may occur due to herniation of the optic nerves into the sella.[17] Varying degrees of hypopituitarism can be demonstrated in 30–40% of cases on detailed testing, but clinically evident hypopituitarism is much less common.[7,16,18] Headaches are present in 50–70% of cases,[7,16] The true incidence of headache is unknown, however, because in many cases the diagnosis is first made during the evaluation of headache (see Chapter 10).

The finding of an empty sella does not exclude the presence of an adenoma in the pituitary tissue lining the wall of the sella. Adenomas secreting GH,[19] ACTH,[20] and prolactin[21,22] coexisting with partially empty sellas have been described in several cases. Obviously, nonsecreting tumors must also coexist with empty sellas in some cases but these small adenomas are probably of no clinical consequence, since the "empty" portion of the sella allows room for considerable expansion before the mass effects would be of concern.

5. Evaluation

All patients with an enlarged sella require a careful endocrine evaluation (see Chapter 11) to exclude hypersecretion syndromes as well as to ascertain deficiencies of pituitary function. Hypopituitarism found in a patient with a nonsecreting adenoma would indicate some degree of aggressiveness on the part of the adenoma and may argue for ablative intervention. The finding of some degree of hypopituitarism does not help in distinguishing between a nonsecreting adenoma and a craniopharyngioma, an empty sella, or other intrasellar lesions. The presence of diabetes insipidus, on the other hand, is more in favor of the lesion's being a craniopharyngioma.[8] Visual-field abnormalities are often seen with adenomas and craniopharyngiomas, but are rarely seen with patients with the empty sella syndrome[7,16] (see Table 1).

Neuroradiographic procedures are almost always necessary to differentiate between a nonsecreting adenoma, an empty sella, a craniopharyngioma, and other lesions. Plain skull films and even polytomography are not usually helpful in this regard except that calcifications are usually seen in craniopharyngiomas and are uncommonly seen in adenomas. However, the lack of any focal erosions is in favor of an empty sella. Computerized tomography (CT) has been found to be helpful in the diagnosis of both the empty sella[23] and craniopharyngiomas.[24] However, tumors with necrotic centers are often difficult to distinguish from empty sellas by CT, and pneumoencephalography is often necessary to make this distinction.[23] Both CT and pneumoencephalography are very helpful in diagnosing suprasellar extension of a tumor (as discussed in Chapters 10 and 14). Arteriography is required to exclude an aneurysm and may be helpful in the evaluation of a meningioma or a chordoma as the cause of the enlarged sella.

Even with complete endocrinological, ophthalmological, and radio-

TABLE 1. Evaluation of the Enlarged Sella Turcia: Useful Features in Differential Diagnosis

	Nonsecreting adenoma	Empty sella	Craniopharyngioma	Other
Hypopituitarism	++	+	++	++
Diabetes insipidus	±	−	++	+
Abnormal visual fields	++	±	++	++
Ballooned sella without erosion	−	++	−	−
Suprasellar extension on CT	+	−	++	++
Calcification	+	−	+++	+

graphic evaluation, it is occasionally very difficult to distinguish between an intrasellar craniopharyngioma and a nonsecreting adenoma. In such cases, only the pathological examination of tissue obtained at surgery will make the correct diagnosis.

6. Therapy

The natural history of nonsecreting adenomas is not well understood, and therefore the therapy directed against such adenomas may vary, depending on the presentation. At present, we favor transsphenoidal surgery for those tumors associated with visual-field abnormalities, significant suprasellar extension (by CT or pneumoencephalography) without visual-field abnormalities, and sphenoid sinus extension. Tumors that remain intrasellar but are large and cause substantial bone erosion may be treated surgically or with irradiation. Adenomas with a great degree of suprasellar extension, a dumbbell shape, or significant lateral extension may require a subfrontal approach. The results achieved by the combination of surgery and irradiation appear to be better than for either procedure used alone,[25,26] and for this reason we usually recommend routine irradiation after the surgical removal of nonfunctioning adenomas (see Chapters 16 and 21). The therapeutic approach to patients with modest sella enlargement due to a nonsecreting adenoma and without visual-field impairment is controversial. The most useful data on the long-term follow-up of such patients come from Sheline.[27] In this series, of eight patients who initially had normal visual fields, three did not develop any change in sella size or visual fields, three had further enlargement of the sella and required treatment after several years, and two developed visual-field defects at 1 and 5 years of follow-up. Of eight patients who initially had abnormal visual fields, the field defects became larger in five, and in three, both the field defects and the sellas enlarged over several years. Because of these findings, we recommend ablative therapy, usually surgery or radiotherapy, for most younger patients with nonsecreting adenomas and sella enlargement on routine skull films but no visual field abnormalities. In older patients or in those with complicating illness, we have adopted a policy of careful observation, including repeated visual-field examinations and sella X-rays at 6-month intervals for the first year, yearly intervals for the next 2 years, and then every 2–3 years thereafter. If the sella enlarges or visual-field defects develop, we then recommend ablative therapy. However, irradiation may also be employed in such patients from the outset. In patients with suspected nonsecreting "microadenomas," we have also adopted a conservative policy of observation with repeat polytomography at yearly intervals for 2 years, then at 2-year intervals for 4 years, and then every 3–5 years thereafter. It is too soon to know how many of these "microadenomas" will enlarge. If after 5 years no enlargement has been found, then a reassessment as to the necessity for repeated tomography will be needed. One potential complication of this conservative approach toward both micro- and macroadenomas is the possibility of hemorrhagic infarction of the tumor resulting in pituitary apoplexy. Although apoplexy usually occurs in the setting of radiotherapy of the tumor, it can happen spontaneously.[28] Such patients usually present with severe headache, visual-field impairment, and occasionally impaired consciousness and vascular collapse. Although corticosteroid administration and surgical decompression are usually successful, deaths have occurred.[28]

7. Summary

Nonsecreting adenomas are the most common pituitary adenomas, and they may be present in up to 20–25% of the population as has been found in autopsy series. Although the larger adenomas often present with visual-field defects and varying degrees of hypopituitarism, these tumors are not infrequently silent and may be picked up only incidentally on skull films taken for other reasons. When evaluating patients with enlarged sellas, endocrine testing may reveal hormone oversecretion or hypopituitarism in varying degrees. However, neuroradiographic procedures such as CT, pneumoencephalography, and arteriography may be necessary to exclude the empty sella syndrome, craniopharyngiomas, and a variety of other lesions that may mimic an adenoma. Therapy of the tumor is always necessary when vision is threatened or when the tumors are very large. With small intrasellar tumors, although a conservative approach may be warranted, careful follow-up with X-rays and visual-field examinations is mandatory to allow ablative therapy should there be signs of tumor enlargement. Finally, sella polytomograms obtained in the course of the evaluation of galactorrhea, amenorrhea, or hypopituitarism may now be able to delineate nonsecreting microadenomas; the natural history of such lesions at present is unknown, and a conservative approach to therapy is indicated.

References

1. R.T. Costello, Subclinical adenoma of the pituitary gland, *Am. J. Pathol.* **12:**205, 1936.
2. W.F. McCormick and N.S. Halmi, Absence of chromophobe adenomas from a large series of pituitary tumors, *Arch. Pathol.* **92:**231, 1971.
3. M.S.F. McLachlan, E.D. Williams, R.W. Fortt, and F.H. Doyle, Estimation of pituitary gland dimensions from radiographs of the sella turcica: A postmortem study, *Br. J. Radiol.* **41:**323, 1968.
4. S. Nader, K. Mashiter, F.H. Doyle, and G.F. Joplin, Galactorrhea, hyperprolactinaemia and pituitary tumours in the female, *Clin. Endocrinol.* **5:**245, 1976.
5. S. Franks, J.D.N. Nabarro, and H.S. Jacobs, Prevalence and presentation of hyperprolactinemia in patients with "functionless" pituitary tumours, *Lancet* **1:**778, 1977.
6. R.B. Geehr, W.E. Allen III, S.L.G. Rothman, and D.D. Spencer, Pluridirectional tomography in the evaluation of the evaluation of pituitary tumors, *Am. J. Roentgenol. Radium Ther. Nucl. Med.* **130:**105, 1978.
7. L.A. Weissberg, E.A. Zimmerman, and A.G. Frantz, Diagnosis and evaluation of patients with an enlarged sella turcica, *Am. J. Med.* **61:**590, 1976.
8. J.E. Kurnick, C.R. Hartman, E.G. Lufkin, and F.D. Hofeldt, Abnormal sella turcica: A tumor board review of the clinical significance, *Arch. Intern. Med.* **137:**111 1977.
9. U. Batzdorf and W.E. Stern, Clinical manifestations of pituitary adenomas: A pilot study using computer analysis, in: *Diagnosis and Treatment of Pituitary Tumors* (P.D. Kohler and G.T. Ross, eds.), p. 17, American Elsevier, New York, 1973.

10. J. Dussault, C. Plamondon, and R. Volpe, Aneurysms of the internal carotid artery stimulating pituitary tumours, *Can. Med. Assoc. J.* **101**:785, 1969.
11. S. Concha, B.P.M. Hamilton, J.C. Millan, and J.D. McQueen, Symptomatic Rathke's cleft cyst with amyloid stroma, *J. Neurol. Neurosurg. Psychiatry* **38**:782, 1975.
12. P.D. Mohr, Hypothalamic-pituitary abscess, *Postgrad. Med. J.* **51**:468, 1975.
13. B.A. Ring and M. Waddington, Primary arachnoid cysts of the sella turcica, *Am. J. Roentgenol. Radium Ther. Nucl. Med.* **98**:611, 1966.
14. J.R. Bartlett, Craniopharyngiomas—a summary of 85 cases, *J. Neurol. Neurosurg. Psychiatry* **34**:37, 1971.
15. A.S. Lichter, W.M. Wara, G.E. Sheline, J.J. Townsend, and C.B. Wilson, The treatment of craniopharygiomas, *Int. J. Radiat. Oncol. Biol. Phys.* **2**:675, 1977.
16. F.A. Neelon, J.A. Gorce, and H.E. Lebovitz, The primary empty sella: Clinical and radiographic characteristics and endocrine function, *Medicine* **52**:73, 1973.
17. M.T. Buckman, M. Husain, T.J. Carlow, and G.T. Peake, Primary empty sella syndrome with visual field defects, *Am. J. Med.* **61**:124, 1976.
18. R. Brisman, J.E.O. Hughes, and D.A. Holub, Endocrine function in nineteen patients with empty sella syndrome, *J. Clin. Endocrinol. Metab.* **34**:570, 1972.
19. M.E. Molitch, G.B. Hieshima, S. Marcovitz, I.M.D. Jackson, and S. Wolpert, Coexisting primary empty sella syndrome and acromegaly, *Clin. Endocrinol.* **7**:261, 1977.
20. A Ganguly, J.B. Stanchfield, T.S. Roberts, C.D. West, and F.H. Tyler, Cushing's syndrome in a patient with an empty sella turcia and a microadenoma of the adenohypophysis, *Am. J. Med.* **60**:306, 1976.
21. T.J. Sutton and J.L. Vezina, Co-existing pituitary adenoma and intrasellar arachnoid invagination, *Am. J. Roentgenol. Radium Ther. Nucl. Med.* **122**:508, 1974.
22. J.N. Domingue, S.D. Wing, and C.B. Wilson, Coexisting pituitary adenomas and partially empty sellas, *J. Neurosurg.* **48**:23, 1978.
23. R. Rozario, S. Hammerschlag, K.D. Post, S.M. Wolpert, and I. Jackson, Diagnosis of empty sella with CT scan, *Neuroradiology* **13**:85, 1977.
24. C.R. Fitz, G. Wortzman, D.C. Harwood-Nash, R.C. Holgate, J.F. Barry, and D.W. Boldt, Computed tomography in craniopharyngiomas, *Radiology* **127**:687, 1978.
25. G.E. Sheline, Treatment of chromophobe adenomas of the pituitary gland and acromegaly, in: *Diagnosis and Treatment of Pituitary Tumors* (P.D. Kohler and G.T. Ross, eds.), p. 201, American Elsevier, New York, 1973.
26. N. Urdanetta, H. Chessin, and J.J. Fischer, Pituitary adenomas and craniopharyngiomas; analysis of 99 cases treated with radiation therapy, *Int. J. Radiat. Oncol. Biol. Phys.* **1**:895, 1976.
27. G.E. Sheline, Untreated and recurrent chromophobe adenomas of the pituitary, *Am J. Roentgenol. Radium Ther. Nucl. Med.* **112**:768, 1971.
28. L.A. Weissberg, Pituitary apoplexy, *Am. J. Med.* **63**:109, 1977.

10

Sellar and Parasellar Lesions Mimicking Adenoma

KALMON D. POST and DAVID L. KASDON

1. Introduction

Many parasellar lesions, tumor and nontumor, may mimic pituitary adenomas clinically, endocrinologically, and radiologically (Table 1). From a review of the Mayo Clinic parasellar lesions series, Thomas and Yoss[1] concluded that the etiological diagnosis of parasellar lesions is not made on clinical grounds, but rather on adjunctive examinations such as blood tests, plain skull X-rays, tomograms, and contrast studies. However, certain clinical patterns do, at times, lead suspicion toward the correct diagnosis, while at other times, even with appropriate tests, the diagnosis may be difficult. For most of these lesions, the treatment of choice is distinctly different from that of a pituitary tumor, and therefore correct diagnosis is of paramount importance. After a brief general discussion of the presenting symptoms and signs of tumors in this region, as well as the radiological manifestations, some specific discussion and examples of these entities will be presented.

2. Symptoms and Signs of Parasellar and Intrasellar Nonpituitary Lesions

Nonpituitary lesions commonly present symptoms of endocrinological abnormality. Unlike pituitary adenomas, which may manifest either hypersecretion or hyposecretion of the pituitary, the nonpituitary lesions have decreased pituitary function, if endocrine abnormalities are present at all. Intrasellar cysts or the empty sella syndrome may bring the patient to the doctor because of pituitary insufficiency, often first manifested by gonadotropin fail-

KALMON D. POST and DAVID L. KASDON • Tufts University School of Medicine; Department of Neurosurgery, Tufts–New England Medical Center Hospital, Boston, Massachusetts 02111. Dr. Kasdon's present address is: Department of Neurosurgery, Wilford Hall Medical Center, Lackland Air Force Base, San Antonio, Texas 78213.

TABLE 1. Classification of Parasellar and Intrasellar Nonpituitary Lesions

I. Cell rest tumors
- a. Craniopharyngioma
- b. Rathke's cleft cyst
- c. Epidermoid (cholesteatoma)
- d. Infundibuloma
- e. Chordoma
- f. Lipoma
- g. Colloid cyst

II. Primitive–germ-cell tumors
- a. Germinoma
- b. Dermoid
- c. Teratoma
- d. Atypical teratoma (dysgerminoma)
- e. Ectopic pinealoma

III. Gliomas
- a. Chiasmatic–optic glioma (astrocytoma, hypothalamic glioma)
- b. Oligodendroglioma
- c. Ependymoma
- d. Infundibuloma
- e. Astrocytoma
- f. Microglioma

IV. Benign lesions
- a. Meningioma (olfactory, tuberculum, diaphragma, sphenoid wing)
- b. Enchondroma

V. Metastatic tumors

VI. Vascular lesions

VII. Granulomatous and infectious
- a. Pituitary abscess, bacterial and fungal
- b. Sarcoid
- c. Tuberculosis
- d. Echinococcal cyst
- e. Mucocele (sphenoid)
- f. Histiocytosis X

VIII. Miscellaneous (CSF-related)
- a. Benign intracranial hypertension (pseudotumor cerebri)
- b. Empty sella syndrome
- c. Arachnoid cyst
- d. Suprasellar–chiasmatic arachnoiditis

ure. Suprasellar lesions, such as arachnoid cysts, meningiomas, and craniopharyngiomas, may present similarly. Failure of growth hormone (GH) secretion and secondary sexual development may be seen in lesions compressing the hypothalamus or the infundibulum.[2] The wasted, underdeveloped, sexually immature child with a hypothalamic tumor (diencephalic syndrome) is perhaps the most dramatic example of endocrine failure from a suprasellar tumor.[3] Abnormalities of the ventromedial and ventrolateral hypothalamus causing abnormalities of appetite-controlling areas can cause syndromes of polyphagia causing massive obesity, or severe starvation.[4] Diabetes insipidus may be the initial symptom in suprasellar lesions that compress the pituitary stalk or the paraventricular region of the third ventricle. More often, vasopressin deficiency is only partial and the patient is aware only of an increased thirst, the presence of diabetes insipidus becoming evident only after water-deprivation studies.[5] Inappropriate antidiuretic secretion causing water retention and severe hyponatremia also occurs.

Occasionally, an intrasellar or suprasellar nonpituitary lesion can present with increased prolactin secretion. Suprasellar meningiomas, craniopharyngiomas, and cystic lesions have been described with elevated prolactin levels thought to be secondary to interference with transport of prolactin-inhibitory factor (PIF).[6] The empty sella syndrome is often associated with hyperprolactinemia, though this may, in some cases, be due to an associated small pituitary adenoma.[7] Adenomas secreting GH,[8,9] ACTH,[10] and prolactin[9,11] coexisting with partially empty sellas have also been described.

The close relationship of the optic nerves, chiasma, and optic tracts to the sella turcica is responsible for the great number of patients with lesions in this location who have visual loss as the presenting symptom.[12] In many instances, the onset of visual loss is insidious and progresses so slowly that it is not noticed until severe field deficits are present. In children, virtual blindness has occurred secondary to compression by lesions such as craniopharyngiomas before the parents or schoolteachers were aware that the child had any visual difficulty whatsoever. Lesions that are anterior to the chiasma, such as meningiomas of the optic nerve sheath, can produce unilateral visual loss. Lesions within the sella, such as the empty sella syndrome and Rathke's cleft cysts, can produce the typical bitemporal field deficit associated with chiasmal distortion from below. Aneurysms, meningiomas, and other lesions in the suprasellar area can present with bitemporal field cuts of the classic superior chiasmal compression variety. Lesions involving the chiasma itself, such as gliomas or arachnoidal adhesions in the chiasmatic cistern from arachnoiditis, may present with bizarre visual deficits. Meningiomas or aneurysms compressing the visual system more posteriorly along the optic tract can produce homonymous hemianopsias that are characteristically incongruous (in contradistinction to the more symmetrical, congruous hemianopsias of occipital lobe lesions). Parasellar lesions can also affect the visual apparatus indirectly because of increased intracranial pressure as with benign intracranial hypertension or with tumors causing obstruction of CSF flow. These lesions can become manifest by transient visual obscurations secondary to the increased intracranial pressure. Papilledema may be found without any field deficit except an increased blind spot (see Chapter 13).

The general signs and symptoms of increased intracranial pressure may also be present. Suprasellar masses that deform or obstruct the anterior third ventricle can produce unilateral or bilateral lateral ventricular enlargement by obstructing either one or both foramina of Monro. This may be the first symptom from anterior third ventricle tumors as diverse as craniopharyngioma, meningioma, and dysgerminoma. Headache may be very prominent. The mechanism of headache in parasellar lesions causing ventricular dilatation is well established; however headache may also be present in parasellar tumors and inflammatory disorders that are too small to cause increased intracranial pressure. In these patients, distortion of the diaphragma or irritation of the parasellar dura may be the cause of bifrontal headache. Similarly, small intrasellar cysts such as Rathke's cleft cysts, empty sella syndrome, and arachnoid cysts in the suprasellar region may present with headache, in the absence of intracranial hypertension.

The deep subfrontal region, including the septal region of the anterior third ventricle, has important connections with the entire limbic system. Mass lesions in this location, therefore, often present with personality change and dementia. This may be as florid as the state of akinetic mutism or as mild as a subtle alteration in spontaneity or a decrease in interest and initiative.[13] The subfrontal tumors in the parasellar region, such as meningiomas, must be considered in the evaluation of any patient with a significant alteration in personality or loss of higher cerebral function. Many lesions in this location also present with anosmia that is undetected by the patient until it is found in a neurological evaluation. The olfactory tracts are in close proximity to the suprasellar region and can easily be compressed by tumors in this location.

3. Radiological Presentation of Intrasellar and Parasellar Nonpituitary Lesions

It is not unusual for asymptomatic sellar and parasellar lesions to be discovered on skull X-rays performed for totally unrelated reasons such as mild head trauma. Whether the lesion is symptomatic or incidental, the changes seen on plain skull X-rays are usually of two types—either bone destruction and enlargement of the sella turcica or abnormal calcification.[14] Not all enlargements of the sella turcica are caused by pituitary tumors. Erosion of the floor of the sella, loss of a clear margin on tomography, and even a double floor can be seen with intracavernous aneurysms, meningiomas of the middle fossa, Rathke's cleft cysts, arachnoid diverticula, and elevated intracranial pressure from any source. Erosion of the top of the dorsum of the sella turcica can be a nonspecific sign of increased intracranial pressure and is commonly seen with lesions of the suprasellar region, either by direct pressure from a tumor or from a dilated third ventricle secondary to obstructive hydrocephalus. Presumably, the increased pressure and the pulsation of the anterior third ventricle are responsible for the erosion of the dorsum in these cases. Erosion of the dorsum can also be seen in lesions that do not cause increased intracranial pressure, such as the empty sella syndrome.[15] Undercutting of the anterior clinoids or elevation of the anterior clinoids can be seen with parasellar aneurysms and optic gliomas, as well as meningiomas of the middle fossa. In most of these situations, the anterior clinoid changes are unilateral. The term "J-shaped sella" should not be used, since it can be a normal developmental structure or it can indicate parasellar lesions.[16] The abnormal, enlarged optic foramen and canal as seen on plain films and tomograms of the optic foramen is a reliable sign for optic and chiasmatic gliomas extending into the canal.

Calcification is often seen in the sellar and parasellar nonpituitary lesions, most commonly with craniopharyngiomas (see Fig. 4). Calcification in the suprasellar region is certainly more common in craniopharyngiomas presenting in children and adolescents than in craniopharyngiomas presenting in adulthood. Linear calcification that is unilateral is often seen in large parasellar aneurysms. These may also be associated with double floor of the sella turcica and extensive erosion at the base of the skull. Meningiomas in the suprasellar region, from either the tuberculum or the diaphragma, can have calcification, as well as enlargement of the sella turcica (see Fig. 10). Chordomas, teratomas, gliomas, and pituitary adenomas may be calcified and can be confused with craniopharyngiomas and meningiomas (see Fig. 1).

The diagnostic usefulness of computerized axial tomographic (CT) scanning in the evaluation of sellar and parasellar lesions has made as important a contribution as it has in other areas of the brain. The empty sella syndrome is often suggested by decreased densities within the sella on CT scanning[17] (see Fig. 19A). In addition, the use of CT scanning without and with subarachnoid metrizamide in the basal cisterns can be diagnostic of an empty sella syndrome (see Fig. 19B). The ability of coronal and sagittal CT scanning to delineate the suprasellar extension of tumors in this location has, in many cases, made pneumoencephalography (PEG) unnecessary (see Fig. 3). As experience is gained with CT scanning utilizing enhanced and nonenhanced scans reconstructed in the transverse, coronal, and sagittal planes, there can be no doubt that the role of PEG in the evaluation of the parasellar lesion will decline. However, until CT reaches the spatial resolution of the PEG, the PEG in conjunction with pluridirectional tomography will still be necessary. Metrizamide CT cisternography may serve to bridge some of the gap between the resolution of standard CT and that of the PEG. Brow-up anteroposterior and lateral PEG with tomograms is still very useful in delineation of parasellar and suprasellar lesions.[18] The empty sella syndrome cannot be diagnosed with certainty except by PEG, and very small lesions may be seen only by PEGs with accurate detail in the region of the chiasmatic cistern.

Angiography is an important diagnostic test in the evaluation of intrasellar and parasellar lesions.[19] The diagnosis of a parasellar aneurysm can be definitely made only with an arteriogram. The vascular blush of the tuberculum or medical sphenoid meningioma, the displacement of the proximal anterior cerebral artery, and the traumatic arteriovenous shunts seen in the carotid cavernous fistula are but a few examples of the advantages of arteriography in evaluation of lesions that might be mistaken for primary pituitary tumors.

4. Specific Lesions of the Parasellar Region

4.1. Craniopharyngioma

Craniopharyngiomas account for 5–10% of brain tumors in children. They arise from embryonic squamous cell rests, the residua from upward migration of stomodeal epithelium to the upper portion of the anterior lobe of

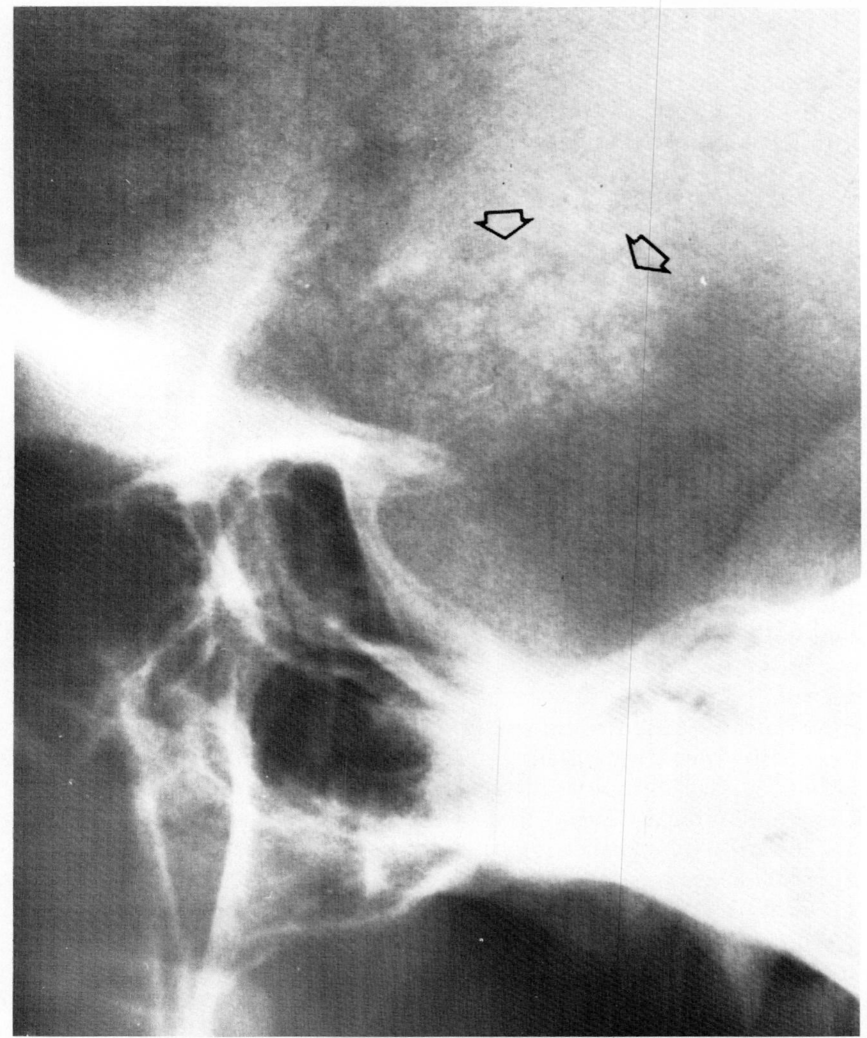

Fig. 1A. Lateral X-ray demonstrating enlargement of the sella with absence of the dorsum sella due to erosion. Note the suprasellar calcification (arrows).

the pituitary gland. Seventy percent arise within the sella, and the remainder above the sella.[3,20] They usually present as a calcific suprasellar tumor with or without erosion of the sella turcica. Craniopharyngioma occurs predominantly in the younger age groups, but may appear in the elderly. Of 313 patients, 27% were over the age of 40 at the time of presentation.[21,23]

The symptoms and signs are usually age-related, but the clinical presentation also depends to a large part on the intra- or suprasellar location of the tumor, the particular anatomy of the optic chiasma (i.e., pre- or postfixed), and the size of the mass. Therefore, some cases may mimic pituitary adenomas more closely than others. Symptoms are grouped: (1) visual; (2) en-

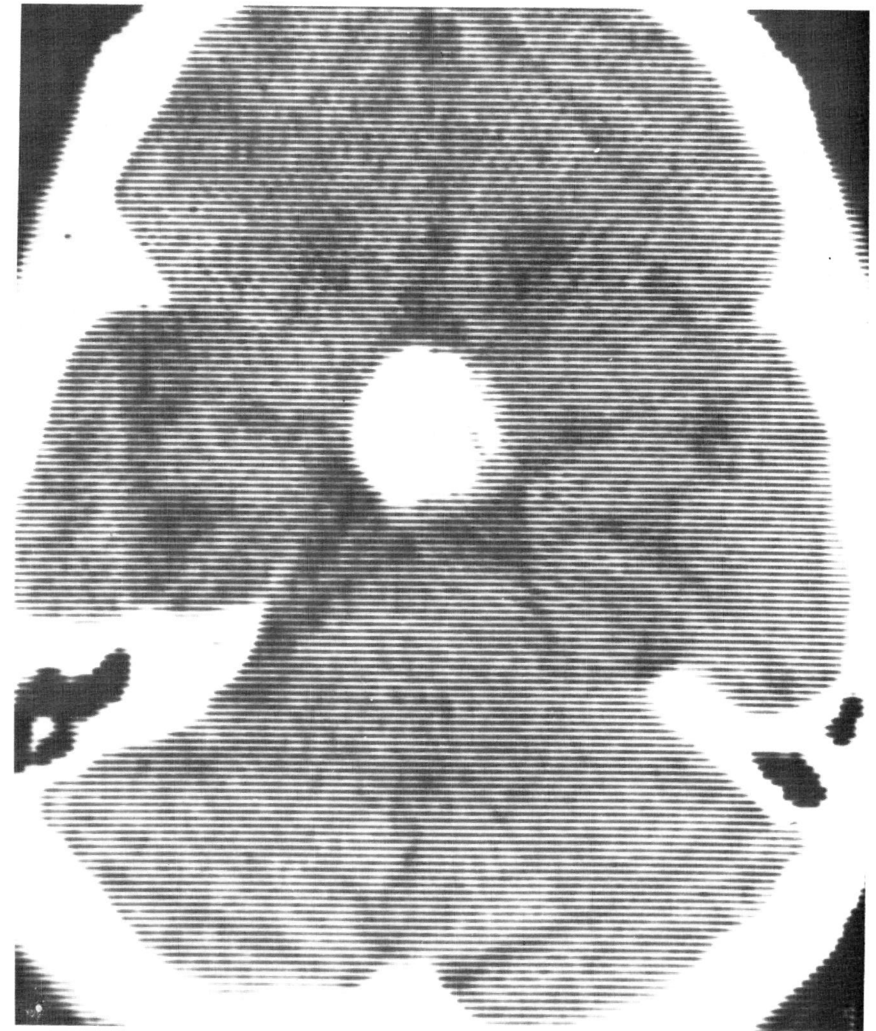

Fig. 1B. Same patient as in Fig. 1A. CT scan of the immediate suprasellar area demonstrating a high-density lesion within the suprasellar cistern. Diagnosis: pituitary adenoma.

docrine; (3) increased intracranial pressure secondary to CSF obstruction; and (4) focal cerebral deficits. Children usually present with increased intracranial pressure, while adults usually present with visual loss.

Approximately 80% of the children had symptoms of increased intracranial pressure in the series reported by Banna[21] and Matson.[3] Headache and vomiting predominated, but papilledema was also noted in 40–55% of these children.[3,22] Sixty percent of children had visual difficulties including acuity loss and field defects.[3,21] In adults, visual failure was seen as the main presenting symptom in about 80% of cases. On examination, however, 93% had visual abnormalities including varying degrees of optic atrophy, papilledema, and field cuts.[21,24,24] In approximately 10% of cases, the optic pathways are normal. The field defect is extremely variable, with changes typical of optic nerve, chiasma, or optic tract pathology. The position of the chiasma, as well as the tumor, dictates the type of field deficit. The most commonly seen, however, is a bitemporal hemianopsia, usually asymmetrical. Extraocular motor nerves III, IV, and VI, as well as the first division of the trigeminal nerve, may occasionally be affected in the cavernous sinus.

Endocrine disturbances are less common. Thirty-eight percent of Matson's[3] 50 patients were of small stature, while only 7% of Banna's[21] patients had stunted growth. Retarded bone age, however, was seen in 41% on X-ray examination. Delayed sexual development is seen in approximately 20%. In children, the visual changes, as well as the endocrinopathies, are often not recognized by their families, and the tumors may reach an enormous size causing CSF obstruction and increased intracranial pressure before medical aid is sought. The most common endocrinopathy of adults is gonadotropin deficiency with either menstrual irregularities, decreased libido, or impotence. Hypothalamic symptoms such as diabetes insipidus, adiposity, somnolence, and hypo- or hyperthemia are also seen.[3,21,25]

In a study by Jenkins *et al.*,[26] 20 patients (6 adults and 14 children and adolescents) with craniopharyngiomas all showed some degree of hypopituitarism. Pituitary–adrenal dysfunction was present in 50%, while all but one had deficiencies of GH and gonadotropins. Serum thyroxine was low in 13 patients, and an additional 6 had an abnormal response of thyroid-stimulating hormone (TSH) to thyrotropin-releasing hormone. Prolactin levels were normal in over half the patients and only moderately elevated in the remainder.[26] We have seen two women recently who presented with amenorrhea–galactorrhea secondary to craniopharyngioma in the suprasellar area (see Case No. 1).

Dementia was seen in approximately 30% of adults.[21,22] It may be minor with slight intellectual impairment or severe with complete disorientation.

By the time craniopharyngiomas have become symptomatic, radiographic studies are almost always abnormal. Retarded bone age has already been noted. An abnormal sella was seen in 50–70% of patients, both children and adults.[2,21,25] The type of sella change is dependent on the origin of the tumor, i.e., intra- or suprasellar. Intracranial calcification is particularly common, with reports of 70–90% in the childhood craniopharyngiomas[24,25] (see Fig. 4) and 40–60% in adults.[24,25] The calcification may be flocculent granuloma or curvilinear, but is not sufficiently characteristic for diagnosis, but if suprasellar in a child, is highly suggestive of craniopharyngioma.[27] In adults, however, pituitary adenomas,[28] meningiomas, gliomas, chordomas, teratomas, and aneurysms may be calcified (Fig. 1).

CT scanning is extremely helpful in differentiating craniopharyngioma from pituitary adenoma because of several features. CT scans of craniopharyngiomas demonstrate frequent calcification, small or large cysts within the mass, occasional low or negative attenuation values because of the cholesterol content, moderate contrast enhancement, occasional scalloped marginal defects, associated hydrocephalus, infrequently sella enlargement, and more likely posterior and superior extension than the anterior and lateral extension seen with adenomas[29] (see Fig. 4). However, even these features may not completely differentiate this tumor from pituitary adenoma or meningioma (see Figs. 1, 2, 4, and 11).

Arteriography may show mass displacement of arteries and a vascular tumor. PEG will usually outline the tumor. Neither test is diagnostic for a craniopharyngioma.

Case No. 1

A 26-year-old teacher had normal menses at age 15 with regular periods until age 17 when she developed oligomenorrhea and significant weight gain. Intermittent headaches were also noted at that time. At age 25, she presented for infertility evaluation and was found to have galactorrhea and hyperprolactinemia of 67 ng/ml (normal: up to 25 ng/ml). Examination was normal except for galactorrhea and obesity. Visual fields were normal. Endocrine studies were normal, other than an elevated prolactin level. Sella tomograms showed an enlarged sella with erosion of the lamina dura (Fig. 2A). CT scan showed a cystic suprasellar mass (Fig. 2B). Craniotomy demonstrated a large suprasellar craniopharyngioma that was then totally removed.

Comment: This patient's history and examination were completely consistent with a prolactin-secreting adenoma. Since the CT scan was more suggestive of craniopharyngioma, a subfrontal, rather than transsphenoidal, surgical approach was performed.

Case No. 2

A 15½-year-old female was thought to be functionally and developmentally normal. During a routine eye examination, it was noted that bitemporal hemianopsia was present. Thereafter, a history of 4–5 years of gradual obesity, mild headaches, primary amenorrhea, and 2 years of galactorrhea was elicited. She had bilateral pallor of her optic discs and a left temporal field defect with a right inferior temporal field defect.

Endocrine evaluation showed a prolactin level of 1018 ng/ml (normal: up to 25 ng/ml), and deficiencies of luteinizing hormone (LH), follicle-stimulating hormone (FSH), and GH.

Skull X-rays and tomograms demonstrated an eroded sella and CT scan showed a large sella and suprasellar mass with some calcification (Fig. 3). A large pituitary adenoma was found and removed transsphenoidally.

Comment: This patient resembles the first patient, demonstrating the potential of craniopharyngiomas to mimic prolactinomas.

Case No. 3

A 6-year-old girl complained of double vision for 2 weeks. It was then learned that for the previous 6 months she had complained of morning headaches and vomiting, which were attributed to nervousness at school. Growth and development were normal. Examination demonstrated normal stature, bi-

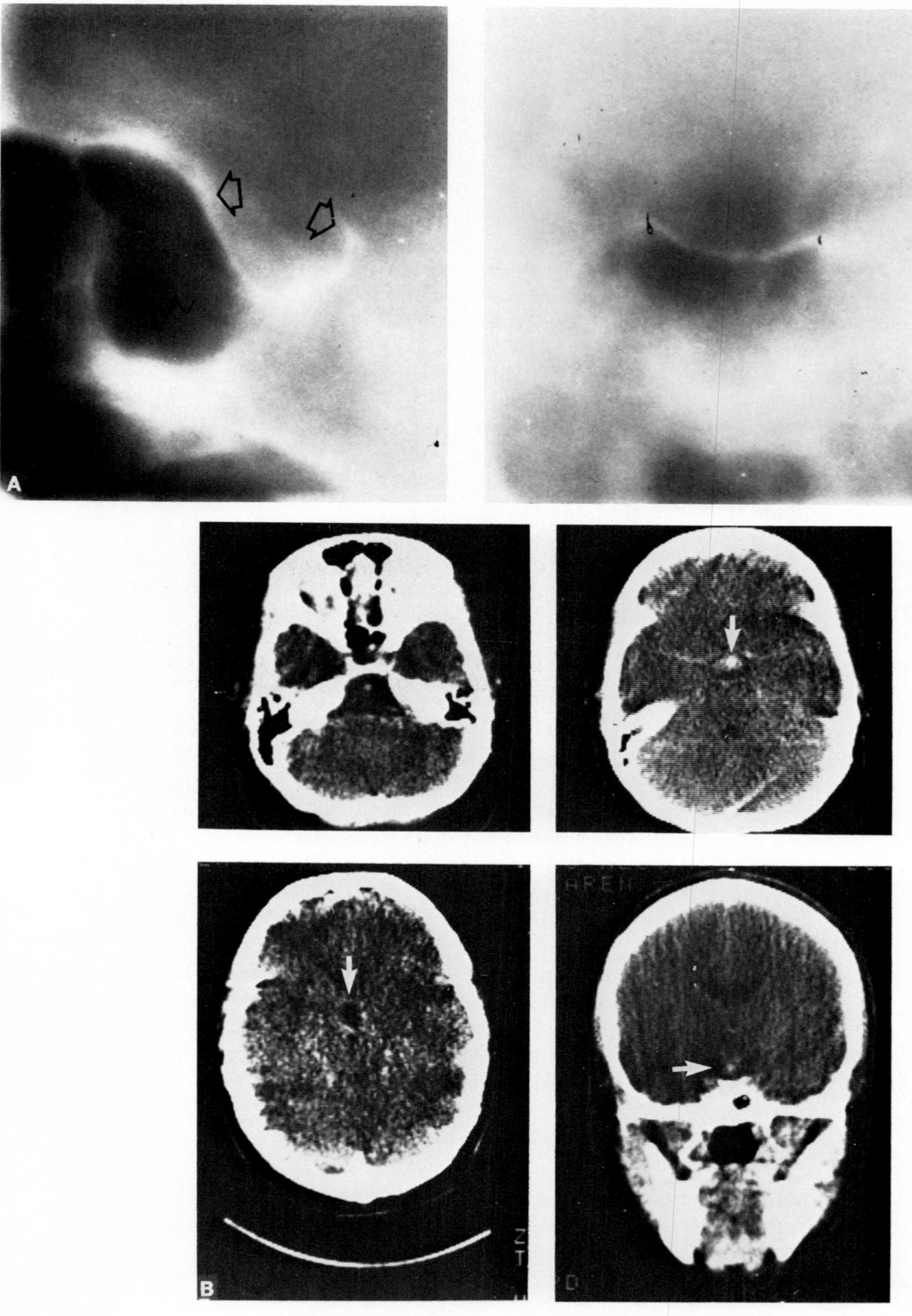
A
B
D

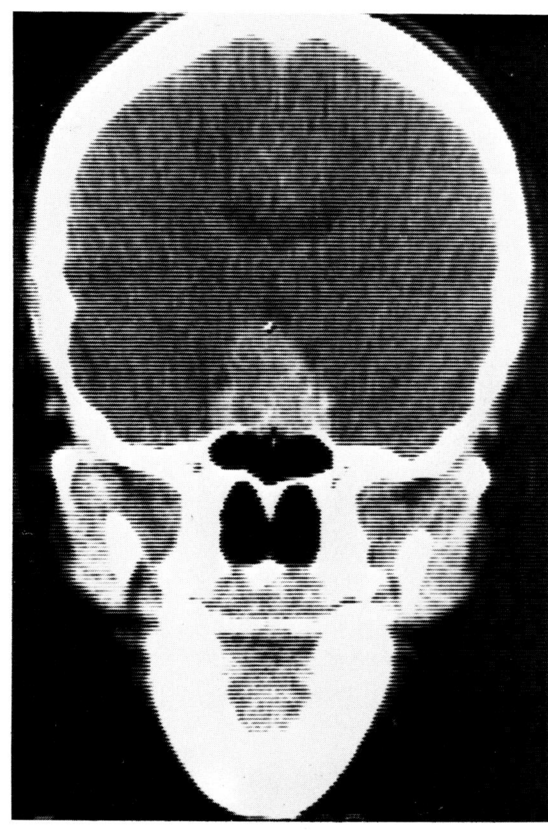

Fig. 3. Enhanced coronal CT scan demonstrating a large enhancing tumor extending out of the sella turcica to indent the third ventricle. Diagnosis: prolactinoma.

lateral papilledema, and a right sixth nerve paresis. Visual fields and acuity were normal.

Evaluation showed suprasellar calcification and sella erosion on skull X-ray (Fig. 4a). CT scan demonstrated a large calcified suprasellar mass extending well into the third ventricle with moderate hydrocephalus (Fig. 4B and c).

Bilateral ventriculoperitoneal shunts were placed prior to a right frontal craniotomy and total removal of the craniopharyngioma. The finding of a prefixed optic chiasma at surgery explained her lack of visual complaints.

Comment: This patient is typical of children presenting with signs and symptoms of increased intracranial pressure who are suffering from the mass effect of craniopharyngioma.

←

Fig. 2. (A) Lateral (*left*) and frontal (*right*) tomography of the sella. The lateral tomogram demonstrates expansion of the opening of the sella (arrows) with erosion of the dorsum sella. The frontal tomogram demonstrates increase in the width of the sella. (B) Horizontal and coronal CT scans after injection of contrast material. Note the contrast-enhancing lesion (arrows) in the suprasellar cistern (*top right*) together with a ringlike enhancement (arrow) at a higher level (*bottom left*). On the coronal scan (*bottom right*), the enhancing lesion in the suprasellar area (arrow) is again demonstrated. Diagnosis: craniopharyngioma.

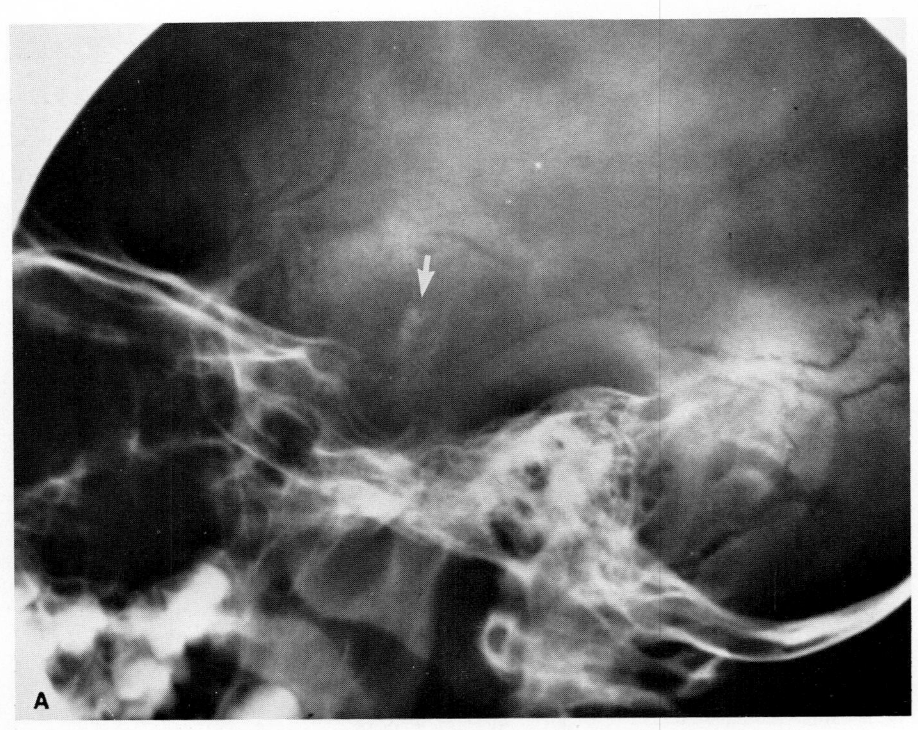
A

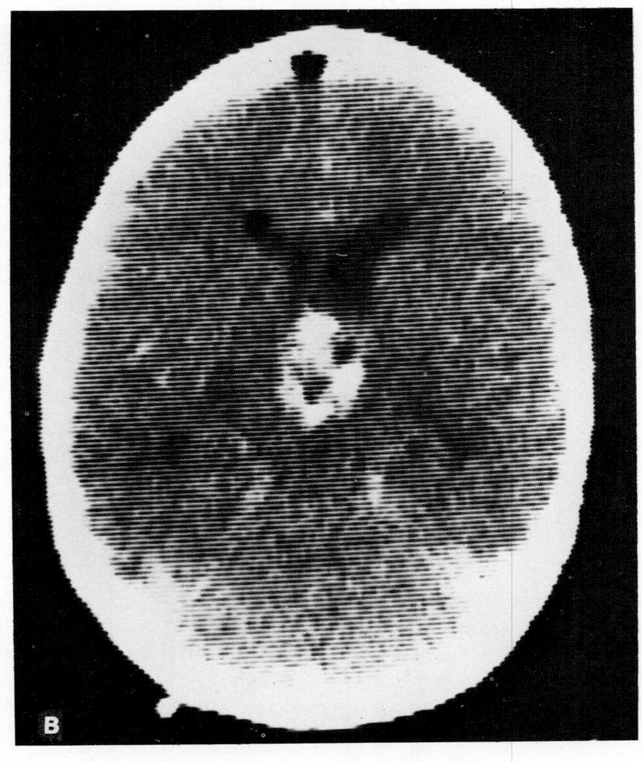
B

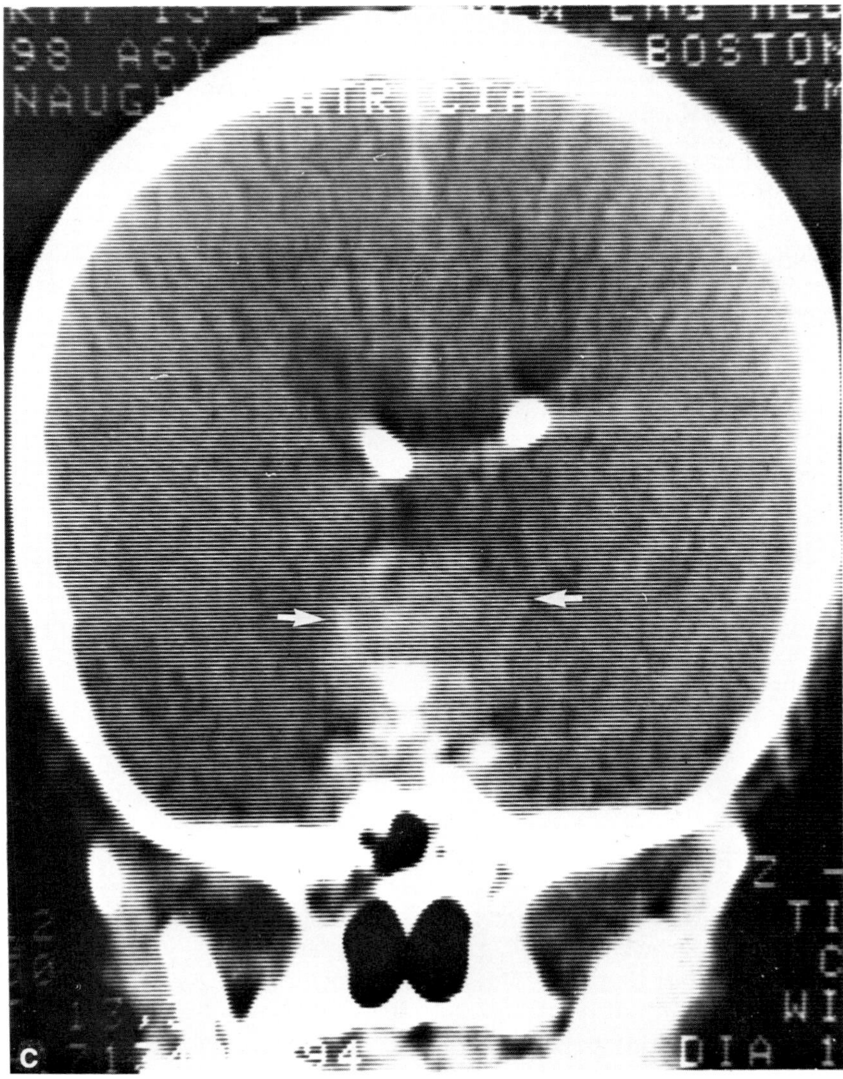

Fig. 4. (A) Lateral skull X-ray demonstrating amputation of the dorsum sella together with suprasellar calcification (arrow). (B) Horizontal CT scan after contrast enhancement demonstrating a calcified, enhancing tumor invading the third ventricle with a minor degree of ventricular enlargement involving the right anterior horn. (C) Coronal CT scan after contrast enhancement. Note the suprasellar extent of the tumor mass (arrows). Suprasellar calcification is also apparent. Shunts are seen in both ventricles. Diagnosis: craniopharyngiomas.

4.2. Suprasellar and Intrasellar Cysts

Arachnoid cysts, epidermoid cysts, Rathke's cleft cysts, optic glioma cysts, and cystic craniopharyngiomas may be seen in the suprasellar region producing signs and symptoms similar to those of pituitary adenoma. Similarly, intrasellar cysts of various etiologies[30–33] occur mimicking pituitary adenoma. Recurrent hemorrhages into the cyst may often be the cause of symptoms.[34]

4.3. Rathke's Cleft Cyst

Cysts derived from Rathke's pouch are found between the pars anterior and the infundibular process in 13–22% of routinely examined pituitary glands.[30,35–37] Generally, they are small and asymptomatic, but occasionally they cause symptoms.[38] The age distribution is wide, 4–72 years, generally occurring between 40 and 60 years.[39] The cyst is usually, but not always, intrasellar.[35,40]

These cysts were classified by Berry and Schlezinger[54] into three groups: (1) those with suprasellar symptoms such as visual impairment or hypothalamic dysfunction; (2) those with hypophyseal dysfunction; and (3) those with no symptoms referable to the hypophyseal region.

The clinical picture can be remarkably similar to that of pituitary adenoma and craniopharyngioma, with visual acuity and field loss, hypopituitarism, headache, and an enlarged sella.

An enlarged sella is common, but lack of calcification was reported to differentiate this from craniopharyngioma[42] (but see Case No. 4 below).

The differentiation of Rathke's cleft cyst from pituitary adenoma is therapeutically important in that the treatment need not be as aggressive as with an adenoma.[38,42,43]

A Rathke's cleft cyst may also be seen in association with pituitary microadenoma.[37,44,45]

Case No. 4

A 49-year-old woman presented with frequently occurring intense frontal and retro-orbital headaches. Twenty years previously, she had suffered a left cerebral infarct during pregnancy. Ten years before this admission, she developed hypopituitarism during her third pregnancy with amenorrhea, loss of axillary and pubic hair, dry skin, increasing fatigue, and cold intolerance. Neurological examination demonstrated a bitemporal superior quadrantic field defect. Preoperative endocrine testing demonstrated deficiencies of TSH, ACTH, GH, FSH, LH, and thyroid function. Skull X-rays showed an enlarged sella with a thickened floor and curvilinear calcification in the suprasellar area (Fig. 5A). A rim of calcification was also seen on the CT scan (Fig. 5C). Cerebral arteriography failed to demonstrate an aneurysm. Pneumoencephalography clearly defined the mass (Figs. 5A and B). At surgery, a Rathke's cleft cyst was found elevating and distorting the optic chiasma and splaying apart the internal carotid arteries (Fig. 5D).

Comment: The similarities between this and craniopharyngioma are striking, and both may readily mimic a pituitary adenoma.

4.4. Arachnoid Cyst

Suprasellar arachnoid cysts are extremely rare. In 1935, Barlow[46] described a patient with a bitemporal hemianopsia and increased CSF pressure

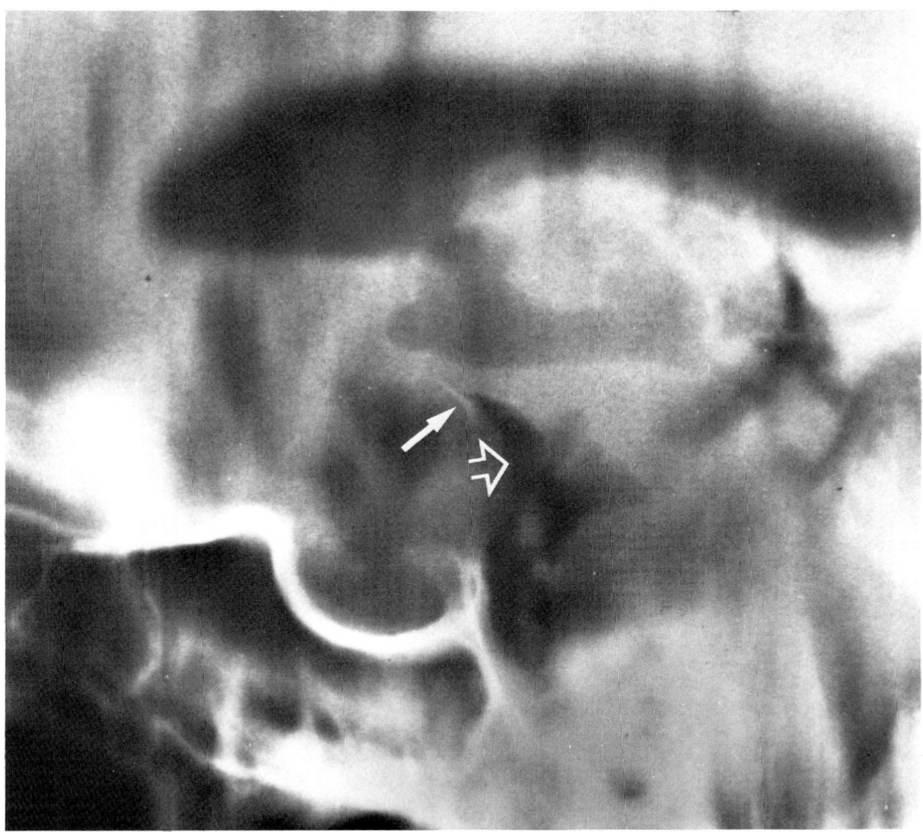

Fig. 5A. Lateral tomographic view at pneumoencephalography demonstrating curvilinear calcification in the dome of a suprasellar tumor (solid arrow). The tumor mass is seen to indent both the interpeduncular cistern (open arrow) and the anterior third ventricle.

who had a cyst composed of arachnoid membrane arising from the sella and compressing the chiasma. Bernard *et al.*[47] described a child who had a suprasellar arachnoid cyst with an inflammatory infiltrate in the wall suggestive of cystic arachnoiditis. Since then, several reports have added only a few cases.[48–51]

The pathogenesis of subarachnoid cysts is speculative and has been summarized recently.[48] Trauma, an adhesive arachnoiditis secondary to infection, congenital maldevelopment of the subarachnoid space, and a ball-valve mechanism have all been considered.

The clinical manifestations are a function of the structure compromised by the mass effect. Visual symptoms from compression of the optic nerves, chiasma, or tracts occur.[48] Hydrocephalus secondary to obstruction of the foramina of Monro is also common.[48,50]

Preoperative diagnosis prior to CT scanning was not reported. PEG may show a suprasellar mass lesion, but without specific characterization. CT scan

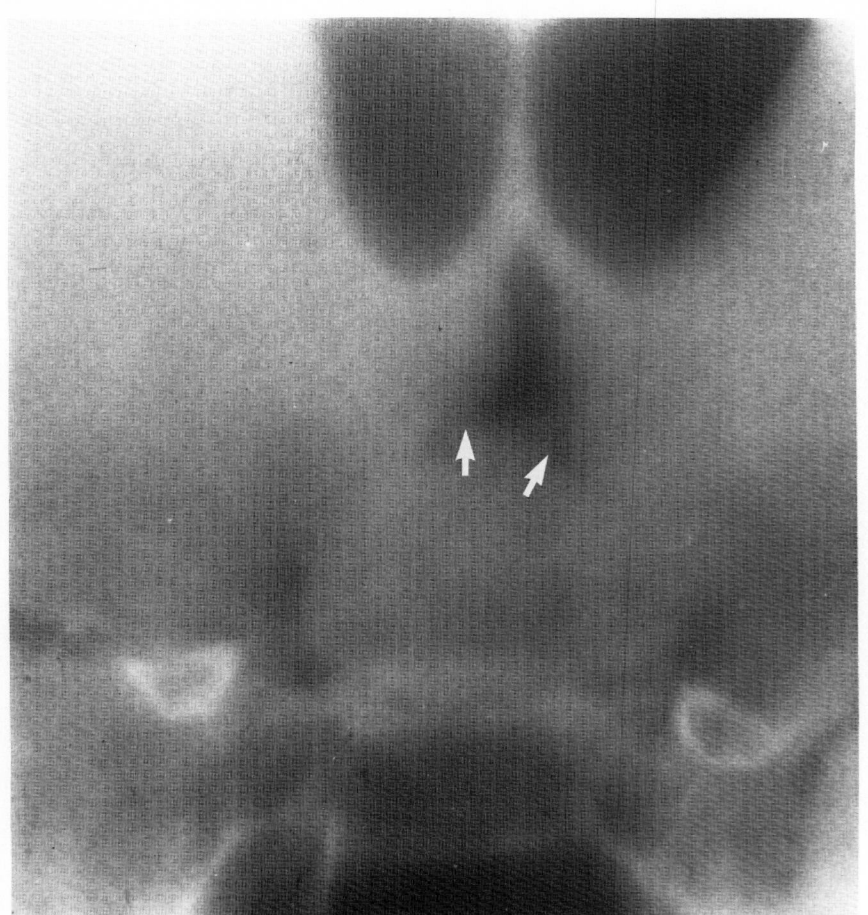

Fig. 5B. Frontal tomographic section, again demonstrating a tumor mass (arrows) invading and indenting the floor of the anterior third ventricle.

demonstrates the cystic nature of the mass, but does not differentiate the type of cyst; surgical diagnosis is definitive.

Case No. 5

A 19-year-old male presented in January 1975 with a 4-year history of headache and vague visual disturbances. Examination was normal, except for visual acuity of 20/25 O.S. and 20/20 O.D. Plain skull X-rays showed a sella with undercutting of the anterior clinoids. PEG revealed considerable enlargement of the lateral ventricles with marked dilatation of what was thought to be the third ventricle. Arteriography revealed only symmetrical ventricular dilatation. A ventriculoperitoneal shunt was placed with resolution of symptoms.

In March 1976, he was readmitted because of several months of progressive visual loss. Fields demonstrated an incongruous left homonymous hemianopsia. Visual acuity was 20/200 O.S. and 20/40 O.D. A CT scan showed a large central area of CSF density in the midline and right subfrontal basal cistern (Fig. 6A). PEG demonstrated a cystlike structure in the suprasellar region, separate from the third ventricle.

Frontal craniotomy revealed a clear, cystlike structure in the subarachnoid space in the right subfrontal region. The cyst also bulged around the right optic nerve, chiasma, and optic tract, extending inferiorly into the sella turcica and interpeduncular fossa (Fig. 6B). There was no communication between the cyst and the third ventricle. The cyst contained clear, colorless fluid. Pathological sections of the cyst wall showed a fibrous connective tissue membrane with mesothelial lining consistent with arachnoid. Subsequently, his vision returned to normal.

Comment: CT scan differentiated this lesion from pituitary adenoma.

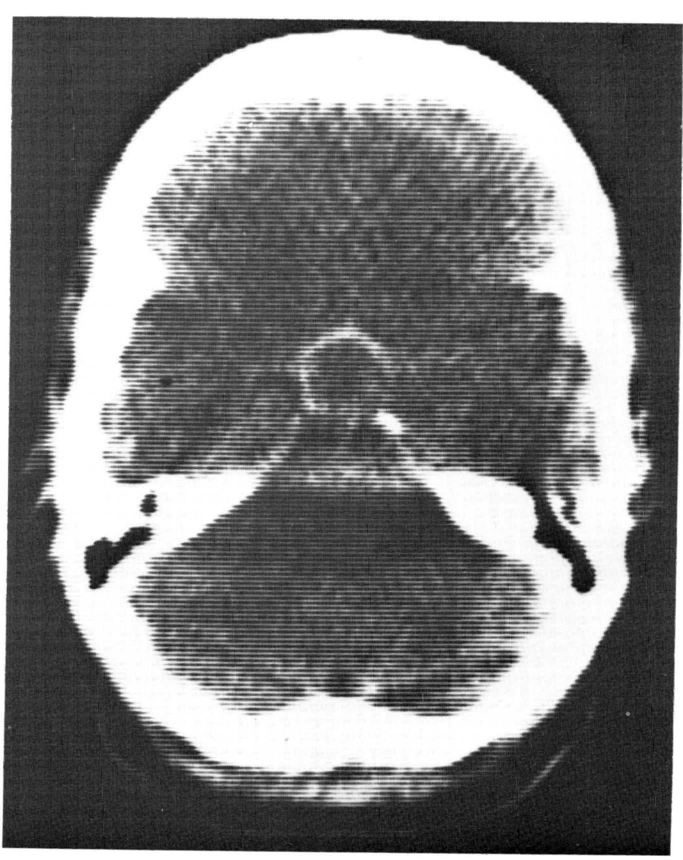

Fig. 5C. Horizontal, nonenhanced CT scan at the skull base demonstrating a ringlike area of calcification in the suprasellar cistern.

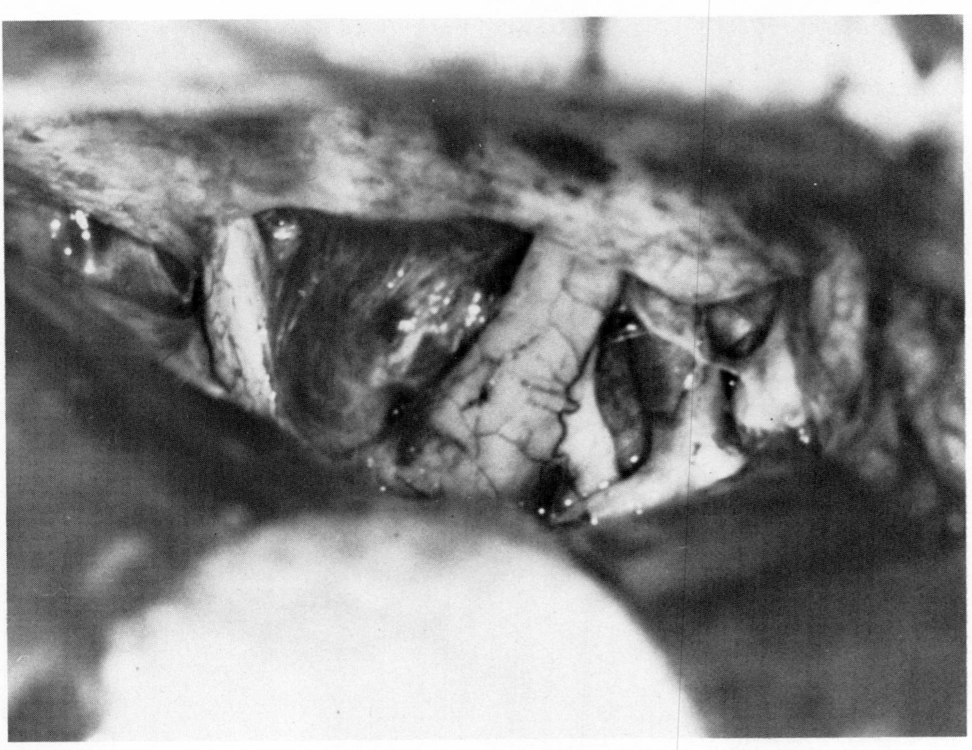

Fig. 5D. Intraoperative view of the suprasellar region through a right frontal craniotomy. Note the suprasellar mass bowing the optic nerves superiorly and laterally, as well as displacing the carotid arteries laterally. Also, note the grooving of the chiasma on the right side by the right anterior cerebral artery. Diagnosis: Rathke's cleft cyst.

However, there may be greater difficulty distinguishing arachnoid cysts from necrotic or cystic adenomas.

4.5. Chordoma

Chordoma is a rare tumor that arises from notochordal remnants in the clivus and usually produces destruction of the basisphenoid.[52] Approximately 35% of chordomas occur in this area with the majority in the 30- to 50-year

Fig. 6. (A) Horizontal, nonenhanced CT scan demonstrating a low-density area in the suprasellar cistern. The lesion is seen to extend out anterolaterally toward the carotid cistern and posterolaterally toward the cerebello–pontine angle cistern. (B) Intraoperative view of the suprasellar region as exposed through a right frontal temporal craniotomy. Note the suprasellar cyst with bowing of the right optic nerve and extension of the cyst above the nerve.

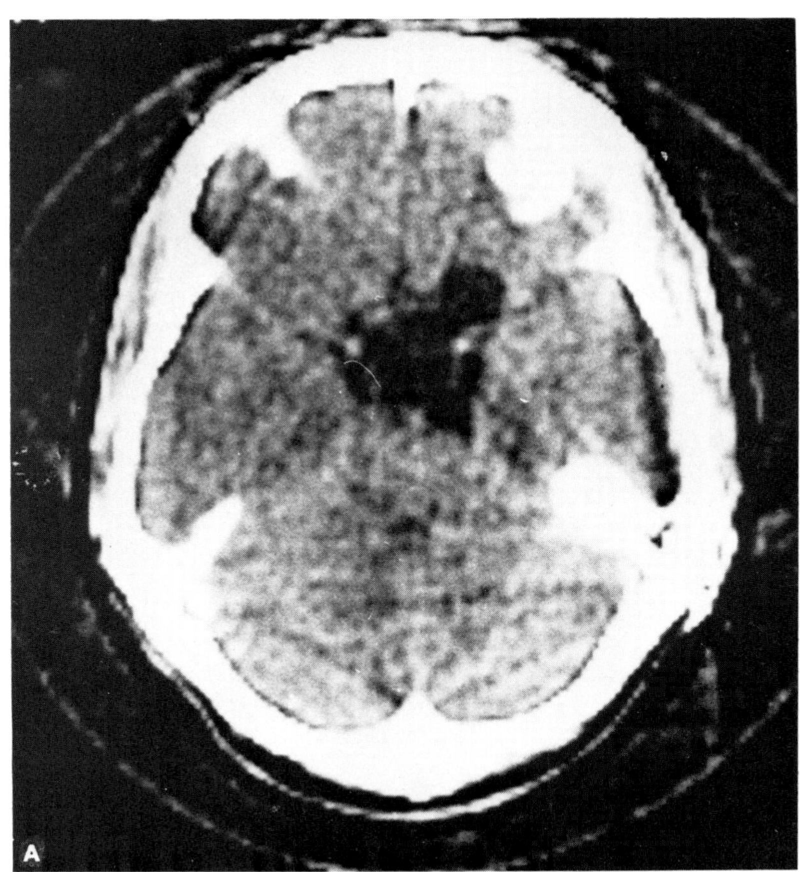
A

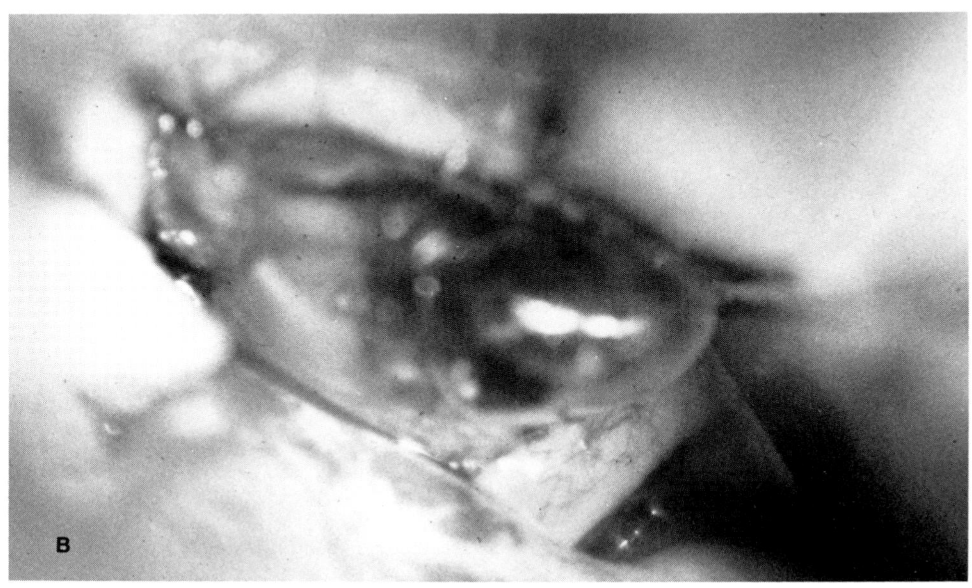
B

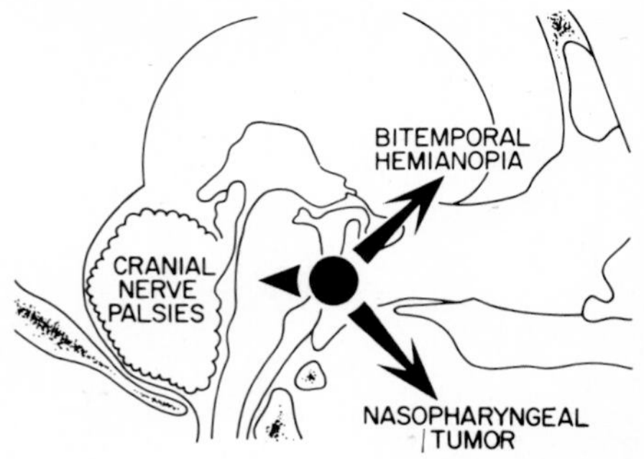

Fig. 7. Diagrammatic representation of potential directions of extension of a clivus chordoma. From Schechter *et al.*[41] Reproduced with the permission of Dr. Schechter.

age group.[53,54] Symptoms depend on the direction of growth of the tumor, as illustrated in Fig. 7.

Clinically, the most common symptoms are headaches, visual disturbances, neck pain, and nasopharyngeal obstruction.[54,55] Diplopia secondary to involvement of cranial nerves III, IV, and VI occurs in approximately one third of cases. Field defects, when they occur, are similar to those seen with pituitary adenoma, while the cranial nerve involvement is most often very asymmetrical. Headaches occur early, whereas endocrine dysfunction is unusual. Posterior fossa mass is usually significant because of signs of brainstem compression, cranial nerve compression, and long tract signs.

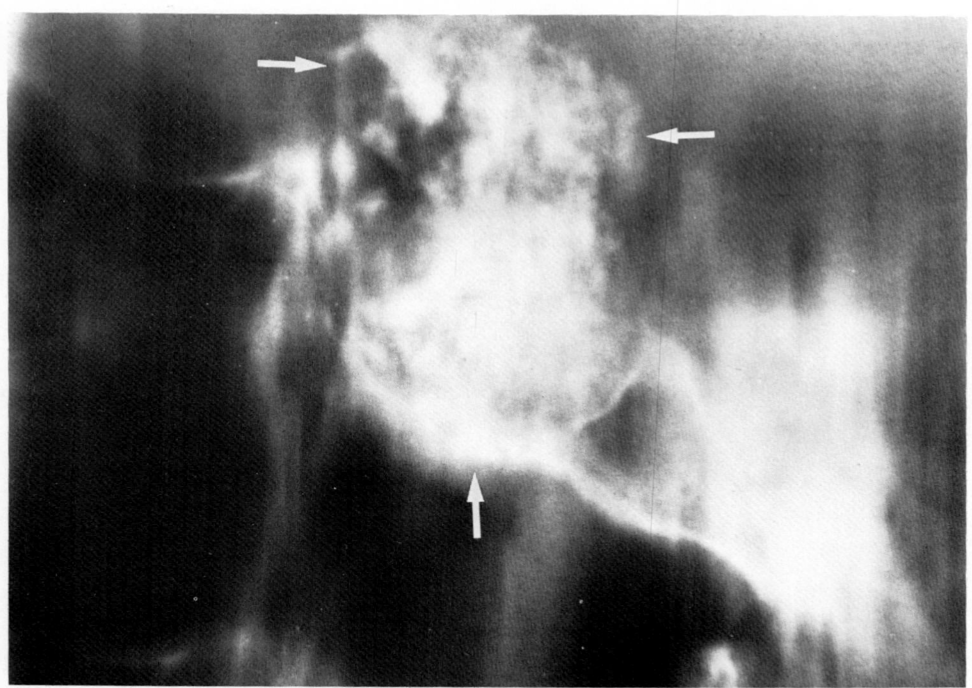

Fig. 8A. Lateral tomogram of the sphenoid and sella region demonstrating large, irregular, craggy calcification (arrows) invading the sphenoid sinus, and clivus with suprasellar extension.

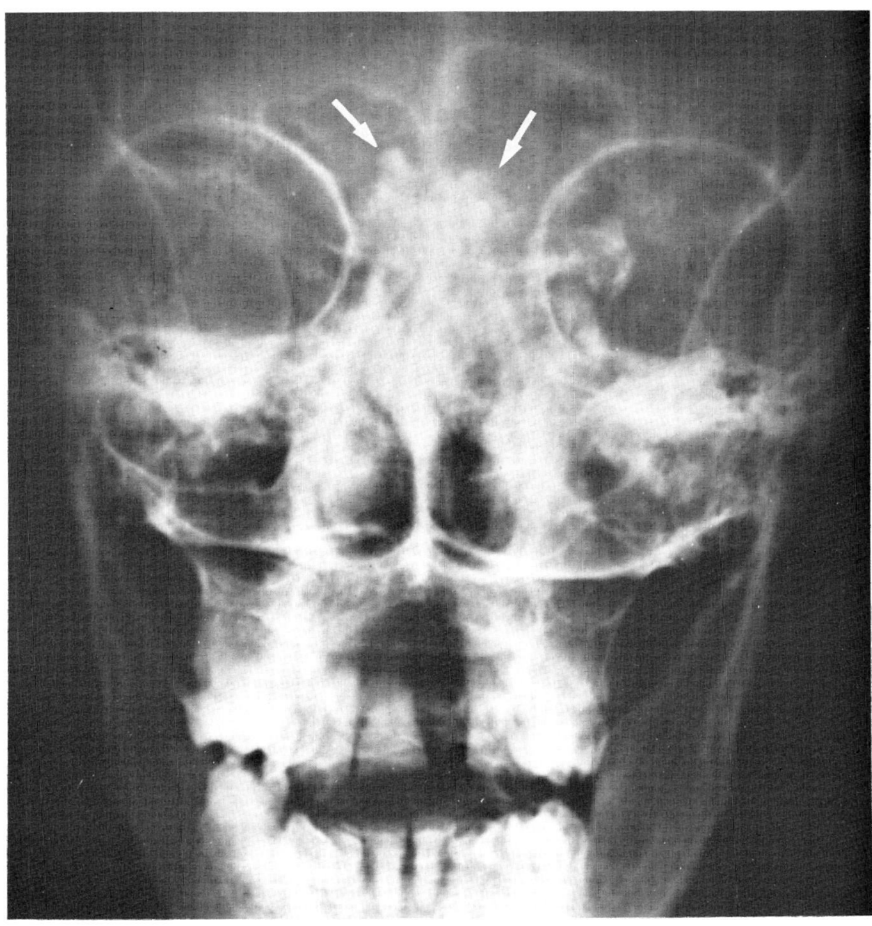

Fig. 8B. Frontal projection, again demonstrating suprasellar calcification (arrows).

Radiologically, bone destruction and calcification are extremely common.[54] Chordomas are usually osteolytic, commence in the spheno-occipital synchondrosis, and extend into the clivus, dorsum sellae, and sella. They may extend along the entire skull base, and laterally into the petrous bones and sphenoid wings with enlargement of the superior orbital fissures. Calcification is seen in one third to one half of cases with either a reticular lacework, a solid nodular mass, a few small 1- to 2-mm flecks, or a cystic type of appearance[54–56] (Fig. 8).

The sella is rarely ballooned as it is with pituitary tumors, and there is no undercutting of the anterior clinoids. The sella floor, however, may be thinned or completely destroyed.[54] Some portion of the sella may be involved in as many as 69% of cases.[42]

Arteriography shows vessel displacement according to the pattern of tumor growth as in Figs. 7 and 8C. A tumor blush is not seen.[41] CT scans will undoubtedly make diagnosis easier.

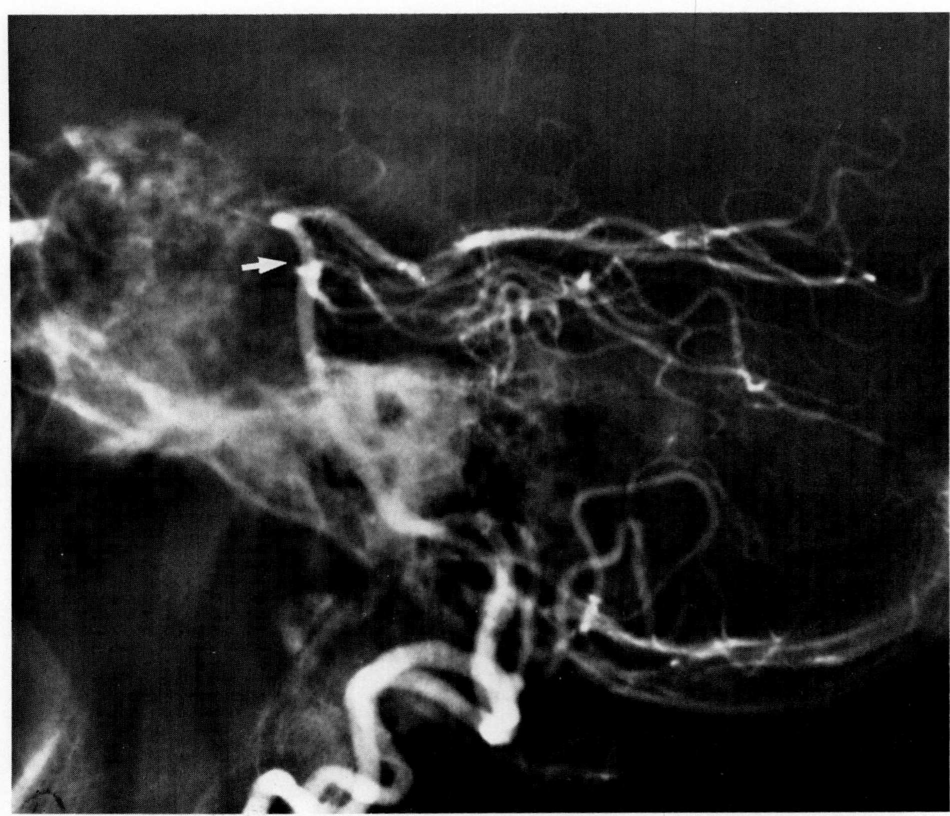

Fig. 8C. Left vertebral angiogram demonstrating that the calcification abuts on the apical basilar artery, causing posterior displacement of the basilar artery away from the clivus (arrow). Diagnosis: chordoma. Courtesy of Dr. Barry Gerald, Memphis, Tennessee.

The location, bone destruction, and calcification usually make differentiation from pituitary adenoma straightforward.

4.6. Suprasellar Germinoma (Atypical Teratoma, Ectopic Pinealoma)

Suprasellar germinomas have been reported as showing a male predominance[57]; however, more recent studies show an equal male/female ratio with a higher incidence in the Japanese population.[58,59] This is also true of suprasellar teratomas.[60]

Three patterns of third-ventricular-region germinoma can be distinguished.[57] Germinomas of the ventral hypothalamus may occur in association with germinoma in the pineal region. It is likely that these are metastatic, but they may possibly represent multifocal origin. Second, they may arise in the anterior third ventricle, and may cause hydrocephalus, involve the hypothalamus, and by extension inferiorly and posteriorly, involve the optic nerves, chiasma, and pituitary. Finally, they may be in the region of the optic chiasma with extension into the sella. Intrasellar germinoma with hypopituitarism has been reported,[61] mimicking intrasellar adenoma.

The common initial symptoms are diabetes insipidus (50%); visual disturbances (17%); headache, nausea, or vomiting (11%); and obesity (5%).[58] Later in the course, diabetes insipidus was seen in 83%, visual disturbances in 78%, headache in 50%, retarded growth in 39%, hypogonadism in 17%, hypothalamic anorexia in 28%, and nausea and vomiting in 11%.[58]

The common visual-field defects were bitemporal hemianopsia, homonymous hemianopsia, and concentric constriction.[20,59] Primary bilateral optic atrophy without papilledema was also seen in many patients.[59]

The occurrence of diabetes insipidus early in the course of the disease warrants special comment. In the review by Camins and Mount[59] of 58 cases, all but 4 patients had diabetes insipidus, in contrast to pituitary adenomas and craniopharyngiomas, where it is not a common phenomenon and rarely occurs before mass evidence of pituitary abnormality. Some cases show hypopituitarism, while others show an elevation of plasma cortisol or LH and FSH.[58] As with other causes of diabetes insipidus, polyuria may appear only after administration of adrenocortical steroids to a patient with associated anterior pituitary deficiency.

Radiographic studies are not diagnostic. Plain skull X-rays show an eroded sella in 20–40% of cases.[58,62] Arteriography and PEG demonstrated a suprasellar mass lesion in the region of the anterior third ventricle. CT scan may show an isodense of hyperdense suprasellar tumor in the suprasellar cistern that can enhance markedly.[63]

Germinomas metastasize within the nervous system in about 10% of cases, and a majority have grossly abnormal CSF. The diagnosis can often be made by the finding of abnormal cells in the CSF. A high measurement of β-human-chorionic gonadotropin (BHCG) in serum or CSF may be helpful diagnostically. Extracranial metastases to the lung have also been reported. This important manifestation should be sought for. If the correct diagnosis can be made clinically, exploratory surgery may be avoided and this very radiosensitive tumor treated by X-ray.[58]

4.7. Dermoid and Epidermoid Tumors

Dermoid and epidermoid tumors are rare developmental tumors. There are no clinical features that distinguish these from other parasellar tumors.

4.8. Optic Nerve Gliomas

Optic nerve gliomas are rare, comprising approximately 2% of orbital tumors in all ages, 3.5% of intracranial tumors in children, and 1% of intracranial tumors in adults.[62] Miller *et al.*[64] describe two distinct groups: an anterior type occurring more commonly in children and a posterior type occurring in adults. The childhood variety usually remains benign,[65] with occasional malignant degeneration.[66,67] The adult type tends to be malignant[68,69] and is rarely diagnosed antemortem.[70]

Approximately 80% of children present at less than 10 years of age,[67,71] with a well-known association with neurofibromatosis.[65,72,73] In children, the most frequent symptoms and signs are loss of vision in 93%, headaches in 36%, and proptosis in 32%.[65] Strabismus accompanied by visual loss also occurs in the majority of those under 10 years of age.[65,74] Unfortunately, visual loss, even if marked, may not be appreciated in very young children. For this reason, involvement of both eyes and the hypothalamus with associated hydrocephalus is present at the time of initial diagnosis.[75] Vision may change rapidly, with deterioration[76–78] or spontaneous improvement in acuity.[79] In adults, initial symptoms may include monocular blurring of vision and retrobulbar pain, thus simulating optic neuritis. The pattern of visual loss indicates chiasmal involvement; within 5–6 weeks, the patient may become totally blind.[68] Patterns of field defects are nonspecific and extremely variable. Central scotoma or measurable depression of the central field was seen in 70% of eyes examined.[80] The long-term course of the field defects and acuity loss may be very static, with the most common pattern of progression being increased density of the central scotoma.[80]

Skull X-rays may show enlargement of the optic foramen, alteration of the sella, or changes from increased intracranial pressure, or they may be entirely normal.[81] An optic foramen greater than 6.5 mm, or a difference of 2.0 mm or greater between the two sides, is abnormal.[56] Transverse tomography of the optic canal may be necessary to detect enlargement, particularly of the cranial end. Calcification is rare, occurring as nodular foci.[70] The sella is normal in most cases with the tumor confined to the orbit, and may also be normal in gliomas involving the chiasma and intracranial portions of the optic nerves. Undercutting of the anterior clinoid process with deepening of the chiasmatic groove may be seen in some cases.

PEG with pluridirectional tomography may show a filling defect of the anterior third ventricle that is indistinguishable from other tumors in this area, though the presence of air between the tumor and the sella would argue against a tumor originating within the sella. The optic nerves or chisma may, however, appear thickened.

CT scanning is now a prime method of diagnosis, since direct visualization of the optic nerves, chiasma, sella, and suprasellar area is possible.

Differentiation of optic nerve glioma from pituitary adenoma is usually not difficult. The young age, marked visual change, intact pituitary function, and radiographic picture are distinct for optic nerve glioma. When the tumor involves the hypothalamus, the radiographic appearances are usually indistinguishable from a hypothalamic glioma. (However, at times in adults, because of the visual field pattern and hypothalamic involvement, it may mimic pituitary adenoma.)

4.9. Hypothalamic Gliomas

Hypothalamic glioma is a rare tumor occurring almost always in early life, often causing the "diencephalic syndrome."[3] Usually, it arises in the anterior hypothalamus, invading the floor of the third ventricle. Pathologically, tumors ranging from extremely low-grade juvenile astrocytoma to grade IV astrocytoma may be seen.[82]

Clinically, failure to grow or gain weight, diabetes insipidus, and visual loss with optic atrophy may be seen. Increased intracranial pressure often occurs late in the disease.[3]

Because of the age and characteristic diencephalic picture, little confusion with pituitary adenoma arises. The sella X-rays are usually normal. CT scanning may demonstrate a suprasellar mass that may enhance after the injection of contrast material. PEG with tomography will demonstrate a mass within the suprasellar cistern accompanied by indentation of the anterior recesses of the third ventricle. When the tumor is large, it can mimic a suprasellar adenoma radiographically, but as already mentioned, the clinical background should be characteristic.

4.10. Microglioma

Case No. 6

A 34-year-old Gravida 4, Para 3 female presented in 1974 with amenorrhea and galactorrhea, a 40-pound weight gain, polydipsia, and mild depression. Her prolactin was 17.3 ng/ml (normal: less than 25 ng/ml). Thyroid studies were slightly low; GH and cortisol were normal. LH, FSH, and estrodiol blood levels were low. Sella tomograms were normal. She was treated with bromocriptine and lergotrile in hope of achieving pregnancy. Galactorrhea ceased, but amenorrhea persisted. Prolactin decreased to less than 1.6 ng/ml. In February 1977, she developed polydipsia, polyuria, right facial weakness, and increasing somnolence. She became confused, losing her way while driving and failing to recognize long-term friends. A CT scan demonstrated a deep right frontal enhancing mass (Fig. 9). The mass was avascular on angiography. CSF cytology showed rare atypical cells, thought to be reticuloendocthelial in origin. A right craniotomy and subfrontal exploration was performed. A deep reddish mucoid-appearing tumor was found and biopsied. The pathology was microglioma.

Comment: Early in her course, this patient was being evaluated for a pituitary microadenoma. The prolactin level of 17.3 ng/ml was not diagnostically elevated. The later development of hypothalamic symptoms clarified the situation, directing attention toward the suprasellar brain.

4.11. Parasellar Meningioma

Parasellar meningiomas can originate from the tuberculum sella, the planum sphenoidale, and the diaphragma sella. They can present as suprasellar masses. Laterally, they grow from the medial sphenoid ridge and cavernous sinus.[83] Intrasellar meningiomas are rare, originating from the arachnoid tissue in a herniated pouch.[62] These tumors are usually seen in adult life with the peak age between 40 and 50 years. Women outnumber men by 4- to 10-fold.[62,84,85] The tumors are usually small, rarely achieving the massive size seen in some pituitary adenomas and craniopharyngiomas.

Visual loss is the predominant initial symptom, with visual blurring in part of a monocular field or a decrease of central visual acuity. Later in the course, bilateral loss of vision is present in almost all patients.[83] An asymmet-

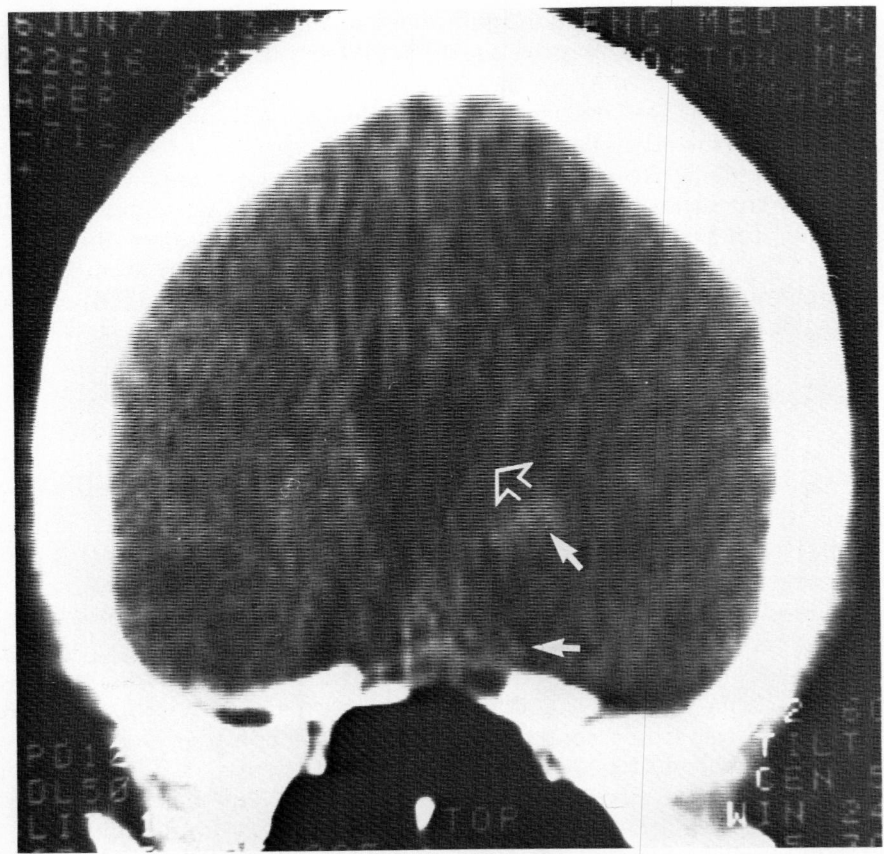

Fig. 9. Coronal CT scan obtained after enhancement. Note the faint enhancing lesion (solid arrows) extending superiorly above the sella to indent the lateral ventricles (open arrow). The tumor mass is extending out laterally to the left side.

rical incongruent variant of a bitemporal hemianopsia, often beginning at the periphery of the field and progressing to blindness, is common.[86,87] The "prechiasmal syndrome" with great variability was noted by Schlezinger *et al.*[88] A posterior chiasmal syndrome is more common with craniopharyngioma, Rathke's cleft cysts, and ectopic pinealomas, but may also be seen with diaphragma sella meningiomas if located slightly posteriorly.[89] The bitemporal hemianopsia defect begins in the macular and extends laterally, but varied combinations of central and peripheral field defects are common.[87,90] The visual symptoms are often confused with retrobulbar neuritis, but with meningiomas, there is no pain on eye movement, and the visual loss is progressive rather than sudden.

Optic atrophy is the predominant funduscopic finding and correlates better with the acuity loss than with the field defect.[83]

Extraocular palsies may be seen with tumor extension into the superior orbital fissure or orbit as well as into the cavernous sinus.[82]

Headaches, both frontal and orbital, are common. Endocrine dysfunction is unusual.[83,84] There may, however, be an increase in the tumor size during menses or pregnancy with alterations of symptoms.[91]

Plain X-ray studies may show hyperostosis of the tuberculum sella, planum sphenoidale, or sphenoid ridge (Fig. 10). The incidence of hyperostosis varies with each tumor, but is most commonly seen with tuberculum sellae meningiomas,[14] occurring in 50% of patients reported by di Chiro and Lindgren.[92] The hyperostosis usually involves the planum, but may extend laterally to the anterior clinoids, optic foramina, or posteriorly into the sella floor. Di Chiro and Lindgren[92] found definite sellar changes in 20%, suggestive changes in 25%, and a normal sella in 55% of patients. Enlargement of the sella in infrequent. The incidence of calcification is low.

CT scans should clearly demonstrate the lesion as well as the hyperostosis[20] (Fig. 11A and B), while arteriography with selective studies and subtraction techniques may show enlarged feeding arteries or a characteristic meningioma blush in about 33% of cases[62] (Fig. 10). PEG will show a filling defect in the anterior third ventricle that is nonspecific.

The differentiation from pituitary adenoma clinically is based on the

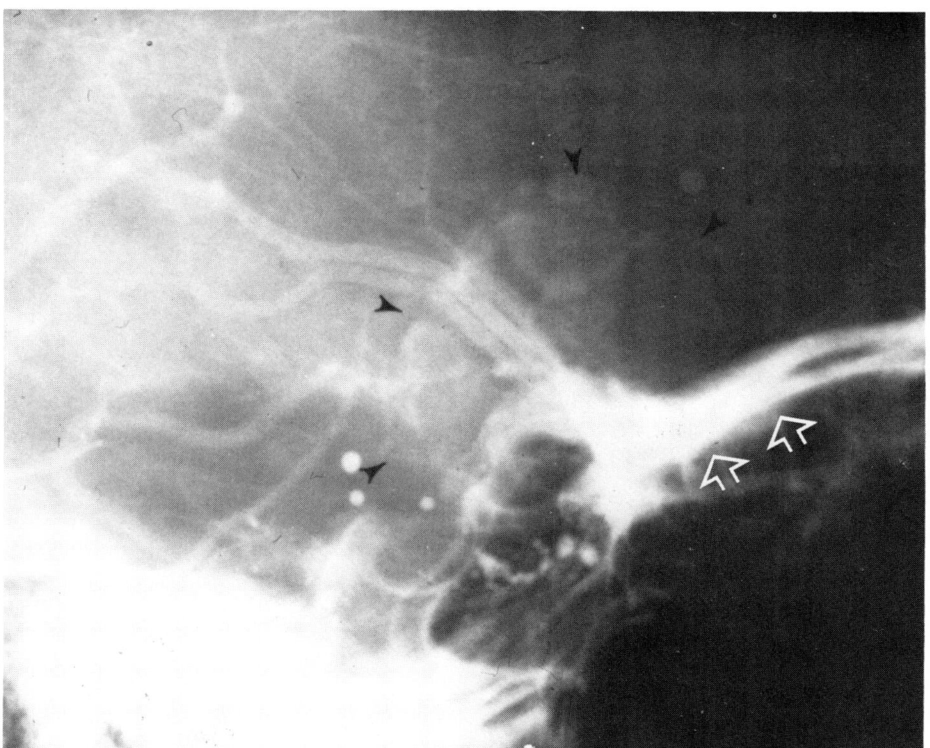

Fig. 10. Right carotid arteriogram, venous phase. Note the homogeneous vascular blush of a tumor (solid arrowhead) above the tuberculum sella and adjacent planum sphenoidale. Note also the hyperostosis involving the planum sphenoidale, extending anteriorly to involve the orbital roofs (open arrows). Diagnosis: meningioma.

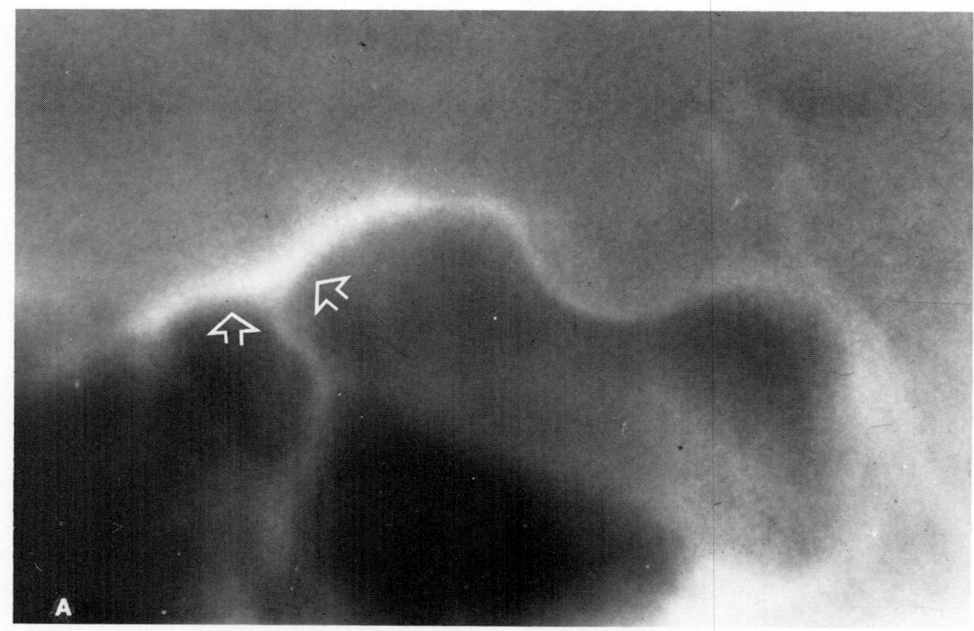

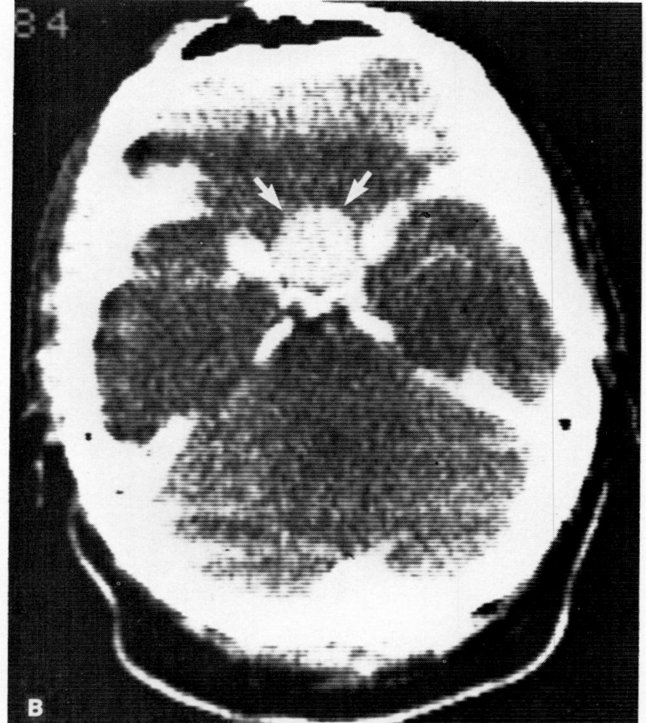

Fig. 11. (A) Lateral tomogram of the sella demonstrating hyperostosis of the planum sphenoidale (arrows). (B) Horizontal enhanced CT scan demonstrating a tumor mass (arrows) anterior to the circle of Willis.

severe visual symptoms and signs with usually intact endocrine function. Radiographically, hyperostosis, a normal-sized sella, and a suprasellar mass on CT and PEG should be definitive.

Case No. 7

A 54-year-old hypertensive engineer had complained of headaches for 7 months. He had noted within the previous month decreased central vision, flashes of light in both eyes, and blurring of his temporal field in the left eye. He described this blurring as a waviness, "like looking at a contour map." Endocrine history was completely negative.

On examination, his visual acuity was 20/20+ in the right eye and 20/40 in the left eye. Amsler grids revealed a bitemporal defect that caused distortion of the lines. Goldmann fields demonstrated a bitemporal field loss. The remainder of his examination was normal.

Skull X-rays and sellar tomography were normal. The CT scan showed a contrast-enhancing lesion in the sellar and suprasellar region (Fig. 11B). Arteriography demonstrated elevation of the A-1 segments of both anterior cerebral arteries and mild lateral displacement of the intracavernous portion of the internal carotid artieries. A tumor blush was not evident.

Because the CT scan indicated that this mass was also intrasellar, a transsphenoidal operation was performed despite the normal tomograms, with the findings of a normal pituitary gland. The following week, through a right frontal craniotomy, a diaphragma meningioma was found and removed. Vision returned to normal.

Comment: This case is typical of suprasellar meningiomas. The normal sella should have suggested the correct diagnosis initially, despite the lack of bone changes or blush on arteriography. The CT scan was probably misinterpreted because a pure sella tomographic cut was not taken. With overlap between the sella and suprasellar region, there appeared to be intrasellar tumor. Eight-millimeter overlapping CT cuts through the sellar region are necessary to assure a pure sella picture. The transsphenoidal route of surgery was chosen because of the significant lower morbidity and mortality as compared with craniotomy. The normal pituitary function would be unusual with a pituitary adenoma of this size.

4.12. Pituitary Metastases

Metastatic disease in the sella or pituitary gland may, on occasion, be confused with a primary tumor. It is usually associated with multiple metastases to bone. The most frequent primary tumors metastasizing to the sella turcica are carcinomas of the breast, bronchus, kidney, and colon. Occasionally, a sellar lesion may be the presenting problem, but usually is part of a metastatic constellation causing no difficulty in diagnosis.

Radiographically, destructive changes are seen in the margins of the sella, but these may be lacking.[93]

The case described below was seen in our clinic.

Case No. 8

A 35-year-old woman presented in May 1975 with complaints of impaired vision in her left eye for 5 months. A left superior temporal quadrantic defect was found on visual-field testing. Her vision deteriorated progressively, and in December 1975 her right eye became affected. Examination showed a bitemporal hemianopsia, right worse than left. Bilateral optic atrophy was noted with acuity 20/40 O.D. and 20/400 O.S. Extraocular movements were full, and the remainder of her examination was normal. Skull X-rays and tomograms showed complete erosion of the sella (Fig. 12A and B); CT scan demonstrated a large enhancing sella and suprasellar mass (Fig. 12C). Arteriography demonstrated a large tumor blush filling the sella, suprasellar cistern, and clinoid region with appropriate vessel displacement (Fig. 12D and E). The meningohypophyseal arteries originating from the internal carotids were enlarged. The initial diagnosis was meningioma, and a right frontal craniotomy was performed with the finding of a very large tumor arising behind the optic nerves and chiasma, compressing them severely, and laterally displacing both carotid arteries. Considerable tumor bleeding limited the procedure. Pathological examination of the specimen showed tumor consistent with pituitary adenoma. Postoperatively, 5000 rads of radiation were given. Endocrine test-

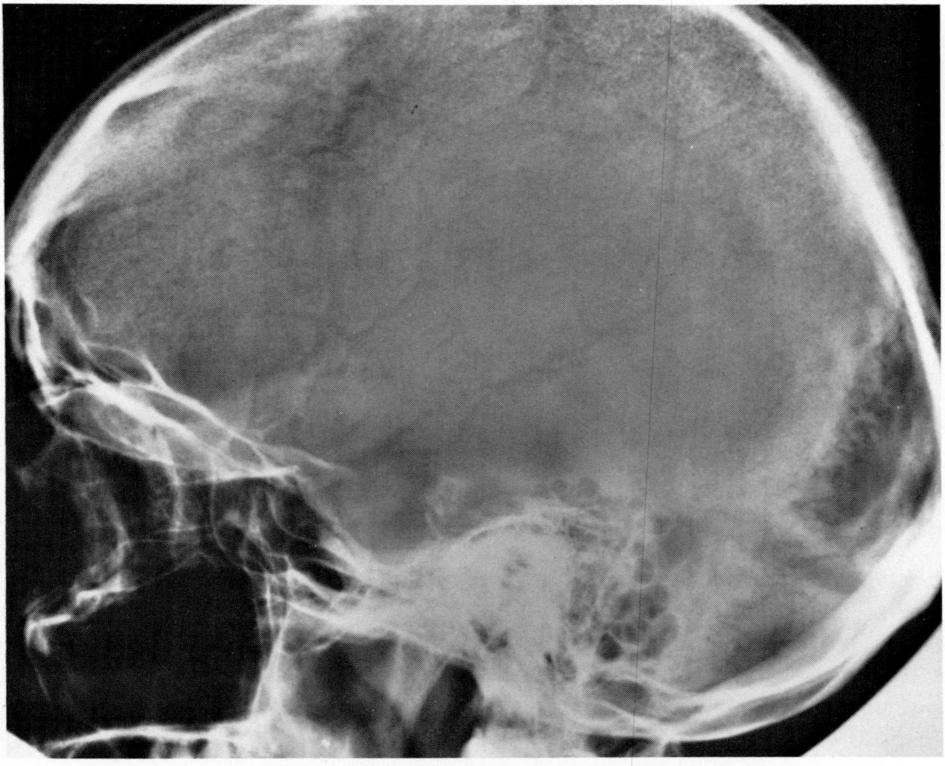

Fig. 12A. Lateral skull X-ray demonstrating a destroyed sella turcica with considerable expansion.

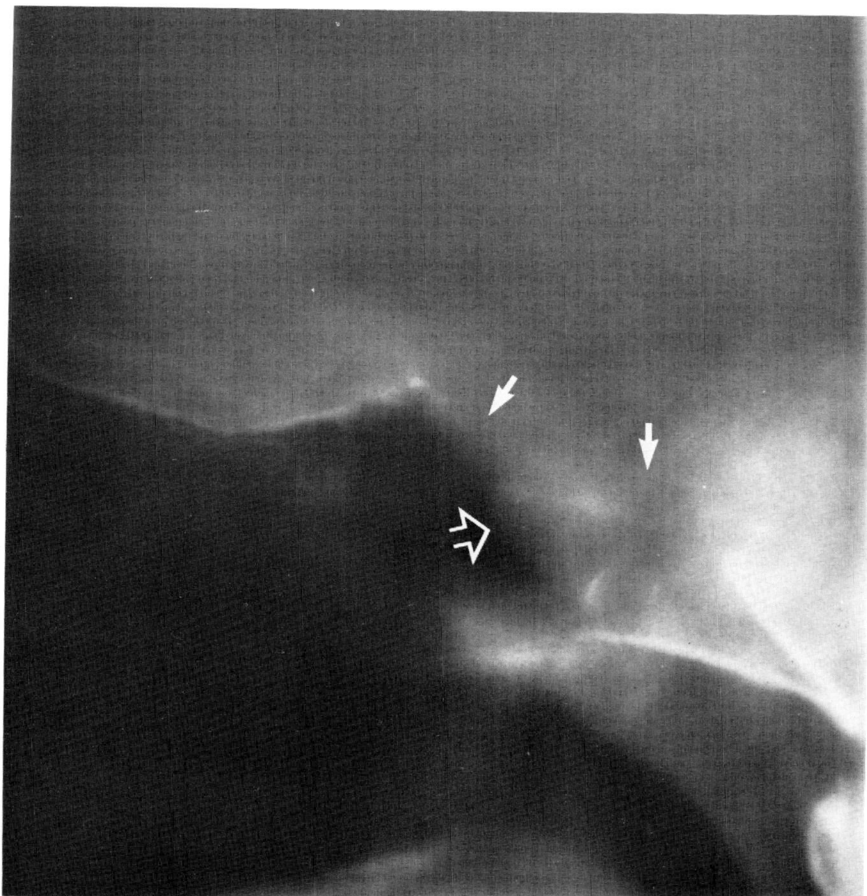

Fig. 12B. Lateral tomogram, again demonstrating considerable destruction of the sella floor (solid arrows) with tumor extending into the sphenoid sinus (open arrow). Note the destruction also of the adjacent clivus.

ing showed panhypopituitarism, and replacement hormones were given. At 5 months after surgery, her acuity had improved to 20/20 O.D. and 20/40 O.S., while visual fields showed only small superior quadrant bitemporal hemianopsia. Repeat CT scan showed resolution of the suprasellar mass; however, 1 month later, she returned with a right sixth nerve paresis. At this time, 12 months after her initial surgery, a transsphenoidal decompression of her tumor was performed; again, the pathology was consistent with pituitary adenoma. There was no mitosis nor any anaplastic cells. Little improvement in the sixth nerve paresis was seen, and she developed, progressively, a right third, fourth, and partial fifth nerve paresis. Shortly thereafter, metastases were appreciated in the liver, and a renal-cell carcinoma was found in the kidney. Review of the previous surgical tissue was consistent with metastasis from this tumor. She expired 2½ years after her initial presentation.

Comment: This case demonstrates an extremely aggressive sellar and

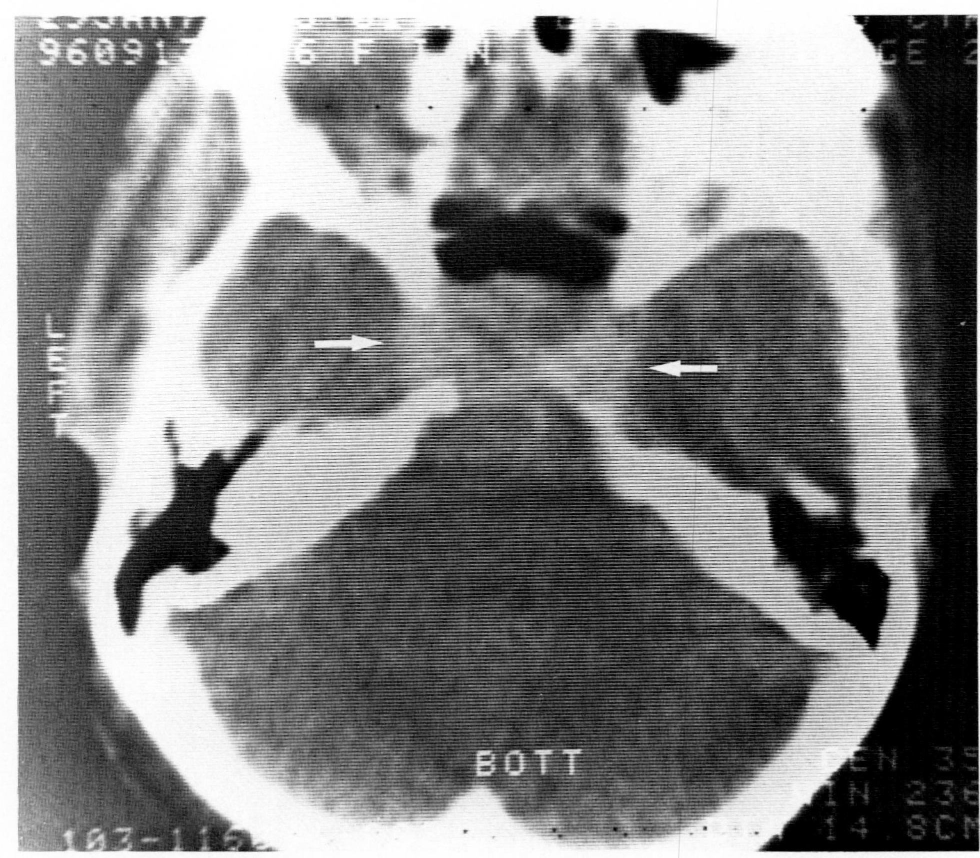

Fig. 12C. Enhanced CT scan demonstrating tumor within the sella and sphenoid sinus. The tumor is seen extending on either side of the sella to involve the cavernous sinuses (arrows).

parasellar tumor, most unusual for pituitary adenoma. The initial extensive bone destruction was a clue to the malignant nature of the tumor, yet the biopsies were read as pituitary adenoma. Renal-cell carcinoma is notorious for the lack of nuclear atypicism and mitosis in many cases. On review of the biopsy material, after the diagnosis of renal-cell carcinoma was established, a tubular pattern of tumor cells was appreciated in the second biopsy. The first biopsy remains histologically indistinguishable from pituitary adenoma, but clearly is the same tumor as that seen in the later biopsy. Metastases must be considered in the differential diagnosis of pituitary adenomas. An isolated lesion in the sella is most unusual, and most metastases are easier to differentiate from adenoma histologically than renal-cell carcinoma.

5. Miscellaneous Tumors

Hypothalamic hamartomas,[94,95] infundibulomas,[96] and myoblastomas[97] also occur in the sellar and parasellar areas. Hypothalamic hamartomas are often associated with precocious puberty, probably due to secretion of luteinizing-hormone-releasing hormone. These tumors are extremely rare and have no specific clinical or radiographic features that distinguish them from other tumors in the sellar and parasellar regions.

6. Aneurysms

A large carotid aneurysm in the sella turcica simulating a pituitary adenoma was reported as early as 1889 by Weir Mitchell.[98] Cushing[99] also reported progressive visual failure and optic atrophy in a patient with a pituitary adenoma as well as an interpeduncular aneurysm; he concluded that the compressive effects of either lesion could be the same, with an aneurysm causing hypopituitarism.

White and Ballatine[100] reviewed 35 cases of intrasellar aneurysm simulating hypophyseal tumors. In their opening paragraph, they state:

> In order for an aneurysm to be mistaken for an adenoma or craniopharyngioma it must expand the sella turcica, interrupt the decussating optic fibers, and compress the pituitary gland. Furthermore, it must do this without telltale bleeding, calcification of its wall, pain in the forehead or ocular palsies from injury to the nerves in the cavernous sinus.

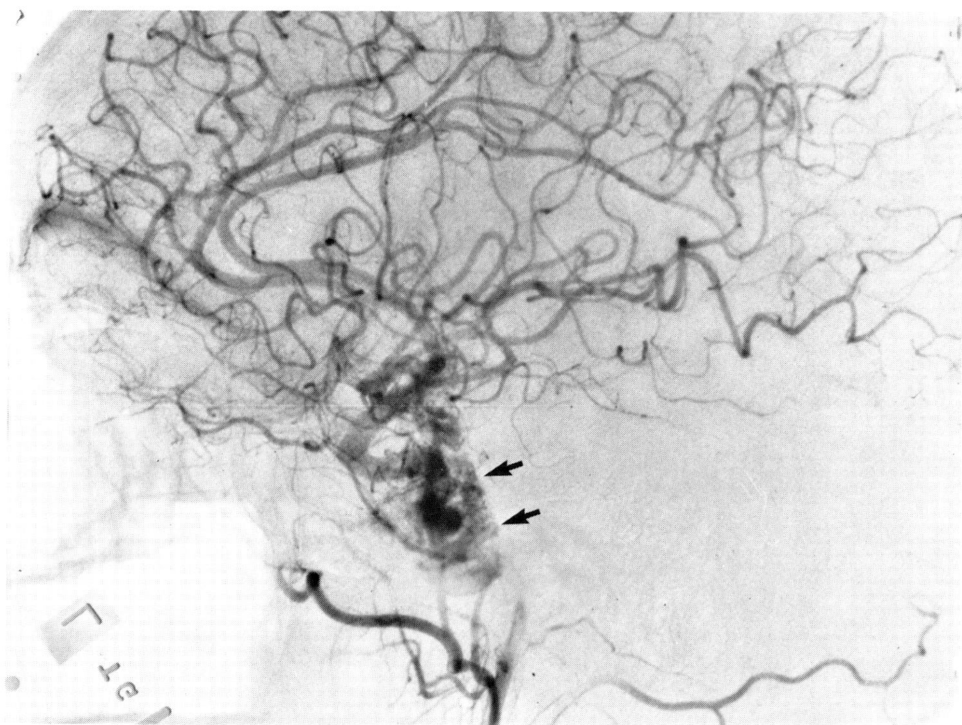

Fig. 12D. Left common carotid arteriogram demonstrating a vascular tumor mass surrounding the petrous and cavernous portions of the internal carotid artery (arrows).

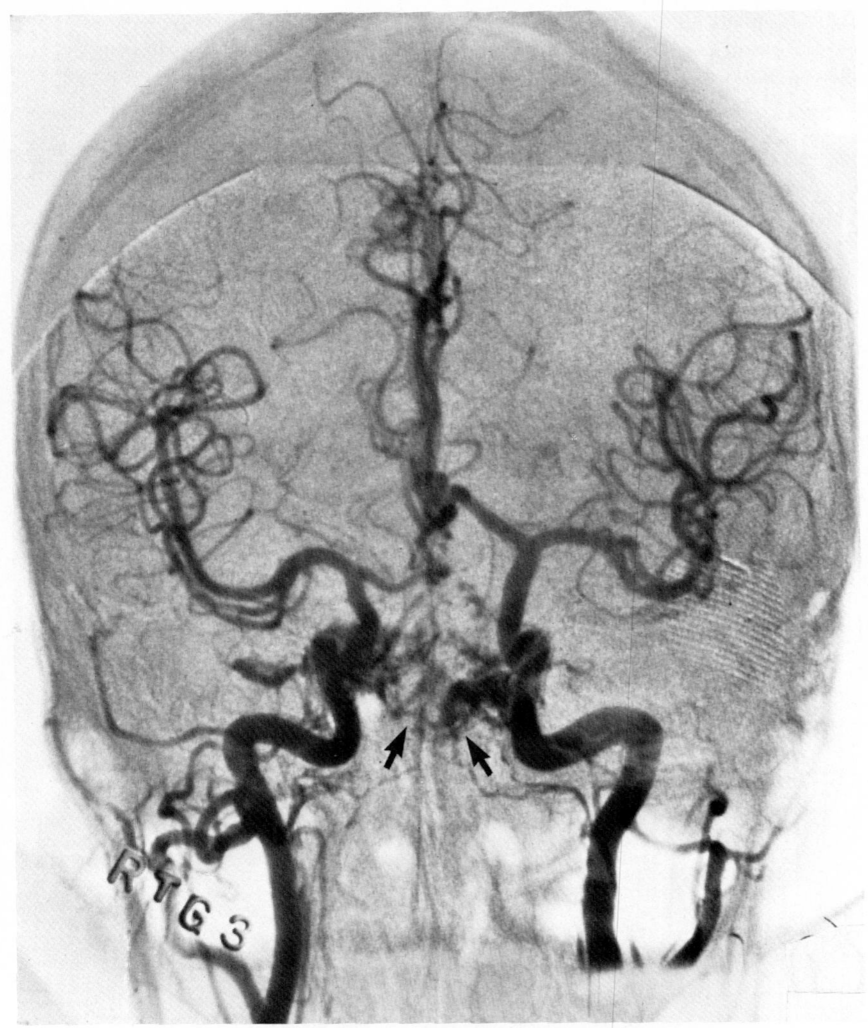

Fig. 12E. Bilateral common carotid arteriograms (superimposed subtraction prints) demonstrating vascular tumor mass between the two petrous and cavernous carotid arteries (arrows). Diagnosis: metastatic renal-cell carcinoma.

Aneurysms may be incidental findings associated with pituitary adenomas[101,102] or suprasellar masses compressing the optic nerve or chiasma or both. They may also rarely be the cause of hypopituitarism.[100,103] Those causing para- and suprasellar signs usually take origin from the proximal intracranial carotid, while those causing direct pituitary compression arise from the infraclinoid carotid with the aneurysm pointing medially into the sella (Fig. 13).

The importance of correct diagnosis is exemplified by White's three cases. The first had a spontaneous rupture the day prior to scheduled craniotomy for pituitary tumor. The second was ruptured during transsphenoidal

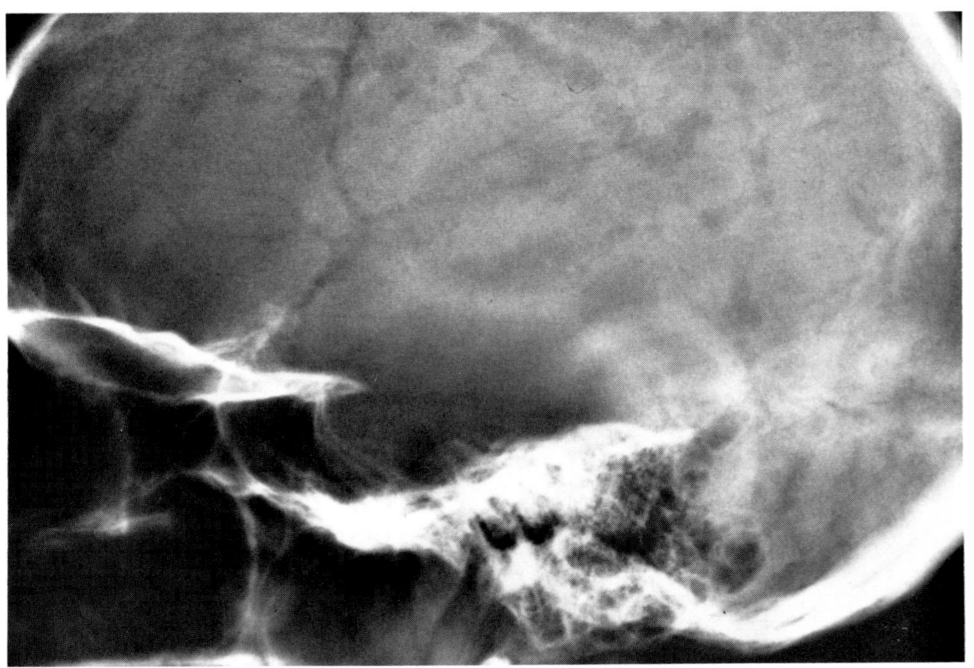

Fig. 13A. Lateral skull X-ray demonstrating enlargement of the sella with erosion of the floor and amputation of the dorsum sella.

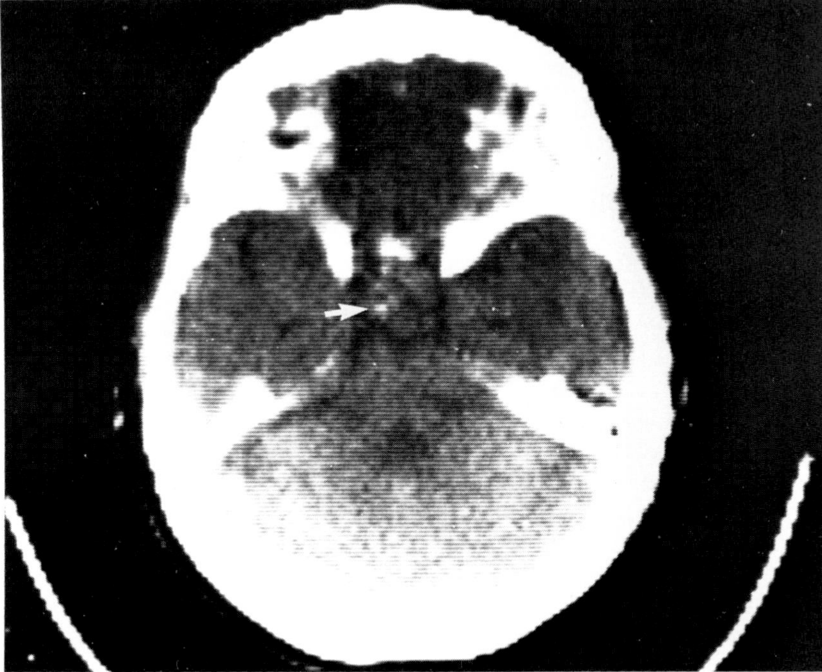

Fig. 13B. Nonenhanced CT scan demonstrating soft tissue mass within the sella. Note the fleck of calcium (arrow).

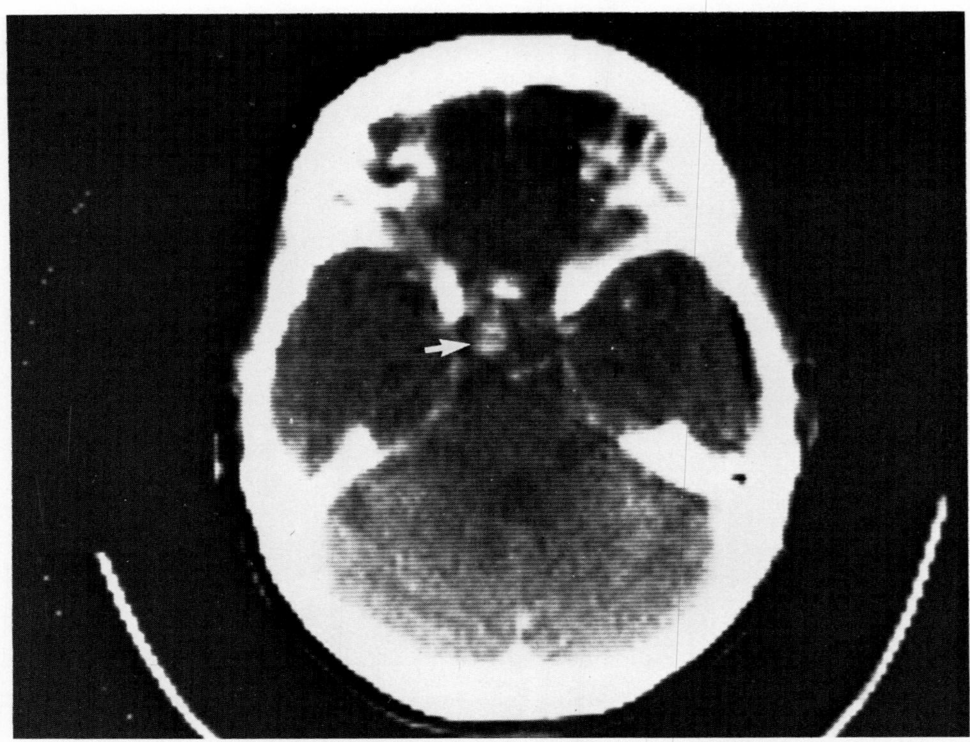

Fig. 13C. CT scan with contrast demonstrating an asymmetrical enhancing lesion within the sella (arrow).

surgery for presumed pituitary adenoma expanding the sella. The third was discovered during a reexploration for recurrent craniopharyngioma.[100]

Intrasellar aneurysms may not yield any visual changes; however, suprasellar aneurysms usually alter the visual fields. Walsh[104] states that the field defects will not differentiate aneurysm from tumor, while Bird *et al.*[105] find that the field loss and temporal profile will help in the diagnosis. Jefferson[106,107] reported that the most characteristic field defects were: "a) a scotomatous homolateral eye, with an overlying homonymous defect in the nasal field of that eye and in the temporal field of the other; b) bitemporal defects only clearly aneurysmal because of inferior quadrantic loss as the earliest sign, or because of the suddenness of development, or because of ocular muscle palsies, as well as pain; c) nasal hemianopsia in the ipsilateral eye." In the series of White and Ballantine,[100] 13 patients had a bitemporal hemianopsia or quadrantanopsia, and 6 had monocular blindness with loss of the temporal field in the opposite eye.

Endocrine disorders may occur, including amenorrhea, impotence, loss of libido, fatigue, somnolence, hypothyroidism, diabetes insipidus, small stature, severe ACTH insufficiency, and obesity.[100,103] The earlier reports were limited in their ability to assay these hormones, but clinical panhypopituitarism has occurred.

Other clinical features suggestive of aneurysm include supraorbital pain, episodes of intense headache, sudden onset of symptoms, and signs of compression of the third, fourth, fifth, and sixth cranial nerves.[62,100]

Radiographic studies of the sella may show classic changes of an enlarged sella secondary to a pituitary tumor. There may be asymmetrical destruction of the sella with erosion of the ipsilateral anterior clinoid.[106] If seen, a rim of calcification in the wall is characteristic, but may resemble a craniopharyngioma (Fig. 5). Arteriography is almost always diagnostic provided the sac is not totally thrombosed as it was in three of White and Ballantine's cases.[100,108] Additionally, the size of the aneurysm may be misleading because of significant amounts of clot within the dome.[109]

CT scans performed immediately after rapid infusion of contrast and during continued maintenance contrast infusion show intense homogeneous blushes. The appearance may be similar to that of a highly vascular meningioma.[29] CT scan, by demonstrating clot within the aneurysm, provides a more accurate evaluation of its size than does angiography. This must be

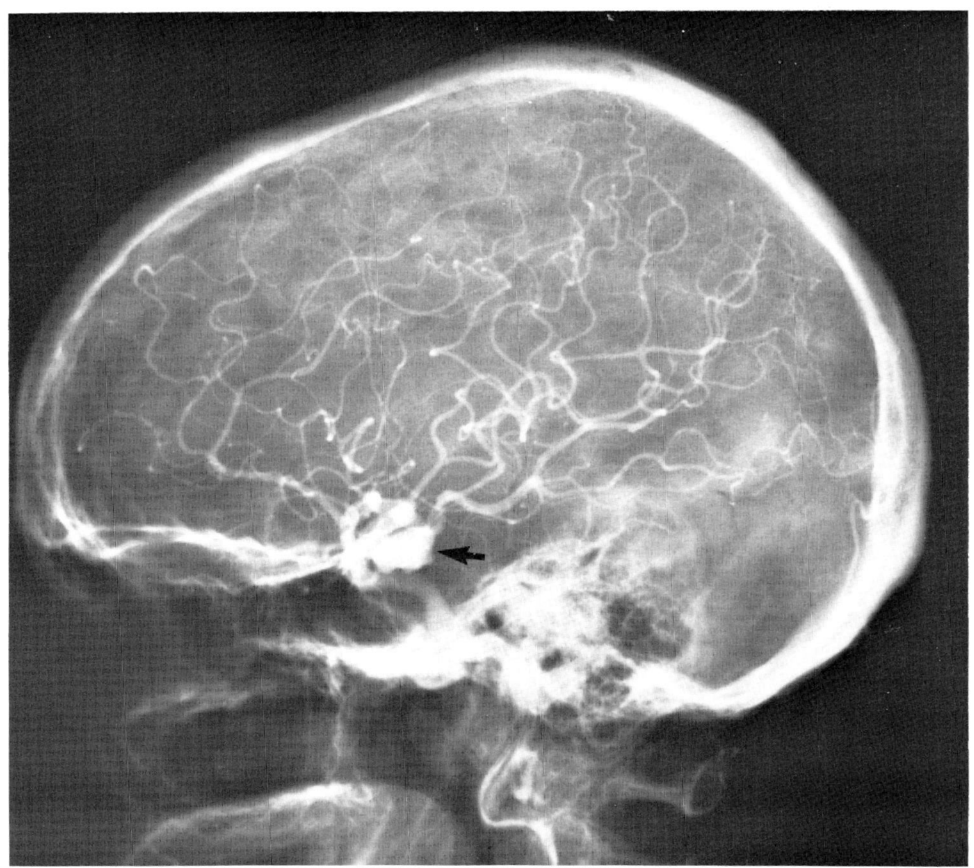

Fig. 13D. Left internal carotid arteriogram demonstrating a large aneurysm (arrow) originating from the terminal internal carotid artery adjacent to the origin of the ophthalmic artery.

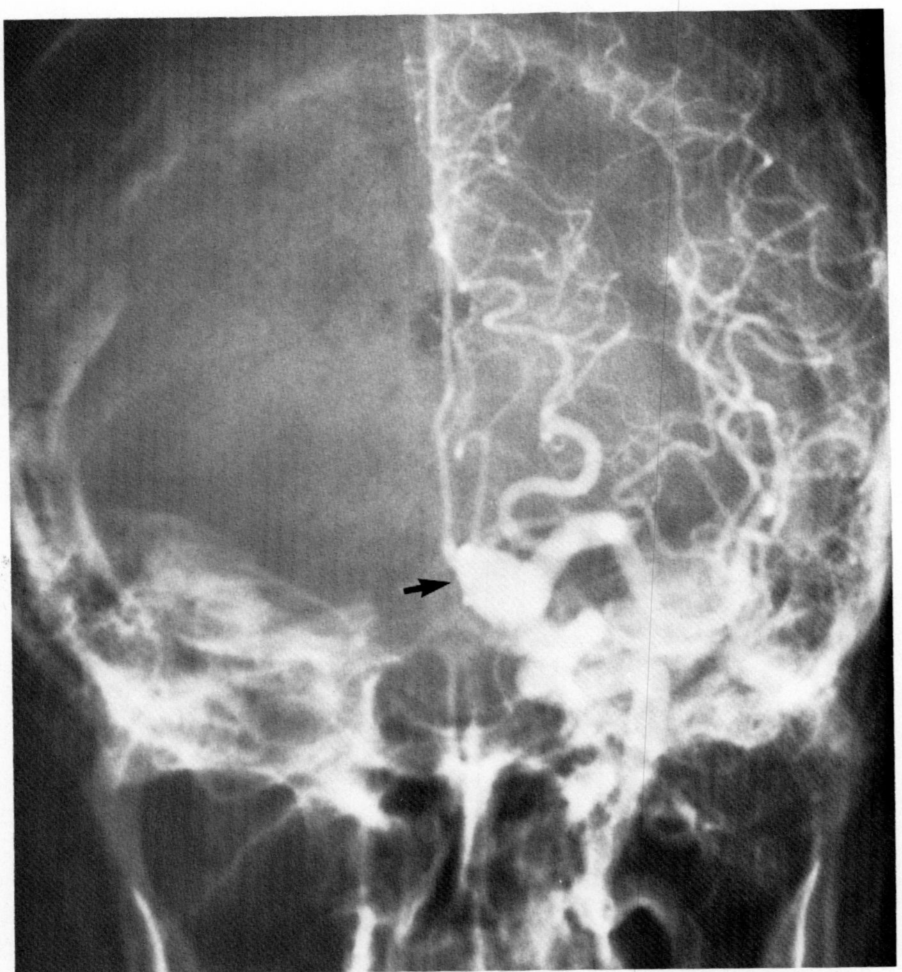

Fig. 13E. (Same patient.) Again, note the large aneurysm extending medially into the sella turcica (arrow).

known because fatal hemorrhage may result if a large aneurysm is inadvertently opened during surgery.

Aneurysms may also be found in conjunction with pituitary adenomas (Fig. 14A and B).

Case No. 9

A 65-year-old woman had a 15-month history of hypothyroidism treated with replacement therapy. Two months prior to referral, she became septic secondary to a urinary tract infection and renal lithiasis. Subsequent testing demonstrated adrenal insufficiency. Neurological examination was normal. Skull X-rays and sella tomograms showed destruction of the sella. A CT scan showed a sellar and suprasellar mass with calcification and asymmetrical en-

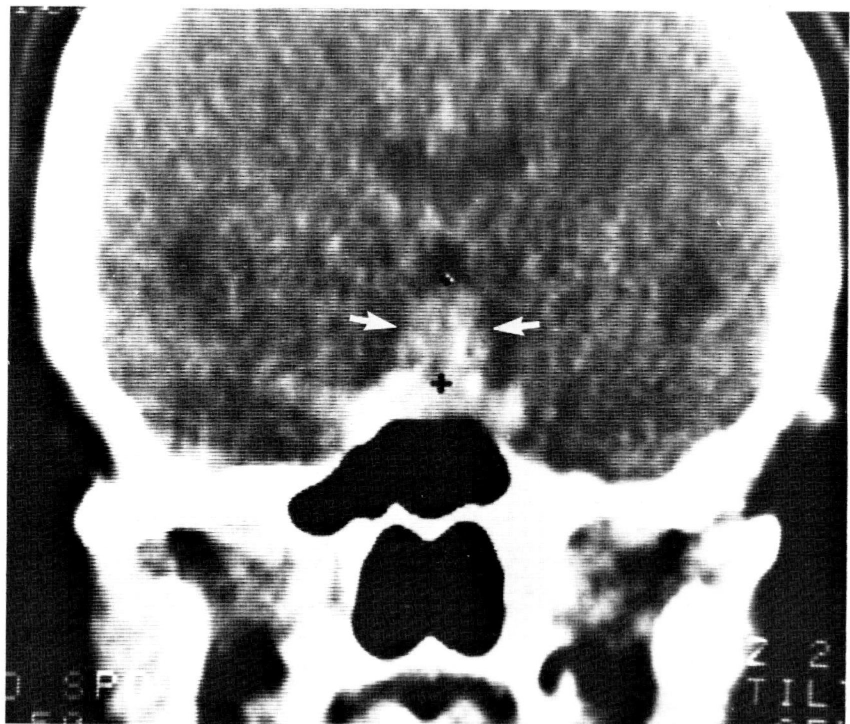

Fig. 14A. Contrast-enhanced coronal CT scan demonstrating a suprasellar mass (arrows) indenting the third ventricle.

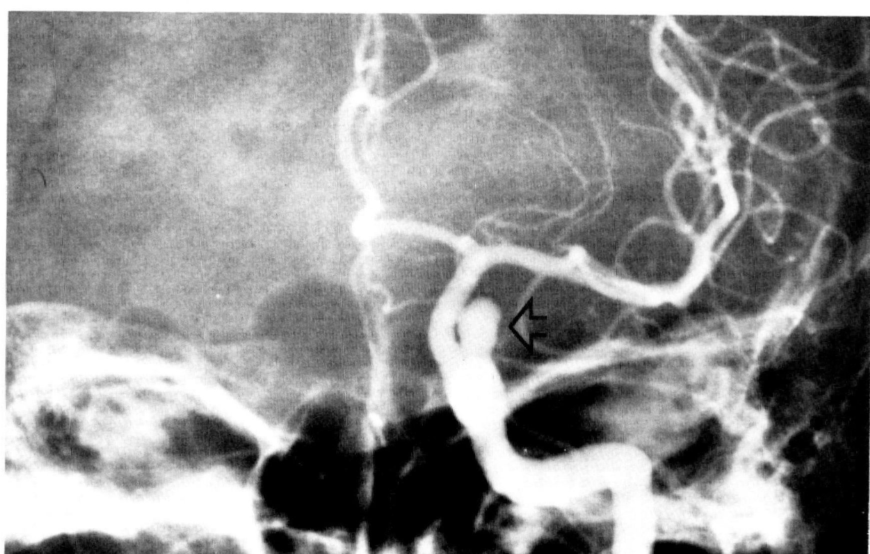

Fig. 14B. Left internal carotid arteriogram demonstrating an aneurysm originating from the cavernous carotid, extending superiorly adjacent to the terminal portion of the internal carotid artery (arrow). Diagnosis: pituitary adenoma and incidental carotid artery aneurysm.

hancement, suggestive of an aneurysm. A carotid arteriogram demonstrated an aneurysm taking origin from the left internal carotid artery just above the cavernous sinus. The aneurysm pointed medially and filled the sella. A left craniotomy was performed and the aneurysm wrapped.

Comment: This patient exemplifies the need for arteriography in non-secreting sellar and parasellar masses to exclude aneurysm. If this patient had been explored via a transsphenoidal route with the anticipation of finding an adenoma, the result could have been disastrous.

7. Pituitary Abscess

Pituitary abscesses may be due to direct extension of adjacent infection in the sphenoid sinuses, cavernous sinus, or CSF, or they may be secondary to a bacteremia. They may also be associated with pituitary adenomas or craniopharygniomas that undergo secondary infection.[110–112] CSF leaks and recurrent meningitis may also be predisposing factors.[113] The infection may be acute, such as with a fulminant meningitis[112] or cavernous sinus thrombosis,[111] or it may be chronic.[110]

Symptoms may be identical to those of pituitary tumors: headache, visual disturbances, endocrinopathy, and diabetes inspidus.[113] The sella is usually enlarged and occasionally destroyed.[114]

Lindholm *et al.*[113] end their review of 18 cases with this statement:

> At present it must be considered impossible to establish the diagnosis pre-operatively. Suspicion of a pituitary or intrasellar abscess should be aroused if signs of an expanding process in the sella are combined with recent episodes of meningitis, rhinorrhea, pleocytosis of the CSF.

However, in a review of 29 cases, Domingue and Wilson[114] suggest that the diagnosis can be made preoperatively. An enlarged sella coexisting with bacterial meningitis, or bacterial meningitis coinciding with a known or suspected pituitary tumor, should alert attention to the possibility of pituitary abscess. Similarly, visual-field defects in a patient with meningitis are suggestive.[114]

8. Granulomatous and Infectious Diseases

8.1. Tuberculosis

Tuberculosis in the central nervous system can present in one of three ways: as tuberculous meningitis at the base, as a tuberculoma in various locations with all the signs of a mass, and as a tuberculous abscess. In the United States, intracranial tuberculoma is found in between 0.7 and 1.4% of all brain tumors.[115] In European countries, it is slightly more common (3–6% of intracranial lesions),[116] and in India, tuberculoma constitutes approximately 20% of tumors.[117] Udani *et al.*[118] studied 600 patients with tuberculous involvement of the central nervous system. Of this group, 8 patients had "hypothalamic–pituitary syndromes." In tuberculous meningitis, a dense plaque-like exudate at the base of the brain can involve the sellar and parasellar region. This may calcify in approximately 3–6% of cases. The pituitary and hypothalamic syndromes seen included Cushing's syndrome, obesity, diabetes inspidus, increased sleep requirement, and precocious sexual development. In some of these cases, a calcified mass (tuberculoma) was demonstrated to cause compression of the pituitary directly, or hypothalamic dysfunction secondary to a dilated third ventricle. Banna *et al.*[116] reported a patient with a large suprasellar mass that was calcified and had a wide dural attachment. Arteriography demonstrated meningeal hypertrophy and the signs of some inflammatory reaction in the anterior cerebral arteries.[116]

It is clear that an avascular tumor, either calcified or not, in the suprasellar region could be difficult to distinguish from a pituitary adenoma with suprasellar extension. Most of the patients with the pituitary or hypothalamic syndromes due to tuberculosis have had other signs of active tuberculosis, although this is not invariably the case. The diagnosis of a tuberculoma in the region may be made only histologically.

8.2. Sarcoid

Sarcoidosis involving the central nervous system is rare, and found in only 18 patients of a total of 450 with sarcoid who were studied by Silverstein *et al.*[119] Although it is uncommon for sarcoid to involve the central nervous system, when it does, there seems to be a predilection for the hypothalamic–pituitary region,[120–122] with a granulomatous or adhesive arachnoiditis and invasion of the floor of the third ventricle. The most common clinical syndrome seen with sarcoid in the hypothalamic region is diabetes insipidus and other signs of hypothalamic insufficiency. There is often optic atrophy and compression of other cranial nerves. Hyperprolactinemia and low GH-secreting reserve have also been described secondary to sarcoid, presumably because of interference with PIF. Intrasellar sarcoid has also been reported, but this is exceedingly rare. Contrast studies and CT scan,[121,123] of hypothalamic sarcoid may resemble suprasellar extension of an adenoma (or any other suprasellar mass). There is usually no bony change in the sella itself, and on angiography the mass is avascular. Although there are usually other signs of sarcoid that help make the diagnosis evident, there are occasional cases reported in which hypothalamic dysfunction was the initial sign of the disease.

8.3. Histiocytosis X

Histiocytosis X is a general term that encompasses three diseases: eosinophilic granuloma, Hand–Schuller–Christian disease, and Letterer–Siwe disease. There seems to be a predilection for hypothalamic involvement when histiocytosis X involves the central nervous system.[124] Hand's original description of the classic presentation in 1893 illustrated a common triad of skull lesions, diabetes insipidus, and exophthalmos. It is now recognized that any endocrinopathy can result.[125] Perhaps one third to one half of all patients with histiocytosis X have diabetes insipidus, and it is often a presenting sign.[126] Presumably, these symptoms are secondary to involvement of the tuber cinereum of the hypothalamus. Atrophy of the pituitary stalk secondary to dural involvement has also been described.[126] Tibbs *et al.*[125] recently reported one case and reviewed eight others of histiocytosis X involving the hypothalamus with granuloma. They found that cerebral involvement was more common in children and that males and females were affected equally. If there are no other signs of histiocytosis X involving other organs, i.e., bone or viscera, then correct preoperative diagnosis might be impossible. Diagnostic studies have shown avascular mass lesions in the region of the hypothalamus that are not calcified and do not blush on angiography. CT scan may demon-

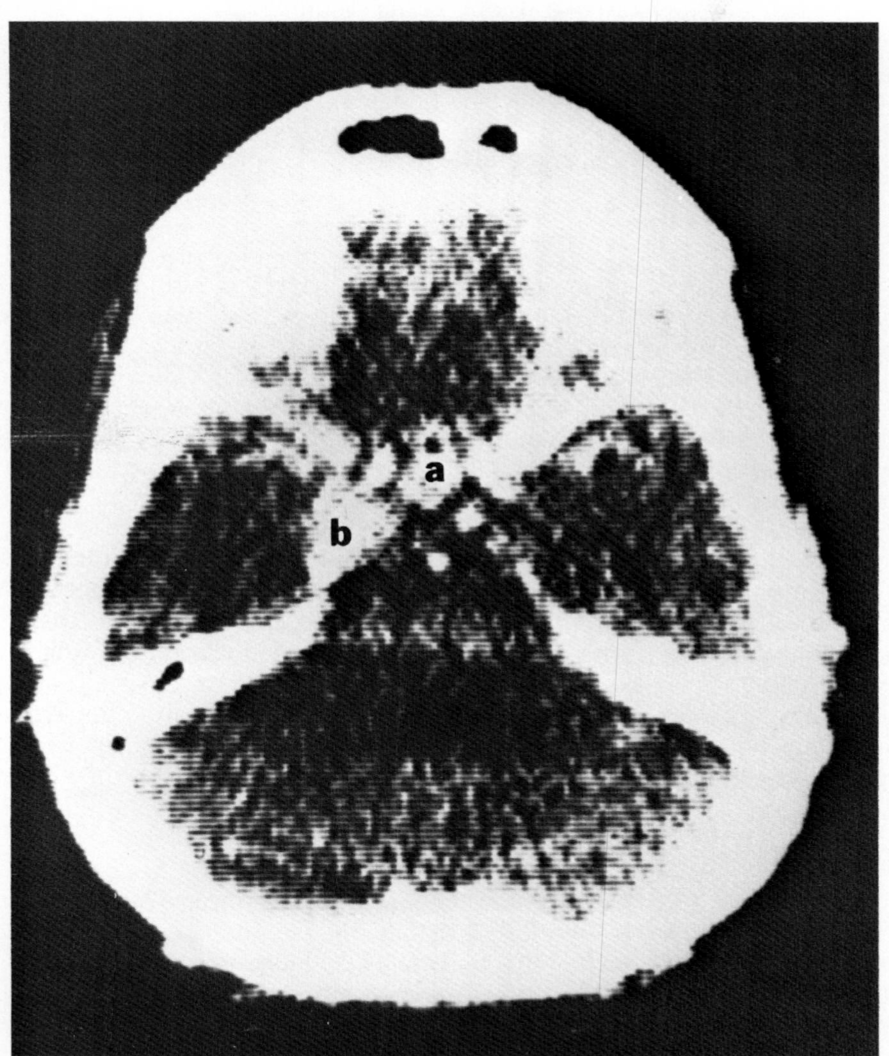

Fig. 15A. Contrast-enhanced CT scan demonstrating suprasellar (a) and parasellar (b) extension of a tumor.

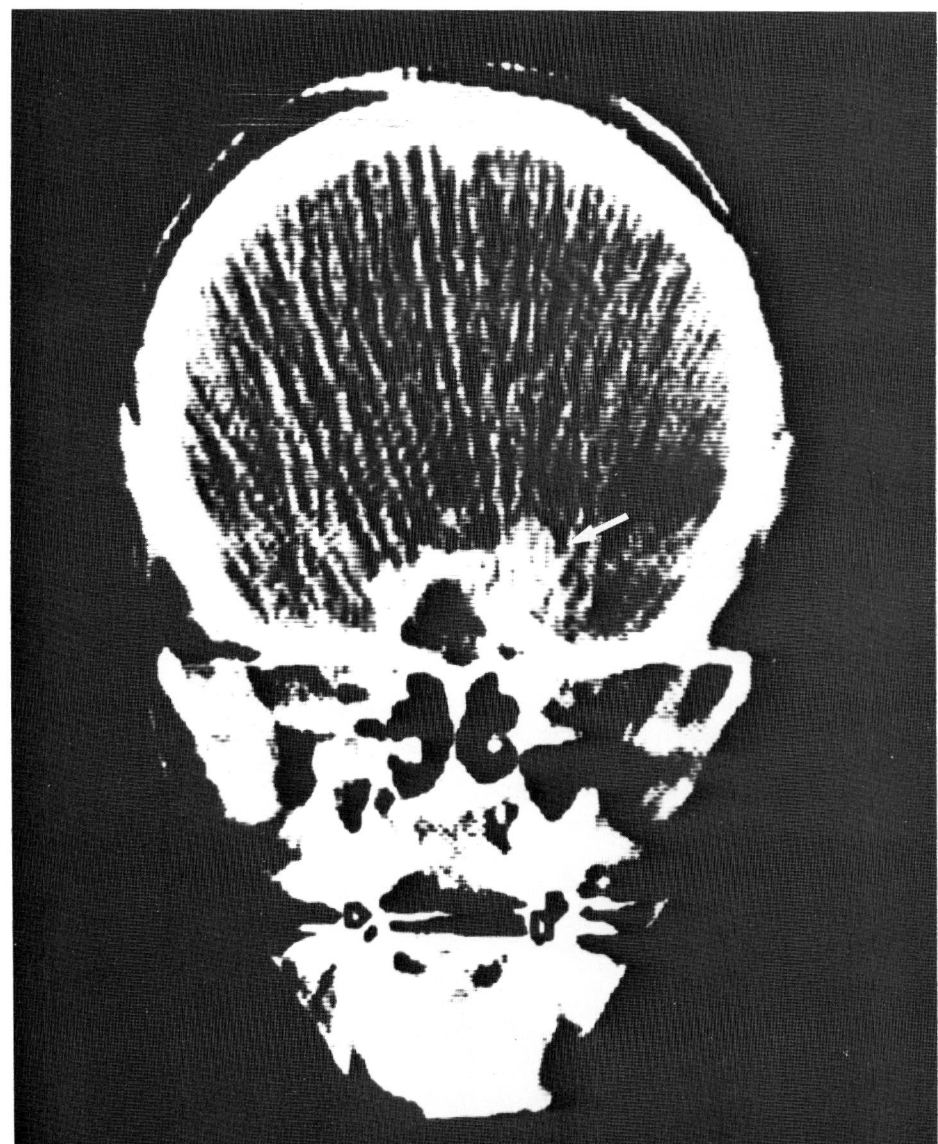

Fig. 15B. Coronal CT scan, again demonstrating the parasellar extent of the tumor (arrow). Diagnosis: eosiniphilic granuloma.

strate an enhancing mass (Fig. 15A and B). Since the treatment of this tumor requires such a small dose of radiation compared to that of a hypothalamic glioma, it is of obvious importance to make a histological diagnosis prior to treatment. Since sellar changes are not commonly seen with hypothalamic involvement by granuloma, it is unlikely that this lesion would be confused with a pituitary adenoma.

Case No. 10

A 29-year-old male had a 2-month history of progressively severe left frontotemporal headaches. Initial examination was unremarkable, and skull X-rays and CT scan were interpreted as normal. Lumbar puncture showed an opening pressure of 195 mm of water with a CSF protein of 70 mg. For 1 month, he noted polyuria and polydipsia, a decreased libido, and poor sexual performance. One week before admission and surgery, he developed left ptosis and diplopia. Examination confirmed a left third and sixth nerve palsy and a left superior quadrantanopsia. Endocrine evaluation confirmed partial diabetes insipidus and partial ACTH and gonadotropin deficiency. A CT scan demonstrated an enhancing sellar and suprasellar lesion with extension toward the left cavernous sinus (Fig. 15A and B). Bilateral carotid arteriograms demonstrated lateral deviation of the intracavernous portion of the carotids bilaterally. PEG failed to outline suprasellar tumor. A transsphenoidal approach to the sella was performed and an intrasellar tumor removed. Pathology was eosinophilic granuloma, and radiation therapy was given in the hope of eliminating the parasellar component.

9. Other Infectious Diseases

Other infectious diseases involving the hypothalamic and pituitary area are extremely rare. Cerebral cysticercosis has been described as a calcified lesion in this region.[127,128] Fungal infection with basal meningitis also can affect the sella and suprasellar structures.

10. Sphenoid Sinus Mucoceles

The etiology of sphenoid sinus mucoceles, first described in 1889 by Berg,[129] is not known, but may represent only an inflammatory occulsion of the draining ostium. There is a cystic accumulation of secretions, which is usually a sterile creamy fluid but occasionally is purulent. The collection expands the sinus, eventually compressing surrounding structures such as the cavernous sinus, pituitary gland, cranial nerves I–VI, and the carotid arteries.[130] There is no specific age preponderance, with a range of 13–75 years in the report of Nugent *et al.*[130]

Sphenoid mucoceles usually evolve over a long period, often years, with nonspecific headaches and relatively late onset of visual loss. The headache is usually severe and localized to the frontal or orbital region, with radiation to the vertex or occiput. Atypical facial pain with paresthesias secondary to irritation of the divisions of the trigeminal nerve may be seen as the mass enlarges posteriorly along the floor of the middle fossa.[131,132]

Visual loss is usually slowly progressive, but may be sudden. Optic neuropathy is most often unilateral, but 7 of 41 were bilateral in the series of Nugent *et al.*[130] Chiasmal type field defects are unusual, seen in only 2 of 41 patients.[130] Exophthalmos is present in about half. The progressive visual loss may be secondary to direct nerve compression by the mass or from scarring caused by an inflammatory reaction. The acute loss may be secondary to vascular compromise of the optic nerve.[131] Diplopia is common, most often from third nerve dysfunction, and less often from fourth nerve dysfunction.

Nugent *et al.*[130] frequently noted a history of previous otolaryngological disease such as sinusitis, intranasal polyps, and nasal discharge, while Kruger *et al.*[133] reported an absence of such history.

Endocrine dysfunction is unusual.[130]

Radiographic evaluation should include tomography demonstrating the superior orbital fissures, optic foramina, ethmoid sinus walls, sphenoid sinus, orbital walls, and sella.[134] Expansion of the sphenoid sinus, usually with intact walls, is found in most cases. The sella is usually involved with erosion of the floor, oftentimes difficult to tell whether from within or without (Fig. 16A and B). Erosion of the optic canal and orbital wall is frequent.[130] Suprasellar extension is unusual, and therefore arteriography and PEG are not revealing. CT scan may demonstrate the lesion.

The primary differences between mucocele and pituitary adenoma are: (1) the chronic, but remitting, course with occasional sudden visual loss, diplopia, and headache; (2) lack of typical bitemporal hemianopsia; (3) lack of pitu-

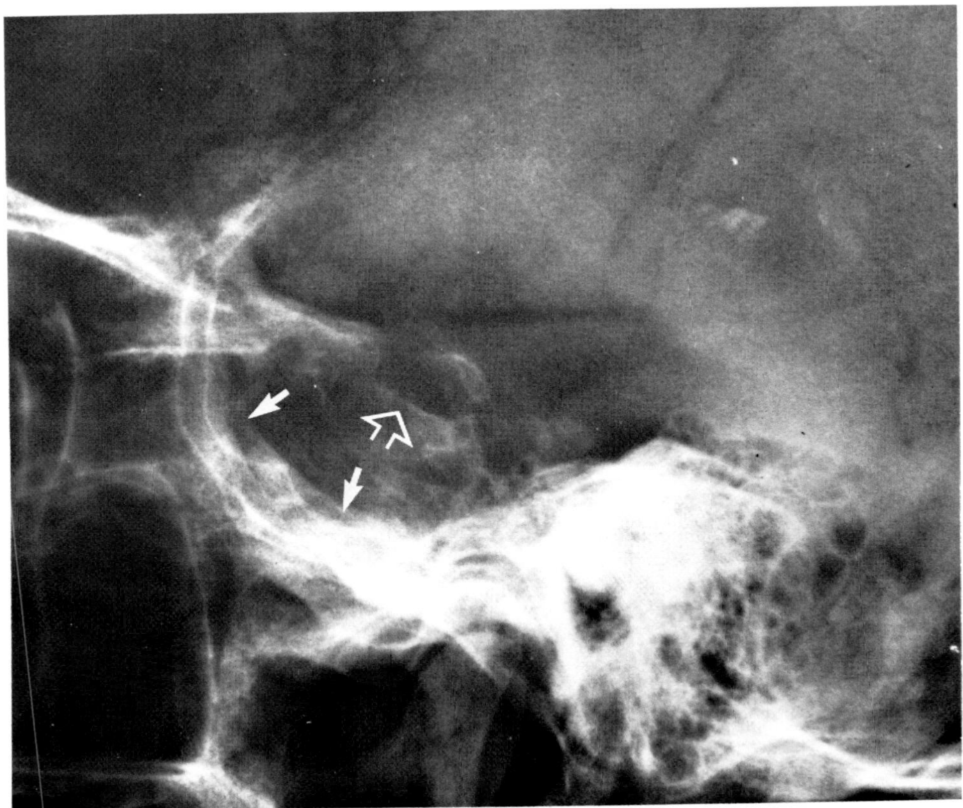

Fig. 16A. Lateral skull X-ray demonstrating an expanded sphenoid sinus (solid arrows) with elevation of the floor of the sella turcica (open arrow).

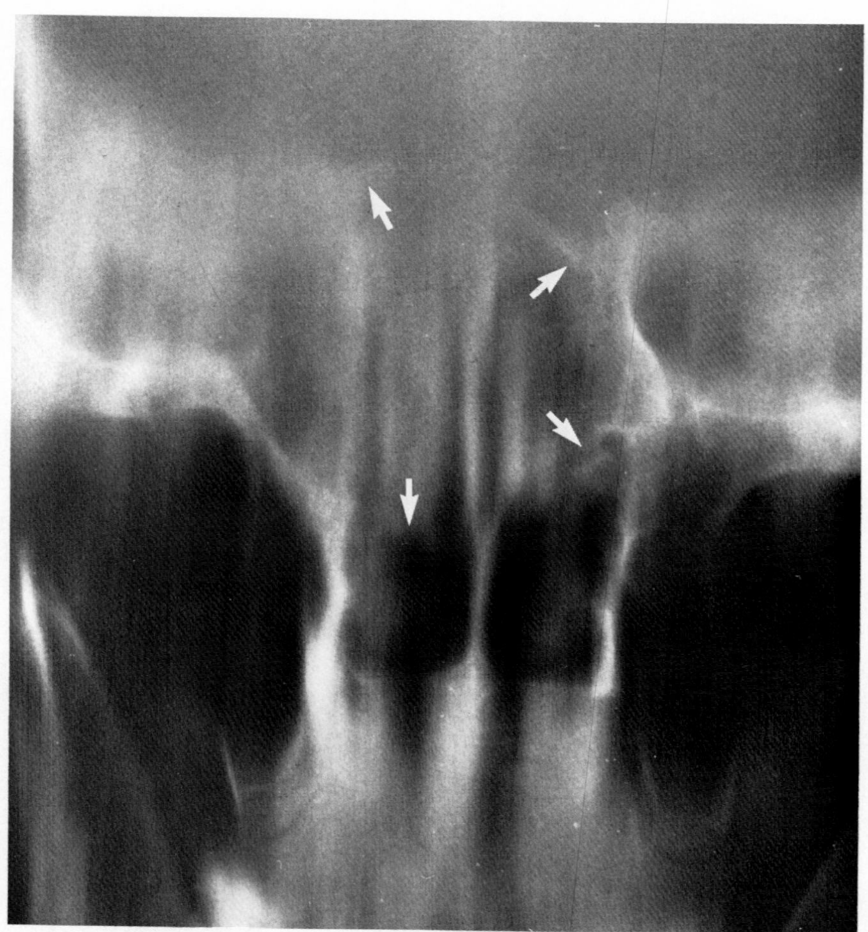

Fig. 16B. Frontal tomogram, again demonstrating expansion of the sphenoid sinus (arrows). Diagnosis: sphenoid sinus mucocele.

itary insufficiency; (4) less frequent ballooning of the sellar or suprasellar extension.[130]

11. Empty Sella

Since the initial description by Busch,[135] the prevalence of the primary empty sella has become extremely well known. Kaufman and Chamberlin[136] reported that 71.9% of diaphragma sellae in 89 autopsies on patients without known endocrine disease were incompetent enough to allow arachnoid herniation. Thirty-seven percent had partially empty sellas and 6.7% had completely empty sellas. A series reported by Bergland *et al.*[137] had a 20% incidence of arachnoid herniation into the sella. Weissberg *et al.*,[138] in a review of the enlarged sella, found the empty sella syndrome to be as common as pituitary adenomas. In this syndrome, the sella is found to be partially filled with CSF (demonstrated as air filling the "empty" space on PEG). The term

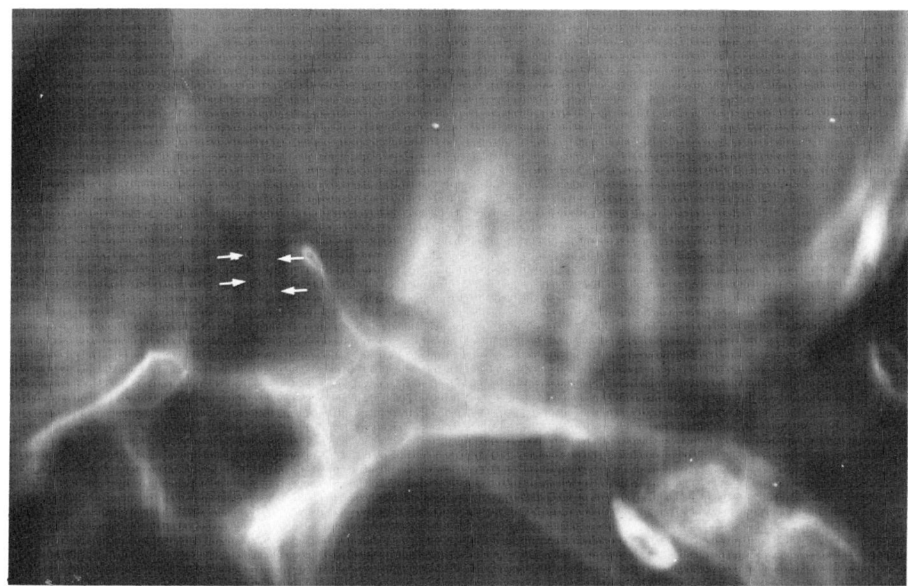

Fig. 17A. Lateral tomogram at pneumoencephalography demonstrating an enlarged sella. Note the defect in the anterior wall of the sella, secondary to surgery. The optic nerve (arrows) is seen herniating into the sella.

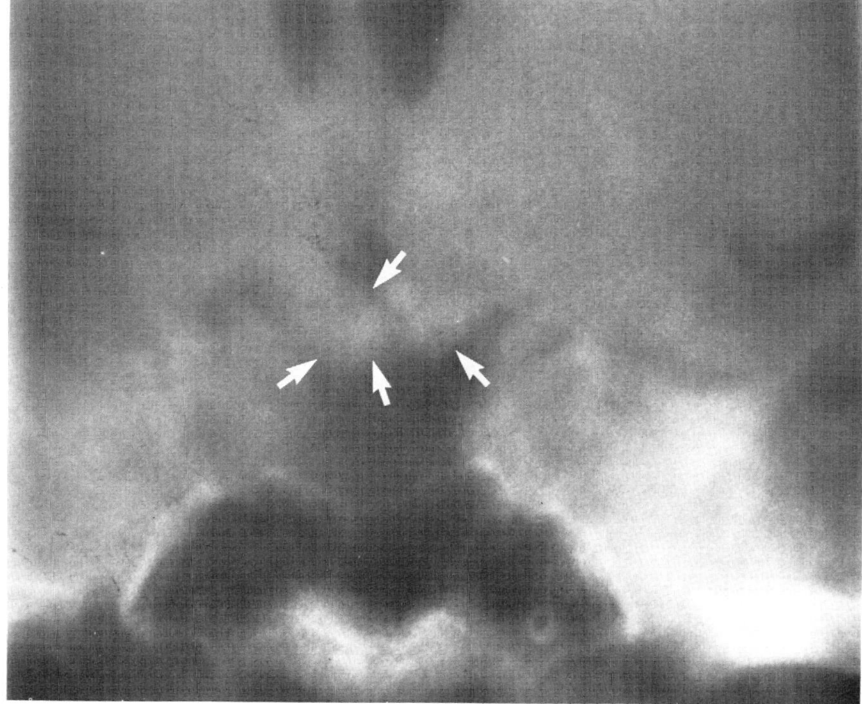

Fig. 17B. Frontal tomogram, again demonstrating the optic nerves (arrows) herniating into the sella. Diagnosis: surgically resected prolactinoma with postsurgical herniation of optic nerves into the sella.

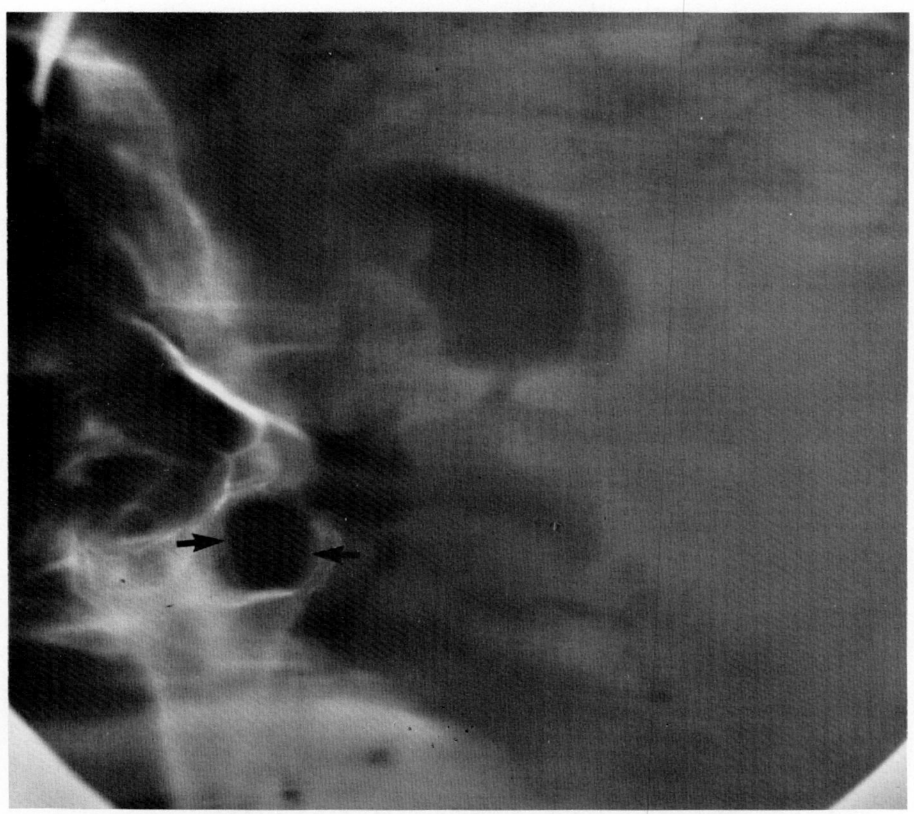

Fig. 18. Lateral tomogram at pneumoencephalography demonstrating air within the sella turcica (arrows). Diagnosis: empty sella.

"intrasellar arachnoidocele" has been recommended.[139] The pathogenesis is still being debated, although it is generally accepted that incompetence of the diaphragma sellae is a prerequisite for evolution of an empty sella.[136,140,141] The diaphragma may be congenitally incompetent[136] or thinned by tumor,[142] increased intracranial pressure,[140,143,144] surgery, or radiation therapy. It is also suggested that this syndrome can develop as a result of spontaneous infarction of a pituitary tumor or a normal pituitary gland.[33,141,143,145] The transmitted pulsations of spinal fluid then cause the arachnoid pouch to expand into the sella, causing a remodeling effect.[140,144,146,147]

The syndrome is far more common in obese females. Varying degrees of hypopituitarism occur in 30–40% on detailed testing, but clinical hypopituitarism is much less common.[138,143,148–150] Headaches, the most common presenting complaint, are present in 50–80%.[138,143,146] Visual-field defects are un-

Fig. 19. (A) Coronal CT scan demonstrating a low-density area within the sella (arrow). (The square box is a region-of-interest marker.) (B) Coronal CT scan after injection of metrizamide into the subarachnoid space demonstrating metrizamide within the sella (arrow). Diagnosis: empty sella.

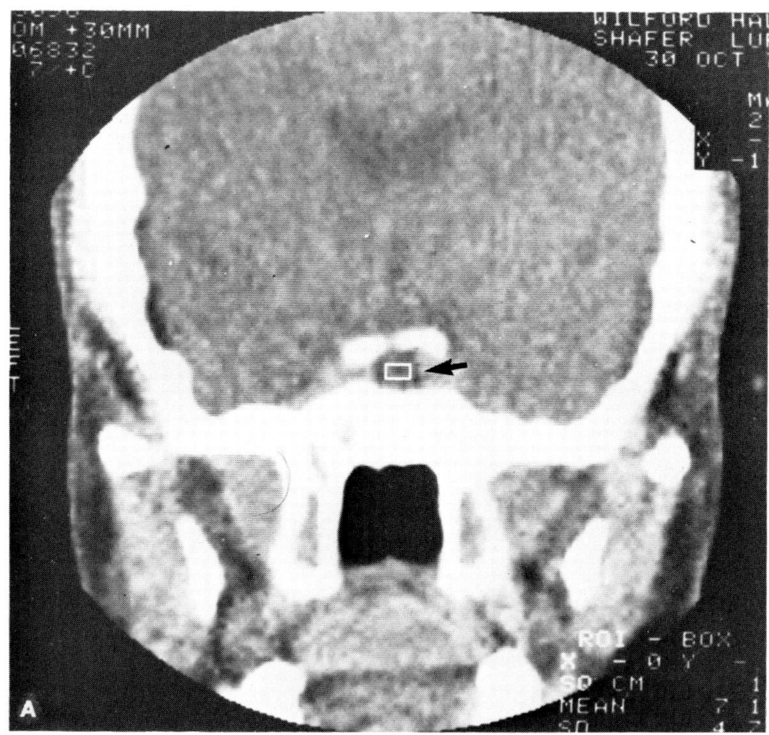
+30MM
SHAFER
30 OCT
ROI - BOX
SQ CM
MEAN
A

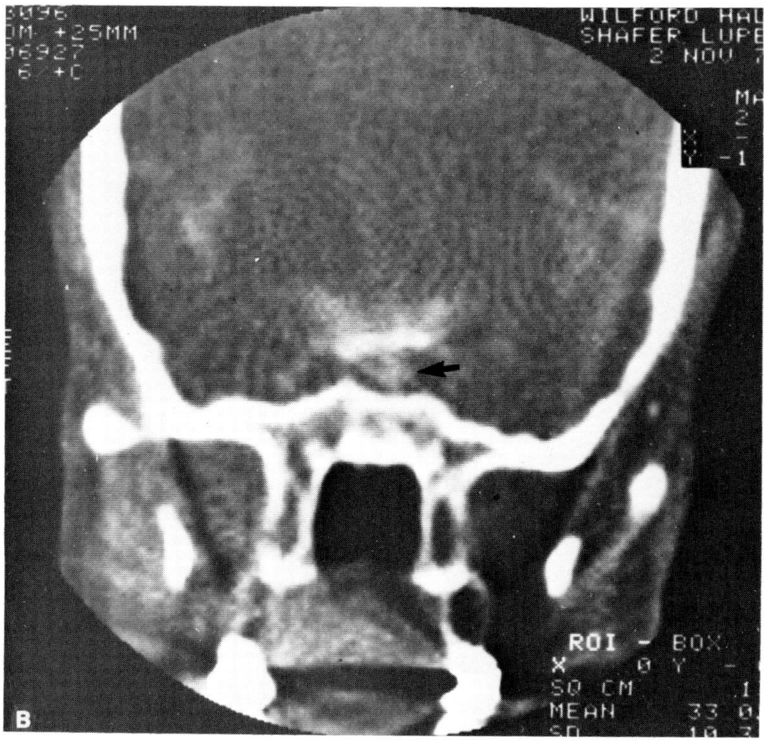
+25MM
WILFORD
2 NOV
ROI - BOX
SQ CM
MEAN
B

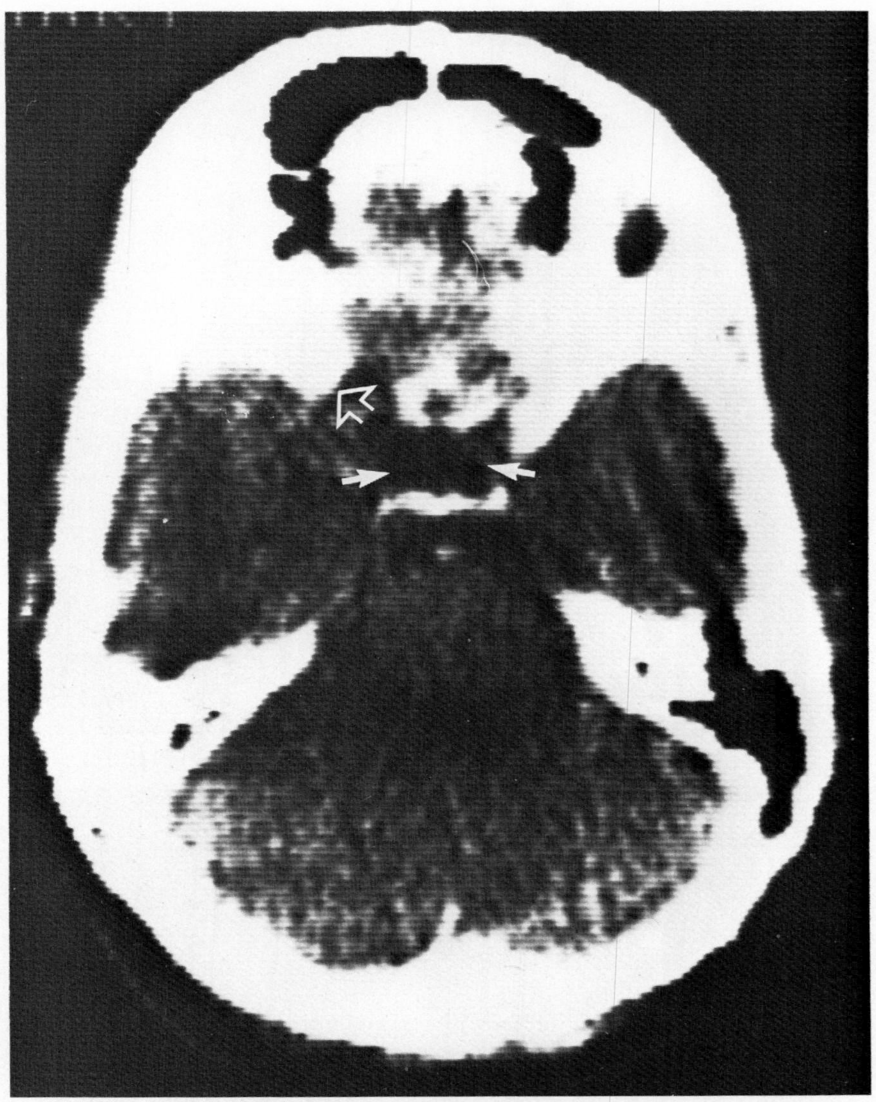

Fig. 20A. Horizontal CT scan demonstrating a low-density area within the sella (solid arrows). Note the erosion of the anterior clinoid process (open arrow).

common and are due to herniation of the optic nerves into the sella[151] (Fig. 17). However, when pseudotumor cerebri is associated with the primary empty sella syndrome,[146] field defects and acuity loss are more likely. In the review by Foley and Posner[146] of 130 cases of primary empty sella, no visual-field abnormalities were present in the absence of increased intracranial pressure.

X-ray examination of the skull fails to differentiate sellar changes caused by an empty sella from those caused by a pituitary adenoma or by increased intracranial pressure.[152,153] Balloon-shaped and cup-shaped sellas are common. A deep sella may be suggestive, but is not diagnostic. The sella is usually symmetrically enlarged without focal erosions, but many cases will have irregularly enlarged sellas with areas of erosion.[140,143] PEG will demonstrate air entering the sella; tomography aids in the diagnosis (Fig. 18). Recently, we have studied a series of empty sella patients with CT scan[17] and found that all cases could be predicted with the CT scan (Fig. 19A). However, three false positives were seen, caused by pituitary tumors with necrotic centers.

The finding of an empty sella by PEG does not exclude the presence of an adenoma in the pituitary gland lining the wall of the sella (Fig. 20). Adenomas secreting GH,[8,9] ACTH,[10] and prolactin[9,11] coexisting with partially empty sellas have been described. In patients with endocrine indications of a secreting pituitary adenoma, a partially empty sella should not preclude the correct diagnosis.[9] In fact, it may be that partial infarction or degeneration in a tumor could be the cause of the partially empty sella.[9] Domingue *et al.*[9] re-

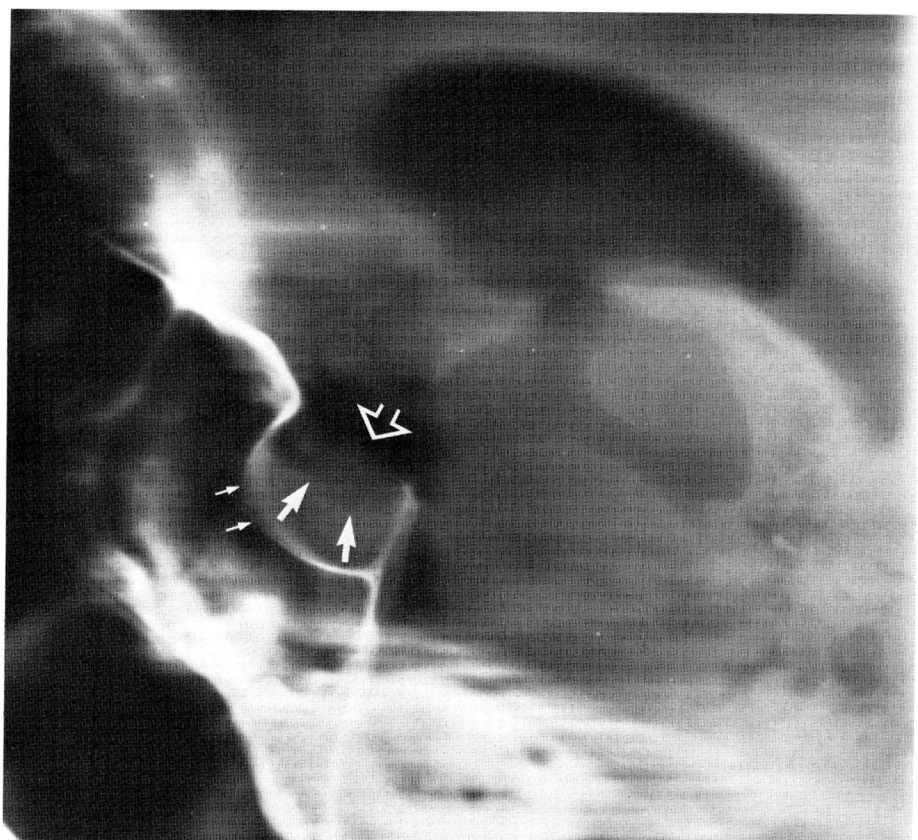

Fig. 20B. Lateral tomogram, again demonstrating a small suprasellar tumor (open arrow). Note also air entering the sella adjacent to the tumor (solid arrows). Furthermore, note the thinning of the floor of the sella (small arrows), indicative of an intrasellar adenoma.

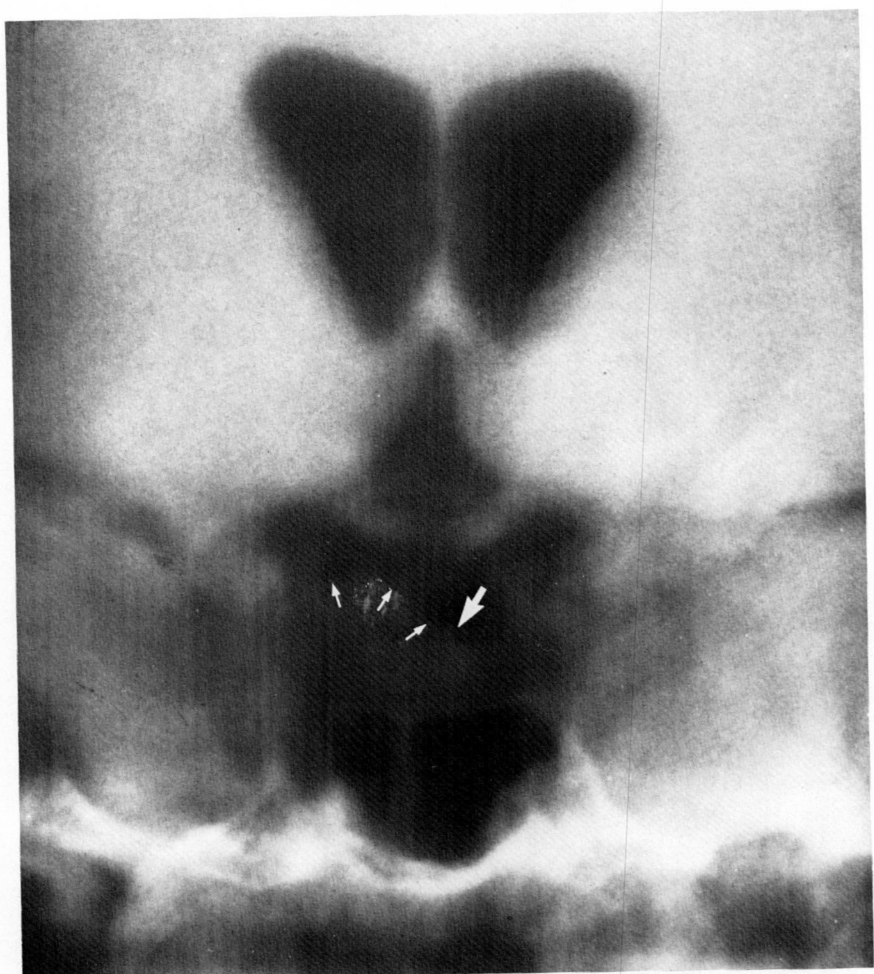

Fig. 20C. Frontal tomographic projection, again demonstrating a suprasellar tumor mass (small arrows) with air entering the sella adjacent to the tumor (large arrow). Diagnosis: empty sella with coexistent prolactinoma.

ported that 17.3% of patients with the syndrome of amenorrhea–galactorrhea and 10% of acromegalic patients had partially empty sellas. Nonsecreting tumors must also coexist with empty sellas in some cases, but these have not been identified.

References

1. M.E. Thomas and R.E. Yoss, The parasellar syndrome: Problems in determining etiology, *Mayo Clin. Proc.* **45:**617–623, 1970.
2. H.G.Bauer, Endocrine and other clinical manifestations of hypothalamic disease: A survey of 60 cases with autopsies, *J. Clin. Endocrinol. Metab.* **14:**13, 1954.

3. D.D. Matson (ed.), *Neurosurgery of Infancy and Childhood*, Charles C. Thomas, Springfield, Illinois, 1969.
4. G.A. Bray and T.F. Gallagher, Jr., Manifestations of hypothalamic obesity in man: A comprehensive investigation of eight patients and a review of the literature, *Medicine* **54:**301, 1975.
5. W.A. Shucart and I. jackson, Management of diabetes insipidus in neurosurgical patients, *J. Neurosurg.* **44:**65–71, 1976.
6. A.G. Frantz, The regulation of prolactin secretion in humans, in: *Frontiers in Neuroendocrinology: 1973* (W.F. Ganong and L. Martini, eds.), p. 337, Oxford University Press, New York, 1973.
7. J.B. Martin, S. Reichlin, and G.M. Brown, Regulation of prolactin secretion and its disorders, in: *Clinical Neuroendocrinology*, pp. 129–145, F.A. Davis, Philadelphia, 1977.
8. M.E. Molitch, G.B. Hieshima, S. Marcovits, I.M.D. Jackson, and S. Wolpert, Coexisting primary empty sella syndrome and acromegaly, *Clin. Endorinol.* **7:**261, 1977.
9. J.N. Domingue, S.D. Wing, and C.B. Wilson, Coexisting pituitary adenomas and partially empty sellas, *J. Neurosurg.* **48:**23, 1978.
10. A. Ganguly, J.B. Stanchfield, R.S. Roberts, C.D. West, and F.H. Tyler, Cushing's syndrome in a patient with an empty sella turcica and a microadenoma of the adenohypophysis, *Am. J. Med.***60:**306, 1976.
11. T.J. Sutton and J.L. Vezina, Co-existing pituitary adenoma and intrasellar arachnoid invagination, *Am. J. Roentgenol, Radium Ther. Nucl. Med.* **122:**508, 1974.
12. D.G. Cogan, *Neurology of the Visual System*, Charles C. Thomas, Springfield, Illinois, 1966.
13. F.M. Skultety, Clinical and experimental aspects of akinetic mutism, *Arch. Neurol.* **19:**1, 1968.
14. S.P. Traub, *Roentgenology of Intracranial Meningiomas*, pp. 54–72, Charles C. Thomas, Springfield, Illinois, 1961.
15. B. Kaufman, The "empty" sella turcica—a manifestation of the intrasellar subarachnoid space, *Radiology* **90:**931, 1968.
16. E.L. Kier, "J" and "omega" shape of sella turcica: Anatomic clarification of radiologic misconceptions, *Acta Radiol.* **9:**91, 1969.
17. R.A. Rozario, S. Hammerschlag, K.D. Post, S. Wolpert, and I. Jackson, Diagnosis of empty sella with CT scan, *Neuroradiology* **13**(3):85, 1977.
18. J.R. Bantson, Relative merits of pneumographic and angiographic procedures in the management of pituitary tumors, in *Diagnosis and Treatment of Pituitary Tumors* (P.O. Kohler and G.T. Ross, eds.), pp. 86–99, Excerpta Medica, Amsterdam, 1973.
19. H. Baker, The angiographic delineation of sellar and parasellar masses, *Radiology* **104:**67, 1972.
20. W.E. Hunt, M.P. Sayers, and D. Yashon, Tumors of the sellar and parasellar area (Chapt. 72), in: *Neurological Surgery, III* (J.R. Youmans, ed.), pp. 1412–1431, W.B. Saunders, Philadelphia, London, and Toronto, 1973.
21. M. Banna, Craniopharyngioma: A review article based on 160 cases, *Br. J. Radiol.* **49:**206–223, 1976.
22. J.R. Bartlett, Craniopharyngiomas—a summary of 85 cases, *J. Neurol. Neurosurg. Psychiatry* **34:**37–41, 1971.
23. R.W. Ross-Russell and J.B. Pennybacker, Craniopharyngioma in the elderly, *J. Neurol. Neurosurg. Psychiatry* **24:**1–13, 1961.
24. H. Krayenbuhl, Hypophysial adenomas and craniopharyngiomas, in: II International Congress of Neurological Surgery, Washington, D.C., *Excerpta Med. Int. Congr. Ser.* **36**(E):10–12, 1961.
25. J.G. Love and T.M. Marshall, Craniopharyngiomas, *Surg. Gynecol. Obstet.* **90:**591, 1950.
26. J.S. Jenkins, C.J. Gilbert, and V. Ang, Hypothalamic–pituitary function in patients with craniopharyngiomas, *J. Clin. Endocrinol. Metab.* **43**(2):394, 1976.
27. D.D. Matson and J.F. Crigler, Management of craniopharyngioma in childhood, *J. Neurosurg.* **30:**377, 1969.
28. A.A. Chambers, R. Lukin, and N. Tsunekawa, Calcification in a chromophobe adenoma, *J. Neurosurg.* **44:**623–625, 1976.
29. T.P. Naidich, R.S. Pinto, M.J. Kushner, J.P. Lin, I.I. Kricheff, N.E. Leeds, and N.E. Chase, Evaluation of sellar and paraseller masses by computed tomography, *Radiology* **120**(1):91–99, 1976.

30. W.M. Shanklin, Incidence and distribution of cilia in the human pituitary with a description of micro-follicular cysts derived from Rathke's cleft, *Acta Anat.* **11**:361–682, 1951.
31. C.A. Fager and H. Carter, Intrasellar epithelial cysts, *J. Neurosurg.* **24**:77–81, 1966.
32. G.F. Rowbotham and P.R.R. Clarke, Colloid cyst of the pituitary gland causing chiasmal compression, *Br. J. Surg.* **44**:107–108, 1956.
33. E.L. Weber, F.S. Vogel, and G.L. Odom, Cysts of the sella turcica, *J. Neurosurg.* **33**(1):48–53, 1970.
34. M. Burnbaum, J.W. Harbison, J.B. Selhorst, and H.F. Young, Blue-domed cyst with optic nerve compression, *J. Neurol. Neurosurg. Psychiatry* **41**:987–991, 1978.
35. G.M. Haas, Chordoma of cranium and cervical portion of spine: Review of literature with report of cases, *Arch. Neurol.* **32**:300–327, 1934.
36. T. Gillman, The incedence of ciliated epithelium and mucous cells in the normal Bantu pituitary, *S. Afr. J. Med. Sci.* **5**:30–40, 1940.
37. S. Shuangshoti, G.M. Netsky, and S.B. Nashold, Jr., Epithelial cysts related to sella turcica, *Arch. Pathol.* **90**:444–450, 1970.
38. S.P. Ringel and O.T. Bailey, Rathke's cleft cyst, *J. Neurol. Neurosurg. Psychiatry* **35**:693–697, 1972.
39. J. Yoshida, T. Kobayashi, N. Kageyama, and M. Kanzaki, Symptomatic Rathke's cleft cyst: Morphological study with light and electron microscopy and tissue culture, *J. Neurosurg.* **47**:451–458, 1977.
40. V.X. Naiken, M. Tellem, and D.R. Meranze, Pituitary cyst of Rathke's cleft origin with hypopituitarism, *J. Neurosurg.* **18**:703–708, 1961.
41. M.M. Schechter, A.L. Liebeskind, and B. Azar-Kia, Intracranial chordomas, *Neuroradiology* **8**:67–82, 1974.
42. J.R. Utne and D.G. Pugh, The roentgenologic aspects of chordomas, *Am. J. Roentgenol.* **74**:593, 1955.
43. S. Concha, B.P.M. Hamilton, J.C. Millan, and J.D. McQueen, Symptomatic Rathke's cleft cyst with amyloid stroja, *J. Neurol. Neurosurg. Psychiatry* **38**:782–786, 1975.
44. W.C. Duffy, Hypophyseal duct tumors: A report of three cases and a fourth case of cyst of Rathke's pouch, *Ann. Surg.* **72**:537–555 and 725–757, 1920.
45. K.M. Trokoudes, P.G. Walfish, R.C. Holgate, K.P.H. Pritzker, M.L. Schwarts, and K. Kovacs, Sellar enlargement with hyperprolactinemia and a Rathke's pouch cyst, *J. Amer. Med. Assoc.* **240**(5):471, 1978.
46. A. Barlow, Suprasellar arachnoid cyst, *Arch. Ophthalmol.* **14**:53–60, 1935.
47. R. Bernard, R. Vigouroux, R. Mariani, N. Pinsard, and H. Pierron, Arachnoidite kystique avec troubles de la vasculairisation carticale, *Pediatrie (Lyon)* **20**:989–992, 1965.
48. D.L. Kasdon, E.A. Douglas, and M.F. Brougham, Suprasellar arachnoid cyst diagnosed preoperatively by computerized tomographic scanning, *Surg. Neurol.* **7**(5):299, 1977.
49. M. Banna, Arachnoid cysts in the hypophyseal area, *Clin. Radiol.* **25**:323–326, 1974.
50. J. Danziger and S. Bloch, Suprasellar arachnoid pouches, *Br. J. Radiol.* **47**:448–451, 1974.
51. R.P. Vigouroux, M. Choux, and C. Baurand, Les kystes arachnoidiens congenitaux, *Neurochirurgia* **9**:169–187, 1966.
52. M.L. Bayoumi, Rathke's cleft and its cysts, *Edinburgh Med. J.* **55**:745–749, 1948.
53. D.C. Dahlin and C.S. MacCarty, Chordoma: A study of 59 cases, *Cancer* **5**:1170–1178, 1952.
54. R.G. Berry and N.S. Schlezinger, Rathke-cleft cysts, *Arch. Neurol.* **1**:48–58, 1959.
55. I. Givner, Ophthalmologic features of intracranial chordoma and allied tumours of the clivus, *Arch. Ophthalmol.* **33**:397–403, 1945.
56. J.M. Taveras and E.H. Wood, *Diagnostic Neuroradiology*, Williams and Wilkins, Baltimore, 1964.
57. N. Kageyama and R. Belsky, Ectopic pinealoma in the chiasmal region, *Neurology* **11**:318–327, 1961.
58. J. Takeuchi, H. Handa, and I. Nagata, Suprasellar germinoma, *J. Neurosurg.* **49**:41, 1978.
59. M.B. Camins and L.A. Mount, Primary suprasellar atypical teratoma, *Brain* **97**:447–456, 1974.
60. J. Takeuchi, K. Mori, K. Moritake, *et al.*, Teratomas in the suprasellar region; report of five cases, *Surg. Neurol.* **3**:247–255, 1975.
61. N.R. Ghatak, A. Kirano, and H.M. Zimmerman, Intrasellar germinomas: A form of ectopic pinealoma, *J. Neurosurg.* **31**:670–675, 1969.

62. J. Hankinson and M. Banna (eds.), *Pituitary and Parapituitary Tumours*, Vol. 6, W.B. Saunders, London, Philadelphia, and Toronto, 1976.
63. T.P. Naidich, R.S. Pinto, M.J. Kuschner, *et al.*, Evaluation of sellar and parasellar masses by computed tomography, *Radiology* **120:**91–99, 1976.
64. N.R. Miller, W.M. Iliff, and W.R. Green, Evaluation and management of gliomas of the anterior visual pathways, *Brain* **97:**743–754, 1974.
65. D.C. Oxenhandler and M.P. Sayers, The dilemma of childhood optic gliomas, *J. Neurosurg.* **48:**34–41, 1978.
66. W.H. Brooks, J.C. Parker, Jr., A.B. Young, *et al.*, Malignant gliomas of the optic chiasm in adolescents, *Clin. Pediatr.* **15:**557–561, 1976.
67. C.B. Wilson, M. Feinsod, W.F. Hoyt, *et al.*, Malignant evolution of childhood chiasmal pilocytic astrocytoma, *Neurology* **26:**322–325, 1976.
68. W.F. Hoyt, L.G. Meshel, S. Lessell, *et al.*, Malignant optic glioma of adulthood, *Brian* **96:**121–132, 1973.
69. C.G. Harper and E.G. Stewart-Wynne, Malignant optic gliomas in adults, *Arch. Neurol.* **35:**731, 1978.
70. R.S. Manor, J. Israeli, and U. Sandbank, Malignant optic glioma in a 70 year old patient, *Arch. Ophthalmol.* **94:**1142–1144, 1976.
71. G. Schuster and G. Westberg, Gliomas of the optic nerve and chiasm, *Acta Radiol.* **6:**221–232, 1967.
72. F.A. Davis, Primary tumors of the optic nerve (a phenomenon of Recklinghausen's disease), *Arch. Ophthalmol.* **23:**735–821, and 957–1022, 1940.
73. D. Marshall, Glioma of the optic nerve, as a manifestation of von Recklinghausen's disease, *Am. J. Ophthalmol.* **37:**15–33, 1954.
74. H.W. Dodge, Jr., J.G. Love, W.McK. Craig, M.B. Dockerty, T.P. Kearns, C.B. Holman, and A.B. Hayles, Gliomas of the optic nerves, *Arch. Neurol. Psychiatry* **79:**607–621, 1958.
75. A.B. Reese, *Tumours of the Eye*, 2nd ed., pp. 532–536, Harper & Row, New York, Evanston, and London, 1963.
76. D.K. Sen and H. Mohan, Glioma of optic nerve (record of an unusual case), *Eye Ear Nose Throat Mon.* **51:**273–275, 1972.
77. W.H. Spencer, Primary neoplasms of the optic nerve and its sheaths: Clinical features and current concepts of pathogenetic mechanisms, *Trans. Am. Ophthalmol. Soc.* **70:**490–528, 1972.
78. I.G. Wong and M. Lubow, Management of optic glioma of childhood: A review of 42 cases, *Neuroophthalmology* **6:**51–60, 1972.
79. H. Eggers, F.A. Jakobiec, and I.S. Jones, Tumors of the optic nerve, *Doc. Ophthalmol.* **41:**43–128, 1976.
80. J.S. Glaser, W.F. Hoyt, and J. Corbett, Visual morbidity with chiasmal glioma, *Arch. Ophthalmol.* **85:**3, 1971.
81. C.B. Holman, Roentgenologic manifestations of glioma of the optic nerve and chiasm, *Am. J. Roentgenol.* **82:**462–471, 1959.
82. D.S. Russell and L.J. Rubinstein, *Pathology of Tumours of the Nervous System*, Edward Arnold, London, 1959.
83. J.D. Trobe, J.S. Glaser, and J.D. Post, Meningiomas and aneurysms of the cavernous sinus: Neuro-ophthalmologic features, *Arch. Ophthalmol.* **96:**457, 1978.
84. F.K. Gregorius, R.S. Hepler, and W.E. Stern, Loss and recovery of vision with suprasellar meningiomas, *J. Neurosurg.* **42:**69, 1975.
85. H. Cushing, The chiasmal syndrome of primary optic atrophy and bitemporal field defects in adults with a normal sella turcica, *Arch. Ophthalmol.* **3:**505–551 and 704–735, 1935.
86. F.D. Grant and T.R. Hedges, Ocular findings in meningiomas of tuberculum sellae, *Arch. Ophthalmol.* **56:**163–170, 1956.
87. H. Hobbs, Tumours and failing vision, *Br. Med. J.* **2:**255, 1962.
88. N.S. Schlezinger, B.J. Alpers, and B.P. Weiss, Suprasellar meningiomas associated with scotomatous field defects, *Arch. Ophthalmol.* **35:**624–642, 1946.
89. W.E. Hunt and C.A. Miller, Parasellar tumors: Variations of a theme, *Clin. Neurosurg.* **25:**425, 1978.
90. H.H. Joy, Suprasellar meningioma: Report of an atypical case, *Trans. Am. Ophthalmol. Soc.* **49:**59–74, 1951.

91. E.R. Bickerstaff, J.M. Small, and I.A. Guest, The relapsing course of meningioma in relation to pregnancy and menstruation. *J. Neurol. Neurosurg. Psychiatry* **21:**89–91, 1958.
92. G. di Chiro and E. Lindgren, Bone changes in cases of suprasellar meningioma, *Acta Radiol.* **38:**133–138, 1952.
93. M. El-S. Mahmoud, The sella in health and disease, *Br. J. Radiol.* **8**(Suppl.):35–57, 1958.
94. D.W.C. Northfield and D.S. Russell, Pubertas praecox due to hypothalamic harmartoma: Report of two cases surviving surgical removal of the tumour, *J. Neurol. Neurosurg. Psychiatry* **30:**166–173, 1967.
95. D.M. Judge, H.E. Kulin, R. Page, R. Santen, and S. Trapukdi, Hypothalamic hamartoma: A source of luteinizing-hormone-releasing factor in precocious puberty, *N. Eng. J. Med.* **296**(1):7, 1977.
96. L. Wolman, Infundibuloma, *J. Pathol. Bacteriol.* **77:**283–296, 1959.
97. A.I. Kobrine and E. Ross, Granular cell myoblastomas of the pituitary region, Surg. *Neurol.* **1:**275–279, 1973.
98. S.W. Mitchell, Aneurysm of an anomalous artery causing antero-posterior division of the chiasm of the optic nerves and producing bitemporal hemianopsia, *J. Nerv. Ment. Dis.* **14:**14–62, 1889.
99. H. Cushing, *The Pituitary Body and Its Disorders: Clinical States Produced by Disorders of the Hypophysis Cerebri,* pp. 97–99, J.B. Lippincott, Philadelphia, 1912.
100. J.C. White and H.T. Ballantine, Jr., Intrasellar aneurysms simulating hypophyseal tumours, *J. Neurosurg.* **18:**34–50, 1961.
101. H.H. Lippman, B.M. Onofrio, and H.L. Baker, Intrasellar aneurysm and pituitary adenoma—report of a case, *Proc. Mayo Clin.* **46:**532–535, 1971.
102. J. Jakubowski and B. Kendall, Coincidental aneurysms with tumors of pituitary origin, *J. Neurol. Neurosurg. Psychiatry* **41:**972–979, 1978.
103. N.E. Cartlidge and D.A. Shaw, Intrasellar aneurysm with subarachnoid hemorrhage and hypopituitarism, *J. Neurosurg.* **36:**640–643, 1972.
104. F.B. Walsh, Visual field defects due to aneurysms at the circle of Willis, *Arch. Ophthalmol.* **71:**15–27, 1964.
105. A.C. Bird, B. Nolan, F.P. Gargano, and N.J. David, Unruptured aneurysm of the supraclinoid carotid artery, *Neurology* **20:**445–454, 1970.
106. G. Jefferson, Compression of the chiasma, optic nerves and optic tracts by intracranial aneurysms, *Brian* **60:**444–497, 1937.
107. G. Jefferson, Further concerning compression of the optic pathways by intracranial aneurysms, *Proc. Congr. Neurol. Surg.* **1:**55–103, 1955.
108. L.A. Raymond and J. Tew, Large suprasellar aneurysms imitating pituitary tumour, *J. Neurol. Neurosurg. Psychiatry* **41:**83–87, 1978.
109. G. Lombardi, A. Passerini, and F. Migliavacca, Intracavernous aneurysms of the internal carotid artery, *Am. J. Roentgenol. Radium Ther. Nucl. Med.* **89:**361–371, 1963.
110. S. Obrador and M.D. Blazquez, Pituitary abscess in a craniopharyngioma: A case report, *J. Neurosurg.* **36:**785–789, 1972.
111. H. de Villiers Hamman, Abscess formation in the pituitary fossa associated with a pituitary adenoma, *J. Neurosurg.* **13:**208–210, 1956.
112. N. Whalley, Abscess formation in a pituitary adenoma, *J. Neurol. Neurosurg. Psychiatry* **15:**66–67, 1952.
113. J. Lindholm, P. Rasmussen, and O. Korsgaard, Intrasellar or pituitary abscess, *J. Neurosurg.* **38:**616–619, 1973.
114. J.N. Domingue and C.B. Wilson, Pituitary abscesses: Report of seven cases and review of the literature, *J. Neurosurg.* **46:**601, 1977.
115. W.A. Sibley and J.L. O'Brien, Intracranial tuberculomas: A review of clinical features and treatment, *Neurology* **6:**157–165, 1956.
116. M. Banna, J. Hankinson, and B.J. Odoris, Interhemispheric suprasellar tuberculoma, *Br. J. Radiol.* **46:**550–553, 1973.
117. B. Ramamurthi and M.G. Varadarajan, Diagnosis of tuberculomas of the brain: Clinical and radiological correlations, *J. Neurosurg.* **18:**1–7, 1961.
118. P.M. Udani, U.C. Parekh, and D.K. Dastur, Neurological and related syndromes in CNS tuberculosis, *J. Neurol. Sci.* **14:**341–357, 1971.

119. A. Silverstein, M.M. Feuer, and L.E. Siltzbach, Neurologic sarcoidosis, *Arch. Neurol.* **12:**1–11, 1965.
120. A.C. Douglas and F.J. Maloney, Sarcoidosis of the central nervous system, *J. Neurol. Neurosurg. Psychiatry* **36:**1024–1033, 1973.
121. H.A. Selenkow *et al.*, Hypopituitarism due to hypothalamic sarcoidosis, *Am. J. Med. Sci.* **238:**456, 1959.
122. J. Colover, Sarcoidosis with involvement of the nervous system, *Brain* **71:**451–475, 1948.
123. C.N. Shealy, L. Kahana, F.L. Engel, and H.T. McPherson, Hypothalamic pituitary sarcoidosis, *Am. J. Med.* **30:**46, 1961.
124. W. Beard, B. Foster, J. Kepes, and R.A. Guillan, Xanthomatosis of the central nervous system, *Neurology* **20:**305–314, 1970.
125. P.A. Tibbs, V. Challa, and R.H. Mortaro, Isolated histiocytosis X of the hypothalamus, *J. Neurosurg.* **49:**929–934, 1978.
126. D. Pressman, R.L. Waldron, and E.H. Wood, Histiocytosis X of the hypothalamus, *Br. J. Radiol.* **48:**176–178, 1975.
127. T.S. Schultz and G.F. Ascherl, Cerebral cysticercosis: Occurrence in the immigrant population, *Neurosurgery* **3:**164–169, 1978.
128. S. Obrador, Cysticercosis cerebri, *Acta Neurochir. (Vienna)* **10:**320–364, 1962.
129. J. Berg, Bidrag till kannedomen om sjukdomarna i nasans bihalor samt till laran om cerebrospinal-vatskas flytning ur nasam, *Nord. Med. Ark.* **21:**1–24, 1889.
130. G.R. Nugent, P. Sprinkle, and B.M. Bloor, Sphenoid sinus mucoceles, *J. Neurosurg.* **32:**443, 1970.
131. J.A. Goodwin and J.S. Glaser, Chiasmal syndrome in sphenoid sinus mucocele, *Ann. Neurol.* **4:**440–444, 1978.
132. D. Petit-Dutaillis, F. Thiebaut, and H. Fischgold, Contribution à l'étude des compressions intracraniennes des nerfs optiques par les abcès ou les mucoceles extradurales d'origine sphenoidethmoidale, *Rev. Neurol. (Paris)* **83:**325–341, 1950.
133. T.P. Krueger, J. McFarland, and A.K. Ommaya, Pyocele of the sphenoid sinus, *J. Neurosurg.* **22:**616–621, 1965.
134. H.M. Simon, Jr., and F.R. Tingwald, Syndrome associated with mucocele of the sphenoid sinus: Report of two cases and their radiographic findings, *Radiology* **64:**538–545, 1955.
135. W. Busch, Die Morphologie der Sella turcica und ihre Beziehungen zur Hypophyse, *Arch. Pathol. Anat.* **320:**437–458, 1951.
136. B. Kaufman and W.B. Chamberlin, Jr., The ubiquitous "sella" turcica, *Acta Radiol. Diagn.* **13:**413–425, 1972.
137. R.M. Bergland, B.S. Ray, and R.M. Torack, Anatomical variations in the pituitary gland and adjacent structures in 225 human autopsy cases, *J. Neurosurg.* **28:**93–99, 1968.
138. L.A. Weissberg, E.A. Zimmerman, and A.G. Frantz, Diagnosis and evaluation of patients with an enlarged sella turcica, *Am. J. Med.* **61:**590, 1976.
139. T.A. Leclercq, J. Hardy, J.L. Vezina, and F. Mercky, Intrasellar arachnoidocele and the so-called empty sella syndrome, *Surg. Neurol.* **3**(5):295, 1974.
140. B. Kaufman, The "empty" sella turcica—a manifestation of the intrasellar subarachnoid space, *Radiology* **90:**931–941, 1968.
141. S. Obrador, The empty sella and some related syndromes, *J. Neurosurg.* **36:**162–168, 1972.
142. R. Mortara and H. Norrell, Consequences of a deficient sellar diaphragm, *J. Neurosurg.* **32:**565–573, 1970.
143. F.A. Neelon, J.A. Goree, and H.E. Lebovitz, The primary empty sella: Clinical and radiographic characteristics and endocrine function, *Medicine* **52:**73–92, 1973.
144. L.A. Weisberg, E.M. Housepian, and D.P. Saur, Empty sella syndrome and complication of benign intracranial hypertension, *J. Neurosurg.* **43:**177–180, 1975.
145. I. Login and R.J. Santen, Empty sella syndrome: Sequela of the spontaneous remission of acromegaly, *Arch. Intern. Med.* **135:**1519–1521, 1975.
146. K.M. Foley and J.B. Posner, Does pseudotumor cerebri cause the empty sella syndrome?, *Neurology* **25:**565–569, 1975.
147. G. Guiot, D. Olson, and F. Hertzog, Kystes arachnoidiens intrasellairs, *Neurochirurgica* **17:**539–547, 1971.

148. R. Brisman, J.E.O. Hughes, and D.A. Holub, Endocrine function in nineteen patients with empty sella syndrome, *J. Clin. Endocrinol. Metab.* **34**:570, 1972.
149. R.H. Caplan and G.D. Dobben, Endocrine studies in patients with "empty" sella syndrome," *Arch. Intern. Med.* **123**:611–619, 1969.
150. G. Faglia, B. Ambrosi, P. Beck-Peccoz, *et al.*, Disorders of growth hormone and corticotropin regulation in patients with empty sella, *J. Neurosurg.* **38**:59–64, 1973.
151. M.T. Buckman, M. Husain, T.J. Carlow, and G.T. Peake, Primary empty sella syndrome with visual field defects, *Am. J. Med.* **61**:124, 1976.
152. X. Bajraktari, Skull changes with intrasellar cisternala syndrome—intrasellar cisternal herniation in "normal" patients with communicating hydrocephalus and intracranial tumors, *Neuroradiology* **17**:35–44, 1978.
153. K. Brismar, X. Bajraktari, R. Goulatia, and S. Efendic, The empty sella syndrome—intrasellar cisternal herniation in "normal" patients with communicating hydrocephalus and intracranial tumors, *Neuroradiology* **17**:35–44, 1978.

III

Clinical Evaluation of Pituitary Tumors

11

Diagnostic Tests for the Evaluation of Pituitary Tumors

IVOR M.D. JACKSON

1. Introduction

Following the description of the technique of radioimmunoassay[1] (RIA) and its application to the measurement of pituitary hormones, disorders of pituitary function could be diagnosed much more readily than before. The subsequent development of a specific RIA for human prolactin[2] (PRL) has revolutionized our means of diagnosing pituitary tumors, for it has become clear that 50–80% of tumors that previously were categorized as inactive chromophobe adenomas actively secrete PRL.[3]

The modern era of clinical neuroendocrinology can, however, be said to date from the isolation of thyrotropin-releasing hormone (TRH) from the mammalian hypothalamus and the establishment of its structure by Guillemin, Schally, and their respective co-workers.[4,5] Subsequently, these two groups described the presence of two other releasing hormones in the hypothalamus: luteinizing-hormone- or gonadotropin-releasing hormone (LH-RH or GnRH) and growth-hormone-release-inhibiting hormone (somatostatin),[6,7] which, like TRH, proved to be simple peptides. With the availability of these substances in pure form, it is widely believed that the development of specific assays for these peptides will allow the clinician to separate hypothalamic from pituitary disorders.[3] Initially, it was proposed that the administration of TRH and LH-RH would permit the differentiation of pituitary from hypothalamic insufficiency, since patients with hypothyrotropic hypothyroidism and hypogonadotropic hypogonadism due to intrinsic pituitary disease should have no increase in pituitary thyroid-stimulating hormone (TSH) or luteinizing hormone (LH) secretion, while an increase in pituitary-hormone secretion might be expected if the thyroidal and gonadal problem resided in the hy-

---

IVOR M.D. JACKSON • Tufts University School of Medicine; Department of Medicine, Division of Endocrinology, Tufts–New England Medical Center Hospital, Boston, Massachusetts 02111.

pothalamus. Unfortunately, neither specific measurements of the hypothalamic hormones in body fluids nor the response of the anterior pituitary to their administration has been as helpful as earlier predicted in the anatomical separation of pituitary from hypothalamic disease (see later). However, the availability of these peptides has afforded a great deal of insight into our understanding of brain–hypothalamic–pituitary disorders, and they may also have a further diagnostic role by virtue of the "paradoxical" responses frequently seen in secretory tumors of the pituitary.

With the development of specific RIAs for TRH, LH-RH, and somatostatin, it became clear that these substances are present in the circulation in low concentrations and are rapidly degraded, thus making their measurement extremely difficult. Furthermore, over 70% of brain TRH lies outside the hypothalamus, and most of somatostatin lies outside the nervous system altogether, suggesting that the hypophysiotropic hormones of the hypothalamus have an extrahypothalamic role—possibly in neuronal transmission—quite unrelated to the regulation of pituitary hormones (for a review, see Jackson[8]). Although it still remains to be determined whether the physiological changes that influence the secretion of the peptide in the hypothalamus operate similarly at extrahypothalamic sites, it seems unlikely at this time that measurement of levels of these hypothalamic peptides in biological fluids can be used to impute dysfunction in the hypothalamus. The only exception to this view would be direct assay of pituitary portal-vessel blood for these substances, and this circulation is inaccessible in intact man.

2. Regulation of Pituitary Secretion

That the anterior pituitary gland is regulated by the hypothalamus is well substantiated. The hypothalamic releasing factors or hormones are synthesized by peptidergic neurons in the hypothalamus, transported to nerve endings in the stalk-median eminence (SME), released into the interstitial space in contiguity with the primary portal capillary plexus, and distributed to the anterior pituitary by means of the portal circulation.[9]

The posterior pituitary hormones are synthesized in the supraoptic and paraventricular nuclei of the hypothalamus, and carried by axonal transport attached to large carrier proteins termed "neurophysins," for storage in the posterior lobe of the pituitary (which is the homologue of the median eminence and *not* of the adenohypophysis). It appears that the hypothalamic peptidergic neurons are in turn regulated by neurotransmitters largely of the monoaminergic variety, dopamine (DA), norepinephrine (NE), and serotonin (5-HT), and that the peptidergic neuron acts as a "neuroendocrine transducer" converting neural information from the brain into chemical information.[10]

The anterior pituitary has been likened to a collection of six independent endocrine glands in one—each gland having its own specific hypothalamic releasing factor(s). However, recent evidence suggests that this may not be so. LH-RH appears to regulate both LH and follicle-stimulating hormone (FSH) secretion. Similarly, TRH induces the release of TSH and PRL, though the evidence suggests that PRL secretion is regulated primarily by inhibitory control through a PRL-inhibitory factor (PIF) (?DA) and that another physiological PRL-releasing factor (PRF) may exist. Somatostatin likewise inhibits the secretion of both growth hormone (GH) and TSH and may be of physiological importance in the regulation of both, though the major regulatory factors appear to be a putative growth-hormone-releasing factor (GH-RF) and TRH, respectively. It has been proposed that adrenocorticotropin (ACTH) is regulated by a corticotropin-releasing factor (CRF).

Four of the pituitary hormones (ACTH, TSH, FSH, and LH) have target glands that produce target hormones that have a direct negative feedback on the pituitary secretion of the tropic hormones. GH and PRL, however, do not mediate their action through a target hormone, though many of the effects of GH may be effected to a great extent through a tissue factor, somatomedin, manufactured in the liver (see Section 5.6).

3. Basal Levels of Pituitary Hormones

The meusurement of the pituitary hormone along with the target hormone is usually helpful in localizing an endocrine deficiency due to a central rather than a peripheral cause. Thus, the presence of hypothyroidism, hypocortisolism, and hypogonadism in the absence of an elevation in circulating TSH, ACTH, and FSH–LH, respectively, points strongly to a hypothalamic–pituitary disorder, since a primary disorder of the target glands causing impaired secretion of the target hormones will normally result in an increased secretion of the pituitary tropic hormones. Measurement of random levels of pituitary hormones *by themselves* are not usually helpful in diagnosis, since the sensitivity of RIA does not permit separation of *normal* from *low* levels, and stimulatory tests are required. This particularly applies to GH, for which no target hormone is readily available for concomitant assay, so that stimulatory tests to determine pituitary reserve are necessary. However, elevated basal levels of pituitary hormones can be helpful in the diagnosis of hyperfunction of the pituitary. Resting fasting levels of serum GH are useful in monitoring a patient with acromegaly before and after therapeutic procedures, and basal morning plasma ACTH levels are invaluable following bilateral adrenalectomy for Cushing's disease and in patients with established Nelson's syndrome (postadrenalectomy pituitary tumor).

4. Tests of Anterior Pituitary Secretion

4.1. Growth Hormone (GH)

Measurement of GH secretion is important in the clinical evaluation of dwarfism and hypopituitarism wherein impaired secretion is being examined and in acromegaly or gigantism wherein the issue of hypersecretion of GH is being determined. In hypopituitarism, GH is often the earliest pituitary hormone to be lost,[11] and in 20 cases of craniopharyngioma reported by Jenkins *et al.*,[12] all but one had deficiences of GH (and gonadotropin), whereas pituitary–adrenal function was preserved in 50% of cases.

Many provocative maneuvers have been utilized to stimulate GH (Table 1), including L-dopa (500 mg p.o.), *insulin-induced hypoglycemia* (0.05–0.3 U/kg body weight intravenously as a bolus), *argininine* (5% solution 0.5 g/kg body weight given intravenously over 30 min), aqueous *vasopressin* (10 pressor units given by intramuscular injection), and crystalline *glaucagon* (1 mg by intramuscular injection). The peak GH rise in normal male controls (increment >5 ng/ml) was achieved at 60 min for all these tests, except for glucagon, in which the peak rise was delayed to 150 min.[13] The most effective stimulus found by Eddy *et al.* [13] was L-dopa and insulin hypoglycemia (95 to 90% positive, respectively, in normal males), but they did not pretreat with estrogen, which is held to be necessary for arginine infusion in males and for GH secretion generally in prepubertal subjects.[14] L-Dopa acts by crossing the blood–brain barrier and being converted to DA and/or NE, which appear to stimulate hypothalamic GH-RF. Insulin-induced hypoglycemia probably acts through both noradrenergic and serotoninergic mechanisms[15] and as a test has the advantage of concomitantly stimulating both PRL and ACTH secretion. Adequate hypoglycemia (>40 mg/dl for 10 min) is required to ensure activation of the pituitary–adrenal axis in normal subjects,[16] though lesser falls in glucose levels are sufficient to trigger GH secretion.

There is evidence of adrenergic modulation of GH secretion, since α adrenergic blockade (phentolamine) and β-adrenergic stimulation (isoproterenol) are capable of suppressing GH secretion in acromegalic subjects.[17] These adrenergic effects on GH secretion appear to be exerted at the hypothalamic level, since *in vitro* studies have failed to demonstrate direct effects of adrenergic agonists or antagonists on pituitary GH release (for a review, see Cryer and Daughaday[17]). Propranolol (a β-adrenergic blocker) potentiates the responses of GH to a wide variety of stimuli including glucagon, suggesting that the latter stimulus also acts via the hypothalamus. However, the peak GH is much delayed and may depend on secondary hypoglycemia.[18] Arginine probably acts through a noradrenergic mechanism in the hypothalamus and also increases the section of PRL as well as insulin (the latter by direct pancreatic stimulation). The site of action of vasopressin (hypothalamic vs. pituitary), which also stimulates ACTH secretion, has not been determined with certainty, and may involve both locations. Vigorous exercise for 20 min has also been reported as a useful noninvasive provocative test for GH secretion in children.[19]

TABLE 1. Tests Utilized to Stimulate GH Secretion

L-Dopa (p.o.)
Insulin (i.v.)
Arginine (i.v.)
Vasopressin (i.m.)
Glucagon (i.m.)
Exercise

TABLE 2. Comparison of Provocative Tests on Serum GH Responses in Acromegaly Compared with Normals

Test	Acromegaly	Normal
Glucose	No change or a rise[a]	Fall
L-Dopa	Fall	Rise
TRH	No change or a rise[b]	No change
LH-RH	No change or a rise[a]	No change

[a]May be blocked by antecedent bromocriptine.
[b]Not blocked by antecedent bromocriptine.

In patients with suspected acromegaly, failure of the serum GH to suppress to normal levels at 2 hr following an oral glucose load (50–100 g) has been considered a criterion of diagnosis. In a series of 50 patients with this condition, only 2 suppressed to less than 5ng/ml.[20] Daughaday *et al.*[20] also found a paradoxical rise of GH in 14% of their cases. This response has also been described in patients with anterior hypothalamic tumors and in other disorders without obvious structural lesions of the hypothalamic–pituitary area, e.g., renal failure and protein calorie malnutrition. L-Dopa, probably due to direct action at the pituitary through its *peripheral* conversion to DA,[21] paradoxically causes a *lowering* of serum GH in acromegaly. TRH and/or LH-RH administration (see also later) frequently stimulates the secretion of GH in acromegaly.[22] It appears that those acromegalics who show a positive response to TRH also demonstrate suppression of GH levels after dopaminergic stimuli.[23] Thus, TRH stimulation of GH secretion in acromegaly might be helpful in the recognition of those patients suitable for treatment with the dopaminergic agonist bromocriptine (see also Chapters 6 and 15). A significant GH response to TRH stimulation, even if it persists after transsphenoidal surgery for acromegaly despite attainment of *normal basal* GH levels, suggests the continued presence of pituitary adenoma tissue secreting GH.[24] On the other hand, the paradoxical GH responses to L-dopa, TRH, and even glucose may disappear after surgery.[25,26] Thus, the altered GH responses in acromegaly (Table 2) do appear to depend on the pituitary adenoma *per se* rather than its hypothalamic connections, and these tests may therefore be used to monitor adequacy of treatment. It should be noted that the GH response to TRH stimulation shows no correlation with TSH rise in acromegaly,[22] and thyroid administration for 1 week does *not* block the TRH-induced GH and PRL release in this condition.[27]

Bromocriptine administration, which may be valuable in the medical management of acromegaly (see Chapter 15), does not block the GH rise induced by TRH or insulin-induced hypoglycemia[28] despite suppression of basal GH levels, but does prevent the GH release induced by LH-RH.[29] These findings suggest that the receptor site for both DA and LH-RH on pituitary adenoma tissue secreting GH may be indentical and separate from the TRH locus.[29] However, since bromocriptine administration blocks the PRL release in acromegaly induced by TRH and LH-RH, it appears that all three substances may share a common receptor locus for PRL release in this pathological condition.[30] Glucose tolerance is frequently much improved on bromocriptine with abolition of the paradoxical GH rise in over 50% of acromegalics demonstrating this response[28,31] (see also Table 2).

4.2. Prolactin (PRL)

In patients with suspected pituitary tumors, an elevated serum PRL may point to a tumor; when lateral X-ray studies show no abnormality, sellar polytomography should be undertaken.[3] However, elevated PRL levels also occur in hypothalamic disease.[32] *TRH administration* (500 μg i.v.) causes PRL secretion from the normal pituitary through direct stimulation of the lactotropes, the peak rise occurring at 15–30 min. *Chlorpromazine* (25 mg p.o. or i.m.) appears to act at the hypothalamic level by blocking dopamine receptors and possibly inhibiting PIF secretion.[33] *L-Dopa* lowers the basal PRL levels of normals as well as patients with varieties of hyperprolactinemia including pituitary tumors.[3] L-Dopa may act both at the hypothalamic and at the pituitary level following decarboxylation to DA. Stimulation and suppression tests in patients with hyperprolactinemia have not proved as useful as originally hoped in distinguishing patients with from those without tumors. However, only 1 of 16 patients with PRL-secreting tumors by Kleinberg *et al.*[34] gave a positive response to TRH, defined as a doubling of the baseline value. Studies in this department have suggested that impaired suppression of PRL following L-dopa occurs in about one third of hyperprolactinemic subjects with a pituitary adenoma (see Chapter 4).

Recently, Fine and Frohman[35] have studied the effect of L-dopa preceded by carbidopa (50 mg q6hr for 24 hr), which produces peripheral dopa decarboxylase inhibition (DDI) but does not cross the blood–brain barrier to cause central DDI. L-Dopa and carbidopa were as effective as L-dopa by itself in lowering PRL in normals, but were *not* effective in patients with prolactinomas. These studies suggest that the inhibition of PRL secretion from pituitary adenomas by L-dopa depends solely on peripheral generation of DA, and further suggests that the carbidopa modification of the L-dopa test may be helpful in the diagnosis of prolactinomas. Further evaluation of this test in subjects with hyperprolactinemia not due to pituitary adenoma is required.

4.3. Adrenocorticotropin (ACTH)

Because of difficulties with the ACTH assay, most dynamic tests of pituitary ACTH secretion have depended on measurements of serum cortisol, which is usually a good reflection of ACTH secretion. A normal diurnal rhythm of the serum cortisol and ACTH—high levels in the morning and low levels in the evening—suggests a normal integrity of the hypothalamic–pituitary–adrenal axis. An altered or disturbed diurnal rhythm occurs in all varieties of Cushing's syndrome, but may also be found in other conditions such as stress, infection, and depression.[36] Circulating total cortisol, but *not* the metabolically active free cortisol, is elevated in both pregnancy and estrogen treatment due to an increase in the plasma "carrier" protein, corticosteroid-binding globulin (CBG). However, in these situations, the cortisol secretion rate[37] is normal. Likewise, urinary levels of free cortisol (normal 20–90 μg/24 hr) are not increased as occurs in Cushing's syndrome.

In evaluating the pituitary–adrenal axis, the adequacy of the adrenal cortex should be confirmed first by preliminary ACTH stimulation with Cortrosyn, β_{1-24} ACTH, 250 μg i.v. or i.m., with measurements of cortisol at 30 and 60 min. This short ACTH simulation test has been shown to accurately reflect the integrity of the hypothalamic–pituitary–adrenal axis, for the peak plasma cortisol during insulin-induced hypoglycemia and the cortisol concentration at 30 min after injection of Cortrosyn show a close concordance ($r = 0.92$).[38]

The adequacy of the hypothalamic–pituitary–adrenal axis can be directly tested by insulin-induced hypoglycemia (see earlier) or by *metyrapone*, which constitutes a feedback challenge. This latter agent blocks production of cortisol (Cd'F') at the level of 11-deoxycortisol (Cd'S') through its action in the adrenal cortex as an inhibitor of 11-hydroxylase. The rise in serum level of Cd'S' reflects the responsiveness of the pituitary and/or the hypothalamus to cortisol deficiency. The test can be performed by administering metyrapone 750 mg p.o. for 6 doses and measuring the increase in the urinary excretion of 17-hydroxycortiscosteroids (17-OHCS) in the urine (normal 2–3 times baseline on the day following the dose), or by giving metyrapone as a single dose (30 mg/kg body weight p.o.) at midnight and measuring the serum cortisol and Cd'S' at 8 A.M. The cortisol level should be suppressed and the 'S' more than 7 μg/dl.[39] Of course, plasma ACTH levels can be measured in place of, or in conjunction with, the cortisol level in the insulin test and the 'S' level in the metyrapone test and constitutes one more direct measurement of anterior pituitary function.[39] Both insulin challenge and metyrapone are satisfactory tests, but the former has the advantage of concurrently testing GH and PRL secretion in addition to ACTH. A further advantage is that patients can be tested while receiving maintenance dexamethasone, whereas the metyrapone test is vitiated by concurrent glucocorticoid administration.[40] On the other hand, there is greater risk to the insulin hypoglycemia test. Other tests used to stimulate the pituitary–adrenal axis include vasopressin (i.m.) (see earlier), and *bacterial pyrogen* (i.v.), which appears to act directly at the pituitary level, and unlike vasopressin is not inhibited by small doses of dexamethasone or morphine.[41] The overnight *dexamethasone suppression* test (1 mg p.o. at midnight) should suppress both the serum cortisol to less than 7 μg/dl and plasma ACTH in normals, but not in patients with Cushing's disease. Dexamethasone (0.5 mg q6hr for 2 days) suppresses urine 17-OHCS, serum cortisol, and plasma ACTH in normal subjects, but not in patients with Cushing's disease. On the other hand, patients with Cushing's disease will usually demonstrate suppression of their pituitary–adrenal axis with high-dose dexamethasone (8 mg/day for 2 days), whereas patients with Cushing's syndrome from other causes (adrenal tumor, ectopic ACTH syndrome) will not show suppression of cortisol production. It should be noted that some patients with authentic Cushing's disease will show "normal suppression" with dexamethasone 0.5 mg q6hr.[42] Such findings appear to reflect *decreased metabolic* clearance of dexamethasone. In contrast, some patients with

Cushing's disease require 16 or even 32 mg dexamethasone daily to suppress the pituitary–adrenal axis. This may be seen in patients with frank pituitary tumors (macroadenomas) as well as in subjects with enhanced metabolism of dexamethasone due to concomitant ingestion of drugs such as diphenylhydantoin or aminoglutethimide that induce hepatic microsmal enzymes that degrade dexamethasone.[43] Some patients with Cushing's disease may appear to show a paradoxical rise in steroid levels to dexamethasone administration. However, such effects may be unrelated to the dexamethasone *per se* and result from an underlying periodic hormonogenesis.[44]

Failure of dexamethasone suppression and of responsiveness to metyrapone but *not* exogenous ACTH may be seen in adrenal nodular hyperplasia,[45] a condition that may result from long-standing tropic hyperstimulation of the adrenal cortex (Cushing's disease).[46] Patients with Cushing's disease have been reported to have an impaired cortisol response to insulin-induced hypoglycemia (suggesting an underlying hypothalamic disorder), a finding that may help to differentiate such cases from obesity[37] and depression,[36] conditions wherein altered cortisol metabolism may be found. However, an occasional patient with bona fide Cushing's disease does show a cortisol rise with insulin.

The metyrapone test has been proposed as the best test to differentiate Cushing's disease from other causes of Cushing's syndrome (for a review, see Besser and Edwards[36]), since in Cushing's disease, but not usually in other types of Cushing's syndrome, metyrapone (750 mg q4hr for 6 doses) results in a massive increase in urine 17-OHCS and plasma Cd′S′. Nevertheless, a brisk response to metyrapone has been reported in a patient with the "ectopic ACTH" syndrome.[47]

TRH has been reported to stimulate ACTH release in some patients with Cushing's disease and Nelson's syndrome.[48] Additionally, administration of cyproheptadine, a serotonin-receptor blocker, reported helpful in the medical management of these disorders (see Chapter 15), to a patient with Nelson's syndrome was associated with skin-lightening, restoration of plasma ACTH circadian periodicity, and *reversal* of the ACTH responsiveness to TRH administration.[49] As with other types of pituitary secretory adenomas, patients with Cushing's disease may show ACTH suppression to dopaminergic stimulation.[50]

Similar to that which has been reported following the selective surgical removal of GH-secreting adenomas, the return of normal cortisol–ACTH dynamics has been reported following transsphenoidal surgery for pituitary microadenomas in Cushing's disease.[51]

4.4. TSH Secretion

Although the TRH stimulation test (200–500 μg i.v.) is valuable in the diagnosis of Graves' disease (characterized by a flat TSH) and occasionally in primary hypothyroidism wherein there is TSH hyperresponsiveness (for a review, see Burger and Patel[52]), its role in the evaluation of hypothalamic–pituitary disease is uncertain (Table 3). While primary hypothalamic disorders, associated with hypothyroidism, frequently demonstrate a TSH peak response

TABLE 3. TSH Responses to TRH in Hypothalamic–Pituitary Disorders

Exaggerated	Flat
Pituitary tumor (occasionally)	Pituitary tumor (frequently)
Hypothalamic disease (frequently)	Acromegaly (occasionally)
GH deficiency (frequently)	"TSH toxicosis" (due to a pituitary adenoma)
"Idiopathic hypopituitarism" in children (very frequently)	Familial hypopituitarism with a large sella turcica in children
"TSH toxicosis" (*not* due to a pituitary, or hypothalamic, tumor)	

that is characteristically delayed to 60 min and primary pituitary disease typically results in an impaired TSH response, anomalies occur so frequently as to undermine the usefulness of this test as a means of anatomically separating hypothalamic from pituitary disorders (see Figs. 1–3). Studies in this laboratory have shown that the exaggerated TSH response has little discriminating power. However, the *absence* of a TRH-induced TSH rise, especially if the patient is hypothyroid, does suggest a primary pituitary disorder with a high degree of probability.[53] Nevertheless, we found that no more than 40% of patients who are hypothyroid from a lesion restricted to the pituitary will have a flat TSH response.[53] Essentially comparable findings have been reported by Snyder *et al.*,[32] who concluded that a TSH response to TRH that is subnormal in magnitude in a patient with secondary hypothyroidism and evidence of a space-occupying lesion suggests that the hypothyroidism is due to pituitary involvement. It has been reported that euthyroid patients with hypothalamic–pituitary disorders may have a normal or supranormal TSH response to TSH but a diminished triiodothyronine (t_3) rise.[54] These workers suggest that a low T_3 response to TRH in some euthyroid patients with hy-

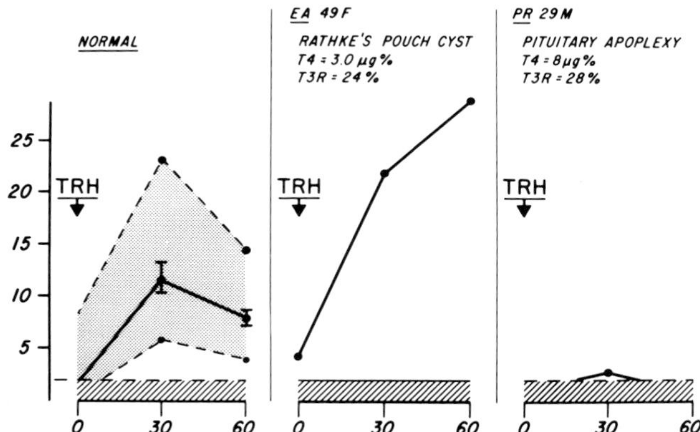

Fig. 1. Examples of the "classic" TSH response to TRH administration. *Left:* mean and range of normal responses; *center:* a delayed exuberant TSH rise in a subject with hypothalamic (or tertiary) hypothyroidism; *right:* an almost flat TSH response in a subject who had sustained a pituitary apoplexy though his 1-thyroxine (T_4) was within normal range. From Cobb *et al.*[53]

pothalamic–pituitary disorders can identify cases of preclinical secondary hypothyroidism possibly due to impaired biological activity of released TSH. The secretion of TSH with impaired biological activity has been reported in patients with hypothalamic–pituitary disease.[55]

In studies recently reported from our laboratory, Cobb *et al.*[56] examined the role of GH in modulating the pituitary thyroid response to TRH administration. We found that subjects with GH deficiency, be it pituitary or hypothalamic in origin, demonstrated an exaggerated TSH rise to TRH with an impaired T_3 response, suggesting that GH suppresses the pituitary thyrotrope cell but is tropic to the thyroid gland. The flat TSH response and presence of a goiter in many patients with acromegaly is consistent with this view.[22]

There is evidence that idiopathic hypopituitarism in childhood associated with a normal or small fossa may be due to a primary hypothalamic disorder, and such subjects do show a TSH response to TRH that is frequently delayed[57] compared with children who have familial hypopituitarism and a large sella turcia,[58] in which the TSH response is flat. The overall evidence in adult patients with lesions in the hypothalamic–pituitary area suggests that attempts to delineate the anatomical involvement of the lesion based on the TSH response to TRH should be made with caution.

An occasional finding that can cause confusion in diagnosis is the presence of a mildly elevated TSH in patients with secondary hypothyroidism.[52] In such subjects, other evidence of pituitary insufficiency must be utilized to make the diagnosis. Diagnostic difficulty in this area can also be increased by the presence of primary hypothyroidism (usually long-standing) associated with enlargement of the pituitary fossa (see Jackson[59] and Chapter 8).

Very occasionally, lesions in the hypothalamic–pituitary area may be associated with elevated TSH levels resulting in thyrotoxicosis.[60] In patients with frank pituitary adenomas, there generally occurs an impaired response to TRH that contrasts with the hyperresponse that is described in TSH-induced

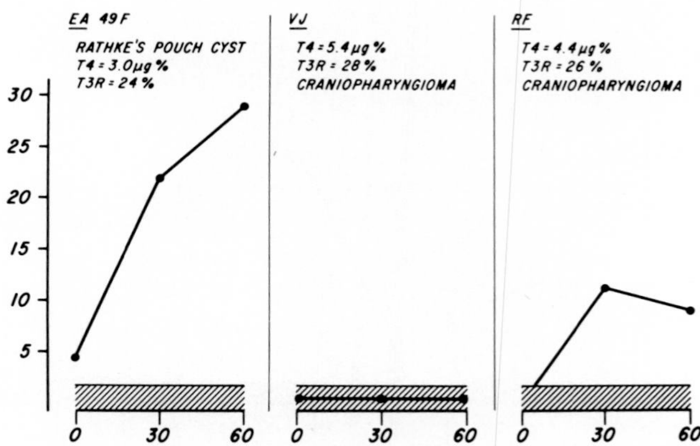

Fig. 2. Examples of the TSH responses to TRH that are obtained in patients with hypothalamic disorders. *Left:* the classic TSH response (also shown in Fig. 1, center); *center:* an absent TSH response in a subject with a craniopharyngioma and borderline hypothyroidism; *right:* a "normal" TSH response in a subject with a craniopharyngioma and hypothyroidism. From Cobb *et al.*[53]

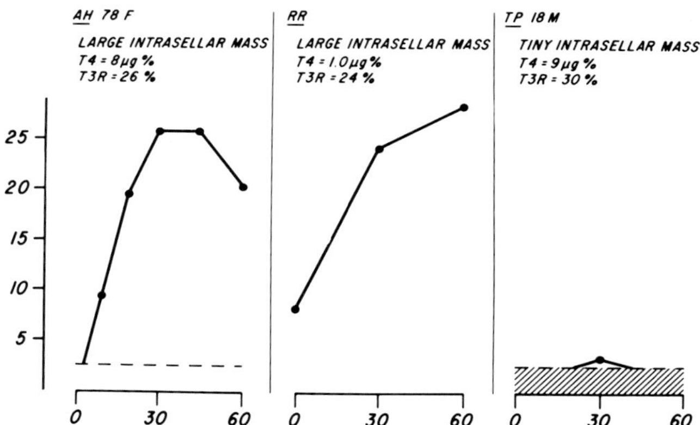

Fig. 3. Examples of the TSH responses to TRH that are obtained in patients with pituitary disease. *Left:* a marked TSH rise in a euthyroid subject with a large intrasellar mass; *center:* a delayed hypersensitive TSH rise in a hypothyroid subject with a large intrasellar mass (but no suprasellar extension); *right:* an almost flat TSH response in a euthyroid subject with a microadenoma. From Cobb *et al.*[53]

thyroxicosis, in which *no* evidence of pituitary tumor is found (Chapters 4 and 8). (See Table 3 for a summary of TSH responses to TRH in hypothalamic–pituitary disorders.)

4.5 Gonadotropin (LH and FSH) Secretion

In males, the presence of a low serum testosterone (<0.3 μg/dl) in association with low circulating gonadotropin levels suggests impaired gonadal function that is of central origin. The administration of *clomiphene citrate* (Clomid) in a dose of 50 mg b.i.d. p.o. for 7 days can be used as a test of the integrity of the hypothalamic–pituitary gonadal axis, since it gives rise to a doubling of the serum LH levels by 7–10 days in normals.[61] The clomiphene challenge appears to operate by displacing gonadal steroids from normal suppression sites in the hypothalamus and pituitary. In females, a similar schedule can be used in patients with amenorrhea, the clomiphene usually being given for 5 days. The LH usually shows a doubling at 5–7 days in those with an intact hypothalamic–pituitary–gonadal axis, and if ovulation is achieved, a midcycle surge of LH is found at 12–15 days following the first clomiphene dose. If the circulating estradiol level is low, which can be determined indirectly by a progesterone withdrawal challenge (Provera 10 mg/day for 3 days followed by withdrawal uterine bleeding in subjects with adequate estrogen priming), no LH rise is usually obtained with clomiphene administration. Some patients in both sexes required a 200 mg/day dose to produce an LH response. Most patients with intrinsic hypothalamic or pituitary disease do not respond to clomiphene (for a review, see Franchimont *et al.*[62]). Clomiphene is generally safe, though occasionally, it gives rise to blurring of vision and depression. It should be avoided in patients with liver disease.

LH-RH (in doses of 25–100 μg i.v.) produces an increase of LH and FSH in normal males and females, the LH rise usually being greater than the FSH except in prepubertal subjects and patients with anorexia nervosa, in whom the FSH response is frequently higher. Although LH-RH administration might be expected to differentiate hypothalamic from pituitary disease,[63] its administration to 155 patients with a variety of hypothalamic–pituitary disorders showed that despite clinical hypogonadism in 137 at the time of testing, only 9 subjects had an absent response to the releasing hormone, and it failed to differentiate between a primary hypothalamic and a primary pituitary disorder.[64] The role of LH-RH testing in the evaluation of hypothalamic–pituitary disease remains uncertain at this time. Theoretically, an absent clomiphene test and a positive LH-RH response should indicate a primary hypothalamic disorder, but exceptions occur so frequently as to undermine the usefulness of this procedure. In some patients with hypothalamic failure, the pituitary gonadotropes will require *repeated* administration of LH-RH to produce an LH rise,[65] so that a single bolus dose may be ineffective. The effect of prolonged administration of LH-RH (400 μg daily i.m. for 5 days) on the gonadotropin response to LH-RH (100 μg single injection i.v.) was studied in a group of patients with pituitary tumors and hypothalamic disorders. A paradoxical fall in response to LH-RH was observed in pituitary disease, whereas an augmented response was observed in a second LH-RH test (100 μg i.v.) after the 5 days' injections.[66] More recently, the role of continuous infusion of LH-RH on gonadotropin secretion in patients with disturbances of the hypothalamic–pituitary–gonadal axis has been studied, but the value of such testing has not been fully determined at this time.

5. Special Tests of Hypothalamic–Pituitary Function

The following tests should not be considered routine, but may occasionally be helpful in difficult diagnostic situations (Table 4).

5.1. Cerebrospinal Fluid (CSF) Pituitary Hormone Levels

Pituitary-hormone levels are occasionally elevated in patients with pituitary tumors, and the presence of increased CSF PRL levels may differentiate (apparently) nonfunctioning pituitary adenomas from the empty sella syndrome, in which the CSF PRL is normal.[67] Studies in our hands have shown that levels of the other pituitary hormones (TSH, FSH, and LH) may be in-

TABLE 4. Special Tests of Hypothalamic–Pituitary Function

CSF pituitary–hormone levels
Measurement of glycoprotein fragments
Sleep EEG studies
Prednisone–TRH reserve test
Cytochemical bioassays of pituitary hormones
Gel chromatography and radioreceptor assays

creased in patients with prolactinomas and that marked elevations of PRL in the CSF are very suggestive of suprasellar extension.[68] Likewise, marked elevation of ACTH in the CSF may be found in Nelson's syndrome with a suprasellar tumor[69] (see also Chapter 12).

5.2. Measurement of Glycoprotein Fragments in Biological Fluids

All the pituitary glycoprotein hormones (TSH, FSH, and LH) and human chorionic gonadotropin (hCG) consist of noncovalently bound alpha (α) and beta (β) subunits. The α subunits of these hormones are indistinguishable by immunoassay, whereas the β subunit is specific. In 60 patients with pituitary adenomas, Kourides *et al.*[70] reported that 5 patients had elevated serum α subunits with a diminished response to TRH and LH-RH (when compared with normal subjects). These workers suggest that an enlarged fossa with such findings may indicate the presence of a pituitary adenoma. An elevated CSF α fragment was also observed in one such patient.

5.3. Sleep EEG Studies

There is evidence that PRL and GH have nocturnal secretory patterns related to the EEG sleep stages. In the former, there is a series of cycles with the nadirs occurring during rapid eye movement (REM) sleep, and in the latter, there is a peak occurring during the first 90 min of sleep lasting 1.5–3.5 hr and related to slow-wave sleep (SWS).[71,72] The normal GH rise after sleep is often absent in acromegaly,[20] and loss of the augmented nocturnal PRL secretion has also been observed in patients with prolactinomas; however, similar findings are also observed in some cases of "functional" hyperprolactinemia.[73] Krieger and Glick[74] have suggested that impaired nocturnal surges of GH and PRL in patients with Cushing's disease bespeak a hypothalamic rather than a pituitary origin for this condition.

5.4. Prednisone–TRH Reserve Test

Using a dual-isotope release method (^{125}I and ^{131}I), endogenous TRH reserve has been assessed by determining the rebound response in thyroidal iodine release (TIR) by measuring urine ^{125}I/^{131}I ratios following withdrawal of pharmacological doses of prednisone (for details see Singer and Nicoloff[75]). These authors found that in patients with hypothalamic or pituitary disorders, there is impairment of TIR, but the two conditions were separated from each other using a TRH stimulation test. Presumably, a normal TRH stimulation test accompanied by a normal TIR implies normality of the hypothalamo–pituitary–thyroid axis.

5.5. Cytochemical Bioassays of Polypeptide Hormones

This method is exquisitely sensitive in the measurement of pituitary hormones, which can be assayed at the femtogram level in serum (for a review, see Bitensky[76]). Using this technique, normal serum levels of LH, TSH, and

ACTH have been clearly differentiated from values in hypopituitary subjects, something that cannot be accomplished with RIA. Cytochemistry is a form of quantitative cellular chemistry in which a microdensitometer is utilized for measuring the amount of precipitated colored reaction product within the cell—in other words, a form of hormone bioassay. At present, this technique is a research tool. The limitation vis-à-vis RIA is the much smaller number of samples that can be processed in unit time and the equipment costs.

5.6. Gel Chromatography and Radioreceptor Assays: Somatomedin C

Circulating pituitary hormones frequently demonstrate molecular heterogeneity on gel chromatography. Since only the monomeric peak of GH is biologically active in a radioreceptor assay (as determined by binding to a rabbit liver membrane), other molecular species of GH, which circulate in acromegalic patients, are incapable of binding to tissue receptors and are probably biologically inactive. Such findings may account for some of the discrepancies occasionally found between immunochemically measured GH levels and clinical severity of the acromegaly.[77]

There is also evidence for circulating fragments of GH that are not detectable by the GH RIA but that may be biologically active.[78] Thus, serum GH levels by RIA could either underestimate or overestimate the GH biological activity in the circulation of patients with acromegaly. The availability of an RIA for somatomedin C may now provide an integrated measurement of the circulating levels of biologically active GH and an improved index of GH secretion. There is also evidence that not all circulating PRL in patients with prolactinoma is biologically active as determined by radioreceptor assay.[79]

6. Posterior Pituitary Function

Tests of vasopressin (antidiuretic hormone, ADH) production are an important adjunct to the evaluation of pituitary function, since the presence of diabetes insipidus suggests that any concomitant anterior pituitary insufficiency results from hypothalamic damage. *Water deprivation* in a normal subject for 8 hr will result in a urine osmolality greater than 800 mosmol/kg, and the plasma osmolality does not rise above 294 mosmol/kg. If the antidiuresis is inadequate, the administration of vasopressin (given as the analogue DDAVP 20 μg intranasally) will produce adequate urinary concentration in subjects with diabetes insipidus that is central in origin. Plasma and urinary measurements of immunoreactive vasopressin can also be done, and such assays can directly separate cases of diabetes insipidus due to vasopressin deficiency from other causes that are nephrogenic, psychogenic, or pharmacological in origin (for a review, see Edwards[80]).

7. Summary and Conclusion

Many tests are available for the evaluation of pituitary function, but it is very important to fashion the test procedures so that they are appropriate to determining the clinical problems. Certain investigations are especially indicated in the evaluation of hypopituitarism, whereas others are of more relevance in presumptive states of pituitary hypersecretion; the procedures considered by this author to be of most value are summarized in Tables 5 and 6. Unfortunately, many metabolic disorders, including obesity, alcoholism, renal disease, and liver disease, endocrine disorders such as primary thyroid and adrenal disease, and drugs, including steroids, anticonvulsants, and tranquilizers, interfere with pituitary function tests and must be borne in mind in the evaluation of pituitary disease (for a review, see Cohen[81]).

Diagnostic difficulties can also ensue if pituitary disease accompanies an end-organ disorder. Long-standing cases of primary hypothyroidism and primary hypogonadism can on occasion lead to pituitary tumor formation, presumably due to unopposed negative feedback at the pituitary (see Chapter 8).

Combined tests for assessment of anterior pituitary function have been proposed. Such procedures involve the simultaneous administration of insulin or arginine along with TRH and LH-RH.[82–84] Although these tests are apparently satisfactory, this author is philosophically opposed to such testing,

TABLE 5. Diagnostic Tests Especially Recommended for the Investigation of Hypopituitarism

Hormone	Test material (adult dosage)	Time of peak serum response	Comments
GH	L-Dopa (500 mg p.o.)	60 min	Very safe; nausea occasionally occurs; GH *falls* in acromegaly, PRL is normally suppressed (see also Table 6).
	Insulin (0.05–0.3 μg/kg body weight i.v.)	60 min	To obtain a maximum response, adequate hypoglycemia must be achieved. ACTH and PRL reserve can be determined simultaneously.
PRL	TRH (500 μg i.v.)	30 min	Very safe. TSH reserve can be determined simultaneously. A GH rise may occur in acromegaly.
	Chlorpromazine (25 mg i.m.)	60–90 min	May produce hypotension and somnolence in hypopituitary or hypothyroid subjects. Tests the hypothalamic reserve for PRL release.
ACTH	Insulin (see under GH above)	30 min for ACTH 60 min for cortisol	See under GH above.
	Metyrapone (30 mg/kg body weight p.o. at midnight) [The longer procedure may also be used (see Table 6).]	9 A.M. for Cd'S' and cortisol and/or ACTH	Safe, but may cause nausea and vomiting. Unlike the insulin challenge, metyrapone testing is vitiated by concurrent glucocorticoid administration.
TSH	TSH (500 μg i.v.)	30–60 min	See also under PRL above. The test does not reliably separate hypothalamic from pituitary hypothyroidism.
Gonadotropins	LH-RH (25–150 μg)	30–60 min	Very safe. A GH rise may occur in acromegaly.
	Clomiphene (50 mg b.i.d. for 5–7 days)	LH at 5–7 days; also in females at 12–15 days for ovulatory surge	In females, can cause ovarian cyst formation and "super-ovulation." Tests the hypothalamic reserve for gonadotropin release.

since in the subsequent evaluation of such patients with, for example, acromegaly, it may not be apparent which agent has stimulated a rise in serum GH.

The availability of the hypophysiotropic hormones (TRH and LH-RH) in pure form has provided a means of directly testing the anterior pituitary gland. However, although the administration of such peptides has provided much insight into the pathophysiology of hypothalamic–pituitary disorders, their value in the individual subject as a means of separating a hypothalamic from a pituitary lesion is limited. In patients with both hypothalamic and pituitary tumors, TRH may cause a normal or delayed exaggerated rise in the serum TSH level. However, a flat TSH response in a patient with secondary hypothyroidism is particularly suggestive of a primary pituitary lesion as the cause of the thyroid insufficiency. With respect to other pituitary tumors,

TABLE 6. Diagnostic Tests Especially Recommended for the Investigation of States of Pituitary Hyperfunction

Hormone	Test material (adult dosage)	Time of maximum serum response	Comments
GH	Glucose (50–100 g p.o.)	120 min	Failure of GH suppression is diagnostic of acromegaly in the appropriate clinical setting.
	L-Dopa (500 mg p.o.)	60–120 min	GH suppression commonly occurs in acromegaly and is suggestive of this diagnosis.
	TRH (200–500 μg i.v.)	30 min	Positive response in acromegaly correlates with therapeutic response to bromocriptine.
PRL	TRH (500 μg i.v.) (see also under PRL in Table 5)	30 min	Failure of PRL rise may occur more frequently in prolactinomas than in other hyperprolactinemic states.
	L-Dopa[a] (500 mg p.o.)	60–120 min	Failure of PRL to fall adequately suggests the presence of a pituitary adenoma.
ACTH	Dexamethasone		
	(i) 1 mg p.o. at 12 midnight	Cortisol and/or ACTH at 9 A.M.[b]	Failure of suppression is a useful screening test for Cushing's syndrome.
	(ii) 0.5 mg q6hr for 2 days	Cortisol and/or ACTH at 48 hr (urine for 17-OHCS and/or "free" cortisol can also be determined)[b]	Failure of suppression suggests Cushing's syndrome.[c]
	(iii) 2 mg q6hr for 2 days	As in (ii)	Suppression occurs in Cushing's disease but not in other causes of Cushing's syndrome.[d]
	Metyrapone (750 mg p.o. q4hr for 6 doses) [The overnight test may also be used (see Table 5).	ACTH and/or Cd'S' at 24 hr (or urine 17-OHCS on the next day)	Marked rise occurs in Cushing's disease but not in other causes of Cushing's syndrome.

[a] Preceded by carbidopa, may be helpful in the diagnosis of prolactinomas (see the text).
[b] In Cushing's syndrome due to adrenal tumor, the ACTH level is already suppressed.
[c] In some patients with Cushing's disease, "normal" suppression occurs.
[d] In some patients with Cushing's disease, higher doses of dexamethasone are required for suppression.

prolactinomas tend to be characterized by a suppressed PRL response, and patients with acromegaly and Cushing's disease may demonstrate a paradoxical rise in serum GH and ACTH, respectively, following TRH administration; these patterns of response can certainly be helpful in diagnostic evaluation of pituitary tumors. LH-RH injection is of little help in the separation of pituitary from hypothalamic lesions as a cause of hypogonadotropic hypogonadism, since absent, normal, and even exaggerated rises of LH can occur in each circumstance. Whether repeat injections or continuous infusions of LH-RH have an important diagnostic facility for pituitary tumors remains to be determined. LH-RH may occasionally cause a rise in GH *and* PRL in some patients with acromegaly. Certainly, whatever hormonal responses are obtained with TRH and LH-RH stimulation, they do potentially provide the physician with a useful means of following the patient and monitoring the effectiveness of therapeutic measures that may subsequently be administered.

References

1. R.S. Yalow and S.A. Berson, Immunoassay of endogenous plasma insulin in man, *J. Clin. Invest.* **39:**1157–1175, 1960.
2. Hwang, H. Guyda, and H. Friesen, A radioimmunoassay for human prolactin, *Proc. Natl. Acad. Sci. U.S.A.* **68:**1902–1906, 1971.
3. A.G. Frantz, Prolactin, *N. Engl. J. Med.* **298:**201–207, 1978.
4. R. Burgus, T. Dunn, D. Desiderio, and G. Guillemin, Structure moleculaire du facteur hypothalamique hypophysiotrope TRF d'origine ovine: Mise en evidence par spectromètre de masse de la sequence PCA-HIS-PRO-NH_2, *C. R. Acad. Sci. (Paris)* **269:**1870–1873, 1969.
5. J. Bøler, F. Enzmann, K. Folkers, C.Y. Bowers, and A.V. Schally, The identity off chemical and hormonal properties of the thyrotropin releasing hormone and pyroglutamyl-histidyl-proline-amide, *Biochem. Biophys. Res. Commun.* **37:**705–710, 1969.
6. A.V. Schally, A. Arimura, A.J. Kastin, H. Matsuo, Y. Baba, T.W. Redding, R.M.G. Nair, L. Debeljuk, and W.F. White, Gonadotropin-releasing hormone: One polypeptide regulates secretion of luteinizing and follicle stimulating hormones, *Science* **173:**1036–1038, 1971.
7. P. Brazeau, W. Vale, R. Burgus, N. Ling, M. Butcher, J. Rivier, and R. Guillemin, Hypothalamic polypeptide that inhibits the secretion of immunoreactive pituitary growth hormone, *Science* **179:**77–79, 1973.
8. I.M.D. Jackson, Extrahypothalamic and phylogenetic distribution of hypothalamic peptides in: *The Hypothalamus* (S. Reichlin, R.J. Baldessarini, and J.B. Martin, eds.), pp. 217–231, Raven Press, New York, 1978.
9. G.W. Harris, Neural control of the pituitary gland, *Physiol. Rev.* **28:**139–179, 1948.
10. R.J. Wurtman, Brain monomamines and endocrine function, *Neurosci. Res. Prog. Bull.* **9:**172–297, 1971.
11. M.T. Rabkin and A.G. Frantz, Hypopituitarism: A study of growth hormone and other endocrine function, *Ann. Intern. Med.* **64:**1197–1966.
12. J.S. Jenkins, C.J. Gilbert, and V. Ang, Hypothalamic–pituitary function in patients with craniopharyngiomas, *J. Clin. Endocrinol. Metab.* **43:**394–399, 1976.
13. R.L. Eddy, P.F. Gilliland, J.D. Ibarra, *et al.*, Human growth hormone release, *Am. J. Med.* **56:**179–185, 1974.
14. A.G. Frantz and M.T. Rabkin, Effects of estrogen and sex difference on secretion of human growth hormone, *J. Clin. Endocrinol. Metab.* **25:**1470–1480, 1965.
15. W.B. Mendelson, L.S. Jacobs, J.D. Reichman, *et al.*, Methysergide suppression of sleep-related prolactin secretion and enhancement of sleep related growth hormone secretion, *J. Clin. Invest.* **56:**690–697, 1975.
16. J. Landon, F.C. Greenwood, T.C.B. Stamp, and V. Wynn, The plasma sugar, free fatty acid,

cortisol and growth hormone response to insulin and the comparison of this procedure with other tests of pituitary and adrenal function, *J. Clin. Invest.* **45**:437, 1966.

17. P.E. Cryer and W.H. Daughaday, Adrenergic modulation of growth hormone secretion in acromegaly: Suppression during phentolamine and phentolamine–isoproterenol administration, *J. Clin. Endocrinol. Metab* **39**:658–663, 1974.
18. M.L. Mitchell, M.J. Byrne, Y. Sanchez, and C.T. Sawin, Detection of growth hormone deficiency: The glucagon stimulation test, *N. Engl. J. Med.* **282**:539–541, 1970.
19. R.E. Johnsonbaugh, D.E. Bybee, and L.P. George, Exercise tolerance test: Single-sample screening technique to rule out growth-hormone deficiency, *J. Am. Med. Assoc.* **240**:664–666, 1978.
20. W.H. Daughaday, P.E. Cryer, and L.S. Jacobs, The role of the hypothalamus in the pathogensis of pituitary tumors in: *Diagnosis and Treatment of Pituitary Tumors* (P.O. Kohler and G.T. Ross, eds.), pp. 26–34, Excerpta Medica, Amsterdam, 1973.
21. F. Cammani, G.B. Picotti, F. Massara, G.M. Molinatti, P. Mategazza, and E.E. Müller, Carbidopa inhibits the growth hormone and prolactin-suppression effect of L-dopa in acromegalic patients, *J. Clin. Endocrinol. Metab.* **47**:647–651, 1978.
22. A. Gomez-Pan, W.M.G. Tunbridge, A. Duns, R. Hall, G.M. Besser, D.H. Coy, A.V. Schally, and A.J. Kastin, Hypothalamic hormone interaction in acromegaly, *Clin. Endocrinol.* **4**:455–460, 1975.
23. A. Liuzzi, P.G. Chiodini, L. Botalla, F. Silvestrini, and E.E. Müller, Growth hormone releasing activity of TRH and GH-lowering effect of dopaminergic drugs in acromegaly: Homogeneity in the two responses, *J. Clin. Endocrinol. Metab.* **39**:871–876, 1974.
24. N.A. Samaan, M.E. Leavens, and R.H. Jesse, Serum growth hormone and prolactin response to thyrotropin-releasing hormone in patients with acromegaly before and after surgery, *J. Clin. Endocrinol. Metab.* **38**:957–963, 1974.
25. K.M. Hoyte and J.B. Martin, Recovery from paradoxical growth hormone responses in acromegaly after trans-sphenoidal selective adenomaectomy, *J. Clin. Endocrinol. Metab.* **41**:656–659, 1975.
26. G. Faglia, A. Paracchi, C. Ferrari, and P. Beck-Peccoz, Evaluation of the results of transsphenoidal surgery in acromegaly by assessment of the growth hormone response to thyrotrophin-releasing hormone, *Clin. Endocrinol.* **8**:373–380, 1978.
27. H.E. Carlson, J.R. Sowers, and R.W. Rand, Lack of effect of thyroid hormones on the growth hormone response to thyrotropin-releasing hormone acromegaly, *Metabolism* **26**:801–805, 1977.
28. L. Belforte, F. Camanni, P.G. Chiodini, A. Liuzzi, F. Massara, G.M. Molinatti, E.E. Müller, and F. Silvestrini, Long term treatment with 2-Br-α-ergocryptine in acromegaly, *Acta Endocrinol.* **85**:235–248, 1977.
29. M. Ishibashi, T. Yamaji, and K. Kosaka, Induction of growth hormone and prolactin secretion by luteinizing hormone–releasing hormone and its blockade by bromergocryptine in acromegalic patients, *J. Clin. Endocrinol. Metab.* **47**:418–421, 1978.
30. M. Ishibashi and T. Yamaji, Effect of thyrotropin-releasing hormone and bromocriptine on growth hormone and prolactin secretion in perfused pituitary adenoma tissues of acromegaly, *J. Clin. Endocrinol. Metab.* **47**:1251–1256, 1978.
31. P.C. Eskildsen, P.A. Svendsen, L. Vang, and J. Nerup, Long-term treatment of acromegaly with bromocriptine, *Acta Endocrinol.* **87**:687–700, 1978.
32. P.J. Snyder, L.S. Jacobs, M.M. Rabello, *et al.*, Diagnostic value of thyrotropin-releasing hormone in pituitary and hypothalamic diseases, *Ann. Intern. Med.* **81**:751–757, 1974.
33. A.E. Boyd, S. Reichlin, and R.N. Turksoy, Galactorrhea–amenorrhea syndrome diagnosis and therapy, *Ann. Intern. Med.* **87**:165–175, 1977.
34. D.L. Kleinberg, G.L. Noel, and A.G. Frantz, Galactorrhea: A study of 235 cases, including 48 with pituitary tumors, N. Engl. J. Med. **296**:589–600, 1977.
35. S.A. Fine and L.A. Frohman, Loss of central nervous system component of dopaminergic inhibition of prolactin secretion in patients with prolactin-secreting pituitary tumors, *J. Clin. Invest.* **61**:973–980, 1978.
36. G.M. Besser and C.R.W. Edwards, Cushing's syndrome, *Clin. Endocrinol. Metab.* **1**:451–490, 1972.
37. I.M.D. Jackson and J.I. Mowat, The hypothalamic–pituitary–adrenal axis in obesity and the effect of prolonged fasting on the cortisol secretion rate, *Acta Endocrinol.* (Copenhagen) **63**:415–422, 1970.

38. J. Lindholm, H. Kehlet, M. Blichert-Toft, B. Dinesen, and J. Riishede, Reliability of the 30 minute ACTH test in assessing hypothalamic–pituitary–adrenal function, *J. Clin. Endocrinol. Metab.* **47**:272–274, 1978.
39. C.D. West and L.I. Dolman, Plasma ACTH radioimmunoassays in the diagnosis of pituitary–adrenal function, *Ann. N.Y. Acad. Sci.* **297**:205–219, 1977.
40. H.S. Jacobs and J.D. Nabarro, Tests of hypothalamic–pituitary–adrenal function in man, *Q. J. Med.* **38**:475–491, 1969.
41. J.S. Jenkins and W. Else, Pituitary–adrenal function tests in patients with untreated pituitary tumors, *Lancet* **2**:940–943, 1968.
42. J.F. Caro, A.W. Meikle, J.H. Check, and S.N. Cohen, "Normal suppression" to dexamethasone in Cushing's disease: An expression of decreased metabolic clearance for dexamethasone, *J. Clin. Endocrinol. Metab.* **47**:667–670, 1978.
43. L.G. Largerquist and F.H. Tyler, Diagnosis and treatment of disorders of the adrenal cortex, *Pharmacol. Ther. C* **1**:259–277, 1976.
44. R.D. Brown, G.R. Van Loon, D.N. Orth, and G.W. Liddle, Cushing's disease with periodic hormonogenesis: One explanation for paradoxical response to dexamethasone, *J. Clin. Endocrinol. Metab.* **36**:445–451, 1973.
45. H.J. Ruder, D.L. Loriaux, and M.B. Lipsett, Severe osteopenia in young adults associated with Cushing's syndrome due to micronodular adrenal disease, *J. Clin. Endocrinol. Metab.* **39**:1138–1147, 1974.
46. D.C. Anderson, P.F. Child, C.H. Sutcliffe, C.H. Buckley, D. Davies, and D. Longson, Cushing's syndrome, nodular adrenal hyperplasia and virilizing carcinoma, *Clin. Endocrinol.* **9**:1–14, 1978.
47. J.C. Nelson and D.J. Tindall, A comparison of the adrenal responses to hypoglycemia, metyrapone and ACTH, *Am. J. Med. Sci.* **275**:165–172, 1978.
48. M. Luria and D.T. Krieger, Response of plasma ACTH to TRF, vasopressin or hypoglycemia in Cushing's disease and Nelson's syndrome, *Clin. Res.* **24**:274A, 1976.
49. D.T. Krieger and E.M. Condon, Cyproheptadine treatment of Nelson's syndrome: Restoration of plasma ACTH circadian periodicity and reversal of response to TRF, *J. Clin. Endocrinol. Metab.* **46**:349–352, 1978.
50. A.L. Kennedy, B. Sheridan, and D.A.D. Montgomery, ACTH and cortisol response to bromocriptine and results of long term therapy in Cushing's disease, *Acta Endocrinol.* **89**:461–468, 1978.
51. A.M. Schall, J.S. Brodkey, B. Kaufman, and O.H. Pearson, Pituitary function after removal of pituitary microadenomas in Cushing's disease, *J. Clin. Endocrinol. Metab.* **47**:410–417, 1978.
52. H.G. Burger and Y.C. Patel, Thyrotrophin releasing hormone—TSH, *Clin. Endocrinol. Metab.* **6**:83–100, 1977.
53. W.E. Cobb, S. Reichlin, and I.M.D. Jackson, The diagnostic value of the TRH test (in prep.), 1980.
54. G. Faglia, C. Ferrari, A. Paracchi, A. Spada, and P. Beck-Peccoz, Triiodothyronine response to thyrotrophin releasing hormone in patients with hypothalamic–pituitary disorders, *Clin. Endocrinol.* **4**:585–590, 1975.
55. V.B. Peterson, A.M. McGregor, P.E. Belchetz, R.S. Elkeles, and R. Hall, The secretion of thyrotrophin with impaired biological activity in patients with hypothalamic–pituitary disease, *Clin. Endocrinol.* **8**:397–402, 1978.
56. W.E. Cobb, S. Reichlin, and I.M.D. Jackson, Importance of growth hormone (GH) in regulating the thyrotropin (TSH) response to thyrotropin releasing hormone (TRH) in patients with hypothalamic–pituitary (HP) disease, *Endocrinology* **103** (Suppl.): T-8, 1978.
57. B.H. Costom, M.M. Grumbach, and S.L. Kaplan, Effect of thyrotropin releasing factor in serum thyroid stimulating hormone: An approach to distinguishing hypothalamic from pituitary forms of idopathic hypopituitary dwarfism, *J. Clin. Invest.* **50**:2219–2225, 1971.
58. J.S. Parks, A. Tenore, A.M. Bongiovanni, and R.T. Kirkland, Familial hypopituitarism with large sella turcica, *N. Engl. J. Med.* **298**:698–702, 1978.
59. I.M.D. Jackson, Pituitary enlargement resulting from primary thyroid disease, *Proc. R. Soc. Med.* **63**:578, 1970.
60. G. Faglia, P. Beck-Peccoz, C. Ferrari, B. Ambrosi, A. Spada, P. Travaglini, and S. Paracchi, Plasma thyrotropin response to thyrotropin-releasing hormone in patients with pituitary and hypothalamic disorders, *J. Clin. Endocrinol. Metab.* **37**:595–601, 1973.

61. R.J. Santen, J.M. Leonard, R.T. Sherins, *et al.*, Short and long term effects of clomiphene citrate on the pituitary–testicular axis, *J. Clin. Endocrinol. Metab.* **33**:970–979, 1971.
62. P. Franchimont, J.C. Valcke, and R. Lambotte, Female gonadal dysfunction, *Clin. Endocrinol. Metab.* **3**:533–536, 1974.
63. A.M. Coscia, N. Fleischer, P.K. Besch, *et al.*, The effect of synthetic luteinizing hormone–releasing factor on plasma LH levels in pituitary disease, *J. Clin. Endocrinol. Metab.* **38**:83–88, 1974.
64. C.H. Mortimer, G.M. Besser, A.S. McNeilly, *et al.*, The LH and FSH releasing hormone test in patients with hypothalamic–pituitary–gonadal dysfunction, *Br. Med. J.* **4**:73–77, 1973.
65. C.H. Mortimer, Clinical applications of the gonadotrophin releasing hormone, *Clin. Endocrinol. Metab.* **6**:167–179, 1977.
66. T. Hashimoto, K. Miyai, T. Uozumi, S. Mori, M. Watanabe, and Y. Kumahara, Effect of prolonged LH-releasing hormone administration on gonadotropin release in patients with hypothalamic and pituitary tumors, *J. Clin. Endocrinol. Metab.* **41**:712–716, 1975.
67. L.L. Schroeder, J.C. Johnson, and M.B. Malarkey, Cerebrospinal fluid prolactin: A reflection of abnormal prolactin secretion in patients with pituitary tumors, *J. Clin. Endocrinol. Metab.* **43**:1255–1260, 1976.
68. B. Biller, K. Post, M. Molitch, S. Reichlin, and I. Jackson, CSF pituitary and hypothalamic hormone concentration in patients with prolactinomas, 45th Meeting of the Program of American Association of Neurological Surgeons, New Orleans, Louisiana, Abstract No. 28, 1977.
69. R.M. Jordan, J.W. Kendall, J.L. Search, *et al.*, Cerebrospinal fluid hormone concentration in the evaluation of pituitary tumors, *Ann, Intern. Med.* **85**:49–55, 1976.
70. I.A. Kourides, B.D. Weintraub, S.W. Rosen, *et al.*, Secretion of alpa subunits of glycoprotein hormones by pituitary adenomas, *J. Clin. Endocrinol. Metab.* **43**:97–106, 1976.
71. Y. Takahashi, D.M. Kipnis, and W.H. Daughaday, Growth hormone secretion during sleep, *J. Clin. Invest.* **47**:2079–2090, 1968.
72. D.C. Parker, L.G. Rossman, and E.F. Vanderlaan, Relation of sleep-entrained human prolactin release to REM–non REM cycles, *J. Clin. Endocrinol. Metab.* **38**:646–651, 1974.
73. R.M. Boyar, S. Kapen, J.W. Finkelstein, *et al.*, Hypothalamic–pituitary function in diverse hyperprolactinemic states, *J. Clin. Invest.* **53**:1588–1598, 1974.
74. D.T. Krieger and S.M. Glick, Growth hormone and cortisol responsiveness in Cushing's syndrome: Relation to a possible central nervous system etiology, *Am. J. Med.* **52**:25–40, 1972.
75. P.A. Singer and J.T. Nicoloff, Assessment of thyrotropin-releasing hormone and thyrotropin reserve in man, *J. Clin. Invest.* **52**:1099–1107, 1973.
76. L. Bitensky, Cytochemical bioassays of polypeptide hormones, *J. Reprod. Fertil.* **51**:287–294, 1977.
77. A.C. Herington, L.S. Jacobs, and W.H. Daughaday, Radioreceptor and radioimmunoassay quantitation of human growth hormone in acromegalic serum: Over estimation by immunoassay and systematic differences between antisera, *J. Clin. Endocrinol. Metab.* **39**:257–268, 1974.
78. W.P. Vanderlaan, M.B. Sigel, R.M.P. Singh, E.F. Vanderlaan, and U.T. Lewis, Radioimmunoassay evidence that 2 chain hGH circulates in blood, Program of the 60th Meeting of the Endocrine Society, Miami, Florida, p. 379, 1978 (Abstract No. 609).
79. P.E. Garnier, M.L. Aubert, S.L. Kaplan, and M.M. Grumbach, Heterogeneity of pituitary and plasma prolactin in man: Descreased affinity of "big" prolactin in a radioreceptor assay and evidence for its secretion, *J. Clin. Endocrinol. Metab.* **47**:1273–1281, 1978.
80. C.R.W. Edwards, Vasopressin and oxytocin in health and disease, *Clin. Endocrinol. Metab.* **6**:223–259, 1977.
81. K.L. Cohen, Metabolic, endocrine and drug-induced interference with pituitary function tests: A review, *Metabolism* **26**:1165–1177, 1977.
82. P. Harsoulis, J.C. Marshall, S.F. Kuku, C.W. Burke, D.R. London, and T.R. Fraser, Combined test for assessment of anterior pituitary function, *Br. Med. J.* **2**:326–329, 1973.
83. J. Rakoff, G. Vandenberg, T.M. Silver, and S.S.C. Yen, An integrated direct functional test of the adenohypophysis, *Am. J. Obstet. Gynecol.* **119**:358–368, 1974.
84. D.C.L. Savage, P.G. Swift, P.G.B. Johnston, D.J. Goldie, and D. Murphy, Combined test of anterior pituitary function in children, *Arch. Dis. Child.* **53**:301–304, 1978.

12

Pituitary Hormone Concentrations in Cerebrospinal Fluid in Patients with Pituitary Tumors

KALMON D. POST, BRUCE J. BILLER, and IVOR M.D. JACKSON

1. Introduction

Adenohypophyseal hormones are frequently detectable in the cerebrospinal fluid (CSF) of patients with pituitary adenomas,[1–9] especially those showing suprasellar extension (SSE).[4,6,7] However, documentation of their presence in CSF of normal subjects is controversial. Some workers readily find anterior pituitary hormones in CSF,[10,11] while others do not.[1,4,6,7,9] It has been proposed that in the normal individual, the blood–brain barrier (BBB) is relatively impermeable to the anterior pituitary hormones and that measurable levels of these substances in the CSF of patients with pituitary tumors indicate a breakdown in the blood–CSF barrier.[4,5,8] However, the possibility that adenohypophyseal hormones are normal constituents of CSF, though present below the limits of sensitivity of available assays, is not excluded. Evidence in favor of this view is provided by studies from Linfoot *et al.*,[7] who reported that growth hormone (GH) levels in CSF of acromegalic patients without SSE correlated with the height of the plasma concentration of GH. Similar findings have also been reported for prolactin (PRL).[12]

In this chapter, we will review previously published evidence concerning the role of anterior pituitary hormones in the CSF and discuss the physiolog-

---

KALMON D. POST • Tufts University School of Medicine; Department of Neurosurgery, Tufts–New England Medical Center Hospital, Boston, Massachusetts 02111. *BRUCE J. BILLER* • Department of Medicine, Massachusetts Institute of Technology, Cambridge, Massachusetts 02139; Department of Medicine, Division of Endocrinology, Tufts–New England Medical Center Hospital, Boston, Massachusetts 02111. *IVOR M.D. JACKSON* • Tufts University School of Medicine; Department of Medicine, Division of Endocrinology, Tufts–New England Medical Center Hospital, Boston, Massachusetts 02111. Reprinted by permission from *Neurobiology of Cerebrospinal Fluid I* (J. Wood, ed.), Plenum Press, New York, 1980.

ical and clinical significance of their presence in this biological fluid. In addition, we will present a summary of our own studies in this area.

2. Factors That Regulate the Presence of Anterior Pituitary Hormones in the Cerebrospinal Fluid

2.1. Molecular Weight

Although the process underlying the formation of CSF is complex,[13] filtration of plasma at the choroid plexus appears to be the most important factor. The CSF content of serum proteins in man is a reflection of the hydrodynamic volume of the protein molecule. For proteins with an overall globular conformation, the CSF concentration correlates with the molecular weight.[12] In keeping with this view, serum/CSF concentration ratios of 237 for albumin (mol. wt. 69,000) and up to 6332 for β-lipoprotein (mol. wt. $> 2 \times 10^6$) have been reported.[14] Since the molecular weight of the adenohypophyseal hormones is less than that of albumin, they should be present in CSF, though detection may be a function of assay sensitivity. In the original studies reported by Assies *et al.*,[2] PRL was not detected in the CSF of normoprolactinemic individuals without pituitary disease. In all cases, the hormone concentration was below the detection limit of the assay used at that time ($<$2.5 ng/ml). However, with a fivefold increase in assay sensitivity, these workers[12] and others[15] have shown that the PRL level of CSF is related to the plasma level in both normoprolactinemic and hyperprolactinemic patients with or without pituitary tumors. GH, which has a molecular weight similar to that of PRL, also appears in the CSF in concentrations related to its level in the peripheral circulation.[16] Indeed, in patients with nonendocrine disease, the PRL plasma/CSF ratio was 6,[12] and was identical to that reported by Schaub *et al.*[6] for GH in 43 normal subjects. Although rat PRL injected intravenously into rabbits entered the CSF,[17] infusion of ACTH[10] and [^{125}I]-ACTH[4] in man have reported not to cross the BBB.

Evidence favoring the integrity of the pituitary–CSF barrier for adenohypophyseal hormones, at least for a pituitary gland not affected by tumor, is provided by studies reported in 12 cases of empty sella syndrome.[18,19] All levels of ACTH, thyroid-stimulating hormone (TSH), luteinizing hormone (LH), follicle-stimulating hormone (FSH), PRL, and GH were at the limits of detectability, and were low despite elevated plasma levels induced by stress, menopause, thyrotropin-releasing hormone (TRH), or LH-releasing factor (LRF).

2.2. Retrograde Transport from Pituitary to Brain

Assies *et al.*[20] studied simultaneous plasma and CSF levels of PRL and human chorionic somatomammotropin (hCS) in six pregnant women without pituitary disease. Plasma and CSF levels were closely correlated for each. Although it was felt that the CSF concentration of a protein hormone depended on the plasma concentration and on its molecular size, the plasma/CSF concentration ratio for hCS (24.6) was significantly different from the PRL ratio (7.2). Since the CSF PRL concentration[21] is higher than would be expected from the concentration in peripheral blood, an additional, but not necessarily alternate, process must be considered. Were pituitary PRL to reach CSF by filtration from blood having a much higher PRL content than peripheral blood, the relative increase in CSF PRL concentration compared with hCS, which is derived solely from the placenta, could be explained.

It has generally been accepted that anterior pituitary secretions drain directly into the cavernous sinuses from lateral hypophyseal veins, and thence into the systemic circulation.[22] Support for this view was provided by the studies of Ganong and Hume,[23] who found high levels of ACTH within the cavernous sinuses of dogs. However, there have been few reports of anatomical studies demonstrating significant veins draining from the anterior pituitary.[24,25]

Many years ago, Szentagothai *et al.*[26] and Torok[27] questioned this concept, and suggested the possibility of retrograde venous transport from pituitary to brain. More recently, elegant anatomical studies by Bergland and his colleagues[24,25,28,29] have reawakened interest in the concept of retrograde vascular transport from the pituitary. Utilizing vascular casts subjected to scanning electron microscopy, Bergland and Page[25] failed to demonstrate lateral hypophyseal veins to the cavernous sinus in the rhesus monkey, but did see Y-shaped confluent pituitary veins joining the pars distalis and the infundibular process to the cavernous sinuses through a common trunk. However, few of these veins were encountered. An arterial supply was found only to the neurophypophysis, and none to the anterior lobe. Numerous anastomotic connections existed between these arteries and a continuous neurohypophyseal capillary bed that connected the infundibulum, infundibular stem, and infundibular process (neurohypophysis). The entire afferent blood supply to the anterior gland was via portal vessels. Many short portal vessels were interposed between the adenohypophysis and the infundibular stem and process, with arrangements that implied alternate efferent routes from the adenohypophysis. This anatomy suggested some circular flow within the gland, i.e., from pars distalis to infundibular process, thence to the infundibulum, and back again to the pars distalis. Efferent routes for the pituitary blood would then be: (1) from adenohypophysis via short portal vessels to neurohypophysis; (2) from adenohypophysis and neurohypophysis to systemic circulation via lateral confluent veins joining the cavernous sinus; (3) from adenohypophysis and infundibular process to hypothalamus via capillaries and portal vessels; (4) to the cerebral arterial system via flow reversal in hypophyseal arteries; (5) to hypothalamus via retrograde axonal transport[30]; and (6) to CSF in the third ventricle and subarachnoid space by tanycyte transport or fenestrations in the portal vessels. From the neurohypophysis, blood may thus drain to the anterior gland, the systemic circulation, or toward the brain, with the most significant vessels suggesting flow toward the brain[24,25] (see Fig. 1). This latter concept was also suggested by the report by Torok[27] of flow within the neurohypophysis going toward the infundibulum and thence to the hypothalamus. Moreover, Oliver *et al.*[31] demonstrated high concentrations of hormones from the pars distalis and pars intermedia in the neurohypophysis, lending support to the circular flow concept.

In a study in sheep,[24] increased concentrations of PRL and GH were found in blood sampled from the internal carotid artery above the level of the

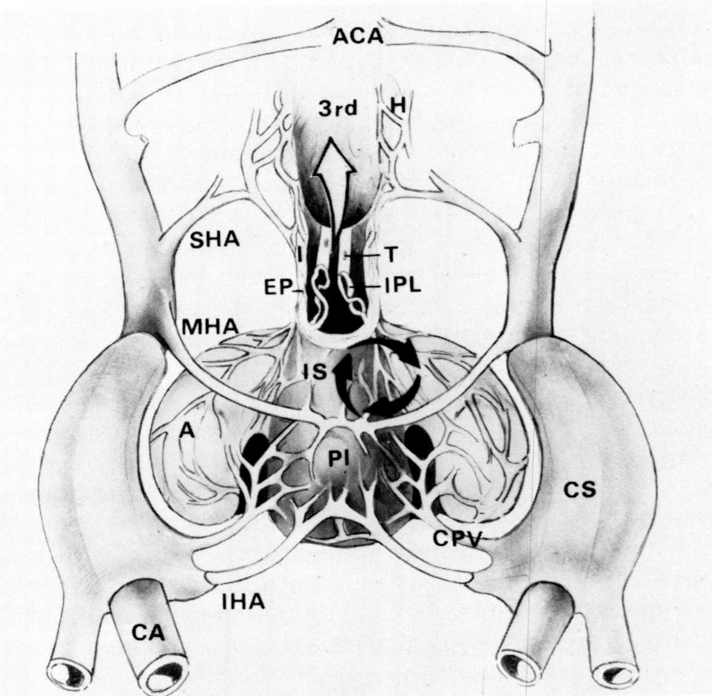

Fig. 1. Pituitary blood circulation. Abbreviations: (A) adenohypophysis; (PI) pars intermedia; (I) infundibulum; (IS) infundibular stem; (H) Hypothalamus; (SHA) superior hypophyseal artery; (MHA) middle hypophyseal artery; (IHA) inferior hypophyseal artery; (CPV) confluent pituitary vein; (CA) carotid artery; (ACA) anterior communicating artery; (CS) cavernous sinus; (T) tanycyte; (3rd) third ventricle; (IPL) internal plexus; (EP) external plexus. The figure demonstrates findings from vascular cast studies visualized posteriorly: Three pairs of arteries serve the neurohypophysis: SHA, MHA, and IHA. They form extensive anastomotic links, but do not pass through the adenohypophysis. Confluent pituitary veins to the cavernous sinus are scant. Numerous short vessels connect the adenohypophysis to the infundibular process, forming a common capillary bed. Within the infundibulum is a thin external plexus and a coiled complex internal plexus. All arterial supply is to the external plexus. Tanycytes are stretched between the internal plexus and the third ventricle. The phenomenon of circular blood flow (solid arrows) within the pituitary could provide tanycytes high concentrations of adenohypophyseal hormones. Tanycyte transport may be toward the third ventricle (outline arrows), delivering hormones to the brain. Reproduced with the kind permission of Dr. Richard M. Bergland.

pituitary gland and also from the sagittal sinus. It was concluded that the neurohypophyseal capillary bed not only received tropic hormones produced in the adenohypophysis, but also, under certain physiological circumstances, delivered those same hormones directly to the brain. Studies by Nakai and Naito[32] in the frog after systemic injection of horseradish peroxidase have shown that the endothelium of the capillaries of the hypophyseal portal vessels was permeable to this substance. It was taken up by pinocytosis of the ependymal tanycytes in the median eminence (ME) and carried by an ascending transport mechanism to be secreted into the third ventricle. The concepts of Bergland and Page applied to the anterior pituitary hormones in mammalian species might similarly allow the ependymal tanycytes to take up pituitary peptides that have reached the ME via retrograde vascular transport for transport to the third ventricle CSF. Alternately, or in addition, the absence of the BBB at the ME[33,34] could allow pituitary hormones to reach the ME from the systemic circulation and subsequently be transported by the ependymal tanycytes to the third ventricle (see Fig. 2A).

2.3. Pituitary Tumors and Cerebrospinal Fluid Secretion

Normal anterior pituitary cells extrude hormone-containing granules primarily at the interface between the cell membrane and the capillaries of the pituitary capillary plexus.[35] But a neoplastic pituitary cell can have multiple sites of granule exocytosis remote from the pericapillary space,[36] as a process termed "misplaced exocytosis" by Horvath and Kovacs.[36] Such misplaced exocytosis could occur because a tumor outgrows its vascular supply, resulting in fewer available pericapillary exocytosis sites, or as a consequence of "dedifferentiation" of the neoplastic cells resulting in an abnormal secretory process.

Pituitary tumors have no capsules as such, but rather are contained by the aponeurotic sheath of the sella.[37] This is bounded superiorly by reflections of the dura that form the diaphragma sellae, with the arachnoid surrounding the aperture of the diaphragma through which the stalk passes.[38] Accordingly, when a tumor extends beyond the diaphragma, only arachnoid separates it from CSF, and via misplaced exocytosis it might release hormone directly into the subarachnoid space. With the distortion of the normal anatomy, either the tumor or the normal gland would be adjacent to the CSF space, and therefore either the tumor hormone or normal gland hormones might be seen in the CSF in elevated concentrations (see Fig. 2B). Such a hypothesis has been proposed by Jordan and co-workers[4,39] to explain their studies. These workers reported increased CSF levels of pituitary hormones only in pituitary tumor patients with SSE. In most instances, but not all, the hormone secreted by the tumor into the peripheral blood appeared in the CSF. Occasionally, more than one hormone was present in the CSF: the abnormally elevated hormone secreted by the tumor along with another, e.g., GH with PRL or a gonadotropin, all of which could be derived from the tumor or adjacent normal tissue. Occasionally, presumably nonfunctional pituitary adenomas were associated with elevated CSF adenohypophyseal hormones supposedly derived from normal tissue, but secretion by the tumor only into the CSF and not into the systemic circulation might have occurred.[40] Surprisingly, the larger-molecular species of PRL ("big" PRL) has been identified in the CSF at concentrations far below that in the plasma, even in patients with tumors showing SSE.[2,39] Such findings are in conflict with the concept of misplaced exocytosis, and favor transport from plasma.

2.4. Other Factors That Might Affect Anterior Pituitary Hormones in the Cerebrospinal Fluid

Large size and lipid insolubility of a substance, factors that will tend to limit the uptake of adenohypophyseal hormones from the systemic circula-

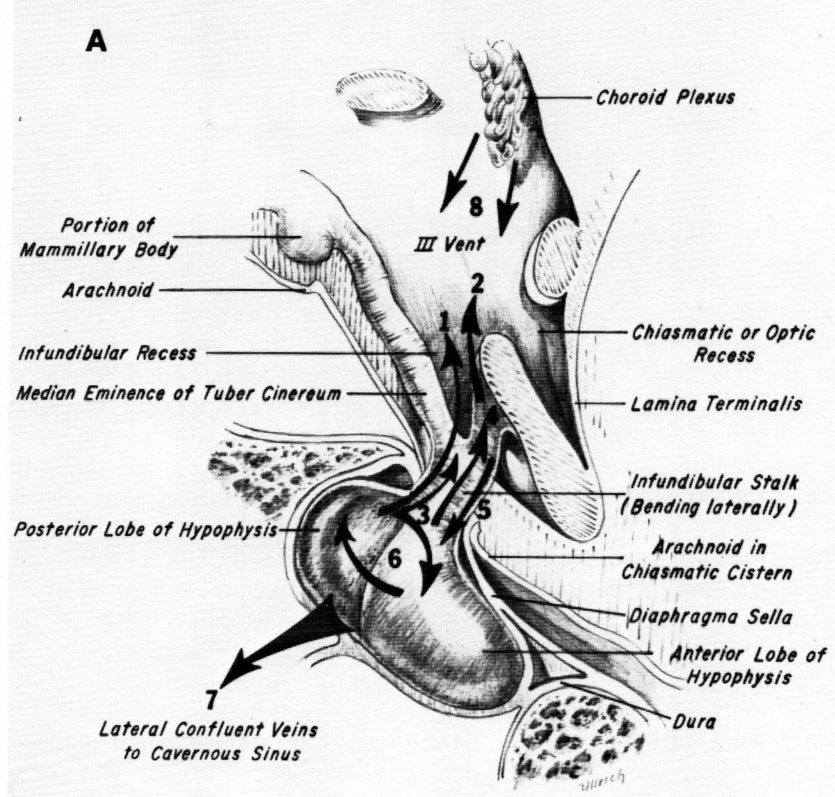

Fig. 2. (A) Representation of the potential pathways for anterior pituitary hormones as discussed in the text: (1) flow in the long portal vessels toward the third ventricle; (2) flow from the tuber cinereum toward the third ventricle; (3) flow in the long portal vessels toward the tuber cinereum; (4) retrograde axonal flow within the stalk; (5) flow down the stalk from the tuber cinereum toward the adenohypophysis; (6) short portal vessel flow between the anterior and posterior gland; (7) venous drainage via the lateral confluent veins toward the cavernous sinus; (8) filtration or secretion of pituitary hormones through the choroid plexus. (B) Representation of the potential pathways for anterior pituitary hormones as discussed in the text (continued): (9) direct secretion from the tumor through the distorted arachnoid, which is mass in direct contrast with the tumor; (10) direct secretion from the tumor into the third ventricle or stalk.

tion, also favor exclusion from transfer across the BBB to the CSF.[41] Although protein binding is not thought to be an important means by which the adenohypophyseal hormones are transported in the blood in contrast to thyroxine and cortisol, any such binding by plasma proteins, either specific or nonspecific, would limit transfer across the BBB.[41] Regardless of the relative contribution of the choroid plexus, the transependymal route from brain parenchyma, or the pial blood vessels,[13] the polypeptide transport system may have a finite capacity. This was illustrated for PRL by Login and MacLeod[17] when they showed that there was a plateau of CSF concentration in rats with PRL-secreting pituitary tumors, despite the presence of up to 38,000 ng/ml in serum.

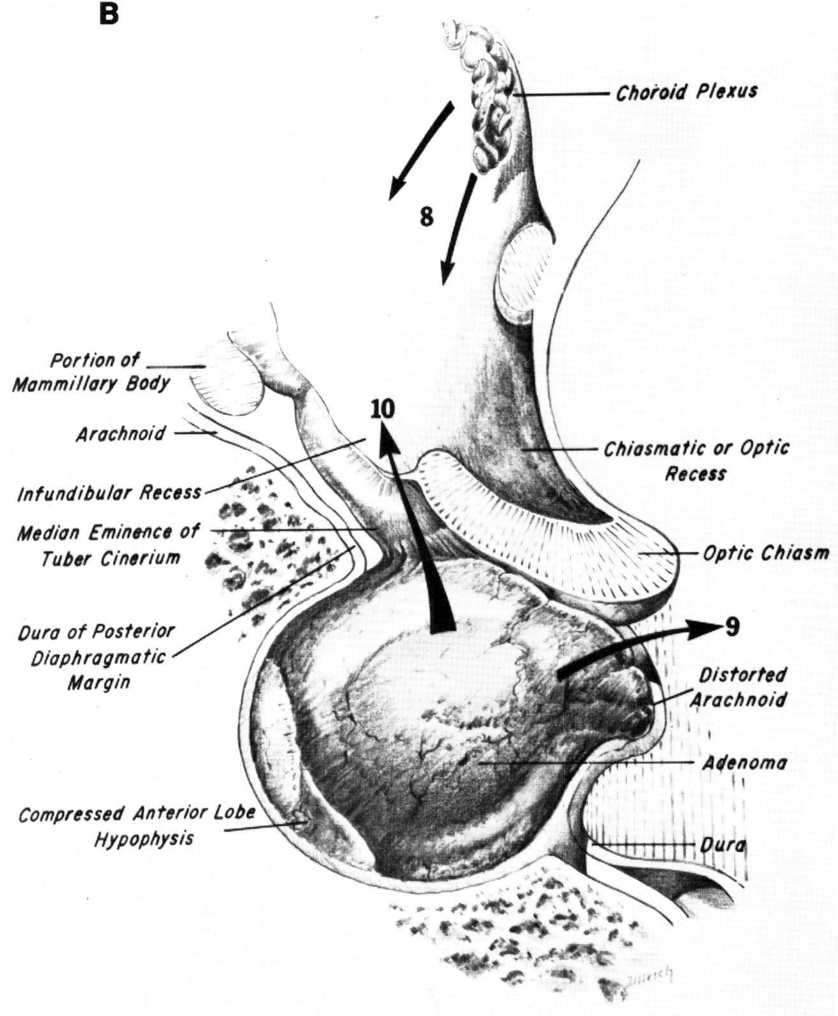

Fig. 2. (*continued*)

3. Functional Role of Anterior Pituitary Hormones in the Cerebrospinal Fluid

The potential importance of the CSF as a link in neuroendocrine control mechanisms[33] has been given increasing recognition. Hormones introduced into the CSF do exert effects on function, but the physiological significance of hormones normally present there is uncertain. Kendall *et al.*[42] found that when a systemically ineffective dose of cortisol was introduced into the CSF ventricular system, the typical stress-related elevation of serum ACTH was prevented or supressed. Similarly, administration of thyroxine caused TSH suppression, perhaps suggesting feedback inhibition. Following injection into the lateral ventricle, TRH, ACTH, thyroxine, and cortisol are concentrated in the ME.[42] Ondo *et al.*[43] also showed that certain compounds in the CSF (such as labeled corticosterone, LH, PRL, and hemoglobin), after injection into the third ventricle, can pass through the ME and enter the hypophyseal blood, while only trace amounts are found in simultaneously obtained arterial blood.

This type of CSF hormonal circulation leads to several interesting hypotheses for short-loop feedback inhibitions. For instance, when PRL is secreted by the pituitary into the systemic circulation, it may then enter the CSF at the choroid plexus, or it might be secreted directly into the CSF. PRL might then circulate in the CSF to a localized receptor area at the infundibular recess of the third ventricle, where it is then transported by tanycyte ependyma to PRL receptors on the dopamine-containing cells of the ME. Here the dopamine [prolactin-inhibitory factor (PIF)] system is activated to complete the loop and regulate the anterior pituitary secretion of PRL.[44] It is possible that the other pituitary hormones may similarly regulate their own secretion through interaction at the hypothalamic level.[45]

There is also much evidence that pituitary hormones may have a role in brain function.[46] PRL[47] and ACTH[48] have been reported to influence behavior in mammals and submammalian vertebrates, and transport from the CSF may be an important route of delivery to specific brain areas.

4. Specific Hormones and the Cerebrospinal Fluid

4.1. Growth Hormone

Wright *et al.*[49] reported 84 cases of acromegaly and showed a significant correlation between pituitary tumor size and serum GH levels. Linfoot *et al.*[7] in 1970, however, published the first report of human GH levels in CSF studied by radioimmunoassay (RIA). They compared the results of 8 normals with 12 acromegalics, 3 of whom had SSE and 1 of whom also had a coexistent partially empty sella. The control GH values were extremely low (mean $<0.09 \pm 0.01$ ng/ml with a range of <0.05–0.12 ng/ml), while the acromegalic patients without SSE had higher levels (mean 0.49 ± 0.11 ng/ml). Simultaneous mean blood GH levels were 0.89 ± 0.30 (range 0.16–1.14 ng/ml) for the normals and 14.1 ± 2.24 ng/ml (range 3.0–26.3 ng/ml) for the acromegalic patients. The acromegalic patients had a CSF GH level 5 times higher and a plasma GH level 16 times higher than the controls, but no significant correlation was appreciated between the CSF and plasma concentrations. However, the 3 patients with SSE of their tumors had a level of GH in their CSF 140–800 times greater than acromegalics whose tumors were confined to the sella. The plasma GH was 16 times higher in the former group, but again no correlation was appreciated between the CSF and plasma levels. This may have just reflected the frequent fluctuations seen in circulating GH both in normals and in acromegalics. After treatment of the tumor with heavy-particle therapy, there was a decrease in both the CSF and the plasma GH, but again without clear correlation between them. In a patient with acromegaly and a partially empty sella, the CSF GH was not higher than in the other patients without SSE. On the basis of these data, Linfoot and colleagues suggested that a breakdown in the blood–CSF barrier accompanying SSE might have been a causative mechanism for increased CSF GH.

In 1972, Thomas *et al.*[9] reported the results of RIA for GH in the CSF of acromegalics using an activated charcoal technique. No GH was detected in the CSF of patients without acromegaly (CSF GH 0.4 ng/ml). GH was measurable in patients with acromegaly (range 0.6–1.2 ng/ml), and in one patient with SSE, the levels were considerably elevated (12.6 ng/ml, while plasma GH was 7.7 ng/ml). They suggested that in conjunction with pneumoencephalography (PEG), CSF GH might be a useful test to diagnose SSE. Thomas and co-workers' series of 18 cases of acromegaly, in contrast to the report of Wright,[49] failed to show any correlation between tumor size and serum GH concentration.

Allen *et al.*[1] in 1974 reported on 26 patients, 3 of whom were acromegalic, who had simultaneous plasma and CSF determinations of ACTH and GH on samples obtained during PEG. There were 17 normal controls in whom a rise in both plasma ACTH and GH was seen during PEG, but without change in CSF levels. The 3 acromegalic patients had both elevated CSF GH and plasma GH, but the patients with SSE had much higher basal CSF GH and CSF ACTH levels than those without SSE. In contrast, 5 patients with nonfunctioning chromophobe adenomas or craniopharyngiomas that extended into the basilar cisterns did not have significant elevation of GH or ACTH in the CSF.

In 1976, Hanson *et al.*[50] reported a case of acromegaly in which baseline plasma GH levels were minimally elevated (11.3 ng/ml) and suppressed partially during a glucose tolerance test (11.3 ng/ml→6.6 ng/ml). However, a markedly elevated CSF GH (23.7 ng/ml; normal <1) was observed in one case. PEG and subsequent craniotomy clearly demonstrated significant suprasellar and parasellar extension. While in the previously cited reports some question could be raised as to the correlation between plasma and CSF levels (because plasma GH was also elevated), this case was unique and suggested disruption of the normal pituitary–CSF barrier.

Jordan *et al.*[4] in 1976 found that only when a pituitary tumor extended beyond the diaphragma sella did the CSF contain elevated levels of pituitary hormones. Moreover, successful treatment resulted in a fall in CSF hormone levels. A total of 83 patients were studied at PEG: 28 with neurological disease, but no evidence of endocrine disease; 49 suspected of harboring pituitary tumors (22 with SSE and 27 without SSE); and 6 with craniopharyngiomas. The control group had a CSF GH of less than 2 ng/ml, and the 27 tumor patients without SSE did not differ significantly from them. One patient without SSE had a coexistent partially empty sella and did not have significant elevation of CSF GH despite this distorted anatomy. All but one of the 22 patients with SSE had elevations of one or more CSF hormones. The hormone actually produced by the tumor was found in elevated CSF concentrations in all cases of SSE except one acromegalic who had increased FSH and LH only. Furthermore, no correlation was found between CSF hormone and plasma hormone levels in patients with SSE, suggesting that a breakdown of a blood–

CSF barrier was unlikely. Rather, it was felt more likely that direct secretion by the tumor into CSF existed, i.e., a disturbed pituitary–CSF barrier. Since 21 of 22 patients with SSE had elevated adenohypophyseal hormone concentrations in the CSF, and 27 tumor patients without SSE had normal GH levels, Jordan *et al.*[4] concluded that CSF GH had value in predicting tumor expansion.

Schaub *et al.*[16] also measured GH concentration in blood and CSF in controls and acromegalic patients. In 43 patients without pituitary disease undergoing PEG, CSF GH was $0.35+0.03$ ng/ml, while plasma GH was 1.95 ± 0.20 ng/ml, giving a plasma/CSF ratio of 6. Twenty-seven patients with diabetic retinopathy had similar values. Ten acromegalic patients without SSE (on lipiodol ventriculography) were studied as well. In 7 acromegalic patients, the CSF GH was consistently more elevated than in the normal subjects (mean 3.35 ± 1.4 ng/ml with a mean plasma/CSF ratio of 11). In one patient, the CSF GH levels were extremely elevated (3850 ng/ml and 250 ng/ml on two samples) and, indeed, were higher than the plasma levels taken simultaneously (78 ng/ml and 27 ng/ml); i.e., the plasma/CSF ratio was less than 1. In 2 acromegalics with SSE, repeated CSF measurements showed markedly increased CSF GH concentration, but lower than basal plasma GH levels (ratio >2). Since elevated GH was seen in the CSF secondary to hypersecreting tumors both with and without SSE, these workers concluded that a breakdown of the BBB from SSE was not necessary. They suggested that an active transport process existed for the secretion of pituitary hormones into the CSF.

4.2. ACTH

Kleerekoper *et al.*[6] were the first to report elevated CSF ACTH levels in patients with Nelson's syndrome. If GH (with a molecular weight of around 21,000) could cross the BBB, then ACTH (with a molecular weight of 4500) should be expected to cross more easily if molecular size were the sole or major determinant of pituitary hormone concentration in the CSF. Both plasma and CSF ACTH were measured in six patients without endocrine disease (CSF ACTH 0–85 pg/ml). In three adrenalectomized patients with high plasma ACTH (113–4500 pg/ml), ACTH was also high in the CSF. The highest value was in a patient with SSE of an ACTH-producing tumor. Kleerekoper and co-workers suggested that ACTH-secreting pituitary tumors did not give rise to very high levels of the hormone in the CSF unless there was SSE of the tumor.

The mean CSF ACTH concentration was 98 pg/ml in a study of 22 patients with nonendocrine disease,[2] a value slightly higher than the mean concentration in simultaneously obtained plasma (74 pg/ml). However, in a subsequent report from the same laboratory,[4] 27 subjects with nonendocrine disease had CSF ACTH levels that were low, a finding that raises questions regarding the specificity of the measurements reported in the two studies.[10] The concentrations of the individual pairs of ACTH values obtained from plasma and CSF were not correlated, suggesting that ACTH did not readily cross the blood–CSF barrier. Studies were also undertaken during a 48-hr ACTH infusion to see whether CSF ACTH levels could be increased by increasing plasma ACTH concentration. Despite the achievement of plasma levels in excess of 10,000 pg/ml, the CSF ACTH concentration remained low. In 2 normal subjects, a single bolus of ACTH labeled with ^{125}I failed to cause a significant increase in CSF [^{131}I] ACTH at either 60 min or 6 hr, suggesting that the blood–CSF barrier was relatively impermeable to ACTH. During infusion of labeled ACTH in cats, a steady-state plasma/CSF radioactivity ratio was reached after 4–6 hr, at which time the concentrations of the labeled ACTH were 100 times higher in plasma than in CSF. These findings supported the view that the blood–CSF barrier is relatively impermeable to ACTH in both man and cat. The relatively high CSF ACTH concentration found in patients with nonendocrine disease indicates that most of the ACTH present entered by a mechanism that bypassed the blood–CSF barrier, such as a direct leak from the pituitary surface into the adjacent basilar cistern or by retrograde transport through the stalk and basal hypothalamus to the third ventricle. Supporting the concept of retrograde transport through the stalk and/or basal hypothalamus to CSF was the finding that in an anencephalic infant who lacked both hypothalamus and pituitary stalk, ACTH was undetectable in CSF, while a concentration of 60 pg/ml was seen in plasma. It should be noted that significant levels of immunoreactive ACTH have been detected in the hypothalamus and other brain locations even in hypophysectomized rats,[51] so that CSF ACTH could be derived from extrapituitary brain sites wherein ACTH may be synthesized *in situ*. Another possibility was that the immunoassay being employed might be measuring fragments of ACTH that possibly entered the CSF more readily than the whole molecule. Supporting the direct-leak theory was one patient with SSE of an ACTH-secreting tumor who showed a CSF ACTH of 3220 pg/ml and a plasma ACTH of 1070 pg/ml. The comparatively higher CSF levels of ACTH as opposed to GH might be due to cell position within the gland.

In a further report from the same group,[1] a series of 26 normal patients and 10 patients with pituitary–hypothalamic disease was described in whom ACTH and GH levels in both CSF and plasma were studied during PEG. Of 3 patients with acromegaly, 2 were seen to have minimal elevation of CSF ACTH, 112–116 pg/ml (normal $<$ 100), while the plasma ACTH was normal. Two patients with Nelson's disease were studied. One patient with SSE had marked plasma ACTH elevation, 1069, pg/ml, but even higher CSF ACTH, 3217 pg/ml. The other patient, without SSE, had elevation of plasma ACTH to 261 pg/ml, while CSF ACTH was 139 pg/ml. Five other patients, 3 with chromophobe adenomas and 2 with craniopharyngiomas, all had normal plasma and CSF ACTH levels even though all 3 patients with chromophobe adenomas had SSE. It was noted that although CSF and plasma ACTH concentrations were about equal, during the stress of PEG only the plasma ACTH rose substantially. However, there may not have been enough time for equilibration between plasma and CSF.

In the 1976 report of Jordan *et al.*,[4] three patients with Nelson's syndrome, all having SSE, had increased ACTH in the CSF. One of these patients also had elevated FSH, LH, and PRL in the CSF, but no correlation between CSF and plasma hormone levels was seen in any patient with SSE. One patient with Nelson's syndrome and SSE had a CSF ACTH level of 3100 pg/ml, and was studied further using [^{125}I] ACTH. At 60 min after intravenous injection, there was no radioactivity in the CSF, suggesting to the authors that the blood–CSF barrier was intact even with SSE, and supporting direction secretion by the tumor into CSF. However, it could be argued that 60 min was not long enough for equilibration after intravenous injection.

Hoffman *et al.*[52] in 1974 described a patient with Nelson's syndrome whose serum and CSF ACTH levels were elevated. They administrated intravenous hydrocortisone and observed that only the serum ACTH was partially suppressed. The CSF ACTH level increased and remained elevated. While the explanation was not clear, the suggestion was made that serum and CSF ACTH were not in equilibrium and that the ACTH might enter the CSF via direct transport from the hypothalamic–pituitary unit.

Thus far, studies have not been done to show a diurnal variation in CSF ACTH as has been shown by Shambaugh *et al*[53] for CSF cortisol (A.M. level: mean 0.68 ± 0.08 mg/100 ml; P.M. level: mean 0.38 ± 0.02 mg/100 ml).

4.3. Prolactin

Clemens and Sawyer[54] clearly demonstrated that PRL can pass the blood–CSF barrier in their studies with rat PRL in the CSF of rabbits. They also concluded that in rats under normal physiological conditions, PRL was present in CSF.

Jimerson *et al.*,[55] Sedvall *et al.*,[56] and Wode-Helgodt *et al.*[57] also confirmed PRL levels in the CSF of humans and found that psychoactive drugs given to psychiatric patients produced predictable changes in CSF PRL. Moreover, the changes were in the same direction as the plasma PRL response to these compounds. The plasma CSF PRL concentrations varied from 5 to 10 in those patients. Since it had been shown for ACTH[10] and insulin[58] that CSF hormone levels respond slowly to an increase in the plasma level and do not mirror the moment-to-moment changes in hormone secretion, this slow equilibration between blood and CSF might account for the low levels of CSF PRL (<1 ng/ml) found in several patients in whom a lumbar puncture was performed 90 min after administration (i.m.) of 25 mg chlorpromazine even though plasma PRL increased 3- to 5-fold.[12] It is possible that sustained and not circadian hormone secretion in hyperprolactinemic tumor tumor patients could be a contributory factor in the increased CSF PRL concentrations reported in such subjects.

In 1974, Assies *et al.*[2] reported that PRL was not detectable in the CSF of patients without pituitary disease who had normal plasma PRL. It was considered that either the hormone was absent or the concentration was below the detection limit of the assay at that time, which was less than 2.5 ng/ml. PRL was measurable, however, in the spinal fluid of several patients with SSE of chromophobe adenomas, and the authors concluded that PRL gained access to the CSF by direct secretional leakage into the third ventricle or basilar cisterns. or both. Assies and co-workers speculated that CSF measurements might be a worthwhile adjunct to PEG in patients with SSE of tumors. Subsequent studies[12] by these workers using a PRL RIA with a sensitivity of 0.5

ng/ml enabled them to demonstrate that PRL was indeed present in the CSF of non-pituitary-tumor patients and that the level was a function of the plasma concentration. They suggested that the entry of the hormones into the spinal fluid occurred via filtration at the choroid plexus with a concentration correlated to molecular size.[12] In their tumor patients, equal plasma and CSF levels of PRL were found in one sixth, while almost half of them had a plasma/CSF ratio of less than 3. In comparison, none of the nontumor patients had a CSF level equal to the plasma level, and almost 90% had ratios greater than 3. In their explanation for these abnormally low ratios, the authors considered the possibility that in the tumor patients with SSE, there was direct secretion or leakage from the tumor into the CSF because of misplaced exocytosis since there was no true tumor capsule.[4] However, since an adenoma is partially bounded by the aponeurotic sheath of the sella and dura, even when it expands above the sella,[3,37] this explanation may be incorrect. Additionally, if there were direct leakage from the pituitary, both "big" and "little" PRL would be expected in the spinal fluid similar to that found in the plasma, pituitary extracts, and pituitary culture media. However, neither Assies *et al.*[12] nor Jordan and Kendall[39] were able to detect substantial quantities of "big" PRL in the spinal fluid, even in patients with SSE, whereas "big" PRL constituted 11–25% of the total plasma concentration. As already discussed, pituitary hormones could reach the CSF by a more direct route, such as retrograde transport via the vessels in the pituitary stalk and ME.[26,28,59]

Assies *et al.*[12] proposed that PRL and presumably other large protein hormones were filtered from the blood into the CSF, the filtration rate being directly proportional to the plasma concentration. They suggested that the filtration process was located in the choroid plexus, but might occur elsewhere in the vicinity of the pituitary gland, the pituitary stalk, or the ME. They concluded that in most patients with PRL-producing tumors with or without SSE, the blood–CSF barrier seemed to be intact and that detectable or high CSF hormone levels *per se* should not be construed as evidence of SSE of the tumor.

Schroeder *et al.*[15] measured PRL in the serum and CSF of control subjects, pregnant women, and patients with pituitary disease. In the 30 control subjects, the mean serum PRL concentration was 7.0 ng/ml and mean CSF prl concentration 1.2 ng/ml. A statistically significant relationship was demonstrated between the serum and CSF PRL levels of 12 hyperprolactinemic patients with pituitary tumors. Additionally, 3 pregnant women were found to have elevated CSF PRL levels, whereas in 15 patients with primary empty sella syndrome and a defective diaphragma sella, low CSF PRL concentrations were found. This latter finding argued against the postulate that disruption of the diaphragma sella by a pituitary tumor significantly influences pituitary hormone concentrations in CSF. Schroeder and colleagues concluded that the CSF PRL concentration was influenced by the serum PRL level, but admitted that other mechanisms besides passive diffusion (i.e., direct secretion of PRL from tumor into CSF) may have determined the CSF PRL levels. Of their tumor patients with SSE, 2 had a higher PRL level in the spinal fluid than in the serum, and in 3 normoprolactinemic tumor patients, 2 had SSE with elevated CSF PRL levels. The possibility that decreased clearance of PRL from the CSF of these patients may have contributed to the elevated levels was also suggested.

Jordan *et al.*[4] reported 13 patients with elevated CSF PRL levels, 12 of whom had chromophobe adenomas and 1 of whom had an embryonal cell carcinoma. There was not felt to be a correlation between CSF and plasma hormone levels in patients with SSE. All had normal CSF proteins. Patients with markedly elevated plasma PRL levels but no SSE had low CSF PRL levels. The conclusion of these authors was that the finding of an elevated adenohypophyseal hormone concentration in the CSF was a sensitive indicator of SSE of a pituitary tumor.

Login and MacLeod[17] reported that rats treated with haloperidol or with implants of PRL-secreting tumors had elevated CSF PRL levels compared to control rats. These levels were commensurate with the serum level of PRL, although there appeared to be an upper limit to the CSF prl concentration (200 ng/ml). They also reported that patients with PRL-secreting pituitary adenomas had elevated CSF hormone levels compared to patients with nonendocrine neurological disease. This CSF elevation, associated with elevated serum PRL, occurred regardless of whether the tumor was intra- or extrasellar, since four of the five patients with PRL-secreting adenomas had totally intrasellar tumors. They concluded that an elevation in CSF PRL should not be used to diagnose SSE, and that the CSF PRL reflected the serum PRL regardless of the cause for the increase. They suggested that entry into the CSF occurred at the choroid plexus via a peptide hormone carrier mechanism with a finite capacity. They raised the possibility that a retarded CSF clearance because of binding, CSF bulk flow, or a less efficient enzyme system might contribute to elevated levels of CSF hormones. The difference between the observations of Login and MacLeod[17] and those of Jordan *et al.*[4] was emphasized again by Login in a letter to the editor of *Annals of Internal Medicine*.[60]

In studies from our own group, Biller *et al.*[61] have reported on 21 patients with PRL-secreting adenomas (19 female and 2 male), 5 of whom had SSE. These were compared with 10 endocrinologically and neurologically normal patients. All patients with hyperprolactinemia had elevated CSF PRL compared to normals (mean 53.7 ng/ml, range 2.6–315.1; normal < 2.5 ng/ml). CSF PRL was markedly elevated in 4 of 5 patients with SSE (mean 211.1 ng/ml, range 124.3–315.1), but in 16 patients without SSE, mean CSF PRL was 15.3 ng/ml (range 2.6–40.5). CSF levels of TSH were elevated compared to normal in 10 of 18 patients with prolactinomas (mean 4.9 μU/ml), but there was no significant difference between tumor patients with and without SSE. Likewise, CSF GH levels were elevated compared to normal in 7 of 18 patients (mean 1.2 ng/ml, range 0.4–3.7), but there was no level that distinguished patients with SSE.

Of 18 patients, 14 had elevations of CSF LH (mean 3.3 mIU/ml, range 1.8–6.0) and 8 had elevations of CSF FSH (mean 3.8 mIU/ml, range 3.3–4.3) compared to normals, but again there was no difference between those with and without SSE. Overall, the frequency of CSF pituitary hormone elevations in this group of 21 patients with PRL-secreting tumors was: PRL, 100%; LH, 77%; FSH, 44%; TSH, 55%; and GH, 38%. Marked elevation of CSF PRL (> 100 ng/ml) was always associated with SSE, although SSE could occur without such marked elevation. Biller *et al.*[61] therefore proposed that CSF PRL levels could be used as an adjunct to other studies to diagnose SSE in patients with prolactinomas.

Supporting Biller and co-workers was the study of Matsumura *et al.*,[62] who found a similar relationship between the CSF/plasma ratio of PRL levels and SSE in PRL-secreting tumors.

4.4. Thyroid-Stimulating Hormone

Since subcutaneous injection of human CSF produced a hyperplasia of the thyroid epithelium of young rabbits, Caulaert *et al.*[63] in 1931 postulated that TSH was present in the CSF. Borell[64] in 1945, studying a variety of mammals, concluded that TSH from the pars distalis reaches the CSF, from where it is absorbed by the choroid plexus. In 1974, Seaich *et al.*[8] reported on a patient with a chromophobe adenoma with SSE who had elevation of CSF TSH by RIA.

Schaub *et al.*[16] in 1977 reported on TSH levels in CSF, finding a normal mean of 2.65±0.2 ng/ml, while plasma levels were 5.95±0.3 μU/ml. There appeared to be a good correlation between CSF and plasma levels for TSH as well as GH, but the regression curves for both were distinctly different and appeared specific for each polypeptide hormone.

4.5. Luteinizing Hormone and Follicle-Stimulating Hormone

The first report of the presence of gonadotropins in the CSF was provided in 1932 by Pighini,[65] who described a substance in the third ventricle CSF with gonadal stimulating properties. Subsequently, in a study of 22 patients harboring pituitary tumors with SSE, 16 had elevation of CSF LH or CSF FSH or both.[4] When these CSF gonadotropin levels were elevated, both were usually seen. This might be expected, since production is probably from a common cell.

Luboshitzky and Barzilai[40] reported on a male patient with a pituitary adenoma, partial hypopituitarism, and normal basal serum FSH and LH, but blunted FSH rise following the administration of LH-releasing hormone (LH-RH). Subsequent assays for CSF LH and FSH showed elevated levels, correctly predicting SSE.

4.6. β-Lipotropin and "β-Melanocyte-Stimulating Hormone"

Until recently, human pituitary β-melanocyte-stimulating hormone (β-MSH) was thought to be a peptide comprising 22 amino acids. However, it now seems likely that human "β-MSH" is an extraction artifact, being a fragment of human β-lipotropin (β-LPH), a 91-amino-acid structure, present not only in the anterior pituitary, but also in other parts of the brain, including the hypothalamus, wherein it may be synthesized.[66] It appears likely that assays purported to measure β-MSH in man are either measuring the whole molecule or a fragment of β-LPH (for a review, see Rees[67]). More recently, evidence has been gathered to suggest that ACTH and β-LPH may be derived from a common precursor molecule and be secreted from the same cell in the anterior pituitary.[68]

With this in mind, Smith and Shuster[69] have reported immunoreactive β-MSH in human CSF. The mean CSF β-MSH was 60.1±8.9 ng/ml (range 0–188) in adult subjects who had CSF removed during routine lumbar puncture, 24 of whom had varying neurological diseases, and 6 of whom had no specific diagnosis. Although simultaneous blood determinations were not performed in these subjects, plasma β-MSH was found to be 16.1±1.1 ng/ml (range 0–33) in a group of normals. There was no obvious association between CSF protein and CSF β-MSH levels, and the significance and source of these levels are unknown.

In a later report,[11] the same group studied plasma β-MSH levels in 19 patients with hypopituitarism, and 5 of these patients had CSF measurements as well. In neither plasma nor CSF were the β-MSH concentrations significantly different from normals, whereas ACTH levels were apparently low. (CSF β-MSH was 78.5±15.8 ng/ml and plasma levels were 23.6±5.6 ng/ml.) This suggests a dissociation between the secretion of β-MSH (or more probably its precursor, β-LPH) and the secretion of ACTH. Moreover, the possibility that the β-MSH in CSF may be derived from extrapituitary sites is suggested by reports of considerable amounts of immunoreactive β-MSH in various regions of the brain, though total brain β-MSH is only about 5% of that of the pituitary.[70] Clearly, the nature of the immunoreactive β-MSH needs to be reexamined with specific measurements of β-LPH.

Data available at present on CSF β-LPH and endorphins will be discussed in a chapter by Bloom and Segal.[71]

5. Extrapituitary Sources of Pituitary Hormones

Evidence now exists demonstrating that anterior pituitary hormones may be synthesized in extrapituitary locations within the brain. Significant amounts of GH and ACTH have been demonstrated in the rat amygdaloid nucleus, and immunoperoxidase staining has demonstrated dense accumulations of the peroxidase antibody to GH complex in amygdala cells.[72] Davis and Gillette[72] reported that the immunoreactive GH content within the amygdaloid nucleus showed a dramatic increase 30 days following hypophysectomy. ACTH has been demonstrated to be widely distributed throughout the limbic system of normal and hypophysectomized animals.[73] TSH has been demonstrated throughout the brain of rats and in the hypothalamic region of the human brain.[74] Finally, α-MSH ($ACTH_{1-13}$) has been demonstrated in appreciable quantities in various regions in the rat brain.[75] PRL has also been demonstrated in brain neurons.[76] With the use of antibodies against rat PRL, fluorescent nerve terminals in many hypothalamic nuclei were seen. These fibers did not disappear after hypophysectomy. These data seem to imply that anterior pituitary hormones can be produced *in situ* in extrapituitary regions of the brain. Whether the hormones produced in these sites contribute to the CSF levels is thus far unknown.

6. Conclusions

The significance and role of anterior pituitary hormones in CSF have been reviewed. Although some reports suggest that anterior pituitary hormones are not present in the normal CSF, the evidence from a number of sources indicates that with increased RIA sensitivity, these peptides can be detected in normal subjects. Since the anterior pituitary hormones are polar and poorly lipophilic, these substances do not readily cross the BBB. It does appear, however, that their presence and concentration in the CSF are a reflection primarily of their molecular weight as well as their concentration in the systemic circulation in patients with a normal hypothalamic–pituitary axis as well as in some patients with pituitary tumors. Failure to see changes in the CSF after infusion of ACTH or after acute elevation of plasma PRL may reflect the slow time of equilibration from blood to CSF, with subsequent retarded clearance. The exclusion of the nontumorous pituitary gland from the brain is also shown by the low levels of CSF pituitary hormones in the "empty sella syndrome."

In some reports, especially in patients with SSE of pituitary tumors, the CSF/plasma ratio is higher than might be expected solely by filtration through the choroid plexus. The possibility of retrograde vascular transport from pituitary to brain has been discussed as a possible mechanism that might account for the higher CSF levels in such patients. Some reports suggest that the presence of anterior pituitary hormones in the CSF indicates SSE of a pituitary tumor with breakdown of the normal pituitary–brain barrier due to the process of misplaced exocytosis. An argument against this view is the failure to find the higher-molecular-weight species of PRL ("big" PRL) in CSF in concentrations approaching that found in the peripheral blood.

Nonetheless, in our own studies of CSF pituitary peptide levels in patients with prolactinomas, we found that a CSF PRL level greater than 100 ng/ml always indicates SSE of a pituitary tumor. Such findings suggest that CSF measurements of pituitary hormones may be helpful diagnostically in certain clinical situations.

Finally, increased recognition of the CSF as a means of regulating neuroendocrine function suggests that the CSF may serve as a conduit in the transfer of anterior pituitary hormones to the hypothalamus for the purpose of regulating secretions through "short-feedback" mechanisms. It is also possible that secretion into the CSF may allow anterior pituitary hormones to reach distant parts of the nervous system to regulate aspects of brain function, including behavior.

References

1. J.P. Allen, J.W. Kendall, R. McGilvra, T.L. Lamorena, and A. Castro, Adrenocorticotrophic and growth hormone secretion: Studies during pneumoencephalography, *Arch. Neurol.* **31:**325–328, 1974.
2. J. Assies, A.P.M. Schellekens, and J.L. Touber, Prolactin secretion in patients with chromophobe adenoma of the pituitary gland, *Neth. J. Med.* **17:**163, 1974.

3. J. Hardy, Trans-sphenoidal microsurgical removal of pituitary microadenoma, *Prog. Neurol. Surg.* **6:**200, 1975.
4. R.M. Jordan, J.W. Kendall, J.L. Seaich, J.P. Allen, C.A. Paulsen, C.W. Kerber, and W.P. Vanderlaan, Cerebrospinal fluid hormone concentration in the evaluation of pituitary tumors, *Ann. Intern. Med.* **85:**49–55, 1976.
5. J.W. Kendall, J.L. Seaich, J.P. Allen, and W.P. Vanderlaan, in: *Brain–Endocrine Interaction II: The Ventricular System* (K.M. Knigge, D.E. Scott, J. Kobayashi, and S. Ishu, eds.), p. 313, S. Karger, Basel, 1975.
6. M. Kleerekoper, R.A. Donald, and S. Posen, Corticotrophin in cerebrospinal fluid of patients with Nelson's syndrome, *Lancet* **1:**74–76, 1972.
7. J.A. Linfoot, J.F. Garcia, W. Wei, R. Fink, R. Sarin, J.L. Born, and J.H. Lawrence, Human growth hormone levels in cerebrospinal fluid, *J. Clin. Endocrinol. Metab.* **31:**230–232, 1970.
8. J.L. Seaich, J.P. Allen, and J.W. Kendall, Diagnostic values of CSF hormone determinations, Abstract presented at the Annual Meeting of the Endocrine Society (Abstract No. 126), June 1974.
9. F.J. Thomas, J.M. Lloyd, and M.J. Thomas, Radioimmunoassay of human growth hormone: Technique and application to plasma, cerebrospinal fluid and pituitary extracts, *J. Clin. Pathol.* **25:**774–782, 1972.
10. J.P. Allen, J.W. Kendall, R. McGilvra, and C. Vancura, Immunoreactive ACTH in cerebrospinal fluid, *J. Clin. Endocrinol. Metab.* **38:**586, 1974.
11. S. Shuster, A. Smith, N. Plummer, A. Thody, and F. Clark, Immunoreactive beta-melanocyte-stimulating hormone in cerebrospinal fluid and plasma in hypopituitarism: Evidence for an extrapituitary origin, *Br. Med. J.* **1:**1318–1319, 1977.
12. J. Assies, A.P.M. Schellekens, and J.L. Touber, Prolactin in human cerebrospinal fluid, *J. Clin. Endocrinol. Metab.* **46**(4):576, 1978.
13. H. Davson, *Physiology of the CSF*, Little, Brown, Boston, 1967.
14. K. Felgenhauer, Protein size and cerebrospinal fluid composition, *Klin. Wochenschr.* **52:**1158–1164, 1974.
15. L.L. Schroeder, J.D. Johnson, and W.B. Malarkey, Cerebrospinal fluid prolactin: A reflection of abnormal prolactin secretion in patients with pituitary tumors, *J. Clin. Endocrinol. Metab.* **43:**1255–1260, 1976.
16. C. Schaub, M.T. Bluet-Pajot, G. Szikla, C. Lornet, and J. Talairach, Distribution of growth hormone and thyroid-stimulating hormone in cerebrospinal fluid and pathological compartments of the central nervous system, *J. Neurol. Sci.* **13:**123, 1977.
17. I.S. Login and R.M. MacLeod, Prolactin in human and rat serum and cerebrospinal fluid, *Brain Res.* **132:**477–483, 1977.
18. R.M. Jordan, J.W. Kendall, and C.W. Kerber, The primary empty sella syndrome, *Am. J. Med.* **62:**569–580, 1977.
19. R.M. Jordan, J.W. Kendall, and J.L. Seaich, CSF hormone studies in pituitary diseases, *Clin. Res.* **24:**143A, 1976.
20. J. Assies, A.P.M. Schellekens, and J.L. Touber, Protein hormones in cerebrospinal fluid: Evidence for retrograde transport of prolactin from the pituitary to the brain in man, *Clin. Endocrinol.* **8:**487–491, 1978.
21. K.D. Bagshawe and S. Harland, Immunodiagnosis and monitoring of gonadotrophin-producing metastases in the central nervous system, *Cancer* **38:**112–118, 1976.
22. G.B. Wislocki, The vascular supply of the hypophysis cerebri of the rhesus monkey and man, *Proc. Assoc. Nerv. Ment. Dis.* **17:**48, 1938.
23. W.F. Ganong and D.M. Hume, Concentration of ACTH in cavernous sinus and peripheral arterial blood in the dog, *Proc. Soc. Exp. Biol. Med.* **92:**721, 1956.
24. R.M. Bergland, S.L. Davis, and R.B. Page, Pituitary secretes to brain, *Lancet* **11:**276–278, 1977.
25. R.M. Bergland and R.B. Page, Can the pituitary secrete directly to the brain? (affirmative anatomical evidence), *Endocrinology* **102**(5):1325–1338, 1978.
26. J. Szentagothai, B. Glerko, B. Mess, and B. Halasz, Hypothalamic control of anterior pituitary, *Budapest Akad. Kiado* **1968:**90.
27. B. Torok, Structure of the vascular connections of the hypothalamohypophyseal region, *Acta Anat.* **59:**84, 1964.

28. R.B. Page and R.M. Bergland, The neurohypophyseal capillary bed: Anatomy and arterial supply, *Am. J. Anat.* **148:**345, 1977.
29. R.B. Page, B.L. Munger, and R.M. Bergland, Scanning microscopy of pituitary vascular casts: The rabbit pituitary portal system revisited, *Am. J. Anat.* **146:**273, 1976.
30. R.D. Broadwell and M.W. Brightman, Entry of peroxidase into neurons of the central and peripheral nervous system from extra cerebral and cerebral blood, *J. Comp. Neurol.* **166:**257, 1976.
31. D. Oliver, R.S. Mical, and J.C. Porter, Hypothalamic–pituitary vasculature: Evidence of retrograde blood flow in the pituitary stalk, *Endocrinology* **101:**598, 1977.
32. U. Nakai and N. Naito, Uptake and bidirectional transport of peroxidase injected into the blood and cerebrospinal fluid by ependymal cells of the median eminence, in: *Brain–Endocrine Interaction II: The Ventricular System* (K.M. Knigge, D.E. Scott, H. Kobayashi, and S. Ishi, eds.), p. 94, S. Karger, Basel, 1975.
33. K.M. Knigge and D.E. Scott, Structure and function of the median eminence, *Am. J. Anat.* **129:**223, 1970.
34. M.G. Farquhar, Origin and fate of secretory granules in cells of the anterior pituitary gland, *Trans. N. Y. Acad. Sci.* **1960:**347–351, 1960.
35. E.M. Rodriguez, in: *Brain–Endocrine Interaction: Median Eminence: Structure and Function* (K.M. Knigge, D.E. Scott, and A. Weindl, eds.), p. 319, S. Karger, Basel, 1972.
36. E. Horvath and K. Kovacs, Misplaced exocytosis, *Arch. Pathol.* **97:**221–224, 1974.
37. J. Hardy, Transsphenoidal microsurgery of the normal and pathological pituitary, *Clin. Neurosurg.* **16:**185–217, 1969.
38. H.D. Kirgis and W. Locke, Anatomy and embryology, in: *The Hypothalamus and Pituitary in Health and Disease* (W. Locke and A.V. Schally, eds.), pp. 57–58, Charles C. Thomas, Springfield, Illinois, 1972.
39. R.M. Jordan and J.W. Kendall, Dissociation of plasma and CSF prolactin heterogeneity, *Clin. Res.* **24:**273, 1976.
40. R. Luboshitzky and D. Barzilai, Suprasellar extension of tumor associated with increased cerebrospinal fluid activity of LH and FSH, *Acta Endocrinol.* (*Copenhagen*) **87**(4):673–684, 1978.
41. W.H. Oldendorf, Blood–brain barrier permeability to drugs, *Am. Rev. Pharmacol.* **14:**239–248, 1974.
42. J.W. Kendall, J.J. Jacobs, and R.M. Kramer, in: *Brain–Endocrine Interaction: Median Eminence: Structure and Function* (K.M. Knigge, D.E. Scott, and A. Weidl, eds.), p. 342, S. Karger, Basel, 1971.
43. J.G. Ondo, R.S. Mical, and J.C. Porter, Passage of radioactive substances from CSF to hypophysial portal blood, *Endocrinology* **91**(5):1239–1246, 1971.
44. R.M. MacLeod and I. Login, Control of prolactin secretion by the hypothalamic catecholamines, *Adv. Sex Horm. Res.* **2:**211–231, 1976.
45. M. Motta, F. Fraschini, and L. Martini, Short feedback mechanisms in the control of anterior pituitary function, in: *Frontiers in Neuroendocrinology* (W.F. Ganong and L. Martini, eds.), pp. 211–254, Oxford University Press, New York, 1969.
46. D. de Wied, Peptides and behavior, *Life Sci.* **20:**195–204, 1977.
47. A.G. Frantz, Prolactin, *Phys. Med. Biol.* **298**(4):201–207, 1978.
48. D. de Wied, Pituitary adrenal system hormones and behavior, Symposium on Developments in Endocrinology, In honour of Dr. G.A. Overbeek, Organon International, Oss, The Netherlands, October 1976.
49. A.D. Wright, M.S. McLachlan, F.H. Doyle, and T. Fraser, Serum GH levels and size of pituitary tumor in untreated acromegaly, *Br. Med. J.* **4:**582–584, 1968.
50. E.J. Hanson, Jr., R.H. Miller, and R.V. Randall, Suprasellar extension of tumor associated with increased cerbrospinal fluid activity of growth hormone, *Mayo Clin. Proc.* **51:**412–416, 1976.
51. D.T. Krieger, A. Liotta, and M.J. Brownstein, Presence of corticotropin in limbic system of normal and hypophysectomized rats, *Brain Res.* **128:**575–579, 1977.
52. J.D. Hoffman, J. Baumgartner, and E.M. Gold, Dissociation of plasma and spinal fluid ACTH in Nelson's syndrome, *J. Am. Med. Assoc.* **228:**491, 1974.
53. G.E. Shambaugh, III, J.F. Wilber, E. Montoya, H. Reider, and E.R. Blonsky, Thyrotrophin-

releasing hormone (TRH): Measurements in human spinal fluid, *J. Clin. Endocrinol. Metab.* **41**(1):131–134, 1975.

54. J.A. Clemens and B.D. Sawyer, Identification of prolactin in cerebrospinal fluid, *Exp. Brain Res.* **21:**399–402, 1974.
55. D.C. Jimerson, R.M. Post, J. Skyler, and W.E. Bunney, Prolactin in cerebrospinal fluid and dopamine function in man, *J. Pharmacol.* **28:**845–847, 1976.
56. G. Sedvall, G. Alfreddson, L.B. Jerkenstedt, P. Eneroth, G. Fyro, C. Harnryd, C.G. Swahn, F.A. Weisel, and B. Wode-Helgodt, Selective effects of psychoactive drugs on levels of monoamine metabolites and prolactin in cerebrospinal fluid of psychiatric patients, *Proceedings of the Sixth International Congress on Pharmacology* **3:**255, 1975.
57. B. Wode-Helgodt, P. Eneroth, B. Fyro, B. Gullberg, and G. Sedvall, Effect of chlorpromazine treatment on prolactin levels in cerebrospinal fluid and plasma of psychotic patients, *Acta Psychiatr. Scand.* **56**(4):280–293, 1977.
58. S.C. Woods and D. Porte, Jr., Insulin and the set-point regulation of bodyweight, in: *Hunger: Basic Mechanisms and Clinical Implication* (D. Novin, W. Wyrwicka, and G. Bray, eds.), p. 273, Raven Press, New York, 1976.
59. E.M. Rodriguez, The cerebrospinal fluid as a pathway in neuroendocrine integration, *J. Endocrinol.* **71:**407–443, 1976.
60. I.S. Login, Spinal fluid prolactin (letter to the editor), *Ann. Intern. Med.* **86:**119, 1977.
61. B. Biller, K.D. Post, M. Molitch, S. Reichlin, and I. Jackson, CSF pituitary hormone concentrations in patients with pituitary tumors, Abstract presented at the American Association of Neurological Surgeons Meeting, New Orleans, Louisiana (Paper No. 28), April 25, 1977.
62. S. Matsumura, S. Mori, H. Yoshimoto, M. Ohta, and T. Uozumi, Endocrinological evaluation of sellar and suprasellar tumor cases (the ninth report)—On the PRL levels in the CSF (author's translation), *No Shinkei Geka* **5**(10):1057–1063, 1977.
63. V.C. Caulaert, M. Aron, and J. Stahl, Sur la presence de l'hormone prehypophysaire excito-secretoire e la thyroide dans le sang et le liquide cephalorachidien et sur sa repartition dans ces milieux et dans l'urine, *C. R. Soc. Biol.* **106:**607–609, 1931.
64. U. Borell, On the transport route of the thyrotropic hormone, the occurrence of the latter in different parts of the brain and its effect on the thyroidea, *Acta Med. Scand.* **161**(Suppl.):1–227, 1945.
65. G. Pighini, Sulla presenza dell'ormone anteipofisario nel "tuber cinereum" nel "liquor" ventricolare dell'uomo, *Rev. Sper. Greniatr. Med. Legale Alienaz. Ment.* **56:**575–622, 1932.
66. S.J. Watson, J.D. Barchas, and C.H. Li, Beta-lipotropin: Localization of cells and axons in rat brain by immunocytochemistry, *Proc. Natl. Acad. Sci. U.S.A.* **74**(11):5155–5158, 1977.
67. L.H. Rees, ACTH, lipotropin, and MSH in health and disease, *Clin. Endocrinol. Metab.* **6:**137–153, 1977.
68. R. Guillemin, Beta-lipotropin and endorphins: Implications of current knowledge, *Hosp. Pract.* **13:**53–60, 1978.
69. A.G. Smith and S. Shuster, Immunoreactive beta-melanocyte-stimulating hormone in cerebrospinal fluid, *Lancet* **1:**1321, 1976.
70. R.J. Carter *et al.*, Unpublished observations.
71. F.E. Bloom and D. Segal, Endorphins in cerebrospinal fluid, in: *Neurobiology of Cerebrospinal Fluid I* (James H. Wood, ed.), Chapt. 45, Plenum Press, New York, 1980.
72. W.J. Davis and R. Gillette, Biologically active pituitary hormones in the rat brain amygdaloid nucleus, *Science* **199:**804–805, 1978.
73. D.T. Krieger, A. Liotta, and M.J. Brownstein, Presence of corticotropin in limbic system of normal and hypophysectomized rats, *Brain Res.* **128:**575–579, 1977.
74. R.L. Moldow and R.S. Yalow, Extrahypophysial distribution of thyrotropin as a function of brain size, *Life Sci.* **22:**1859–1864, 1978.
75. C. Oliver and J.C. Porter, Distribution and characterization of alpha-melanocyte-stimulating hormone in the rat brain, *Endocrinology* **102**(3):697–705, 1978.
76. K. Fuxe, T. Hokfelt, P. Eneroth, J.A. Gustafsson, and P. Skett, Prolactin: Localization in nerve terminals of the rat hypothalamus, *Science* **196:**899–900, 1977.

13

Ophthalmological Evaluation of Pituitary Adenomas

JOHN W. GITTINGER, Jr.

1. Visual Involvement in Pituitary Adenomas

When pituitary adenomas present as mass lesions, visual involvement is the rule. Decreased acuity and field loss occur less regularly when the tumor presents with endocrinological manifestations such as acromegaly, galactorrhea, amenorrhea, and Cushing's syndrome. Because of their secretory activity, these tumors become manifest while they are still small. A tumor arising in the sella must be quite large and have significant extrasellar extension before impinging on the visual pathways; consequently, visual-field testing is not a sensitive screening method for small pituitary tumors. When adenomas causing field defects are approached intracranially, the usual finding is a grossly distorted chiasm stretched over a large tumor (see Chapter 16, Fig. 2).

Since only large pituitary adenomas with extrasellar extension compress the chiasm, most patients with pituitary adenomas and visual-field defects will have abnormal sella turcicas on plain skull films.[1] Conversely, the presence of chiasmal field defects in a patient with a radiologically normal sella suggests a process other than pituitary adenoma. Cushing[2] called attention to a "chiasmal syndrome" of bitemporal field defects, optic atrophy, and normal sella as being typical of meningiomas arising from the tuberculum sellae. As is often true in medicine, there is no absolute rule, and cases of pituitary adenomas with apparently normal sellas are reported. Deficiencies in the diaphragma sella associated with a well-developed sphenoid sinus roof preventing inferior expansion is a suggested explanation for the early suprasellar growth in these cases.[3]

In the largest series of pituitary adenomas in the literature, 1000 cases from the Mayo Clinic, 70% had visual-field defects.[4,5] In 42% of these cases,

JOHN W. GITTINGER, Jr. • Tufts University School of Medicine; Department of Ophthalmology, Division of Neuro-ophthalmology, Tufts–New England Medical Center Hospital, Boston, Massachusetts 02111.

visual symptoms were the presenting complaint. The importance of obtaining a visual field during the evaluation of unexplained visual loss in an adult cannot be overemphasized. Frequently, patients with pituitary adenomas or other chiasmal lesions are followed for years with mistaken diagnoses such as chronic optic neuritis, amblyopia, refractive error, or low-tension glaucoma before the correct diagnosis is made.[6] The usual explanation for such errors is failure to obtain or misinterpretation of appropriate visual-field and radiological studies.[7] Beneficial response to antiinflammatory steroids alone is not an adequate criterion to distinguish visual loss as a result of optic neuritis from that associated with pituitary adenoma. A case of pituitary adenoma in which ACTH therapy caused a dramatic improvement in acuity, thus obscuring the correct diagnosis for 18 months, has been reported.[8]

2. Visual-Field Testing

The testing of the visual field may be performed with degrees of sophistication varying from simple confrontation to quantitative perimetry with complicated machines like the Goldmann or Tubinger perimeter. Many clinicians still prefer to use the tangent screen with white and colored test objects or projected lights. In skilled hands, there is probably little difference in the sensitivity of the methods. The advantage of the quantitative perimeters, however, is that they allow testing under rigidly standardized conditions and thus are particularly well adapted to following improvement or deterioration. The decreased variability in the stimulus may also be an advantage in the detection of early defects. For a description of one technique of assessing visual fields in patients with suspected chiasmal compression, see the Appendix (Section 11).

Whatever techniques are used, there are certain characteristics of fields adequate to evaluate a patient with suspected chiasmal compression from pituitary adenoma that should be emphasized. Since the central field (within 30° of fixation) tends to be affected earlier and more extensively than the peripheral field, an examination in which only the peripheral field is studied is inadequate. At least two central isopters should be obtained with particular attention paid to the vertical meridian above fixation [see the Appendix (Section 11), Fig. 21].

There is an unfortunate tendency to treat a visual-field chart like an X-ray and to impart to it a precision that is often unjustified. The clinician who does not perform his own fields should be wary of attaching too much significance to minor variations. The visual field is a subjective test and may yield artifacts due to patient fatigue or confusion as to what is expected. Often a repeat field examination performed by a physician aware of the clinical implications of the abnormal findings will clarify the situation.

2.1. Visual Criteria in the Management of Pituitary Adenomas

Preservation of vision is a major goal of the treatment of pituitary adenomas. Because of the use of combined therapies and because of differing indications for determining modalities of therapy, it is difficult to know whether any regimen has advantage over the others in terms of improving visual prognosis. It is even hard to determine whether modern diagnostic and therapeutic techniques result in an improved visual prognosis. In the Mayo Clinic series, collected between 1935 and 1972, visual improvement after therapy was observed in 61.4% of patients[4]; 7.3% worsened. Klauber *et al.*[9] report a remarkably similar percentage with visual improvement—62% of their patients collected between 1967 and 1974. A comparison of the degree of visual improvement seen in 71 patients who had transfrontal craniotomies for pituitary adenomas performed at the Mayo Clinic between 1950 and 1958 with 62 patients (45 with pituitary adenomas) who had transsphenoidal procedures at the same institution between 1972 and 1975 reveals that the median visual loss of the patients in the older series preoperatively was 40.5% and in the more recent series 17%.[10,11] Postoperatively, the median visual loss was 22% in the older series and 3% in the more recent. Thus, visual loss was more severe in the older series preoperatively and the eventual visual result was poorer, but the amount of visual improvement, expressed as a percentage of total visual function, is very nearly the same—18.5% in the older series and about 14% in the recent series. These series illustrate the difficulties that arise in attempting to compare the efficacy of present vs. past therapy, even when the cases are from the same institution and have been assessed by the same methods.

Of the patients in the Mayo Clinic series, 42% presented with visual complaints.[4] Wray[12] found that only 20% of her patients collected between 1974 and 1976 came to medical attention because of visual loss. Endocrinological findings and headache were more common complaints. Since a larger percentage of cases are now detected because of these symptoms, often at a time when the tumor is small and does not impinge on the visual pathways, the visual prognosis of the population of patients with pituitary adenomas is improved. On the other hand, there is no direct evidence at present that current therapeutic regimens result in a better visual prognosis for a patient who presents with visual loss than for his counterpart ten or twenty years ago. We can conclude, however, that a large majority of patients who are treated either have visual improvement or remain unchanged. An occasional patient loses vision during therapy either as a result of the treatment or because of enlargement or recurrence of the tumor.

The question arises as to how frequently a patient with a known pituitary adenoma should have visual fields performed. This decision, within broad limits, should lie with the physician primarily responsible for the patient's care. A rule that has been followed by many clinicians is a yearly field examination after an initial normal field. In the postoperative period, a field should be obtained as soon as the patient is able to cooperate. The recommended frequency after this varies from institution to institution. Hollenhorst at the Mayo Clinic performs a field at 3 months and at 1 year, and then yearly.[13] Burde at Barnes Hospital suggests intervals of 3 months for 1 year, 6 months for 2 or 3 years, and then yearly.[13] Glaser at the Bascom Palmer Eye Institute recommends monthly fields for 6 months and then yearly fields.[14] The schedule of visual-field testing should probably depend on the patient and his tumor. A patient who has had a small adenoma removed with no preoperative field defect should obviously be examined less frequently than a patient with significant field and acuity loss.

There has been some controversy about the necessity of frequent visual-field examinations during radiotherapy. Concern as to the possibility of acute deterioration during radiotherapy has occasionally prompted requests for daily field examinations. Both Hollenhorst and Hoyt[4] state that they have never seen such paroxysmal field loss, and fields performed at the beginning, middle, and end of radiotherapy are probably adequate.

When there is continued deterioration of vision in the postoperative or postirradiation period, there may be a recurrence of the tumor. If this is not demonstrated, an empty sella syndrome may also explain visual loss. Here, the chiasm herniates toward the space in the sella left after the removal of the tumor.[15] The diagnosis has been made by pneumoencephalography, but now can often be demonstrated on computed tomography (CT) scan. Treatment is directed toward supporting the chiasm from below.[16] There is also the possibility that radiotherapy may damage the visual pathways.[17] A relationship to therapeutic fractions above 250 rads/day has been suggested.[18] Usually, this diagnosis is one of exclusion, and the possibility of a nonspecific optochiasmic arachnoiditis must also be considered.

2.2. Visual Evoked Potentials (VEPs)

Visual evoked potentials (VEPs) are obtained by subtracting out the EEG from the electrical activity recorded from occipital skin electrodes. With the use of a computer averager, only those potentials that relate to the activity of the visual system produced by a changing light or patterned stimulus remain. A normal VEP reflects the functional integrity of the visual pathways up to the calcarine cortex. Abnormalities of the VEP occur in various lesions of the visual pathways and in fact may be the only sign of these lesions. VEPs have become a clinically useful tool in detecting otherwise subclinical demyelination of the optic nerve.[19]

Some application of this technique to the evaluation of patients with compressive lesions of the optic nerve and chiasm has been made. Halliday reports eight patients with pituitary adenomas, all of whom had abnormal VEPs in one or both eyes.[20] Five of these patients had eyes with normal acuity but an abnormal VEP, suggesting that this technique may be valuable as a screening test for compressive involvement of visual pathways. The availability of an objective method to make this determination would be particularly useful in patients in whom perimetric data are unreliable. The abnormality seen in VEPs in patients with compressive lesions is a distortion of the waveform rather than the prolongation of latency seen in patients with demyelination of their optic nerve. The VEP may improve or return to normal once the compression is relieved, and this has been used as a technique for intraoperative monitoring of optic nerve and chiasmal function to assure adequate surgical decompression.[21]

3. Chiasmal Syndromes

Pituitary adenomas are the most common cause of chiasmal syndromes, but many other etiologies must be considered. Craniopharyngiomas and meningiomas are the tumors that most often enter the differential diagnosis. Many other mass lesions (see Chapter 10)—aneurysms or dilated ectatic vessels, metastatic disease, gliomas, chordomas, nasopharyngeal carcinomas, dysgerminomas—also occasionally affect the chiasm. Less commonly, inflammatory or infiltrative diseases such as syphilis, sarcoid, or arachnoiditis produce visual loss. Intrasellar abscesses or sphenoid sinus mucoceles have on occasion been reported to mimic pituitary tumors.[22,87] Ischemic chiasmal lesions are rare but may occur in association with systemic arteritis.[23] Trauma, toxins, demyelinization and anomalies may also involve the chiasm.[24,88]

An unusual form of chiasmal compression occurs as a consequence of internal hydrocephalus caused by blockage of cerebrospinal fluid outflow. The third ventricle dilates and acts as a suprasellar mass and may produce both field loss and ocular motor signs. In this instance, the chiasmal syndrome is a false localizing sign, since the true pathology lies in the ventricular system.[25]

Because of the many types of lesions and the various mechanisms by which they may produce visual loss, it is difficult to use the ocular findings to do more than simply localize a lesion to the region of the chiasm. Nevertheless, by the application of knowledge of the anatomical relationship of the chiasm and of the fiber tracts it contains, clinically useful information is obtained from visual-field examinations. Many authors have reviewed the localizing value of patterns of field loss in terms of the anatomy of the chiasm.[10,14,26–32]

3.1. Relationships of the Chiasm

The optic chiasm or chiasm (from the Greek letter chi or "χ") is a plate of neural tissue approximately 4 mm thick, 13 mm wide, and 8 mm long that lies at the junction of the floor and the anterior wall of the third ventricle.[30] Approximately 53% of the axons in both optic nerves decussate to form the median bar of the chiasm.[31] The cell bodies of these decussating axons are located in the retina nasal to the fovea of each eye. They carry visual input from the temporal visual field of that eye. The existence of a partial decussation was first postulated by Issac Newton.[32] This partial decussation allows all sensory information from the right or left visual fields of both eyes to be represented in the contralateral side of the brain.

The relationship of the chiasm to the pituitary fossa, and thus its vulnerability to expanding masses originating there, is subject to anatomical variation[33] (Fig. 1). Considerable emphasis has been placed on the position of the chiasm in the anteroposterior plane. Schaeffer[34] first pointed out that in 9% of anatomical specimens, the chiasmal bar overlies the tuberculum sellae. This is called a *prefixed chiasm*. In 11% the bar is over the dorsum sellae; this is a *postfixed chiasm*. In the remaining 80%, the chiasm lies directly over the pituitary fossa (see Chapter 19, Fig. 3). Of equal importance clinically is the separation of the chiasm from the pituitary fossa in the vertical plane. The

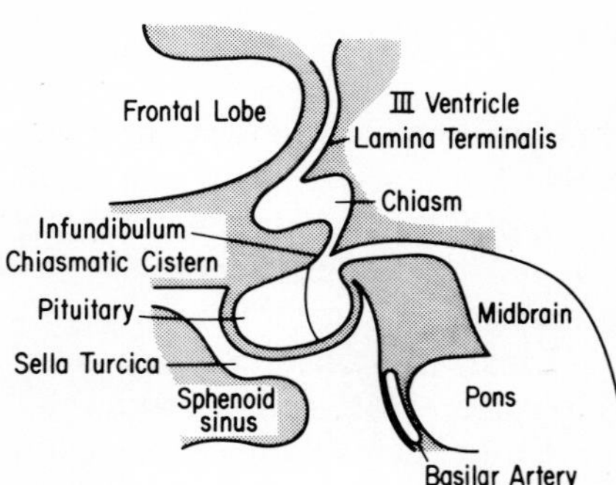

Fig. 1. Sagittal section through the region of the chiasm showing its relationships.

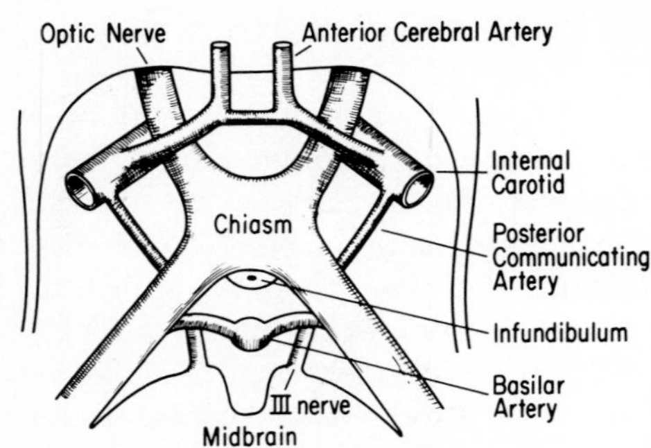

Fig. 2. Diagrammatic representation of the relationships between the chiasm and the circle of Willis as seen from above.

chiasm does not usually cap the pituitary fossa, but rather lies up to 1 cm above it, tilting forward as much as 45° from the horizontal.[30]

The optic chiasm, nerves, and tracts pass through the circle of Willis (Fig. 2). The anterior part of the arterial circle (including the anterior cerebral arteries and arterior communicating artery) is above the chiasm, and the posterior part (including the posterior cerebral, posterior communicating, and basilar arteries) is below the visual pathways. The internal carotid arteries are inferior to the optic nerves at the point where the ophthalmic arteries originate. They then pass laterally to the nerves and chiasm. The vascular supply of the chiasm is complex and may arise in part from all the vessels mentioned except the small anterior communicating artery. Bergland and Ray[35] distinguished a superior and an inferior group of arteries supplying the chiasm and observed that the median bar containing the decussating fibers was supplied only by the inferior group. This may have a functional significance and will be mentioned again later.

3.2. Axonal Arrangement in the Anterior Visual Pathways

To explain the field defects and ophthalmoscopic signs of pituitary adenomas, the arrangement of axons in the anterior visual pathways must be considered. The studies of Hoyt and co-workers[36–38] have contributed greatly to understanding these relationships. Hoyt made discrete lesions on the retina of the macaque monkey with a xenon photocoagulator. Histologically, there was complete destruction of ganglion cells and nerve fibers within these lesions. After 2 weeks were allowed for axonal degeneration to occur, the animals were sacrificed, and sections of the optic nerves, chiasm, and tracts were examined using a stain specific for degenerating axons. Thus, it was possible to trace the axons originating in or passing through the retinal lesions into the optic nerve chiasm and optic tract.

These studies showed that the chiasm consists for the most part of macular projections, (Fig. 3). In fact, in Hoyt's pathological specimens, only thin areas of anterior and posterior inferior chiasm were free of macular fibers. Hoyt also demonstrated that a segregation of small axons derived from macu-

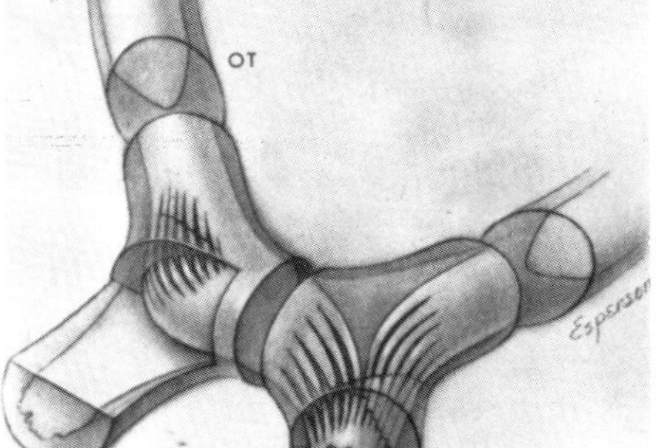

Fig. 3. A reconstruction based on degeneration studies of the macular projections through the chiasm. (OT) Optic tract; (ON) optic nerve. Reprinted with permission from Hoyt and Luis,[37] *Arch. Ophthalmol.* **70:**69, copyright 1963, American Medical Association.

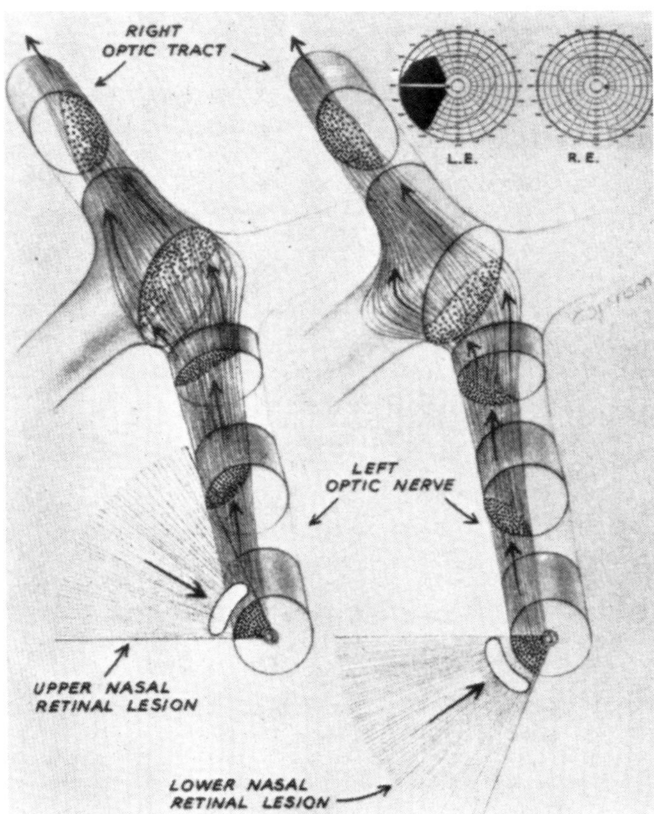

Fig. 4. A reconstruction of the projections of the nasal retina through the chiasm based on degeneration studies. Note that the fibers from the lower nasal retina project forward into the contralateral optic nerve. This is the knee of Von Wilbrand. Reprinted with permission from Hoyt and Luis,[36] *Arch. Ophthalmol.* **68:**94, copyright 1962, American Medical Association.

lar ganglion cells is a prominent phenomenon in the primate chiasm.[37] The early involvement of central fields and acuity in chiasmal compression is characteristic.[39] This may be a result either of the predominance of macular representation or of selective vulnerability of small axons to compression.[30]

These studies also confirmed the presence of a group of axons consisting of crossed inferior quadrant extramacular fibers extending into the posterior part of the optic nerve—the knee of Von Wilbrand, (Fig. 4). A lesion in the posterior optic nerve or anterior chiasm involving these fibers produces a central or hemianopic scotoma in the ipsilateral eye and a superior temporal defect in the opposite eye. A paracentral scotoma with hemianopic or quadrantic features is called the "junction scotoma" of Traquair and suggests a lesion at the chiasmal termination of the optic nerve.[40] Dysfunction confined to this anatomical site can be seen with pituitary adenomas, but is more common with meningioma or aneurysm.[41]

4. Patterns of Visual Loss

4.1. Bitemporal

Bitemporal field loss is the most common pattern observed in patients with pituitary adenomas (Fig. 5). The median bar of the chiasm is the only place in the visual system where a single lesion can produce bitemporal defects. The mechanism by which a compressive lesion selectively involves these decussating fibers is still the subject of debate. Since the axons for the superior field pass in the inferior optic nerve and chiasm, compression from below would be expected to produce a defect involving the entire upper field, called an "altitudinal defect." Such superior altitudinal defects are rarely observed, and in fact there is a tendency for the superonasal field to be spared

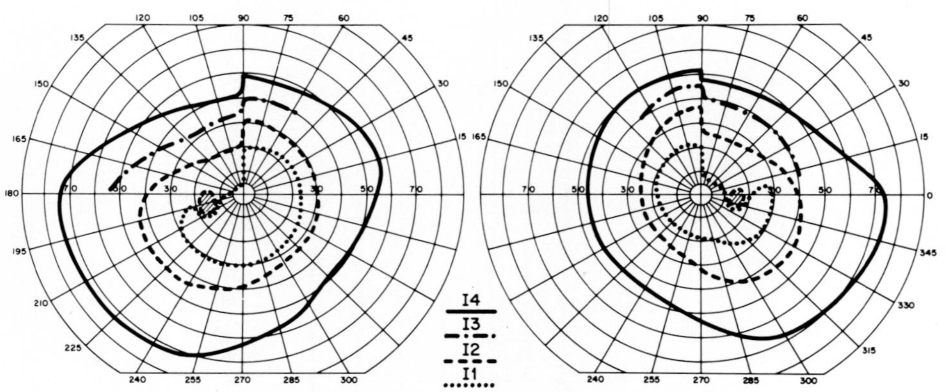

Fig. 5. An idealized bitemporal superior field defect showing how the depression of isopters tends to respect the vertical meridian above fixation (the center of the chart). The defect is greater for smaller isopters.

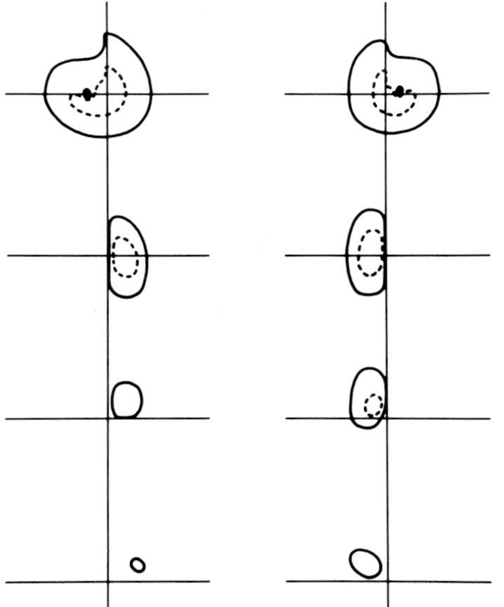

Fig. 6. Characteristic progression of field loss with chiasmal compression from pituitary adenomas. Not until the other three quadrants are affected does the field loss cross the vertical meridian above fixation.

even when the entire inferior field is involved, (Fig. 6). Thus, compression alone seems to be an inadequate explanation for the visual-field defects observed with pituitary adenomas. Bergland and Ray[33] explain this on the basis of their observations that the chiasmal bar is entirely supplied by an inferior group of arteries that become involved with a pituitary adenoma early in its suprasellar extension. Hoyt[30] states that the pattern of arterial supply cannot be invoked to explain this selective involvement, for compression by tumor would be unlikely to exceed the perfusion pressures of arteries. He believes that a more likely explanation is that the compression of venous channels and capillary networks produces a stagnant anoxia and results in conduction block in the visual pathways.

An alternative hypothesis offered by O'Connell is that the topography and attachments of the chiasm are such that expanding tumors selectively produce tension on the crossing fibers.[42] He supports this suggestion by demonstrating in cadavers that a section of the median bar of the chiasm and medial parts of the optic nerve produce more gaping incisions than laterally placed lesions. An even simpler explanation is suggested by Hedges, who found that a balloon placed in the sella of a cadaver produced selective stretching of superior fibers in the median bar of the chiasm. He compares this to bending a finger, where the upper skin becomes taut and the lower less stretched.[98]

Whatever the mechanism by which the field loss is produced, the clinical utility of this tendency to spare the vertical meridian above fixation is clear. When a temporal visual-field defect fails to cross the vertical meridian, this favors a compressive lesion. Hoyt[30] cautions that this respect for the vertical meridian is not invariable. Younge[43] points out that even in lesions posterior to the chiasm there may be tilting of the field up to 10° across the midline, and this phenomenon should be considered before early superonasal field loss is diagnosed.

A surprisingly common asymmetrical pattern of visual loss in pituitary adenomas is complete blindness in one eye with a temporal defect in the opposite eye. Eighty-one cases (8.1%) presenting in this way were included in the Mayo Clinic series.[5] Cogan[44] states that this pattern is as characteristic of chiasmal involvement as are bitemporal defects. The frequency of such severe visual loss confirms that many patients are unaware of their deficit.

4.2. Bitemporal Hemianopic Scotomata

The usual pattern of visual loss involves both central and peripheral fields. Occasionally, only the central field is affected, producing an island of visual loss called a *scotoma* (Fig. 7). Traquair[40] described scotomatous bitemporal hemianopia as characteristic of chiasmal lesions. He thought that this pattern of field loss indicated a more rapidly growing tumor than those causing nonscotomatous bitemporal hemianopia.[40] This opinion has been supported by the finding at surgery of hemorrhagic cysts, suggesting recent rapid expansion, in four of a series of eight patients with scotomatous defects.[45]

Hoyt[30] finds that bitemporal hemianopic scotomata are rare and, when present, suggest a mass behind the chiasm. Huber[46] quotes an incidence of 3.5% and comments on the rarity of this pattern in his experience. Wilson and Falconer,[28] however, found bitemporal hemianopic scotomata in 24 of their 50 patients with pituitary adenomas, but state that they considered the pattern of postoperative regression of the field in classifying the preoperative defect. This may have artifactually elevated the reported incidence. Pneumoencephalography performed on Wilson and Falconer's patients demonstrated that the apices of the tumors were behind the chiasm. This confirms the

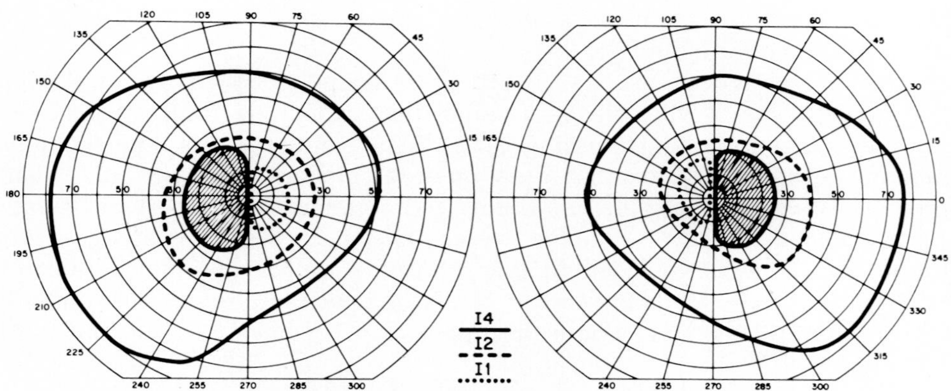

Fig. 7. An idealized bitemporal hemianopic scotomatous pattern. In this and other representations of the visual field, scotomata are represented by a pattern of lines surrounded by an isopter. This indicates that the stimulus defining that isopter is not seen within this area of the field.

clinical impression that bitemporal hemianopic scotomata are particularly seen in the prefixed chiasm where compression is occurring from behind.

4.3. Monocular Visual-Field Defects

Despite the predilection for bitemporal or at least bilateral visual-field involvement in pituitary adenomas, monocular deficits occur in a significant proportion of cases. In the Mayo Clinic series, 9% of patients with visual-field defects had involvement of only a single eye.[4] This was most often (33 of 61 cases) a superior temporal defect. A unilateral temporal defect suggests the possibility of chiasmal involvement.

Monocular visual-field loss may result in an initial confusion with other pathological processes. Central scotomata are often initially attributed to optic neuritis and arcuate defects to glaucoma. The occurrence of a central scotoma alone in a patient with pituitary tumor is a rare event, occurring in perhaps 1% of cases.[4] Little *et al.*[47] suggest that this is most frequent with a rapidly expanding lesion. Because central scotomata occur in compressive lesions, radiological studies are mandatory in the evaluation of the patient with presumed retrobulbar optic neuritis. As has been emphasized above, the sella is enlarged in most patients in whom a pituitary adenoma is the etiology; however, Asbury[48] reports a case with a central scotoma, normal sella, and pituitary adenoma. Careful attention to the vertical meridian in perimetric examination may assist in distinguishing compression from neuritis in cases of monocular visual loss.[49]

The pathophysiological basis for optic nerve involvement in pituitary adenoma may be selective growth of the tumor anteriorly, the presence of a postfixed chiasm with exposure of an unusually long intracranial portion of the optic nerve, or a particular vulnerability of the vascular supply to the posterior portion of the optic nerve. Schneider *et al.*[50] report a patient with markedly asymmetrical field loss who at surgery had an area of apparent infarction on the superior optic nerve at the junction with the chiasm. They call this "prechiasmal infarction" and attribute it to the fragility of the anastomotic vascular supply to the anterior chiasm. Selective optic nerve involvement could also be explained by its compression against the anterior cerebral artery as it passes over the posterior optic nerve, against a dural band connecting the anterior clinoid processes, or against the roof of the optic canal. This type of compression is also offered as an explanation for the occasional observation of inferior altitudinal hemianopias in patients with mass lesions in this region.[51]

The anatomical association of axons as they enter the optic nerve is the basis for the arcuate scotomata or nerve fiber bundle defects seen particularly with glaucoma but also with optic neuritis. Hoyt[52] demonstrated that adjacent axons remain anatomically associated until they are within the chiasm. This observation provides a neuroanatomical basis for the occasional arcuate scotoma seen with pituitary adenomas compressing the chiasm.[53] An arcuate defect that is relatively specific for a chiasmal lesion is the hemianopic temporal arcuate scotoma extending from the blind spot to the vertical midline[54] (Fig. 8).

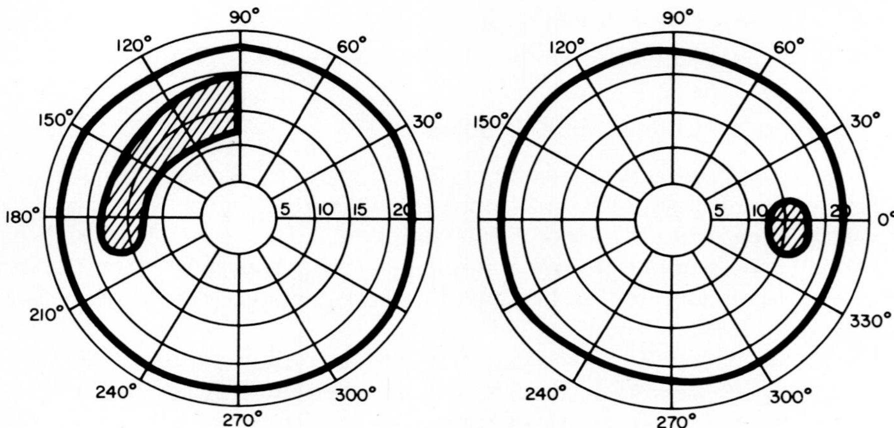

Fig. 8. A hemianopic temporal arcuate scotoma in the left eye as would be seen on a tangent screen with a 1-mm test object at 2 m. The fact that the scotoma ends at the vertical meridian distinguishes it from the more commonly seen arcuate scotoma of anterior optic nerve disease.

4.4. Binasal Field Loss

Chiasmal compression may rarely present as binasal field loss. True binasal hemianopias respecting the vertical midline are almost never observed.[44] Rather, two separate lesions produce an irregular nasal involvement. Relatively common causes of binasal field loss seen clinically are glaucoma, chronic papilledema, and drusen of the optic nerves. O'Connell and Du Boulay[55] suggest that when binasal field loss is seen with a mass in the chiasmal region, this is due to the superior uncrossed fibers in the optic nerves being compressed against the anterior cerebral arteries.

5. Causes of Bitemporal Hemianopia Other Than Chiasmal Lesions

Occasionally, a patient will present with bitemporal field loss that is a result of two separate lesions in the optic nerve or retina. Testing artifacts may also produce a false localizing bitemporal hemianopia.

Congenital anomalies of the optic disk and retina, such as occur in nasal fundus ectasia[56] or the tilted disk syndrome,[57] may produce bitemporal field defects. These defects can usually be distinguished from true chiasmal field loss because they do not respect the vertical meridian but slope across from the superotemporal to the superonasal field, (Fig. 9). There are two possible explanations for this appearance of the visual fields. In the tilted disk syndrome, the inferior retina is more myopic than the superior retina because of ectasia of the globe. Increasing the myopic correction used for testing may result in improvement of the defect. Graham and Wakefield,[58] however, found persistent field loss even when compensation was made for the refractive state and suggested an associated local inferior retinal hypoplasia. Progressive tem-

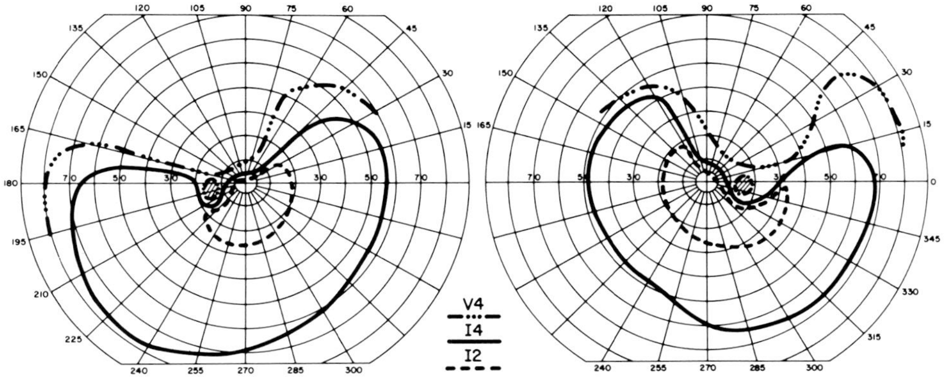

Fig. 9. A bitemporal pattern of field loss that could be mistaken for chiasmal compression but is actually due to bilateral optic nerve disease. Note that the isopters slope across the vertical meridian into the superonasal field.

poral-field loss can occur when patients with anomalous disks develop glaucoma, a process usually associated with nasal-field defects.[59] As an illustration of the diagnostic difficulties that sometimes occur, Keane[60] reports a case of an apparently anomalous disk on the side of a monocular scotomatous temporal-field defect in which work-up revealed a pituitary adenoma.

Cogan[44] mentions the possibility that ischemic optic neuropathy can be confused with chiasmal lesions.

Case Report

A 51-year-old man presented with a history of gradually decreasing vision over a 3-week period in the right eye. On examination, the visual acuity in the right eye was 20/200 and in the left eye was 20/20+2. An afferent pupillary defect was present on the right. Fundus examination revealed optic atrophy of the right eye; the left disk appeared normal. Goldmann fields revealed constriction of all isopters in the right eye with a superotemporal field defect to large isopters. In the left eye, there was a superotemporal depression in the central field (Fig. 10). The possibility of chiasmal compression was considered; however, plain skull films and a CT scan were normal.

Subsequently, information was obtained from physicians who had examined the patient at the time of his visual loss that there was disk swelling inferiorly in the right eye. A diagnosis of ischemic optic neuropathy had been made. No clear cause of the superotemporal depression in the left eye was ever determined.

Comment. Even without the history, the probability that this patient's field loss was not due to a chiasmal lesion should have been appreciated because the whole field in the right eye is constricted and the superior depression slopes across the vertical meridian. Some variability in response was present, since the perimetrist was unable to demonstrate a blind spot in the right eye.

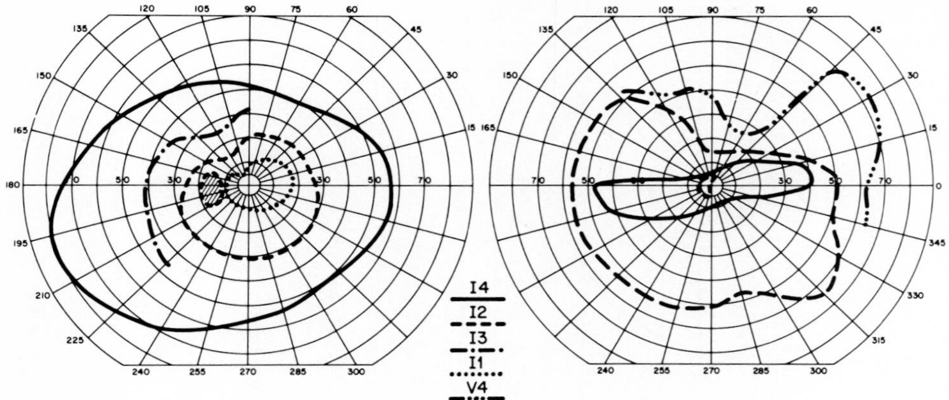

Fig. 10. A false bitemporal hemianopia.

In the examination of the central visual fields, correction for refractive error should be made with appropriate lenses. The effect of not making this correction is to flatten the island of vision, decreasing the increment of sensitivity of the macula over the periphery.[61] Especially with kinetic perimetry, this may result in artifacts in the central isopter that are indistinguishable from early chiasmal compression but that disappear when an appropriate lens is used.

Case Report

A 65-year-old woman was evaluated because of suspected pituitary calcification. She was bilaterally aphakic and wore both hard and soft contact lenses. On her initial examination, her corrected visual acuity was 20/20−1 in the right eye and 20/30−3 in the left eye. Visual fields revealed some constriction of isopters with a bitemporal hemianopia to small isopters tht respected the vertical meridian in the right eye and crossed it by 15° in the left eye (Fig.

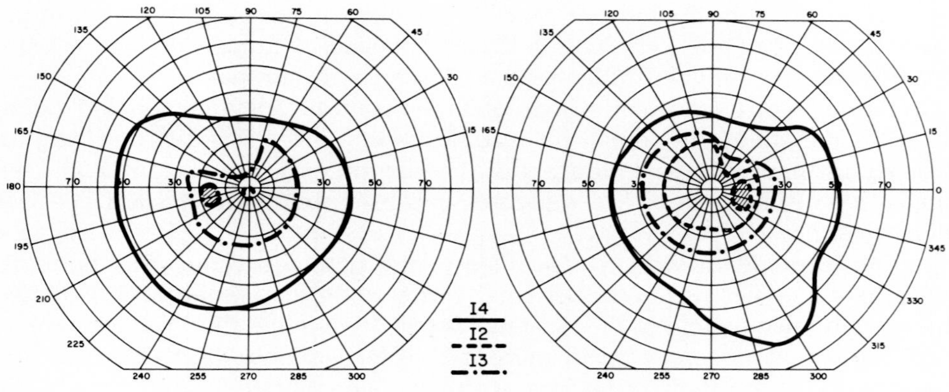

Fig. 11. Artifactual bitemporal hemianopia due to a refractive scotoma produced by contact lenses.

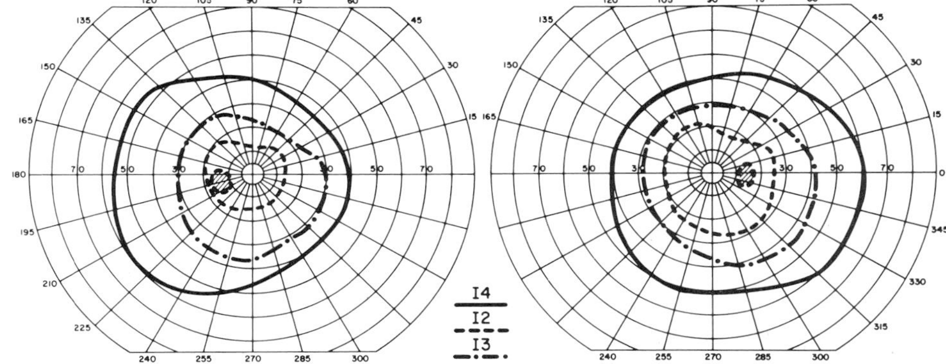

Fig. 12. Fields of the same patient as in Fig. 11 with a larger contact lens in place.

11). Because it was noted on slit-lamp examination that her hard contact lenses rode inferiorly and nasally in both eyes, a second set of fields was done with her larger soft contact lenses in place. The bitemporal field defect completely disappeared, revealing normal fields (Fig. 12). Subsequent work-up included a negative CT scan. The radiopaque material in the region of her sella was felt to be dye from a previous myelogram.

Riise[62] reviewed 34 cases in which a bitemporal hemianopia was not attributable to a mass lesion. Anomalies of the optic disk and retina were the most common cause. Other etiologies—glaucoma, drusen of the optic nerve, sectorial pigmentary retinal degeneration, papilledema, toxic optic neuropathy, trauma, and multiple sclerosis—were also identified. Choroidal folds with or without associated papilledema have also been observed to produce bitemporal field loss.[63] In some cases, there may actually be pathology at the chiasm; for example, trauma and multiple sclerosis have been identified as noncompressive chiasmal syndromes.[24] Most probably represent false localization. An occasional patient has no identified etiology.

6. Sensory Phenomena Associated with Chiasmal Compression

Only a few patients with chiasmal compression complain of field loss as long as acuity is normal. Other subjective sensory phenomena are sometimes associated with visual loss due to chiasmal compression. Weinberger and Grant[64] described complex visual hallucinations in patients with pituitary adenomas. Difficulties with depth perception occur and have been attributed to postfixational blindness[65]; that is, a patient with a complete bitemporal hemianopia has an expanding wedge of blind field beyond fixation where the two temporal defects are overlapping (Fig. 13).

Bitemporal hemianopias may also produce intermittent diplopia in the

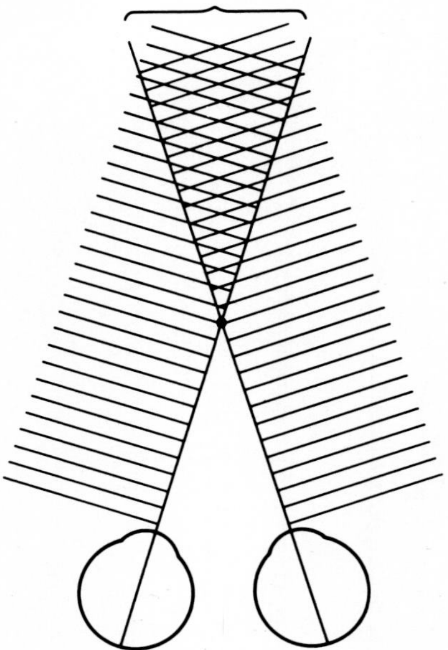

Fig. 13. Wedge of blind field as a result of overlapping temporal-field defects.

absence of ocular motor paresis—nonparetic diplopia.[66] This is apparently a result of loss of fusional stabilization from the normal overlapping of fields, a phenomenon called "hemifield slide."[6]

Case Report

A 54-year-old engineer had complained of headaches for 7 months. He had noted within the past month decreased central vision, flashes of light in both eyes, and blurring of his temporal field in the left eye. He described this blurring as a waviness, "like looking at a contour map."

On examination, his visual acuity was 20/30+ in the right eye and 20/40 in the left eye. Amsler grid testing revealed a bitemporal defect that caused distortion of the lines. Goldmann fields demonstrated bitemporal field loss. A skull film was normal with no enlargement of the bony sella. A CT scan showed a contrast-enhancing lesion in the sella and suprasellar regions (see Chapter 10, Fig. 11). While he was being evaluated in the hospital, his vision deteriorated suddenly. At emergency surgery, a suprasellar meningioma with its origin on the diaphragma sella was found. Total removal was accomplished with return of visual acuity to 20/20 and marked improvement of visual fields.

Comment. The sensory phenomenon in this case is called *metamorphopsia*. Metamorphopsia is a distortion of the visual environment usually seen in macular disease. A type of metamorphopsia can also be seen in cortical disease.[67] Neither of these mechanisms seems to apply here, and the explanation of their occurrence in a patient with chiasmal compression remains problematical.

7. Ophthalmoscopy in Pituitary Adenomas

Compression of the chiasm producing visual loss may also result in retrograde axonal degeneration producing optic atrophy. Papilledema is rare in pituitary adenomas; the occurrence of papilledema in a patient with chiasmal field defects suggests an etiology other than pituitary adenoma. Suprasellar tumors such as craniopharyngiomas in children often present with papilledema, since they are in a position to obstruct cerebrospinal fluid flow.

The appearance of optic atrophy by routine ophthalmoscopy is a late sign in chiasmal compression; its absence does not militate against this diagnosis. In the Mayo Clinic series, only 34% of eyes had disk pallor, while 67% of eyes had field defects.[4] Before optic atrophy appears, there may be early changes in the appearance of the peripapillary nerve fiber bundle layer due to drop-out of axons.[68] These defects, described as "guttering," can best be appreciated with red-free light and photographically.[69] Lundstrom and Frisén[70] studied seven eyes of patients with chiasmal compression from pituitary adenoma using these techniques. They found that some degree of nerve fiber damage could be identified in all cases studied, including one in which no field defect could be recognized. The potential application of this method, especially to patients who are unable to cooperate for accurate visual-field studies, represents an area for further study.

Hoyt *et al.*[71] have also called attention to a specific pattern of optic atrophy that occurs when decussating axons are lost. These axons originate in the retina nasal to fixation and enter the disk largely nasally and temporally. Axons originating in the temporal retina that do not decussate enter the disk largely superiorly and inferiorly. Thus, when only decussating axons are affected, the pattern of optic atrophy is medially and laterally, so-called "bow-tie" or "butterfly" optic atrophy (Fig. 14).

8. Ocular Motor Involvement in Pituitary Adenomas

In comparison with the frequency of visual loss, ocular motor palsies as an isolated initial manifestation of pituitary tumors are uncommon. Neetens

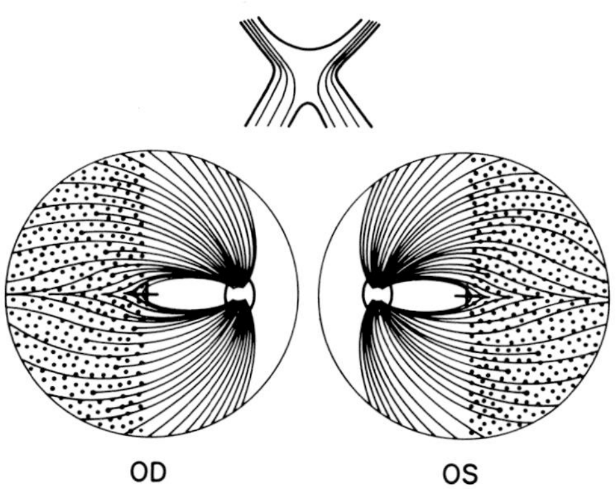

Fig. 14. Pattern of nerve fiber distribution in the retina when decussating axons have been lost. Only the superior and inferior portions of the disk have a preserved axonal compliment, producing the appearance of "bow-tie" or "butterfly" optic atrophy.

and Selosse[72] found only about 50 cases of this type reported. Involvement of the third, fourth, or sixth cranial nerve occurs more frequently in conjunction with other signs of the tumor. In the Mayo Clinic series, single or multiple ocular motor palsies were found in only 46 of 1000 cases.[4] Generally, ocular motor palsies signify a large or invasive tumor and are thus a bad prognostic sign.[72] They may be relatively more frequent in those pituitary adenomas associated with Cushing's syndrome.[73]

The third nerve is involved most often; sixth- and fourth-nerve palsies occasionally occur. Selective involvement of the ocular motor nerves in the adjacent cavernous sinus may be an anatomical consequence of particularly well-developed sellar diaphragms and associated structures obstructing the usual path of suprasellar growth.[74] Robert *et al.*[75] reported that of nine patients with ocular motor palsies associated with pituitary tumors, three had normal fields. This suggests a preferential lateral rather than suprasellar path of extension.[75] They also noted normally reactive pupils in four of their seven patients with third-nerve involvement and cautioned against confusion of this entity with diabetic third-nerve palsies where pupillary reactions are characteristically spared.

8.1. See-Saw Nystagmus

A dramatic and rare ocular motor abnormality sometimes associated with pituitary adenomas and other parasellar tumors is see-saw nystagmus.[76] A conjugate clockwise then counterclockwise rotation of the eyes at from 150 to 300 cycles/min is observed with elevation of the intorting eye and depression of the extorting eye. This produces the appearance of the two eyes riding a see-saw over the nose (Fig. 15). Nystagmus consisting only of torsional movements without vertical excursions is reported and probably represents a *forme fruste* of see-saw nystagmus.[77]

The mechanism causing see-saw nystagmus is unclear. One group of patients with this ocular motility disturbance have had bitemporal hemianopias due to tumor, trauma, or developmental defects,[78] suggesting the presence of an underlying sensory release phenomenon perhaps related to hemifield slide

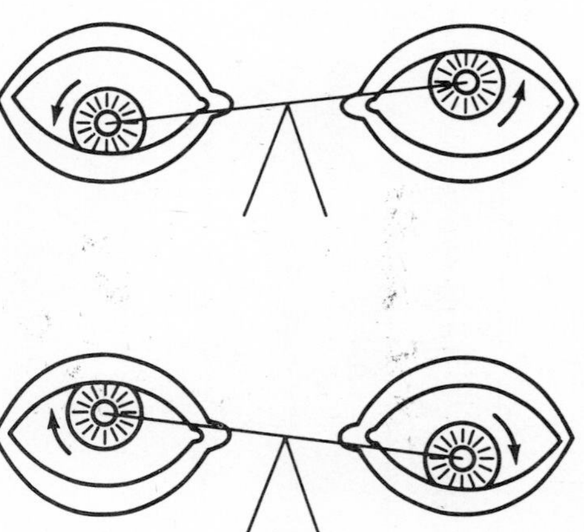

Fig. 15. Diagrammatic representation of the eye movements in see-saw nystagmus.

as described above. On the other hand, see-saw nystagmus has been seen with vascular disease of the upper brainstem in patients without bitemporal hemianopias, and it is possible that in those cases with bitemporal hemianopia, the nearby brainstem is affected.[79,80] Thus, while see-saw nystagmus is not specific to tumors compressing the chiasm, its presence should prompt appropriate studies.

9. Pituitary Apoplexy and Its Variants

Ocular motor palsies are a prominent feature of what has been called "pituitary apoplexy."[81] The sudden development of ophthalmoplegia, visual loss, and headache may be indicative of rapid enlargement of a pituitary adenoma.[82,83] There is some debate over what should be called pituitary apoplexy. David *et al.*[84] discuss a group of patients who developed ophthalmoplegia without visual loss and consider pituitary apoplexy as "a syndrome produced by any sudden enlargement of a preexisting pituitary adenoma." The term pituitary apoplexy was originally applied to spontaneous infarction of nontumorous pituitaries producing hypopituitarism, and some authors prefer to restrict it to this usage.[85] Whatever terminology is used, various clinical pictures suggestive of spontaneous tumor enlargement or shrinkage do occur.

Case Report

A 57-year-old man was followed for refractive error with visual acuity of 20/16.7 in the right eye and 20/20+1 in the left eye and full fields to confrontation. He developed coryzal symptoms and then had the sudden onset of severe vertex and bitemporal headaches (after a coughing spell) associated with nausea and vomiting. Immediately afterward, he noted blurring of vision temporally in both eyes. This was improving somewhat over the next week, but he presented for examination.

His visual acuity was 20/20 in each eye. A bitemporal field defect was present (Fig. 16). Skull films showed an eroded sella, and a CT scan demon-

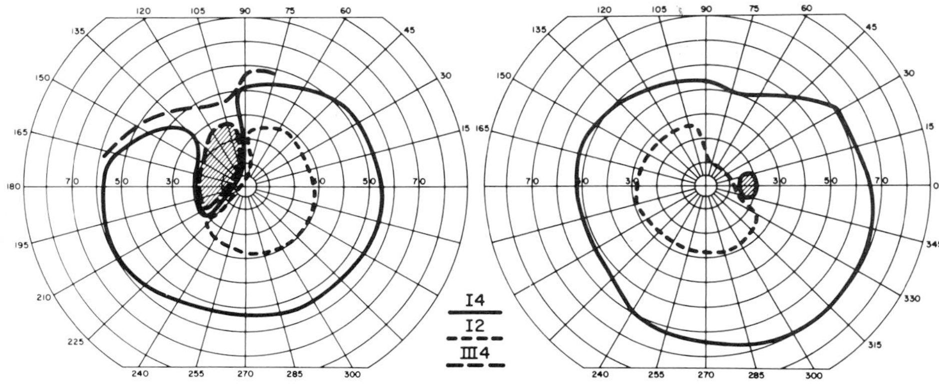

Fig. 16.

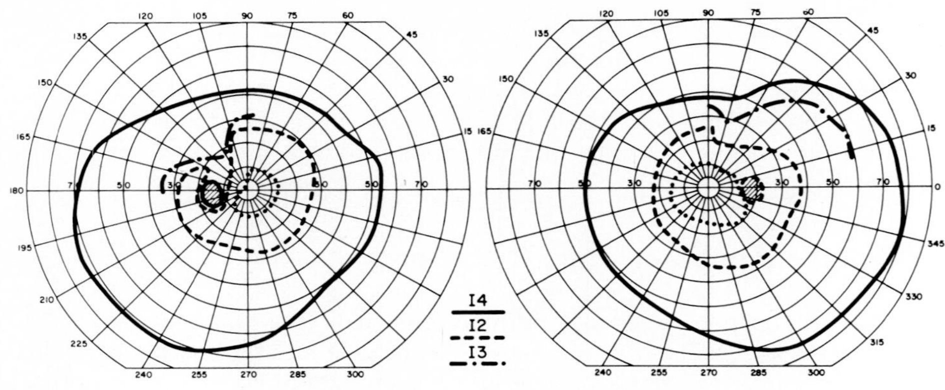

Fig. 17.

strated a large suprasellar lesion with calcification in its most anterior portion and an area of decreased density interpreted as suggesting a cystic or necrotic area.

Transsphenoidal surgery revealed pituitary adenoma, as expected, and his visual fields improved postoperatively (Fig. 17).

Comment. The association of upper respiratory infections with tumor enlargement has been previously noted.[83] Coughing causes a rapid change in the intracranial pressure, presumably compromising the tumor's vascular supply.

Case Report

A 44-year-old woman presented with amenorrhea, galactorrhea, elevated prolactin and abnormal sella tomograms. A tangent-screen examination dem-

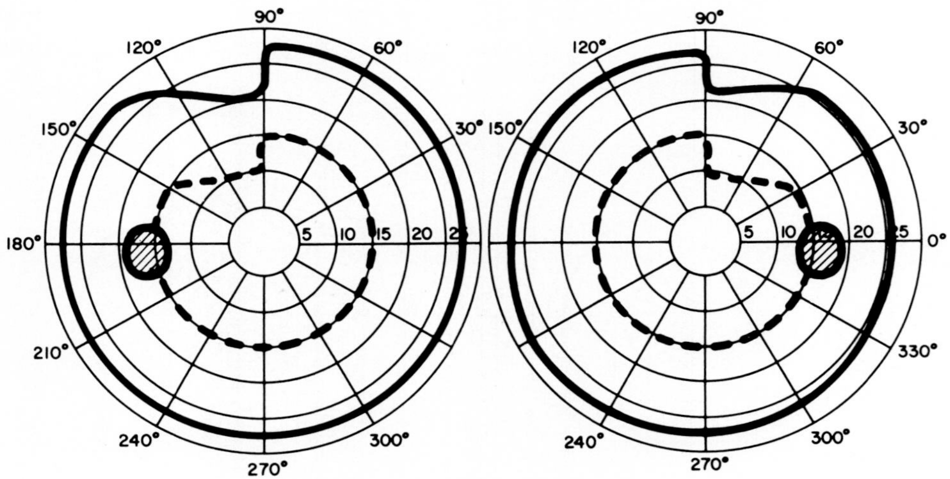

Fig. 18.

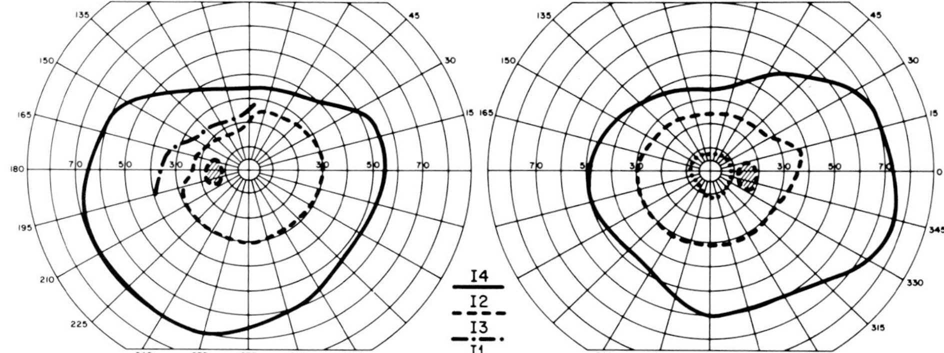

Fig. 19.

onstrated definite superotemporal depression to a 1/1000 and 1/2000 white test object and to a 10/1000 and 10/2000 red test object (Fig. 18). Her visual acuity was 20/25 − in the right eye and 20/25 + in the left eye. Over a 6-month period, there was enlargement of her temporal field defects. She was referred for evaluation. A CT scan in both the horizontal and coronal planes with and without contrast was normal. Goldmann visual fields demonstrated only a slight superior temporal depression in the left eye to the smaller isopters (Fig. 19). The right eye was normal. A reexamination 1 month later found 20/15 − 1 vision in the right eye and 20/15 − 2 in the left eye. Visual fields were now normal (Fig. 20). The patient, a physician's wife, decided not to proceed with pneumoencephalography. The diagnosis of spontaneous shrinkage of pituitary adenoma was suggested to explain the visual improvement.

Comment. Senelick and Van Dyk[8] coined the phrase "subclinical" pituitary apoplexy to describe similar cases. The spontaneous infarction of a pituitary adenoma may occasionally be therapeutic in acromegaly.[86]

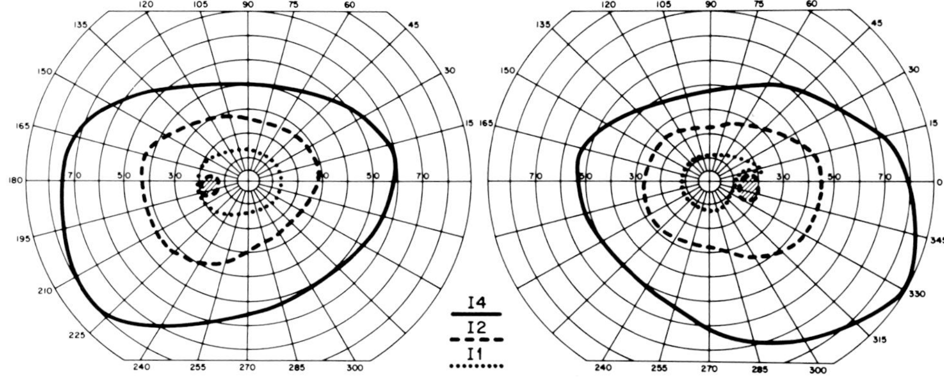

Fig. 20. Normal Goldmann fields showing only baring of the blind spot (not usually considered significant) to the smallest isopter in the right eye.

10. Summary

The development of sophisticated endocrinological tests and radiological techniques should not obscure the fact that many patients with pituitary adenomas present with visual loss or complaints and that visual morbidity is one of the most significant considerations in the management of all patients with lesions in the region of the chiasm. Ophthalmological evaluation to include visual-field testing should be part of the workup of every patient suspected of having a pituitary adenoma.

11. Appendix: Perimetric Techniques

The schema of visual-field testing that follows is based on the use of the Haag-Streit 940 ST Goldmann perimeter. The purpose of this discussion is not to provide a complete manual of perimetry, but rather to describe one technique for the assessment of visual fields in patients known or suspected to harbor a pituitary adenoma. For a more complete discussion of quantitative perimetry in neuroophthalmological diagnosis, the interested reader is referred to the reviews by Enoksson[89] or Ellenberger.[90]

After an accurate visual acuity and refraction are obtained, the subject is seated at the perimeter in a darkened room with one eye occluded. With the eye constantly fixating centrally, a light of size I (¼ mm^2) and intensity 4e (0.1 Lambert) is brought slowly—less than 5°/sec—from the periphery along a meridian until the subject signals its presence.[91] The point in the visual field at which this occurs is recorded on a chart by means of a pantographic arm. This process is repeated along meridians 15° apart until a set of points said to represent an *isopter* of peripheral visual field is obtained. The actual size of the isopter will vary with the age, refractive state, and alertness of the patient, but the shape is very constant in normal subjects.[92] If there is a localized constriction of this peripheral isopter or if the isopter is unusually small, a larger III–4e (4 mm^2) or V–4e (64 mm^2) stimulus is used to obtain a second peripheral isopter.

Next, the refraction that best corrects the eye at 30 cm (the radius of the Goldmann perimeter) is inserted into a lens holder. A I–2e (¼ mm^2, 0.01 Lambert) stimulus is brought in from the periphery until it is recognized. This process is repeated at meridians 30° apart except around the vertical meridian above fixation, where 15° or even smaller intervals are used. If this isopter does not pass outside the blind spot, the complete I–3e isopter is also obtained. Otherwise, a partial I–3e (¼ mm^2, 0.03 Lambert) isopter including the superotemporal field and crossing the vertical meridian is taken. The corrective lenses are removed for any parts of the isopters outside 30° from fixation.

The limits of the blind spot are outlined with an appropriate stimulus (I–4e, I–3e, or I–2e). A I–1e (¼ mm^2, 0.003 Lambert) isopter will also be taken if it is large enough, since the variation in isopters smaller than 5° from fixation in their largest extent may be such that they are difficult to interpret (Fig. 21). To look for scotomata, the I–1e or I–2e stimulus is projected inside its corresponding isopter and moved slowly across the field while the subject

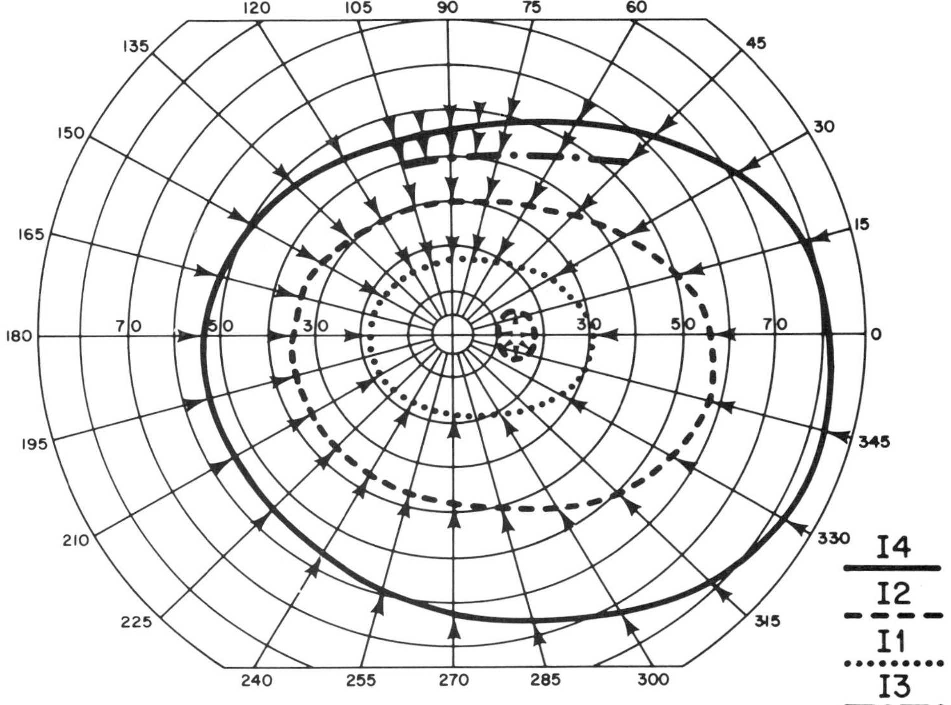

Fig. 21. A strategy, sometimes called selective perimetry, showing the points determined (arrows) in a kinetic field for the evaluation of a normal patient for chiasmal compression. Note the concentration of points around the vertical meridian superiorly and the use of a partial I–3e isopter. Usually, the I–1e target produces a smaller isopter, and a smaller stimulus (the 0–1e) might also be used if the responses were as good as those diagrammed to produce an isopter within 20° of fixation.

maintains central fixation and constantly signals its presence. The subject is instructed to stop signaling when the stimulus is no longer visible. This should occur only when the stimulus leaves the isopter or enters the blind spot or when the examiner turns the stimulus off. Otherwise, a pathological scotoma has been discovered. (Note also that the central 2° of the perimeter are taken up by a fixation device. Simple adjustment of the perimeter[91] allows this area to be tested.)

The same procedure is repeated for the other eye. If the field is abnormal, additional isopters or partial isopters may be necessary to define the defect. Obtaining the visual field should require less than 30 min in a reasonably cooperative subject. Longer examinations may result in patient fatigue, which adversely affects the accuracy of responses.

This is the usual technique of obtaining visual fields and is called *kinetic perimetry*; that is, the visual stimulus is moving. Two other available methods to test the visual fields on the Goldmann perimeter are *suprathreshold static perimetry* and *threshold static perimetry*. Suprathreshold static perimetry is usually used in conjunction with kinetic perimetry. In a normal visual field, all the points inside an isopter (with the exception of the normal blind spot) should be sensitive to the target used to obtain the isopter. If this is not true, then a depression of the visual field, called a *scotoma*, is present. The blind spot is an example of a scotoma. Small scotomata lying between kinetic isopters may be missed. To search for such scotomata, the perimetrist projects a suprathreshold stimulus at a number of points within its isopter and asks the patient to recognize its presence.

Threshold static perimetry consists of projecting a test stimulus that is below the threshold of recognition at a particular point in the field.[93] The brightness of the test stimulus is increased in steps until it is seen; thus, a threshold is determined. This process is repeated at a number of points in the visual field until a profile of the sensitivity of the visual system is obtained. The pattern of presentation is usually *meridional*—that is, along a meridian such as the horizontal—or *circular*—a given eccentricity from fixation. A 15° circular static consists of a set of points 15° from fixation and thus includes the blind spot. Another possible presentation is to test a series of points scattered throughout the visual field.

The major advantages of threshold static perimetry are that small scotomata that are undetectable by kinetic perimetry are recognized[94] and that defects found on kinetic perimetry can be defined more precisely to allow follow-up. This latter advantage has led some perimetrists to take a single meridional static through the most defective part of the kinetic field in patients with pituitary adenomas.[70] Ellenberger[90] reports a case in which 35° circular static fields detected early bitemporal field loss not seen on kinetic perimetry, The disadvantage of threshold static perimetry is that it requires a very cooperative patient and is somewhat tedious for both subject and examiner.

11.1 Color Visual Fields

The use of colored test objects for visual-field testing in chiasmal lesions deserves comment. When a tangent screen is used, white test objects smaller than 1 mm in diameter are impractical, but the isopter obtained by a white test object of this size with the tangent screen 2 m away from a normal individual may extend beyond 30° temporally, that is, exceed the size of the entire tangent screen.[40] A convenient way of decreasing the strength of the visual stimulus on a tangent screen is to use a colored test object, allowing smaller isopters to be obtained. Traquair[40] felt that the field was never altered for color stimuli without being altered for appropriate white stimuli. White test objects can be used to produce smaller isopters on a tangent screen by increasing the testing distance, changing the background (usually black), or decreasing the illumination.

On modern projection perimeters, neutral-density filters are capable of reducing the brightness of the projected stimulus even below the threshold for central vision. The perimetrist can thus easily obtain isopters in a normal field of almost any desired size, and therefore colored stimuli are rarely used.

Despite Traquair's admonition, however, some clinicians feel that there may be qualities of color fields other than reduced stimulus value that will prove useful in the evaluation of chiasmal lesions. Bartoli and Liuzzi[95] found that kinetic Goldmann perimetry using a monochromatic red light produced isopters that defined defects more clearly than similar-sized white-light isopters in six patients with pituitary adenomas. This contradicts the earlier observations of Enoksson,[96] who found conformity between colored and white isopters in ten cases of chiasmal compression.

There is agreement, however, that as an adjunct to perimetry, comparison of color saturation may be helpful in discovering depression of the central visual field. Red or blue-green test objects are presented either simultaneously[49] or sequentially[97] on either side of fixation, and the subject is asked to compare their saturations or note a change in saturation. When bitemporal color desaturation is discovered, this points to a chiasmal lesion in the same sense as bitemporal field defects.

References

1. A. Huber, Roentgen diagnosis vs. visual field, *Arch. Ophthalmol.* **90:**1, 1973.
2. H. Cushing, The chiasmal syndrome of primary optic atrophy and bitemporal field defects in adults with a normal sella turcica, *Arch. Ophthalmol.* **3:**505–551, and 704–735, 1930.
3. J.C. Johnson, M. Lubow, T. Banerjee, and D. Yashon, Chromophobe adenoma and chiasmal syndrome without enlargement of the bony sella, *Ann. Ophthalmol.* **8:**1043, 1977.
4. R.W. Hollenhorst and B.R. Younge, Ocular manifestations produced by adenomas of the pituitary gland: Analysis of 1000 cases, in: *Diagnosis and Treatment of Pituitary Tumors* (P.O. Kohler and G.T. Ross, eds.), pp. 53–68, Excerpta Medica, Amsterdam, 1973.
5. R.W. Hollenhorst and B.R. Younge, Ocular manifestations of intrasellar and suprasellar tumors, in: *Symposium on Neuro-ophthalmology: Transactions of the New Orleans Academy of Ophthalmology,* pp. 191–207, C.V. Mosby, St. Louis, 1976.
6. T.K. Lyle and P. Clover, Ocular symptoms and signs in pituitary tumours, *Proc. R. Soc. Med.* **54:**611, 1961.
7. A.J. Segal and R.S. Fishman, Delayed diagnosis of pituitary tumors, *Am. J. Ophthalmol.* **79:**77, 1975.
8. R.C. Senelick and H.J.L. Van Dyk, Chromophobe adenoma masquerading as corticosteroid-responsive optic neuritis, *Am. J. Ophthalmol.* **78:**485, 1974.
9. A. Klauber, P. Rasmussen, and J. Lindholm, Pituitary adenoma and visual function, *Acta Ophthalmol.* **56:**252, 1978.
10. E.R. Laws, Jr., J.C. Trautmann, and R. W. Hollenhorst, Jr., Transsphenoidal decompression of the optic nerve and chiasm: Visual results in 62 patients, *J. Neurosurg.* **46:**717, 1977.
11. H.J. Svien, J.G. Love, W.C. Kennedy, M.Y. Colby, Jr., and T.P. Kearns, Status of vision following surgical treatment for pituitary chromophobe adenoma, *J. Neurosurg.* **22:**47–52, 1965.
12. S.H. Wray, Neuro-ophthalmologic manifestations of pituitary and parasellar lesions, *Clin. Neurosurg.* **24:**86, 1977.
13. R.M. Burde, J.S. Glaser, R.W. Hollenhorst, A. Jampolsky, N.J. Schatz, G.B. Udvarhelyi, and H.J.L. Van Dyk, Round table discussions, *Symposium on Neuro-ophthalmology,* in: *Transactions of the New Orleans Academy of Ophthalmology,* p. 353, C.V. Mosby, St. Louis, 1976.
14. J.S. Glaser, Topical diagnosis: The optic chiasm, in: *Clinical Ophthalmology,* Vol. 2 (T.D. Duane, ed.), Chapt. 6, pp. 1–17, Harper and Row, New York, 1976.
15. W.M. Lee and J.E. Adams, The empty sella syndrome, *J. Neurosurg.* **28:**351, 1968.
16. K. Welch and J.C. Stears, Chiasmapexy for the correction of traction on the optic nerves and chiasm associated with their descent into an empty sella turcia—Case report, *J. Neurosurg.* **35:**760, 1971.
17. N.J. Schatz, S. Lichtenstein, and J.J. Corbett, Delayed radiation necrosis of the optic nerves and chiasm, in: *Neuro-ophthalmology VIII* (J.S. Glaser and J.L. Smith, eds.), p. 131, C.V. Mosby, St. Louis, 1975.

18. J.R. Harris and M.B. Levene, Visual complications following irradiation for pituitary adenomas and craniopharyngiomas, *Radiology* **120:**167, 1976.
19. S. Sokol, Visual evoked potentials, in: *Electrophysiologic Approaches to Neurologic Diagnosis* (M. Aminoff, ed.) Churchill Livingstone, New York (in press).
20. A.M. Halliday, E. Halliday, A. Kriss, W.I. McDonald, and J. Mushin, The pattern-evoked potential in compression of the anterior visual pathways, *Brain* **99:**357, 1976.
21. M. Feinsod, J.B. Selhorst, W.F. Hoyt, and C.D. Wilson, Monitoring optic nerve function during craniotomy, *J. Neurosurg.* **44:**20–31, 1976.
22. Y. Goldhammer, J.L. Smith, and B.M. Yates, Mycotic intrasellar abscess, *Am. J. Ophthalmol.* **78:**478, 1974.
23. K.F. Lee, N.J. Schatz, and P.J. Savino, Ischemic chiasmal syndrome, in: *Neuro-ophthalmology VIII* (J.S. Glaser and J.L. Smith, eds.), p. 115, C.V. Mosby, St. Louis, 1975.
24. N.J. Schatz and N.S. Schlezinger, Noncompressive causes of chiasmal disease, in: *Symposium on Neuro-ophthalmology: Transactions of the New Orleans Academy of Ophthalmology*, p. 90, C.V. Mosby, St. Louis, 1976.
25. R.H. Osher, J.J. Corbett, N.J. Schatz, P.J. Savino, and L.S. Orr, Neuro-ophthalmological complications of enlargement of the third ventricle, *Br. J. Ophthalmol.* **62:**536, 1978.
26. A. Kestenbaum, *Clinical Methods of Neuro-ophthalmic Examination*, Grune and Stratton, New York, 1946.
27. D.O. Harrington, *The Visual Fields: A Textbook and Atlas of Clinical Perimetry*, C.V. Mosby, St. Louis, 1976.
28. P. Wilson and M.A. Falconer, Patterns of visual failure with pituitary tumors, *Br. J. Ophthalmol.* **52:**94, 1968.
29. F.B. Walsh and W.F. Hoyt, *Clinical Neuro-ophthalmology*, Williams and Wilkins, Baltimore, 1969.
30. W.F. Hoyt, Correlative functional anatomy of the optic chiasm—1969, *Clin. Neurosurg.* **17:**189, 1970.
31. C. Kupfer, L. Chumbley, and J. deC. Downer, Quantitative histology of optic nerve, optic tract and lateral geniculate nucleus of man, *J. Anat.* **101:**393–401, 1967.
32. C.W. Rucker, The concept of a semidecussation of the optic nerves, *Arch. Ophthalmol.* **59:**159, 1958.
33. R.M. Bergland, B.S. Ray, and R.M. Torack, Anatomical variations in the pituitary gland and adjacent structures in 225 human autopsy cases, *J. Neurosurg.* **28:**93, 1968.
34. J.P. Schaeffer, Some points in the regional anatomy of the optic pathway, with especial reference to tumors of the hypophysis cerebri and resulting ocular changes, *Anat. Rec.* **28:**243, 1924.
35. R. Bergland and B.S. Ray, The arterial supply of the human optic chiasm, *J. Neurosurg.* **31:**327, 1969.
36. W.F. Hoyt and O. Luis, Visual fiber anatomy in the infrageniculate pathway of the primate: Uncrossed and crossed retinal quadrant fiber projections studied with Nauta silver stain, *Arch. Ophthalmol.* **68:**94, 1962.
37. W.F. Hoyt and O. Luis, The primate chiasm: Details of visual fiber organization studied by silver impregnation techniques, *Arch. Ophthalmol.* **70:**69, 1963.
38. W.F. Hoyt and R.C. Tudor, The course of the parapapillary temporal retinal axons through the anterior optic nerve: A Nauta degeneration study in the primate, *Arch. Ophthalmol.* **69:**503, 1963.
39. M. Chamlin and L.M. Davidoff, The 1/2000 field in chiasmal interference, *Arch. Ophthalmol.* **44:**53, 1950.
40. H.M. Traquair, *An Introduction to Clinical Perimetry*, 4th ed., C.V. Mosby, St. Louis, 1944.
41. A.C. Bird, Field loss due to lesions at the anterior angle of the chiasm, *Proc. R. Soc. Med.* **65:**519, 1972.
42. J.E.A. O'Connell, The anatomy of the optic chiasma and heteronymous hemianopia, *J. Neurol. Neurosurg. Psychiatry* **36:**710, 1973.
43. B.R. Younge, Midline tilting between seeing and nonseeing areas in hemianopia, *Mayo Clin. Proc.* **51:**563, 1976.
44. D.G. Cogan, *Neurology of the Visual System*, Charles C. Thomas, Springfield, Illinois, 1966.
45. K. Sugita, O. Sato, T. Hirota, R. Tsugane, and N. Kageyama, Scotomatous defects in the central visual fields in pituitary adenomas, *Neurochirurgica* **18:**155, 1975.

46. A. Huber, *Eye Symptoms in Brain Tumors,* 2nd ed., C.V. Mosby, St. Louis, 1971.
47. H.L. Little, J.W. Chambers, and F.B. Walsh, Unilateral intracranial optic nerve involvement: Neurosurgical significance, *Arch. Ophthalmol.* **73:**331, 1965.
48. T. Asbury, Unilateral scotoma as the presenting sign of pituitary tumor, *Am. J. Ophthalmol.* **59:**510, 1965.
49. J.D. Trobe and J.S. Glaser, Quantitative perimetry in compressive optic neuropathy and optic neuritis, *Arch. Ophthalmol.* **96:**1210, 1978.
50. R.C. Schneider, F.C. Kriss, and H.F. Falls, Prechiasmal infarction associated with intrachiasmal and suprasellar tumors, *J. Neurosurg.* **32:**197, 1970.
51. D. Schmidt and K. Bührmann, Inferior hemianopia in parasellar and pituitary tumors, in: *Neuro-ophthalmology IX* (J.S. Glaser, ed.), p. 236, C.V. Mosby, St. Louis, 1977.
52. W.F. Hoyt, Anatomic considerations of arcuate scotomas associated with lesions of the optic nerve and chiasm: A Nauta axon degeneration study in the monkey, *Bull. Johns Hopkins Hosp.* **111:**58, 1962.
53. T.P. Kearns and C.W. Rucker, Arcuate defects in the visual fields due to chromophobe adenomas of the pituitary gland, *Am. J. Ophthalmol.* **45:**505, 1958.
54. J.D. Trobe, Chromophobe adenoma presenting with a hemianopic temporal arcuate scotoma, *Am. J. Ophthalmol.* **77:**388, 1974.
55. J.E.A. O'Connell and E.P.G.H. Du Boulay, Binasal hemianopia, *J. Neurol. Neurosurg. Psychiatry* **36:**697, 1973.
56. D. Riise, Nasal fundus ectasia, *Acta Ophthalmol.,* Suppl. 126, 1975.
57. S.E. Young, F.B. Walsh, and D.L. Knox, The tilted disk syndrome, *Am. J. Ophthalmol.* **82:**16, 1976.
58. M.V. Graham and G.J. Wakefield, Bitemporal visual field defects associated with anomalies of the optic discs, *Br. J. Ophthalmol.* **57:**307, 1973.
59. A.J. Chadwick, Inversion of the disc and temporal field loss in chronic simple glaucoma, *Br. J. Ophthalmol.* **52:**932, 1968.
60. J.R. Keane, Suprasellar tumors and incidental optic disc anomalies, *Arch. Ophthalmol.* **95:**2180, 1977.
61. C. Maguire, Ametropia in the visual field, *Trans. Ophthalmol. Soc. U.K.* **91:**663, 1971.
62. D. Riise, Neuro-ophthalmological patients with bitemporal hemianopsia, *Acta Ophthalmol.* **48:**685, 1970.
63. L. Frisén and M. Holm, Visual field defects associated with choroidal folds, in *Neuro-ophthalmology IX* (J.S. Glaser, ed.), p. 248, C.V. Mosby, St. Louis, 1977.
64. L.M. Weinberger and F.C. Grant, Visual hallucinations and their neuro-optical correlations (review), *Arch. Ophthalmol.* **23:**166, 1940.
65. T.H. Kirkham, The ocular symptomatology of pituitary tumors, *Proc. R. Soc. Med.* **65:**517, 1972.
66. H. Nachtigäller and W. F. Hoyt, Störungen des Scheindruckes bei bitemporaler Hemianopsie und Verschiebung der Sehachsen, *Klin. Monatsbl. Augenheilkd.* **186:**821, 1970.
67. M. Critchley, The problem of visual agnosia, *J. Neurol. Sci.* **1:**274, 1964.
68. L. Frisén and W. F. Hoyt, Insidious atrophy of retinal nerve fibers in multiple sclerosis: Funduscopic identification in patients with and without visual complaints, *Arch. Ophthalmol.* **92:**91–97, 1974.
69. N.M. Newman, Ophthalmoscopic observation of the retinal nerve fiber layer, *Trans. Am. Acad. Ophthalmol. Otolaryngol.* **83:**OP–786, 1977.
70. M. Lundstrom and L. Frisén, Atrophy of the nerve fibers in compression of the chiasm: Degree and distribution of ophthalmoscopic changes, *Acta Ophthalmol.* **54:**623, 1976.
71. W.F. Hoyt, E.N. Rios-Montenegro, M.M. Behrens, and R.J. Eckelhoff, Homonyous hemioptic hypoplasia *Br. J. Ophthalmol.* **56:**537, 1972.
72. A. Neetens and P. Selosse, Oculomotor anomalies in sellar and parasellar pathology, *Ophthalmologica* **175:**80, 1977.
73. R.L. Rovit and T.D. Duane, Eye signs in patients with Cushing's syndrome and pituitary tumors, *Arch. Ophthalmol.* **79:**513, 1968.
74. L.M. Weinberger, F.H. Aden, and F.C. Grant, Primary pituitary adenoma and the syndrome of the cavernous sinus: A clinical and anatomic study, *Arch. Opthalmol.* **24:**1197, 1940.
75. C.M. Robert, Jr., J.A. Feigenbaum, and W.E. Stern, Ocular palsy occurring with pituitary tumors, *J. Neurosurg.* **38:**17, 1973.

76. J.M. Fein and R.D.B. Williams, See saw nystagmus, *J. Neurol. Neurosurg. Psychiatry* **32:**202, 1969.
77. T.D. Sabin and J.A. Poche, Pure torsional nystagmus as a consequence of head trauma, *J. Neurol. Neurosurg. Psychiatry* **32:**265, 1969.
78. G.V. Davis and J.P. Shock, Septo-optic dysplasia associated with see-saw nystagmus, *Arch. Ophthalmol.* **93:**137, 1975.
79. R.B. Daroff, See-saw nystagmus, *Neurology* **15:**874, 1965.
80. E.J. Arnott and S.J.H. Miller, See-saw nystagmus, *Trans. Ophthalmol. Soc. U.K.* **90:**491, 1970.
81. D. Brougham, A.D. Heusner, and R.D. Adams, Acute degenerative changes of adenomas of the pituitary body with special reference to pituitary apoplexy, *J. Neurosurg.* **7:**321, 1950.
82. S.P. Meadows, Unusual clinical features and modes of presentation in pituitary adenoma, including pituitary apoplexy, in: *Neuro-ophthalmology IV* (J.L. Smith, ed.), p. 178, C.V. Mosby, St. Louis, 1968.
83. P.L. Rovit and J.M. Fein, Pituitary apoplexy: A review and reappraisal, *J. Neurosurg.* **37:**280, 1972.
84. N.H. David, F.P. Gargano, and J.S. Glaser, Pituitary apoplexy in clinical perspective, in: *Neuro-ophthalmology VIII* (J.S. Glaser and J.L. Smith, eds.), p. 140, C.V. Mosby, St. Louis, 1975.
85. J.P. Conomy, J.H. Ferguson, J.S. Brodkey, and H. Mitsumoto, Spontaneous infarction in pituitary tumors: Neurologic and therapeutic aspects, *Neurology* **25:**580, 1975.
86. A.L. Taylor, J.L. Finster, P. Raskin, J.B. Field, and D.H. Mintz, Pituitary apoplexy in acromegaly, *J. Clin. Endocrinol. Metab.* **28:**1784, 1968.
87. M.G. Alper, Mucoceles of the sphenoid sinus: Neuro-opthalmic manifestations, *Trans. Am. Ophthalmol. Soc.* **74:**53, 1976.
88. L.J. Streletz and N.J. Schatz, Transsphenoidal encephalocele associated with colobomas of the optic disc and hypopituitary dwarfism, *Neuro-ophthalmology VII* (J.L. Smith and J.S. Glaser, eds.), p. 78, C.V. Mosby Company, St. Louis, 1973.
89. P. Enoksson, Perimetry in neuro-ophthalmological diagnosis, *Acta Ophthalmol.*, Suppl. 82, 1965.
90. C. Ellenberger, Jr., Modern perimetry in neuro-ophthalmic diagnosis, *Arch. Neurol.* **30:**193, 1974.
91. *Goldmann Perimeter 940: Instructions for Use,* Haag-Streit AG, Switzerland.
92. L. Frisén and M. Frisén, Objective recognition of abnormal isopters, *Acta Ophthalmol.* **53:**378, 1975.
93. E.L. Greve, Static perimetry, *Ophthalmologica (Basel)* **171:**26–38, 1975.
94. G.L. Portney and M.A. Krohn, The limitation of kinetic perimetry in early scotoma detection, *Ophthalmology* **85:**287, 1978.
95. F. Bartoli and L. Liuzzi, Laser perimetry: Diagnostic application in six cases of pituitary chromophobe adenoma, *Acta Ophthalmol.* **51:**841, 1973.
96. P. Enoksson, A study of the visual fields with white and coloured objects in cases of pituitary tumour with especial reference to early diagnosis, *Acta Ophthalmol.* **31:**505–515, 1953.
97. L. Frisén, A versatile color confrontation test for the central visual field: A comparison with quantitative perimetry, *Arch. Ophthalmol.* **89:**3, 1973.
98. T.R. Hedges, Preservation of the upper nasal field in the chiasmal syndrome: An anatomic explanation, *Trans. Am. Ophthalmol. Soc.* **67:**131, 1969.

14

The Radiology of Pituitary Adenomas—An Update

SAMUEL M. WOLPERT

1. Introduction

Prior to the utilization of sellar tomography in patients with intrasellar tumors, adenomas less than 10 mm in diameter were seldom detected radiographically. The application of pluridirectional and, more recently, computed tomography (CT) of the sella to the workup of these patients has revolutionized their management. Patients with tumors ranging in size from 5 mm in diameter to large supra- and parasellar masses can now be medically or surgically managed entirely on the basis of tomography, CT of the sella, the endocrine findings, and the visual-field examination. Pneumoencephalography (PEG) is now seldom indicated in these patients, though on occasions, particularly when an empty sella is suspected, the definitive diagnosis is achieved by PEG. Even more recently, a water-soluble contrast agent, metrizamide, for subarachnoid space opacification has been introduced. The agent can be maneuvered into the suprasellar cisterns, and the use of metrizamide cisternography with CT may eliminate PEG in the few instances in which it is still presently indicated (see Chapter 10, Fig. 19).

The recognition that many pituitary tumors can be detected when they are small and confined to the sella and that many of these tumors secrete prolactin in excessive amounts has alerted the physician to the high prevalence of prolactinomas. Recent reports have shown that prolactinomas can account for between 60 and 70% of pituitary adenomas.[1–3] Newer histopathological techniques have also shown that the old classification of chromophobe adenomas, eosinophilic adenomas, and basophilic adenomas is not acceptable since, on pathological analysis, many patients with one type of tumor can be shown to harbor elements of the other types. An improved clas-

SAMUEL M. WOLPERT • Tufts University School of Medicine; Department of Radiology, Section of Neuroradiology, Tufts–New England Medical Center Hospital, Boston, Massachusetts 02111.

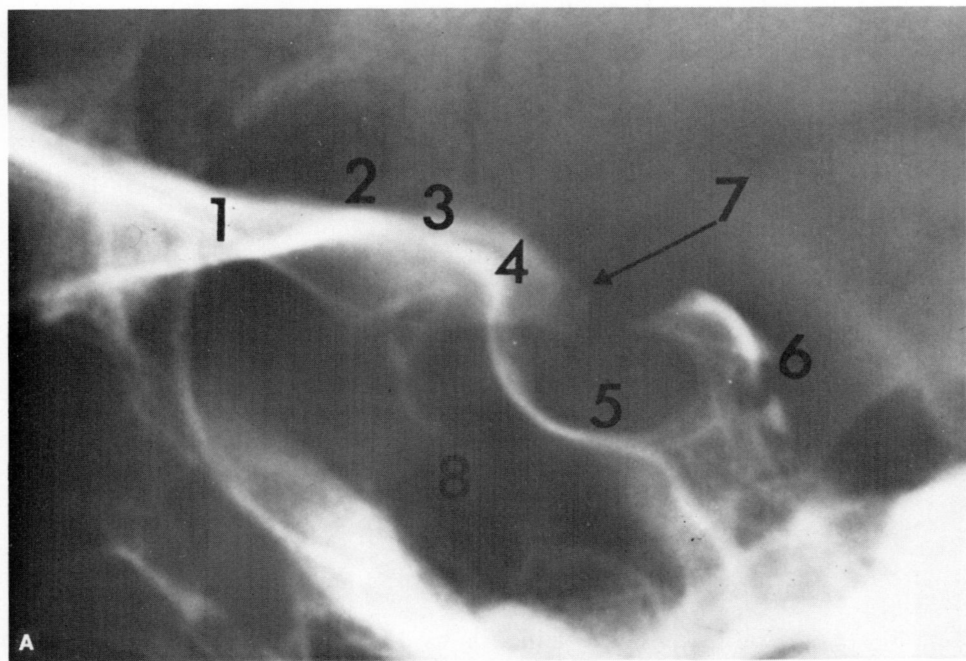

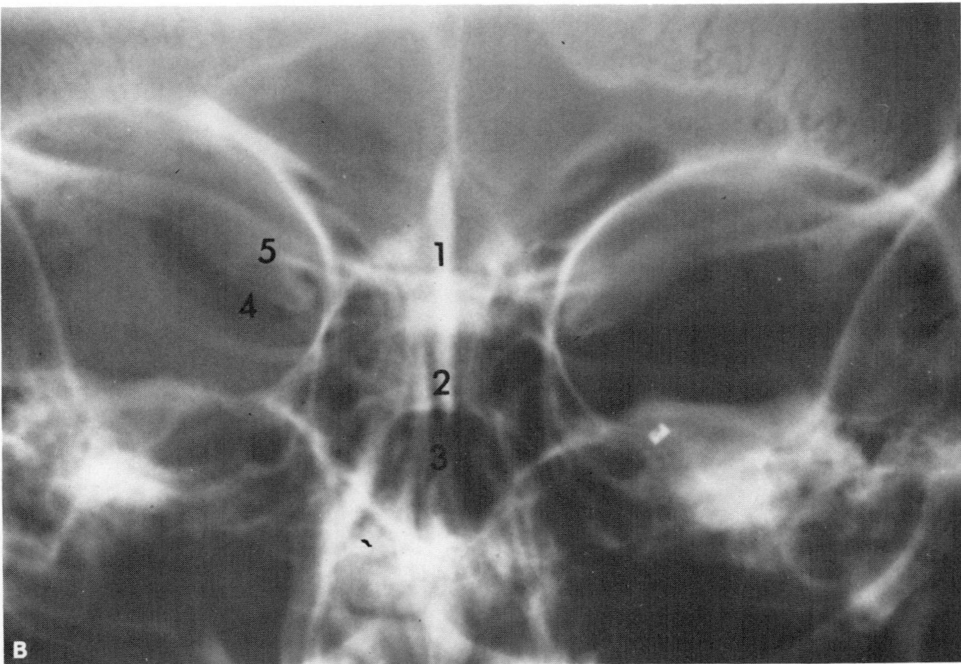

Fig. 1. (A) Skull X-ray, lateral projection. Note the planum sphenoidale (1), limbus sphenoidale (2), sulcus chiasmaticus (3), tuberculum sellae (4), sellar floor with distinct lamina dura (5), dorsum sellae (6), anterior clinoid processes (7), and sphenoid sinus (8). (B) Caldwell projection. Note the planum sphenoidale (1), floor of sella (2), sphenoid sinus (3), sphenoidal fissure (4), and inner one-third of sphenoidal ridge (5).

sification divides pituitary adenomas into secretory and nonsecretory tumors, depending on the presence or absence of hormone output. Within this classification, the common secretory tumors are prolactin-secreting tumors, growth hormone (GH)-secreting tumors, and adrenal corticotropic hormone (ACTH)-secreting tumors. Patients with these tumors often present with endocrine symptomatology due to elevated serum levels of the secreted hormone. Such tumors are often still quite small, and only sellar tomography may demonstrate a radiographic abnormality. Patients with nonsecretory tumors or with tumors producing insufficient hormone to elevate serum hormone levels may not seek medical attention until the tumors have enlarged sufficiently to cause visual-field abnormalities or hypopituitarism. In such patients, an abnormal sella can usually be detected on plain films.

2. Plain Films of the Sella Turcica

The radiological examination of a patient with a suspected adenoma should be systematically carried out, and should commence with a coned-down lateral view of the sella to assess its profile and a Caldwell frontal view to assess the width of the sella. On the lateral projection, superimposition of the two anterior clinoid processes ensures a true lateral view with no rotation (Figs. 1A and 2). The elements of the sellar profile should be systematically

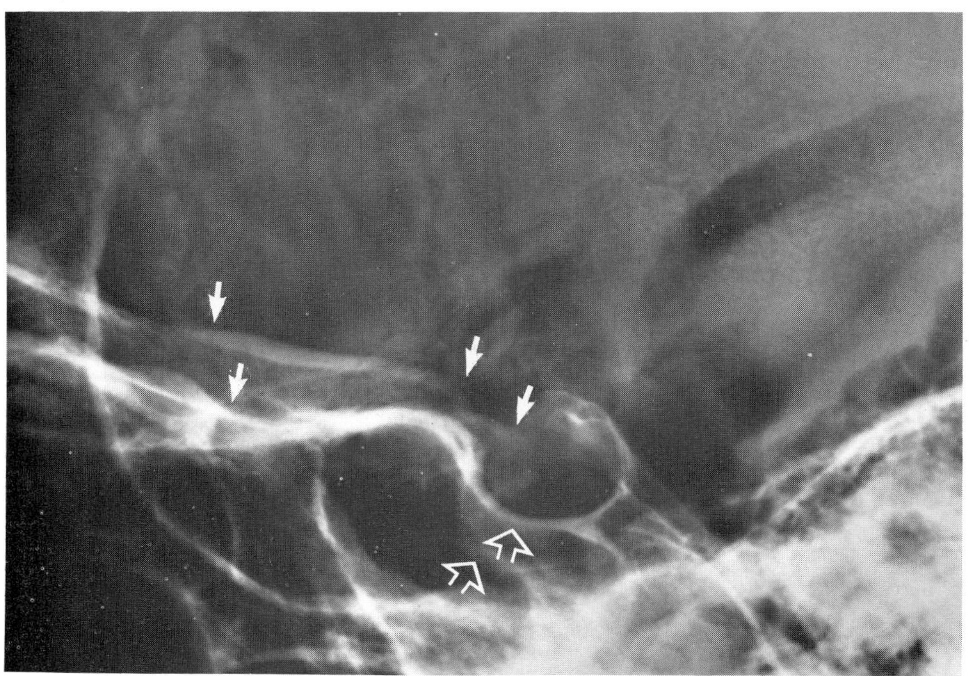

Fig. 2. Rotated lateral view of sella. Note that the two anterior processes and orbital roofs (solid arrows) are not superimposed. The apparently depressed sellar floor (open arrows) may be due to the obliquity of the X-ray. Repeat X-rays of the sella are needed to determine whether or not the floor is depressed.

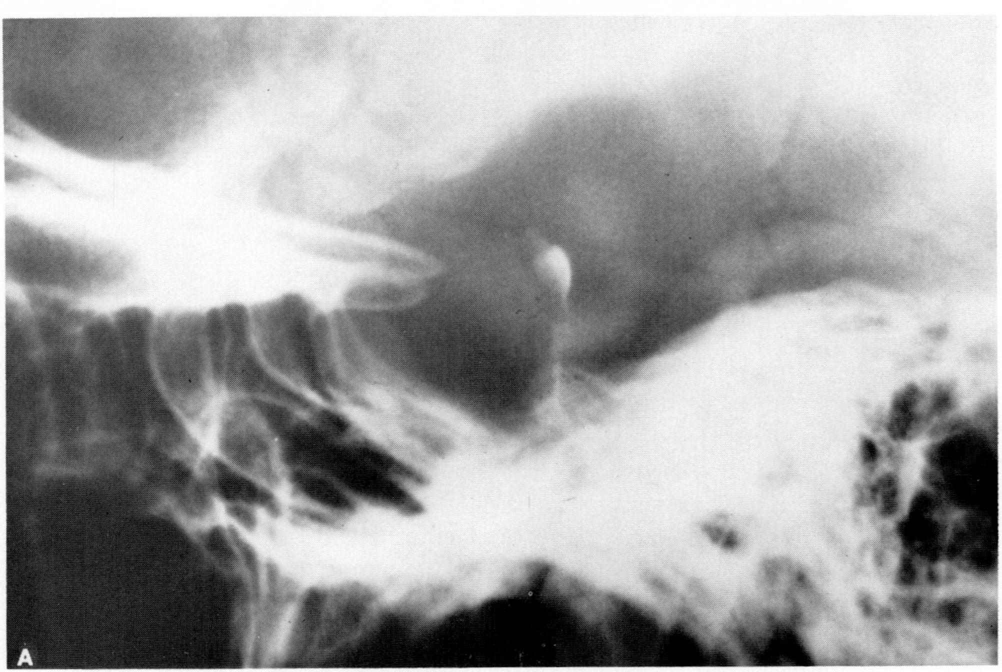

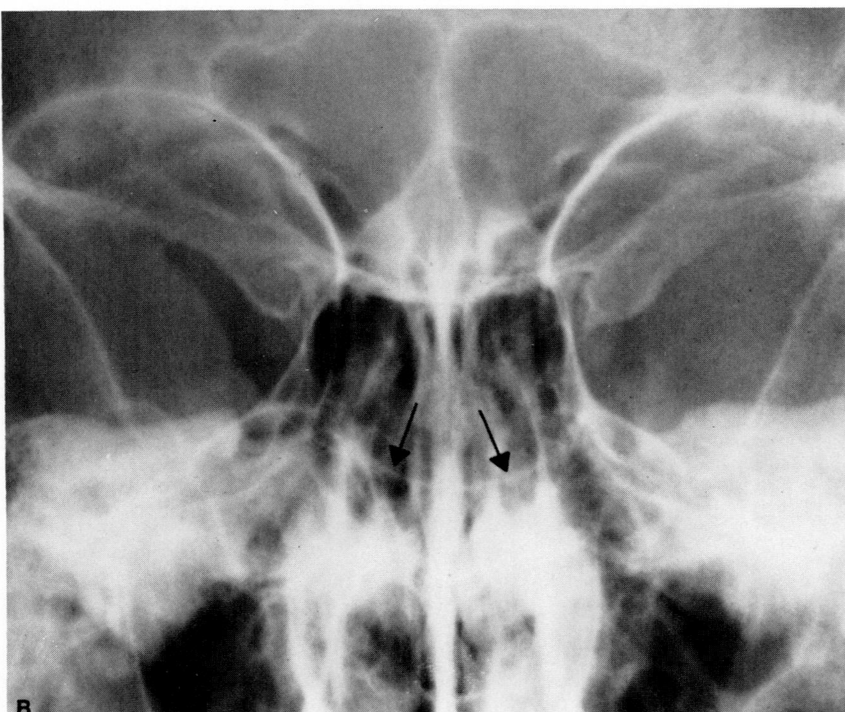

Fig. 3. (A) Skull X-ray, lateral projection. The sella is enlarged, and the dorsum sellae is thinned. (Note: Caution is necessary in the interpretation because of the slight rotation.) (B) Caldwell projection. The floor of the sella (arrows) is thinned. Diagnosis: Pituitary adenoma.

assessed by identifying, in order, the planum sphenoidale, the limbus sphenoidale, the sulcus chiasmaticus, the tuberculum sellae, the lamina dura of the floor of the sella, and the dorsum sellae. In addition, the anterior clinoid processes, sphenoid sinuses, and retropharyngeal space should be inspected. On the Caldwell frontal view, the lesser wings of the sphenoid bone and the planum sphenoidale should be initially identified. Below the planum sphenoidale lies the floor of the sella, which forms part of the roof of the sphenoid sinus. The superior orbital fissures below the lesser wings of the sphenoid bone can also be seen (Fig. 1B). A frontal half-axial (Towne's projection) is a useful view for further evaluation of the dorsum sellae. In a steeply angled Towne's projection, the dorsum sellae is projected through the foramen magnum.

The size of the normal sella turcica is particularly variable. Though measurements of the sellar volume are available, an overall impression of sellar size provides a more certain index of abnormality in a patient suspected of harboring a pituitary adenoma. The radiological changes that should be sought for in patients with adenomas include: enlargement of the sella, erosion of its floor, thinning of the dorsum sellae, loss of the lamina dura forming the floor of the sella, erosion or elevation of the anterior clinoid processes, a double floor of the sella, soft-tissue densities within the sphenoid sinus, and supra- or intrasellar calcium (Fig. 3).

3. Tomography of the Sella Turcica

Even if any of the changes described above are present on the plain films, it is still necessary to carry out pluridirectional tomography, since if a transsphenoidal adenomectomy is to be carried out, the surgeon needs information about the configuration of the sphenoid sinus and its septa. Tomography may also reveal tumor growth into the sphenoid sinus (see Fig. 8) or show an unsuspected lesion of the sphenoid sinus such as a polyp, mucocele (see Chapter 10, Fig. 16), or inflammatory mucosal thickening.

Variations in the degree of sphenoid sinus pneumatization are easily defined by tomography (see Figs. 6 and 9). The sellar floor is also subject to many variations such as prominent sinus septations and carotid artery indentations, both of which may mimic intrasellar tumors (Figs. 4 and 24). Tomography is of considerable help in identifying these variations.[4,5]

Since the majority of patients being evaluated today for suspected pituitary adenomas are presenting when the adenoma is still small, abnormalities are usually not seen on the plain films. In these patients, pluridirectional tomography may reveal changes in the floor of the sella that will suggest the presence of an adenoma.[6] These alterations, which can be missed if tomography at 1-mm intervals in the lateral plane and at 2-mm intervals in the frontal plane is not carried out, include thinning, erosion, and focal ballooning of the sella, usually anteriorly and inferiorly (Figs. 5 and 7–9). The borderline between the diagnosis of the normal and abnormal sella may be difficult.[7] It has been estimated that the adenoma must be at least 5 mm in diameter before tomographic changes can be seen. When the tumor is large, considerable destruction of the sella is usually present (Fig. 10A).

For the results of the different types of therapy (medical, surgical, and radiation) to be compared, a classification of the type and degree of sellar destruction is necessary. Hardy[8] has classified the sella turcica changes into two main groups, the enclosed and the invasive types (Fig. 11). With the enclosed type (Grade I), the tumor remains confined to the sella, the sellar floor is always intact (although it may bulge unilaterally), and the sella is not enlarged (see Fig. 5). In a second variety of the enclosed type (Grade II), the sella is enlarged, but again the floor is intact (see Fig. 6). With the invasive adenoma, the tumor has eroded the floor of the sella with possible herniation of the pathological tissue into the sphenoid sinus (see Figs. 7–10). Again, two varieties are described—localized (Grade III) and generalized (Grade IV) erosion of the floor.

Hardy[8] furthermore suggested that there is a topographic localization for secreting microadenomas within the pituitary gland. He suggested that GH-secreting adenomas are situated laterally, and ACTH-secreting adenomas are situated centrally, within the gland. Other investigators, however, have not confirmed these findings.

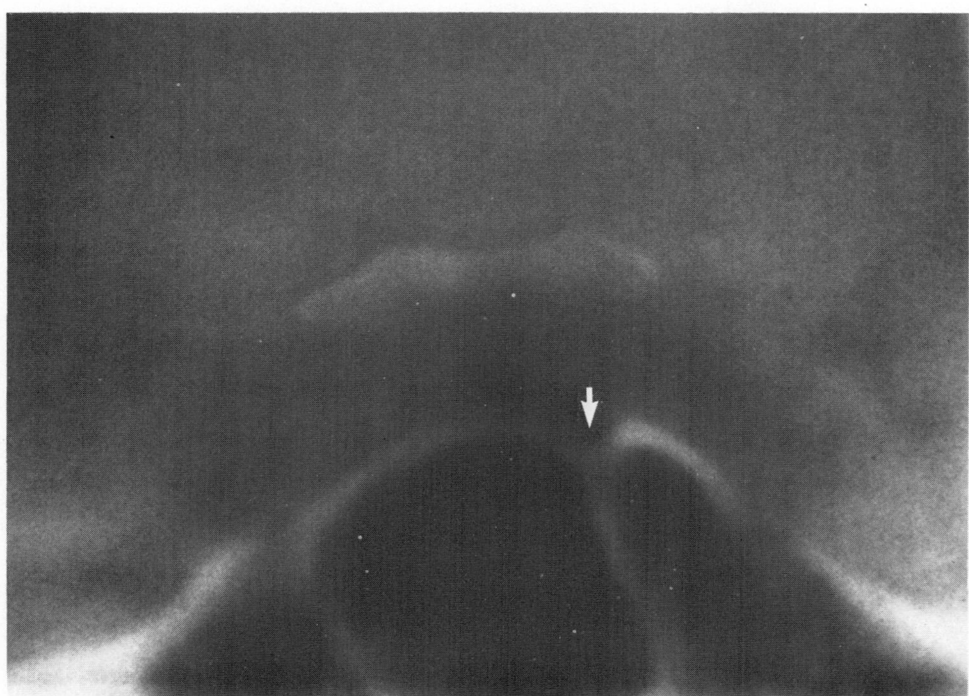

Fig. 4. Anteroposterior tomogram demonstrating a depression in the sellar floor (arrow) at the insertion of the sphenoid sinus septum. On the lateral projection, the floor of the sella may be defective at this point and mimic an erosion.

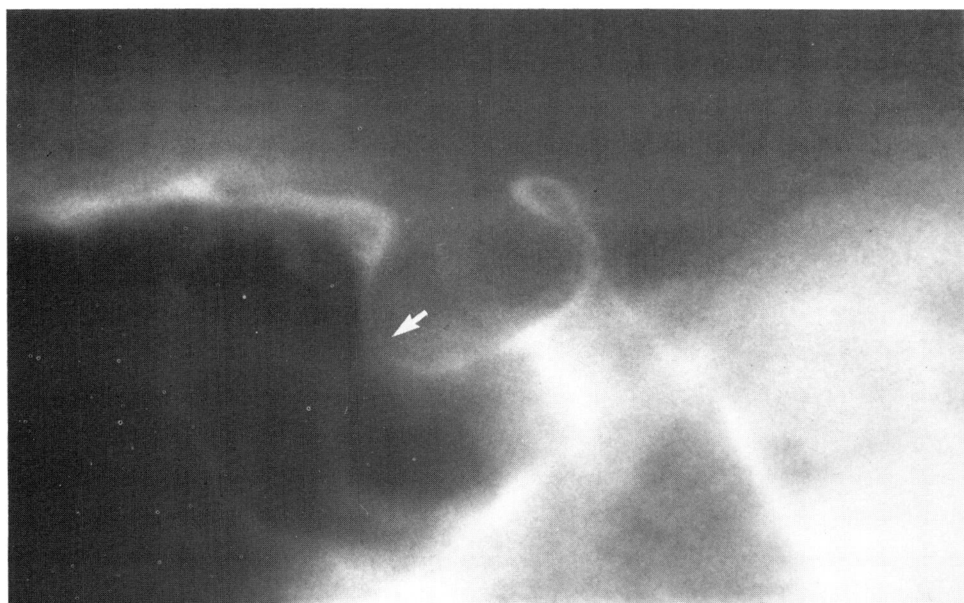

Fig. 5. Lateral tomogram demonstrating bulging of the sella anteroinferiorly (arrow) with marked thinning of the lamina dura. Diagnosis: Prolactinoma.

4. Radiological Investigation of Patients with Suspected Prolactinomas

At the Tufts–New England Medical Center, we have evaluated the results of the radiological studies in a series of 140 consecutive patients who presented with galactorrhea thought to be due to prolactinomas (Table 1). Patients were preselected to exclude such conditions as menstruation, ingestion of tranquilizing drugs or contraceptive pills, and hypothyroidism. The pa-

TABLE 1. Analysis of 140 Consecutive Patients with Galactorrhea

Group[a]	Number of patients	Tumors at surgery	Negative surgery	Empty sella	Medical or DXT Rx	Being followed
I	51	36	3[b]	3	3	6
II	19	—	—	3	—	16
III	17	—	1	2	—	14
IV	53	—	—	—	—	53

[a]Group I: abnormal tomograms (see the text) and elevated serum prolactin levels (>25 ng/ml); Group II: abnormal tomograms and normal serum prolactin levels; Group III: normal tomograms and elevated serum prolactin levels; Group IV: normal tomograms and normal serum prolactin levels.

[b]In two patients, the prolactin levels decreased and the galactorrhea disappeared after surgery.

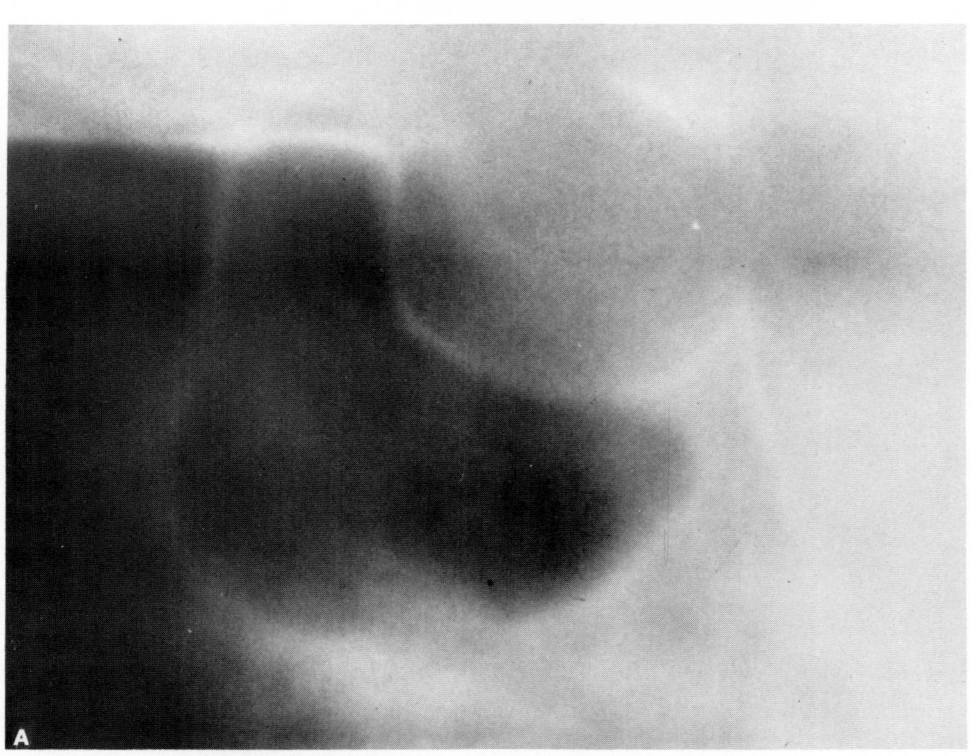
A

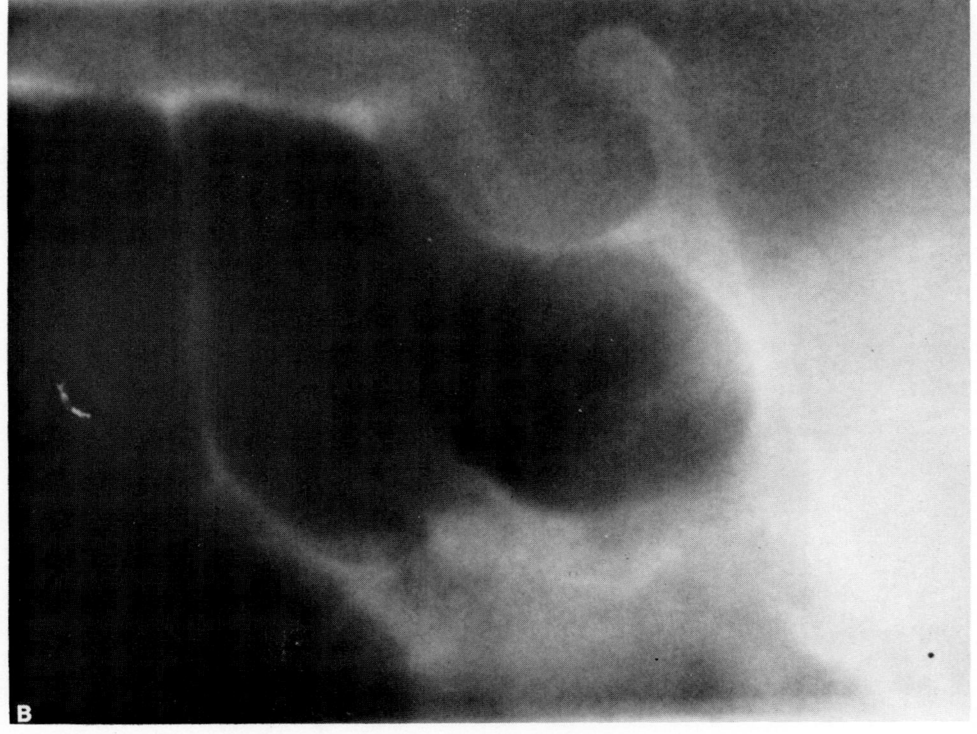
B

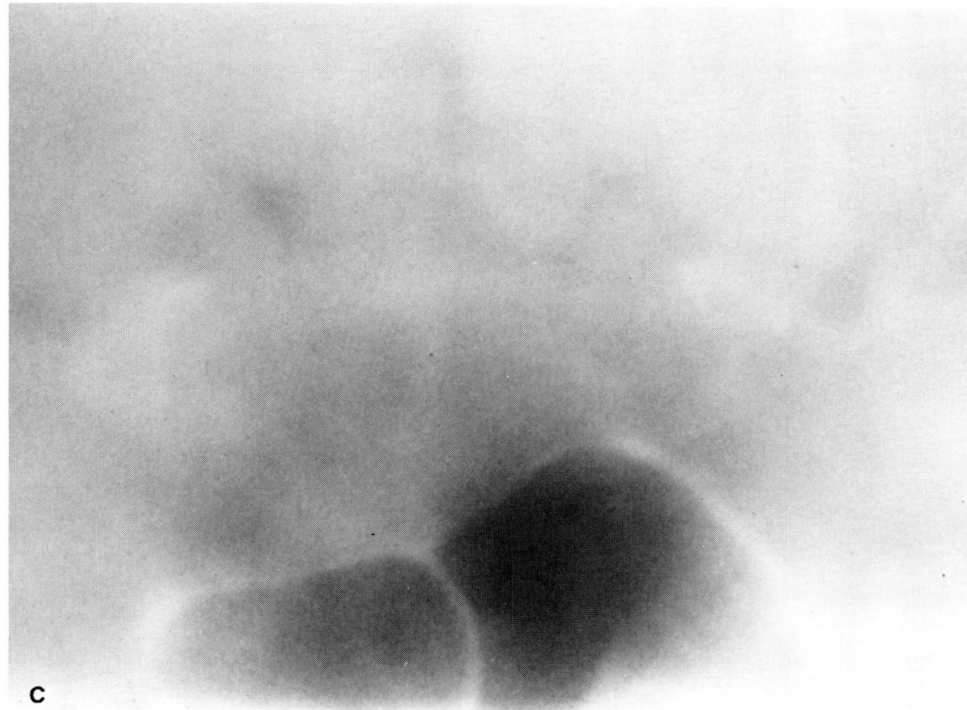

Fig. 6. (A) Lateral tomogram to the right of the midline demonstrating enlargement of the sella. (B) Tomogram to the left of the midline demonstrating a normal-sized sella. (C) Frontal tomogram. Note the asymmetrical enlargement of the right side of the sella. Diagnosis: Pituitary adenoma.

tients were divided into the following four groups:

Group I: Patients with abnormal tomograms and elevated serum prolactin levels (>25 ng/ml)—51 patients.
Group II: Patients with abnormal tomograms and normal serum prolactin levels—19 patients.
Group III: Patients with normal tomograms and elevated serum prolactin levels—17 patients.
Group IV: Patients with normal tomograms and normal serum prolactin levels—53 patients.

4.1. Value of Tomography

Tomography was abnormal in 70 of the 140 patients. Surgery was carried out on 39 patients in Group I and 1 patient in Group III. Tumors were surgically verified in 36 patients (all in Group I). In 4 patients, no intrasellar tumor was identified at surgery, but in 2 of these patients (both in Group I), decrease of the prolactin levels to normal levels and disappearance of galactorrhea indicated that the tumors may have been present prior to surgery. In the other 2 patients, both the galactorrhea and elevated serum prolactin have persisted

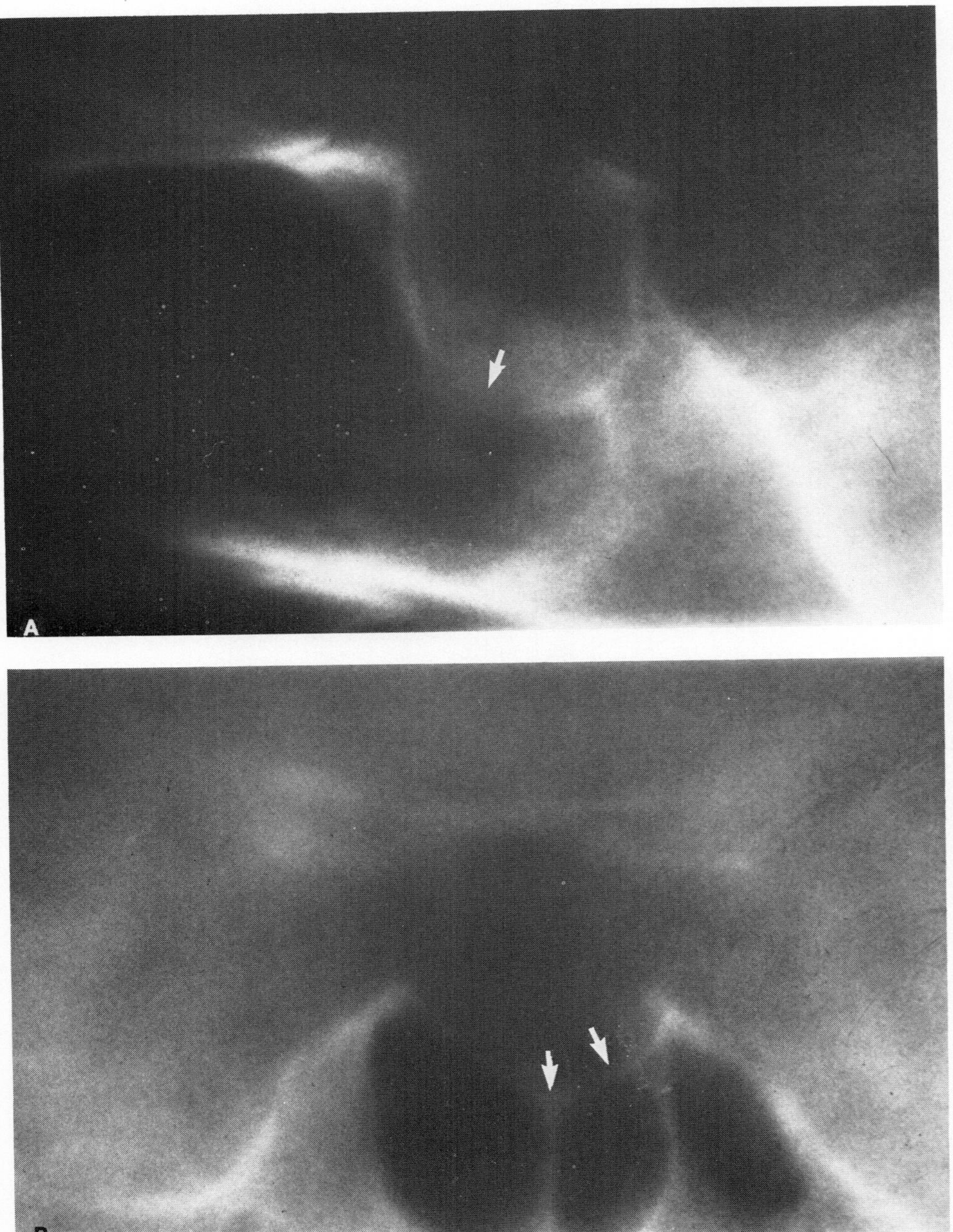

Fig. 7. (A) Lateral tomogram demonstrating bulging of the sella inferiorly with a break in the lamina dura (arrow). (B) Frontal tomogram demonstrating bulging of the sella inferiorly (arrows). (C) CT demonstrating a low-density area (arrows) within the sella. (D) Pneumoencephalogram, lateral tomogram. The chiasmatic cistern (arrows) is normal without evidence of an empty sella. Diagnosis: Necrotic prolactinoma confirmed at surgery.

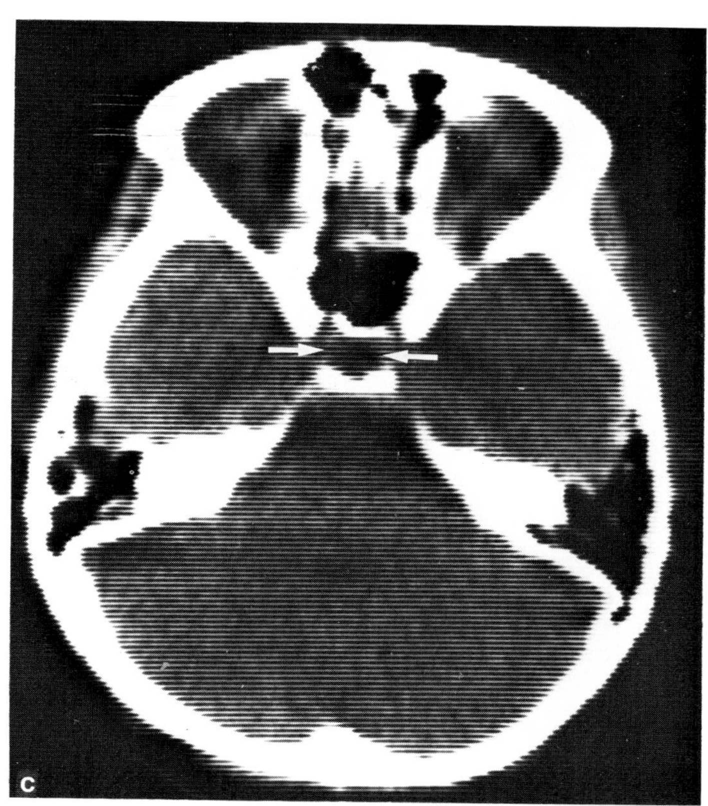
C

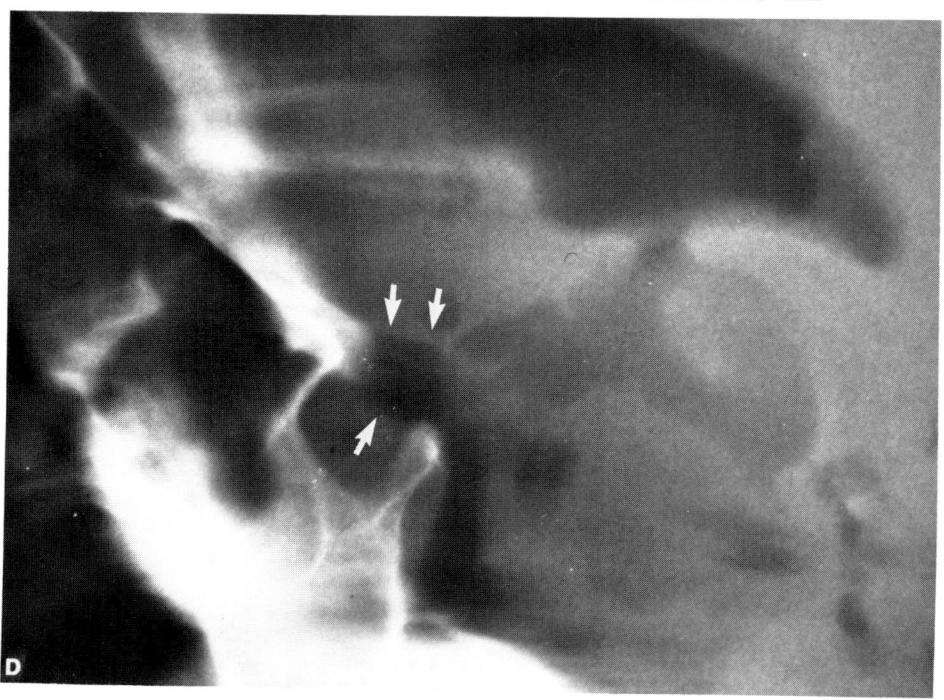
D

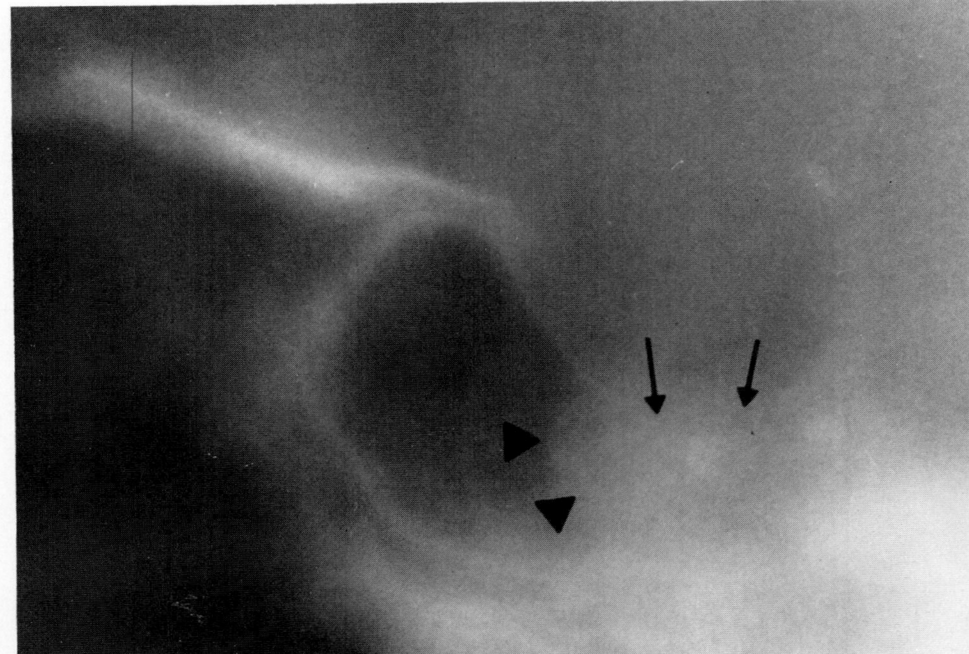

Fig. 8. Lateral tomogram. The sella is enlarged, and there is erosion of the floor of the sella (arrows) with a tumor mass (arrowheads) extending into the sphenoid sinus. Diagnosis: Prolactinoma with extension into sphenoid sinus.

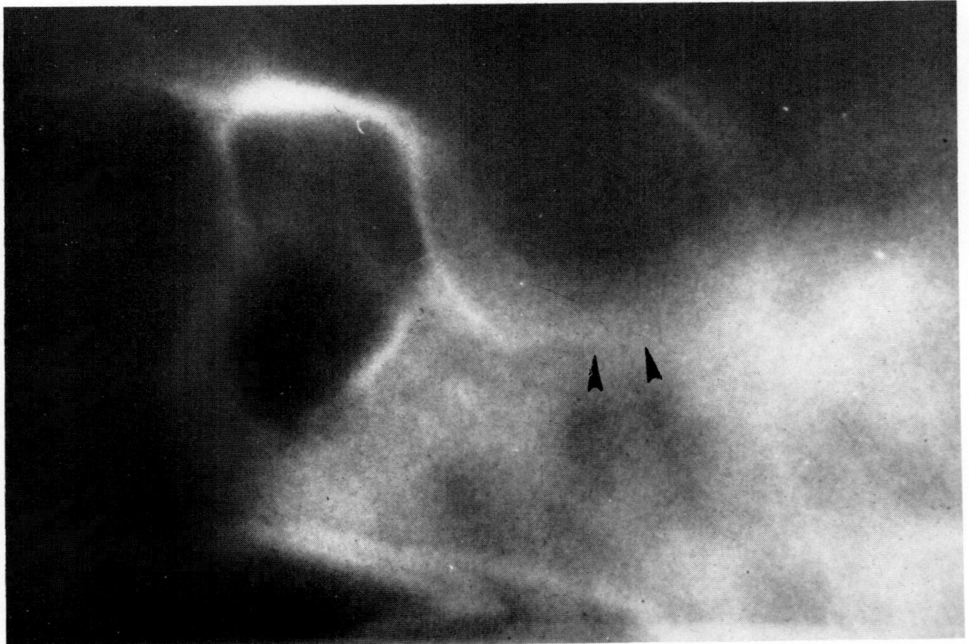

Fig. 9. Lateral tomogram. There is enlargement of the sella with erosion of the floor posteriorly (arrowheads). The sphenoid sinus is relatively poorly pneumatized (compare with Fig. 6A). Diagnosis: Pituitary adenoma with presphenoid type of pneumatization of sphenoid sinus.

since surgery. In 6 patients in Groups I and II and 2 in Group III, empty sellas were diagnosed by PEG.

Twenty-five patients are still suspected of harboring adenomas because of abnormal tomograms. None of these patients has been operated on. It is possible that some of these patients, particularly those with borderline abnormal sellas and normal serum prolactin levels, do not harbor adenomas. Long-term follow-up evaluations of the sellas and the serum prolactin levels will ultimately clarify this group.

In all 36 patients with tumors confirmed by surgery, tomography was abnormal. Similarly, others have found the incidence of tomographic abnormalities in patients with *surgically confirmed* hypersecreting pituitary tumors to be close to 100%.[8–10] Thus, in almost all cases, the patient with galactorrhea, elevated serum prolactin, and tomographic evidence of tumor can be assumed to be harboring an adenoma.

4.2. Value of Computed Tomography

Since the adenoma may extend through the diaphragma sellae into the suprasellar or parasellar cisterns even without a demonstrable visual-field defect and also since pituitary adenomas may coexist with an empty sella, further radiological investigations other than plain films and pluridirectional tomography are often necessary. Until recently, PEG with tomography was the preferred method of assessing supra- and parasellar extension and of diagnosing an empty sella (see Chapter 10, Fig. 17). However, with the advent of CT, PEG can, in many instances, be replaced by CT.[11–15] In our practice, we have come to rely increasingly on the CT scan (always including contrast enhancement), and air studies are seldom necessary. Sellar enlargement and erosion, necrotic and solid intrasellar tumors, empty sellas, and extension of tumors into the sphenoid sinus or suprasellar cisterns have all been detected by CT (Figs. 7 and 12–17).[14]

CT has been carried out in 94 of our 140 patients presenting with galactorrhea. Our CT technique is to overlap the scans to ensure that the sella and suprasellar cisterns are completely evaluated.* Abnormalities were found in 26 patients (28%) (Table 2).

The most frequent abnormality seen on the CT scan, a low-density area

* All scans were obtained with the Delta 50 Slow Scanner, utilizing the 13-mm collimator.

TABLE 2. Results of Computed Tomography in 94 Patients with Galactorrhea

Group	Number of patients	Low density	Sella enlarged	Tumor in sphenoid sinus	Suprasellar tumor	Intrasellar tumor	Normal
I	46	10	5	2	2	1	26
II	13	6	—	—	—	—	7
III	11	—	—	—	—	—	11
IV	24	—	—	—	—	—	24
TOTALS:	94	16	5	2	2	1	68

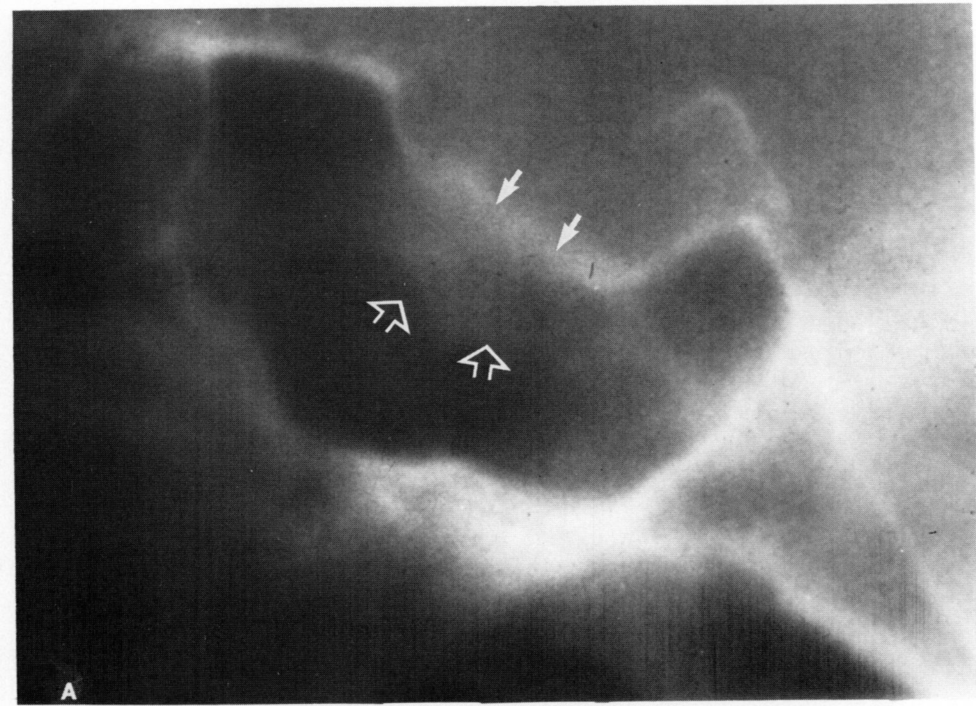

Fig. 10. (A) Lateral tomogram. In addition to enlargement of the sella, there is considerable erosion of the sellar floor (solid arrows) with a soft-tissue mass within the sphenoid sinus (open arrows). (B) Metrizamide CT cisternogram. A filling defect (arrows) is present in the opacified suprasellar cistern. Diagnosis: Pituitary adenoma with asymmetrical localization.

within the sella, was found in a total of 16 patients (Figs. 7 and 17). Since the scan thickness with our present scanner is 13 mm, for a low-density area to be called abnormal, the sella must have a height of at least 13 mm. If its height is less than 13 mm, any low-density area may be due to partial-volume averaging of the sella with the sphenoid sinus or suprasellar cistern. Suprasellar tumors were seen in only 2 of the 94 patients (both in Group I). CT also demonstrated an enlarged sella in 5 patients, a tumor within the sphenoid sinus in 2 patients, and an enhancing intrasellar tumor in one patient.

Since CT provides useful information only in patients with abnormal tomograms, we have discontinued carrying out CT scans in patients in Groups III and IV. However, when a scanner with thinner collimation becomes available to us, we will resume scanning this type of patient since it has been recently shown that intrasellar adenomas can be detected by thin section CT, probably even in Group III patients.[16]

4.3. Value of Pneumoencephalography

In 22 of the 94 patients who had CTs, PEG was carried out to expand on and elucidate the CT appearances. PEG was carried out in 12 of the 16 pa-

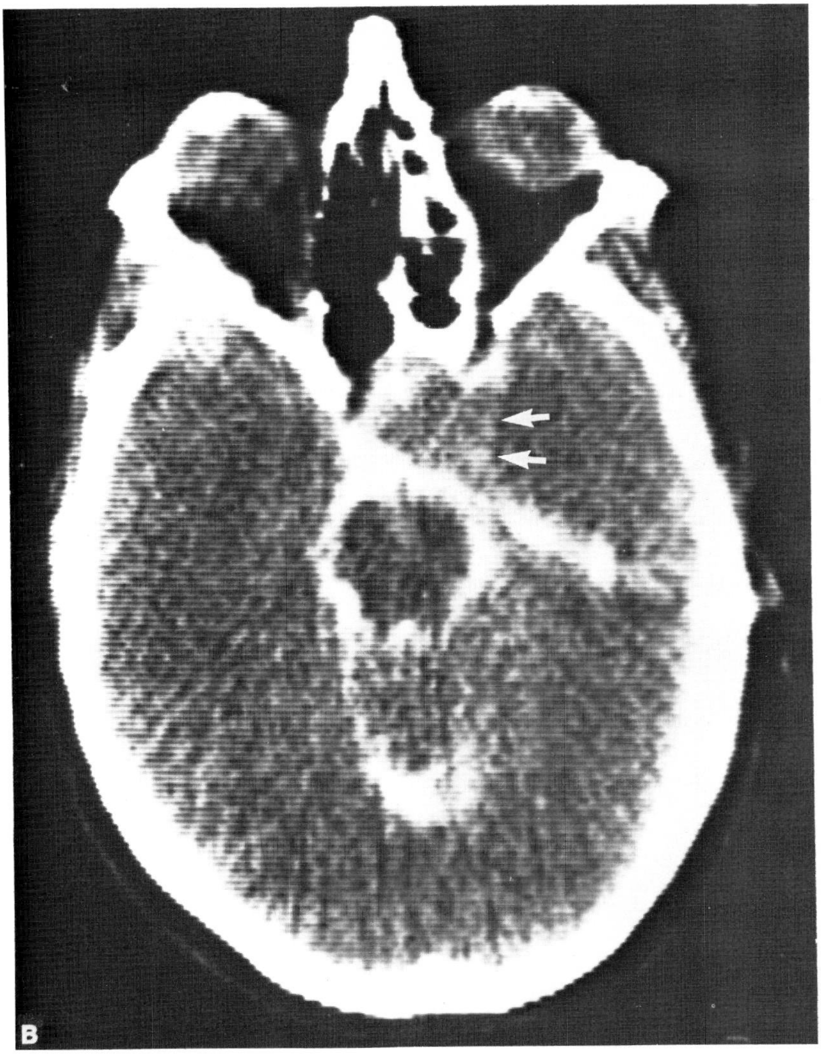

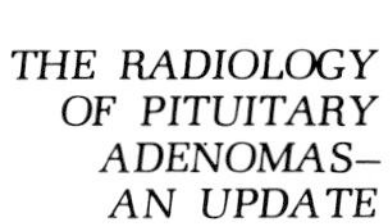

Fig. 10. *(continued)*

tients with low-density areas within the sella, with the anticipation of finding empty sellas (Table 3). Surprisingly, empty sellas were found in only 4 patients (see Chapter 10, Figs. 17 and 18). PEG was normal in 5 of the remaining 8 patients, and in 3 patients, suprasellar tumors were found.

Surgery carried out on the 4 patients (all in Group I) with normal PEGs revealed necrotic tumors in all. Thus, our data suggest that in a patient with galactorrhea and with a sella measuring at least 13 mm in height, a low-density area within the sella is as likely to be due to a necrotic tumor as to be due to an empty sella.[15] Furthermore, it has been shown that the empty sella and an adenoma are not mutually exclusive and can coexist[17] (see Chapter 10, Fig. 20).

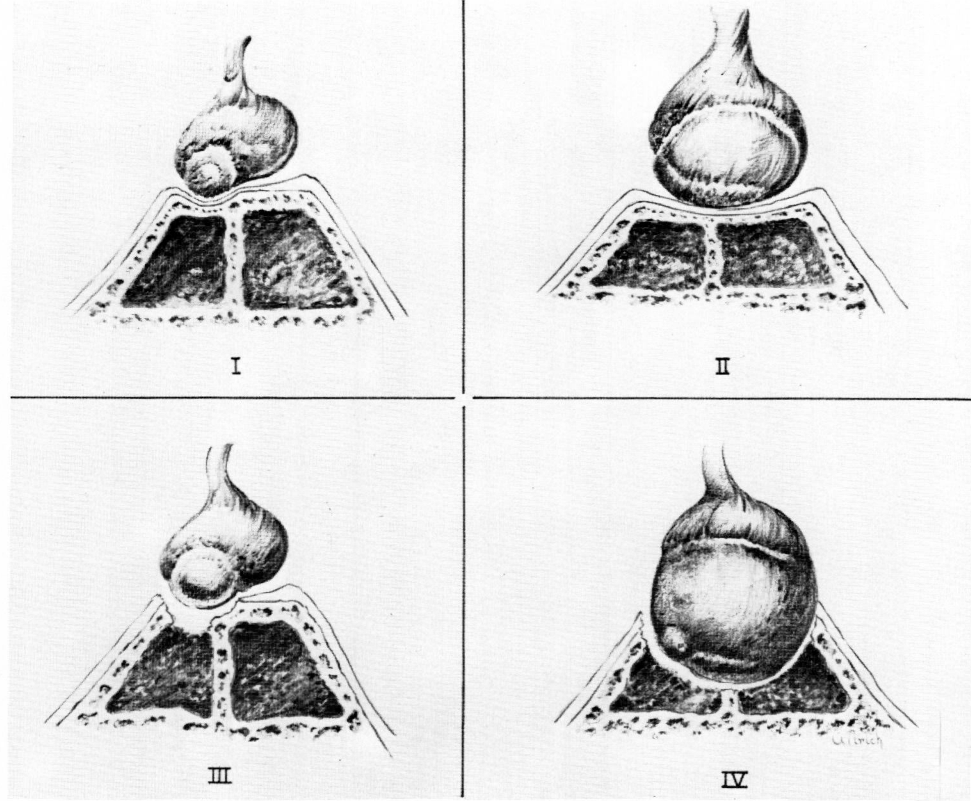

Fig. 11. Diagram demonstrating scheme for evaluating the extent of tumor growth. Grade I: focal bulging of sellar floor with no expansion. Grade II: diffuse bulging of sellar floor with sellar expansion. Grade III: focal erosion of sellar floor with no expansion. Grade IV: diffuse erosion of sellar floor with sellar expansion.

Empty sellas were also found by PEG in 4 other patients, 3 with normal CTs and 1 with an enlarged sella on CT. Of the remaining 6 patients who underwent PEG, in 4 both the CTs and PEGs were normal, in 1 patient the CT showed an enlarged sella with normal PEG, and in 1 patient both PEG and CT demonstrated a suprasellar tumor.

The role of PEG in our series has been to expand on the appearances of the CT scan—identifying the empty sella and delineating it from the necrotic tumor. In carrying out PEG, we endeavor to outline both the anterior third ventricle and the basal cisterns. Utilizing tomography, excellent detail of the suprasellar structures such as the interpeduncular, chiasmatic, and carotid cisterns, the supraclinoid carotid arteries, the optic chiasm, and the two anterior recesses of the third ventricle is obtainable (see Figs. 7D and 19). PEG also has a role in identifying small suprasellar tumors not seen on CT (Fig. 20). This occurred in 3 of our 140 patients with galactorrhea (all in Group I). Furthermore, identification of the optic chiasm is important if the patient is to undergo proton-beam therapy (Fig. 21).

The indications for PEG have been reduced yet further by the recent introduction of metrizamide CT cisternography.[18] The technique is to inject a water-soluble contrast agent, metrizamide, into the subarachnoid space via lumbar puncture and maneuver the contrast agent into the basal cisterns, which are then examined by CT (see Fig. 10B). Since the contrast resolution of CT is considerably greater than that of standard tomography, a dilute solution of metrizamide is adequate. Tumors not seen by standard CT scanning can be seen by metrizamide CT cisternography. The combined use of the newer thin-section collimators with metrizamide cisternography may completely eliminate pneumoencephalography, especially if coronal and sagittal CT images are obtained. Unfortunately, however, metrizamide CT cisternography delivers substantial radiation to the patient, and since the majority of these patients are young, this may constitute a health hazard that cannot be ignored.

It may be questioned whether it is necessary to demonstrate minor degrees of suprasellar extension of pituitary adenomas since, during transsphenoidal exploration, the degree of suprasellar tumor extension can be appreciated and that portion removed. If, initially, substantial suprasellar tumor is present, the CT scan will usually identify the tumor, and a decision as to a transsphenoidal or subfrontal approach can be made easily.

TABLE 3. Correlative Value of Pneumoencephalography and Computed Tomography

Group	CT[a]	Pneumoencephalography[a]	Follow-up
I	Low density	Slight SS extension	Necrotic adenoma
	Low density	Normal	Necrotic adenoma
	Low density	Normal	Necrotic adenoma
	Low density	Normal	Necrotic adenoma
	Low density	Slight SS extension	Craniopharyngioma
	Low density	Normal	Necrotic adenoma
	Low density	Empty sella	—
	Low density	Normal	Proton-beam therapy
	Low density	Slight SS extension	Negative exploration
	Enlarged sella	Normal	Adenoma
	SS tumor	SS tumor	Adenoma
	Normal	Normal	Proton-beam therapy
	Normal	Normal	Adenoma
	Normal	Normal	Adenoma
	Enlarged sella	Empty sella	—
	Normal	Empty sella	—
II	Low density	Empty sella	—
	Low density	Empty sella	—
	Low density	Empty sella	—
III	Normal	Normal	—
	Normal	Empty sella	—
	Normal	Empty sella	—

[a] (SS) Suprasellar.

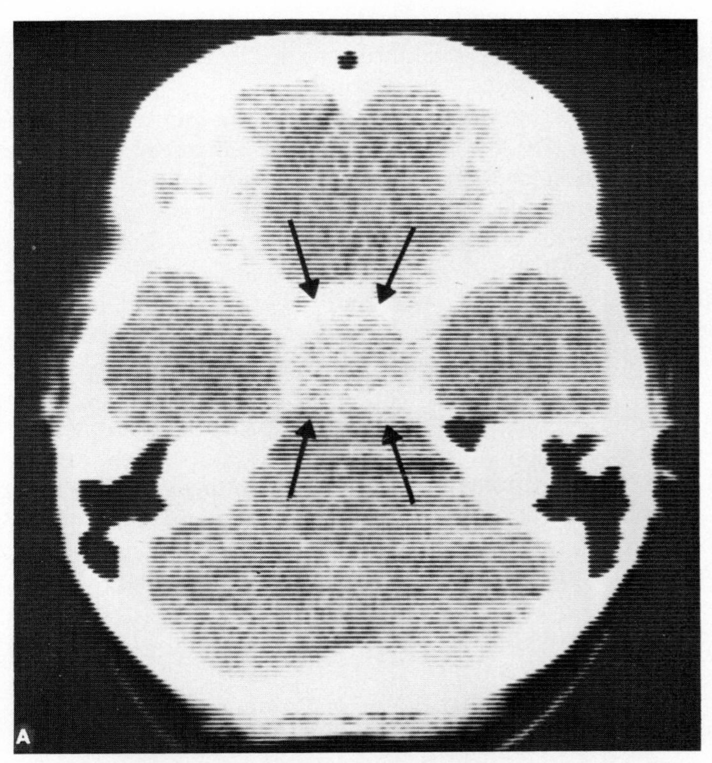

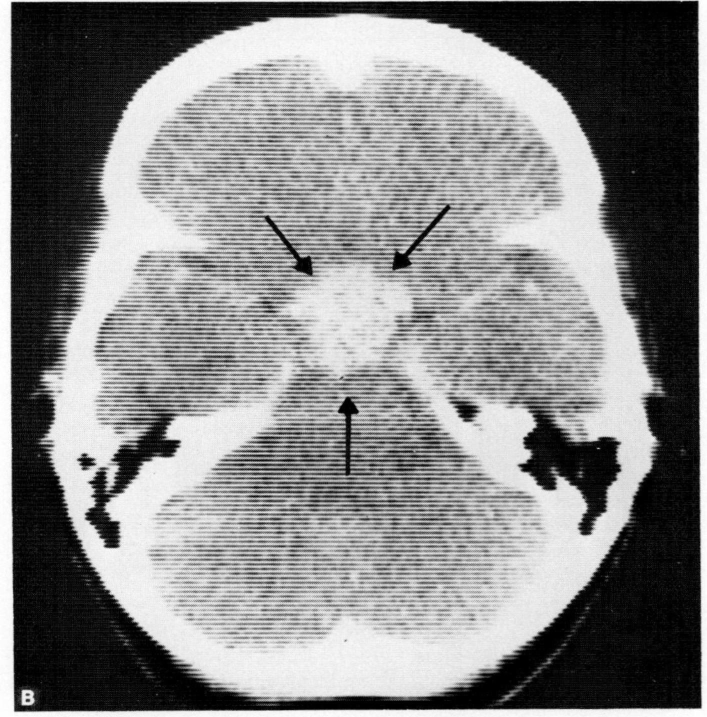

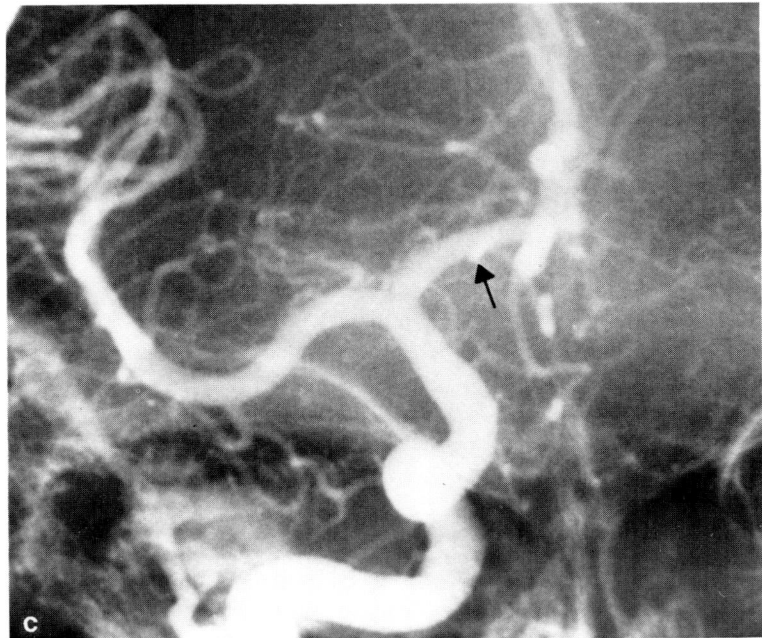

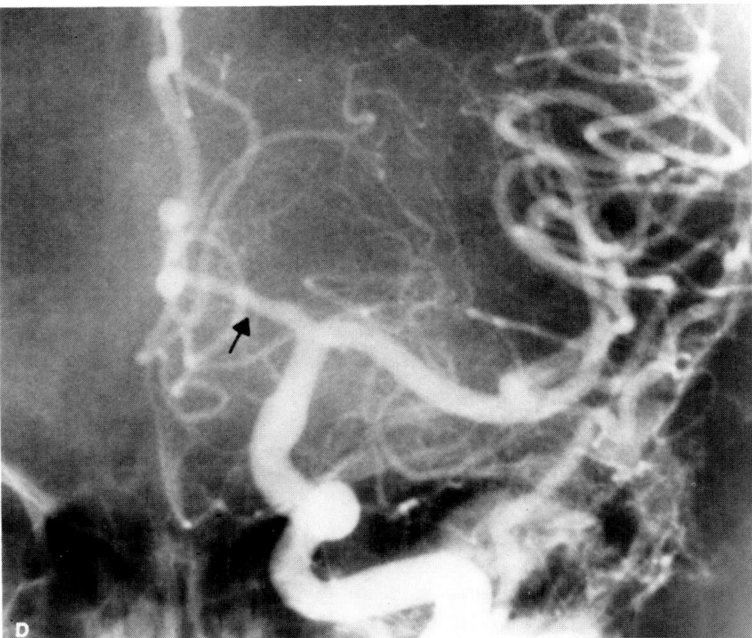

Fig. 12. (A) CT scan, contrast-enhanced. Note the enlargement of the sella turcica (arrows) with contrast-enhancing tumor within it. (B) Scan obtained 13 mm cephalad to Fig. 12A. A large suprasellar contrast-enhancing lesion (arrows) is seen. (C, D) Bilateral carotid angiogram demonstrating slight elevation of both proximal anterior cerebral arteries (arrows). Diagnosis: Pituitary adenoma.

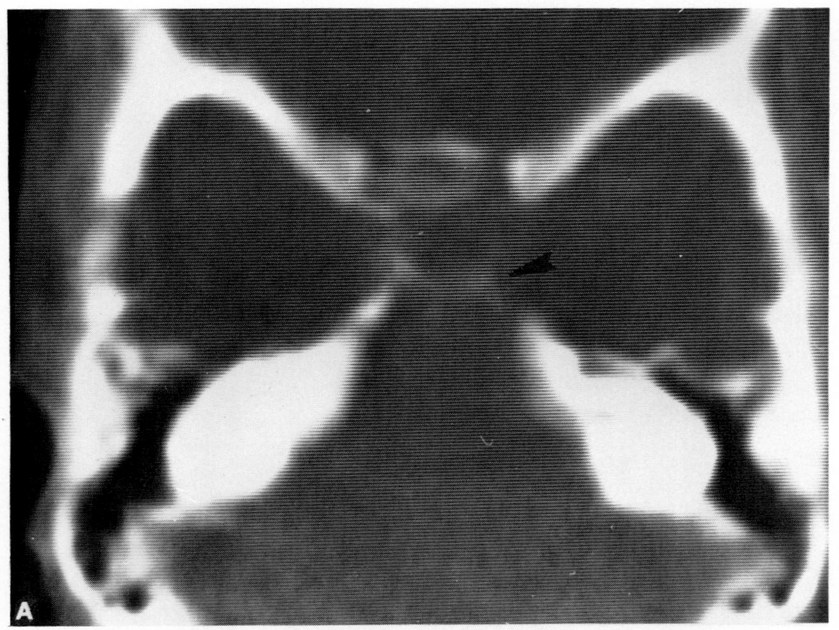

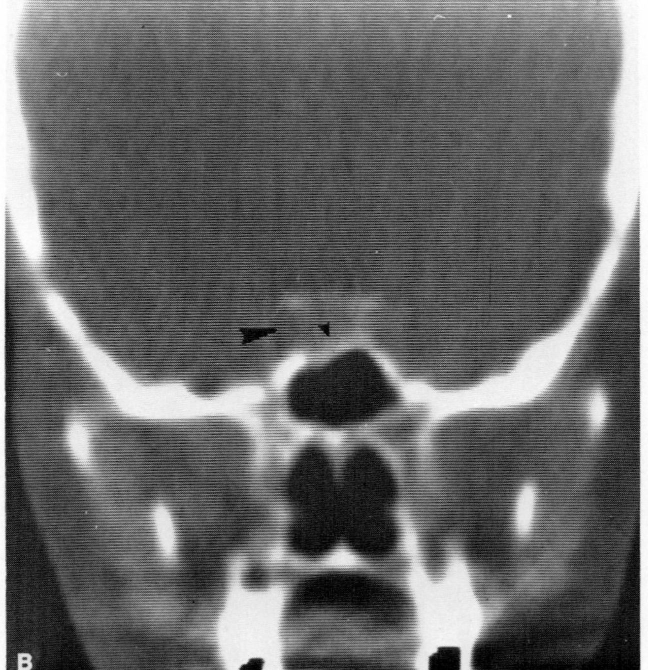

Fig. 13. (A) CT scan of the skull base demonstrating erosion of the lateral margin of the dorsum sellae (arrowhead). (B) Coronal plane CT scan demonstrating erosion of the lateral margin of the dorsum sellae (large arrowhead) and asymmetrical depression of the floor of the sella (small arrowhead). Reproduced from Wolpert *et al.*,[14] with the permission of *CT: The Journal of Computed Tomography*.

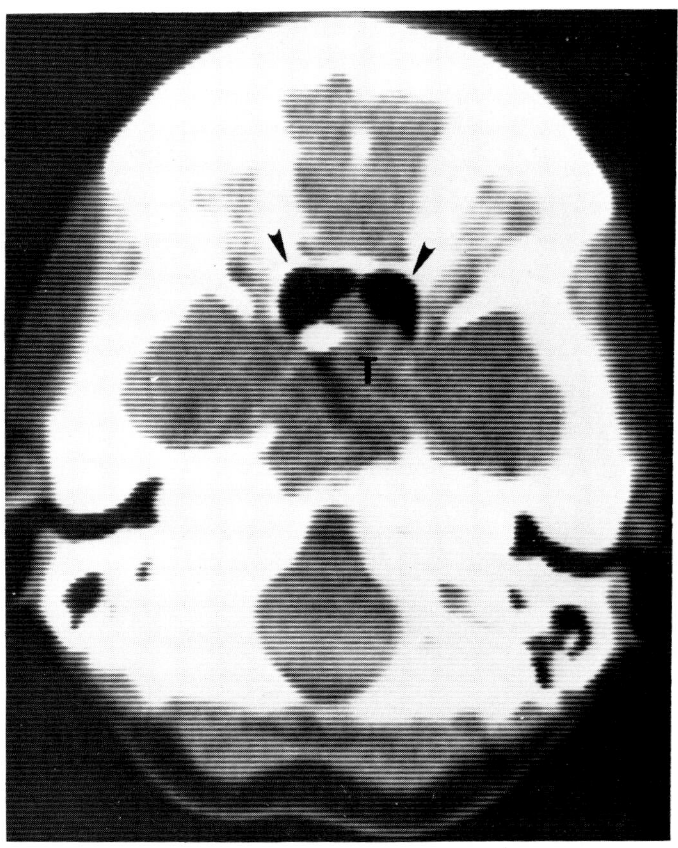

Fig. 14. CT scan of the skull base demonstrating a tumor (T) within the sphenoid sinus (arrowheads). Diagnosis: Pituitary adenoma. Reproduced from Wolpert *et al.*,[14] with the permission of *CT: The Journal of Computed Tomography.*

5. Radiological Investigation of Patients with Tumors Other Than Prolactinomas

Whereas prolactinomas causing galactorrhea (often accompanied by amenorrhea) have become recognized as a common clinical entity, many pituitary tumors may be nonsecretory or may secrete GH or ACTH. Overproduction of GH results in acromegaly with excessive growth of skeletal tissue and is manifested on the skull X-ray by thickening of the skull vault with increased bone density, enlargement of all paranasal sinuses, and proliferation of the mastoid air cells. The changes in the sella on tomography are identical to those seen with prolactinomas. When sella turcica enlargement and prognathism accompany the skull-vault changes, the diagnosis is easily established.

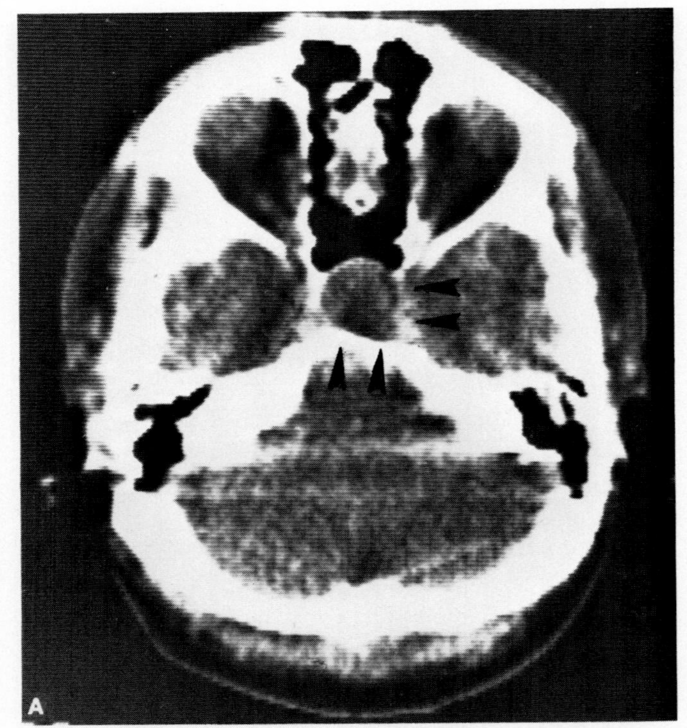
A

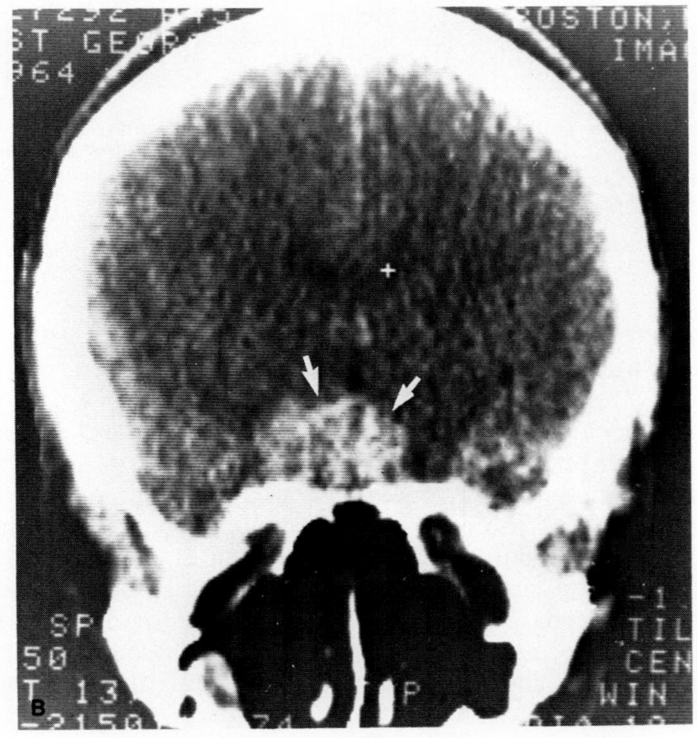
B

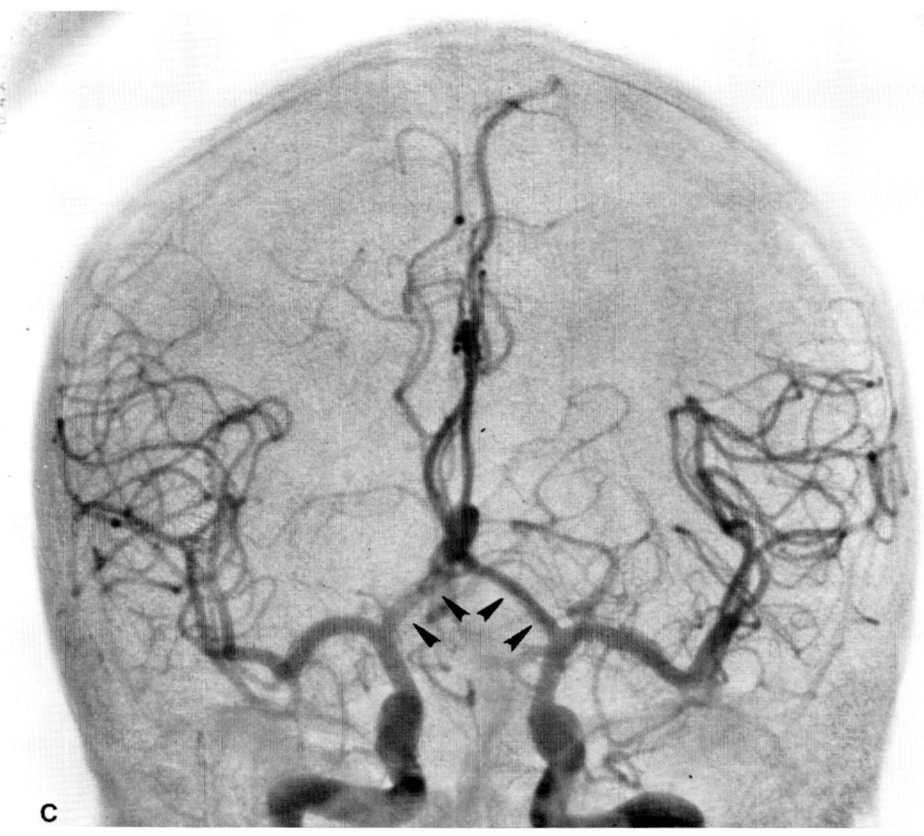

Fig. 15. (A) CT scan demonstrating asymmetrical enlargement of the sella turcica (arrowheads). (B) CT scan, coronal plane after contrast enhancement, demonstrating a vascular suprasellar tumor (arrows). (C) Carotid angiograms, arterial phases, superimposed subtraction films demonstrating elevation of both proximal anterior cerebral arteries (arrowheads). Diagnosis: Intrasellar adenoma with suprasellar extension.

Abnormal secretion of pituitary ACTH results in Cushing's disease. In 12 of 20 patients in one series, changes consistent with a microadenoma were seen on polytomography.[9] Similar changes have recently been described in patients with primary end-organ failure.[20]

When a nonfunctioning intra- or suprasellar tumor is suspected, the initial radiological workup should include plain films of the sella, pluridirectional sellar tomography, and CT. Further evaluation should always include angiography to exclude an aneurysm as a cause of the abnormal studies.

Spontaneous hemorrhage into large suprasellar tumors can occur and usually presents as a surgical emergency with acute headache, bilateral loss of vision, and ophthalmoplegia. CT can play a vital role in this entity by detecting on an unenhanced scan a high-density area within a suprasellar tumor (see Fig. 18).

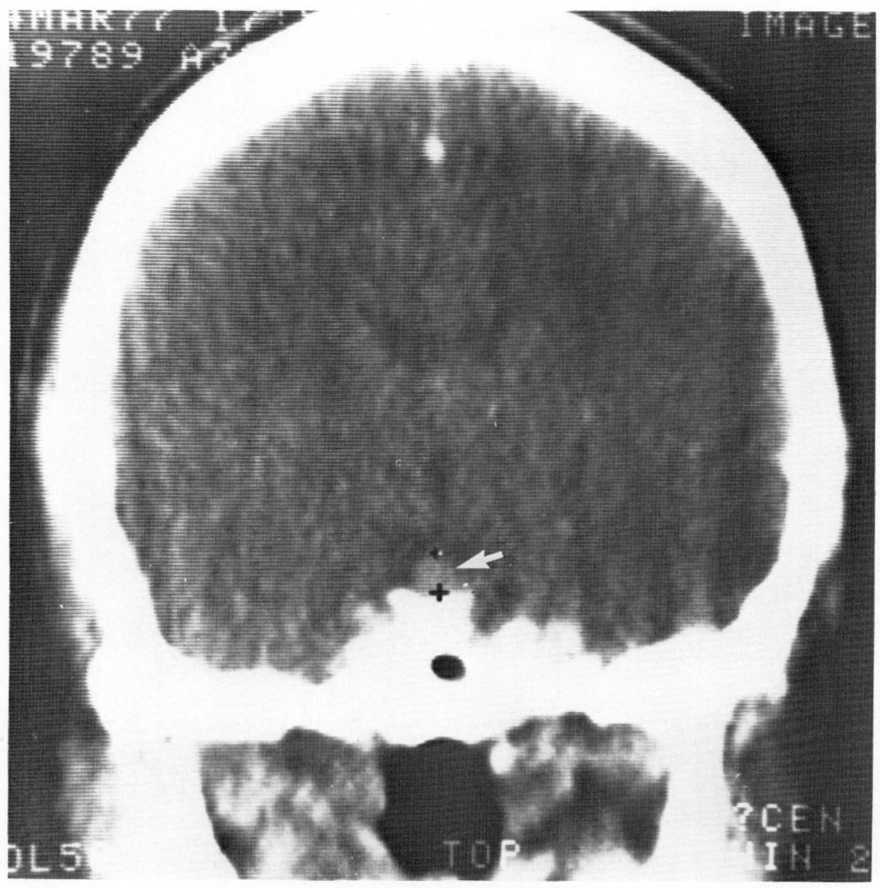

Fig. 16. CT scan, coronal plane after contrast enhancement, demonstrating a small (8 × 5 mm) suprasellar tumor (arrow). Diagnosis: Suprasellar adenoma.

5.1. Value of Angiography

The role of angiography in the evaluation of the patient with an enlarged sella is multifold. If a CT scan shows lateral extension of an adenoma, the cavernous carotid arteries are usually laterally displaced. The relationship of the tumor to the carotid arteries can then be of importance to the surgeon, particularly if a transsphenoidal approach is contemplated. With suprasellar extension of an adenoma, the terminal segments of the internal carotid arteries may be stretched and the proximal segments of the anterior cerebral arteries may be elevated (see Figs. 12 and 15). Magnification angiography of the sella has been used to demonstrate intrasellar and suprasellar tumors.[21] The pituitary gland is supplied by the meningohypophyseal and inferior hypophyseal branches of the internal carotid artery, and the enlargement of these vessels may be seen in patients with pituitary tumors (Fig. 22).

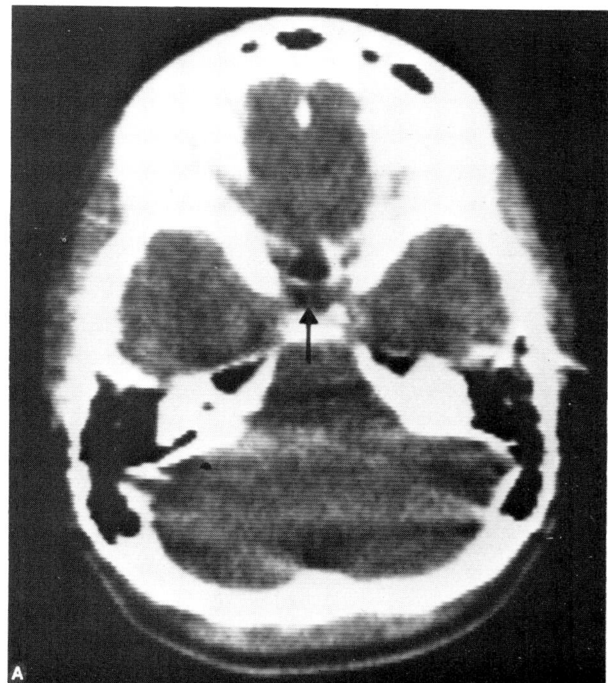

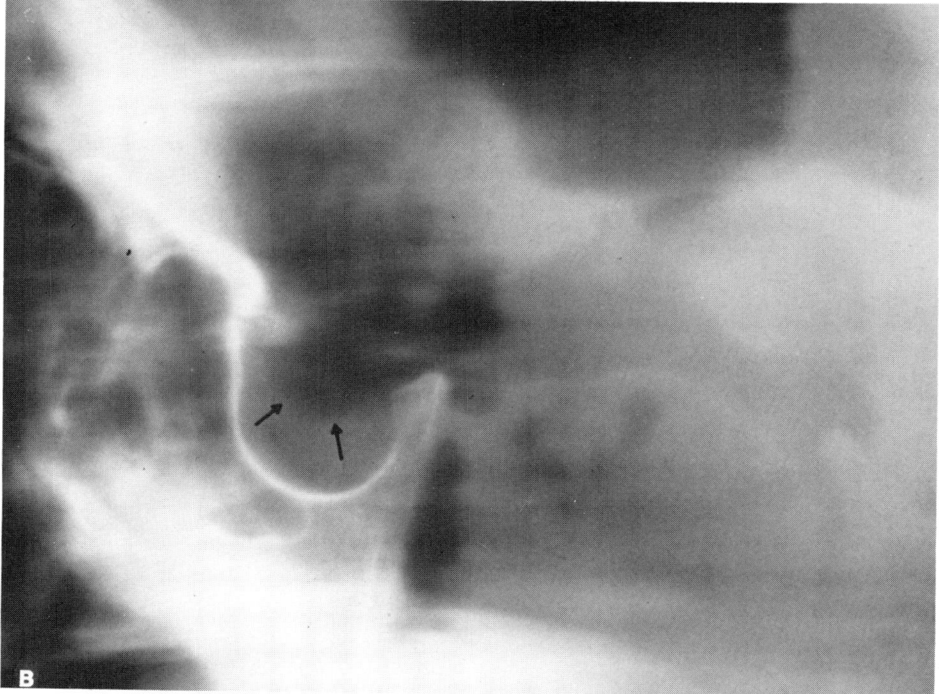

Fig. 17. (A) Nonenhanced CT scan. A low-density area (arrows) is present within the sella turcica. (B) Pneumoencephalogram, lateral tomogram. Air is seen extending into the sella turcica (arrows). Diagnosis: Empty sella.

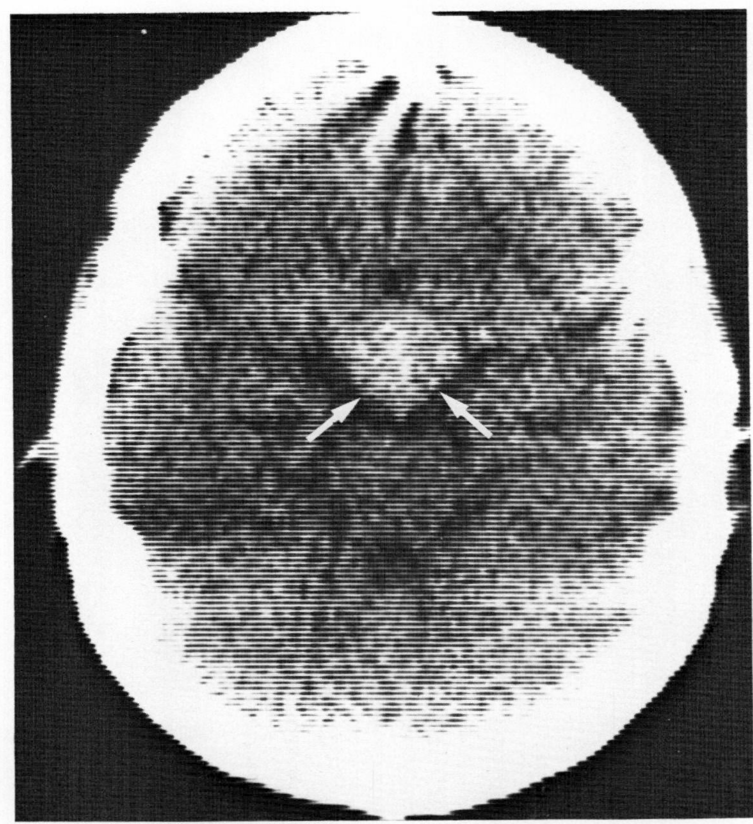

Fig. 18. CT scan, nonenhanced, in a patient presenting with an acute headache. Note the high-density lesion (arrows) indicating hemorrhage into a suprasellar tumor. Diagnosis: Hemorrhage into a suprasellar adenoma.

5.2. Differential Diagnosis of Pituitary Adenomas

Enlargement of the sella can be due to a meningioma originating from the diaphragma sellae, the planum sphenoidale, or the inner third of the lesser sphenoid wing. Enlargement, however, is unusual, and hyperostosis is seen more frequently and can be detected in 50% of the cases[22] (see Chapter 10, Fig. 10). Angiography can permit the specific diagnosis of a meningioma to be made. The tumors in these locations can envelop the carotid arteries and can also extend posteriorly into the pontine and cerebellopontine angle cisterns. While CT demonstrates such extension, vertebral angiography provides information about the precise displacement of the posterior cerebral arteries, the superior cerebellar arteries, the basilar artery, and the anterior inferior cerebellar arteries. On occasion, an adenoma may become invasive and may mimic the angiographic appearances of a meningioma. Whether true malignancy can occur in an adenoma has been questioned, and some workers consider that cellular pleomorphism and a few mitotic figures should not be equated with clinical malignancy.[23] It is better to characterize these tumors as "invasive."

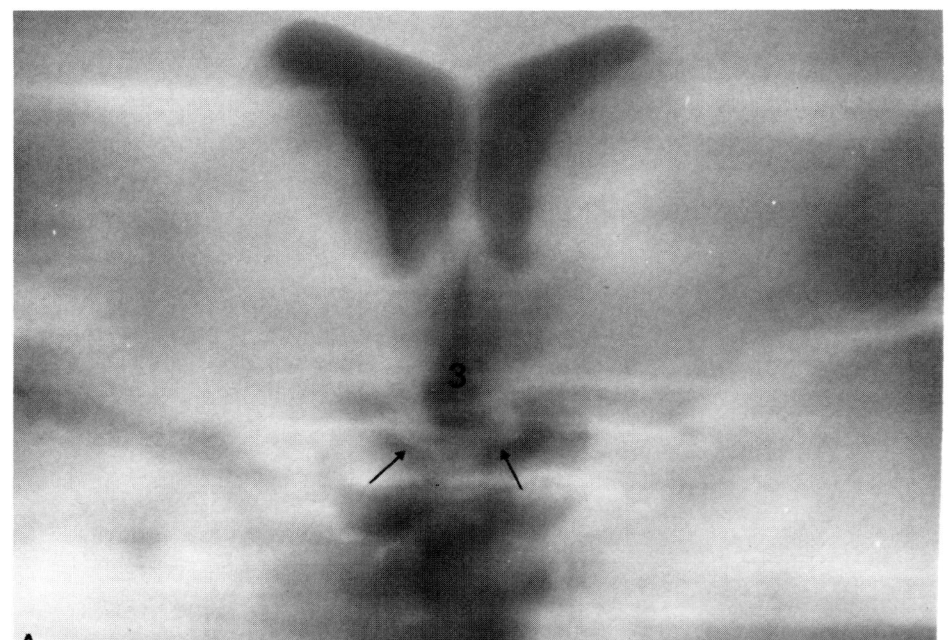

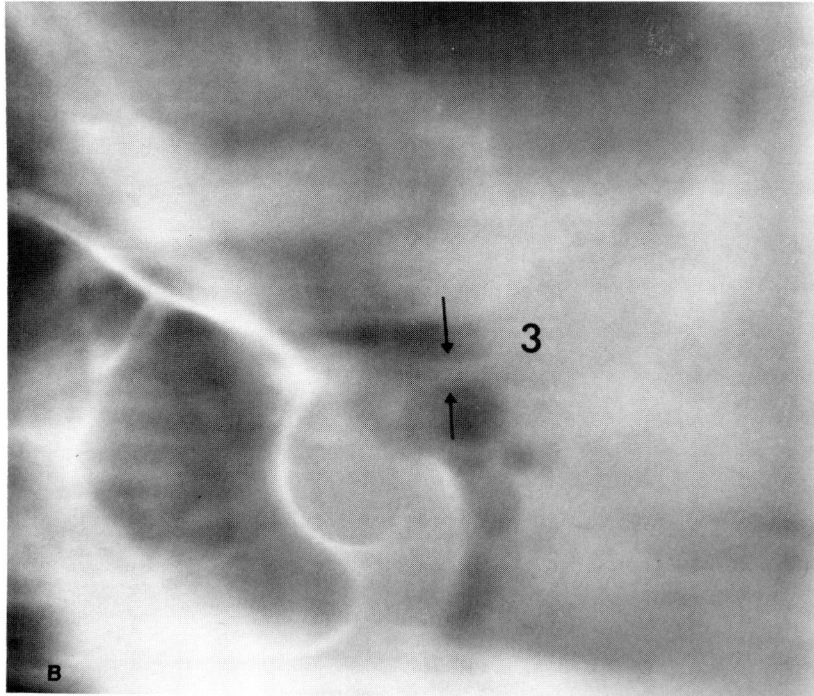

Fig. 19. (A) Pneumoencephalogram, frontal tomogram. Note the optic chiasm (arrowheads), the third ventricle (3), and the anterior horns. (B) Lateral projection. The optic chiasm (arrows) is outlined by air in the chiasmatic cistern. The anterior third ventricle is well defined.

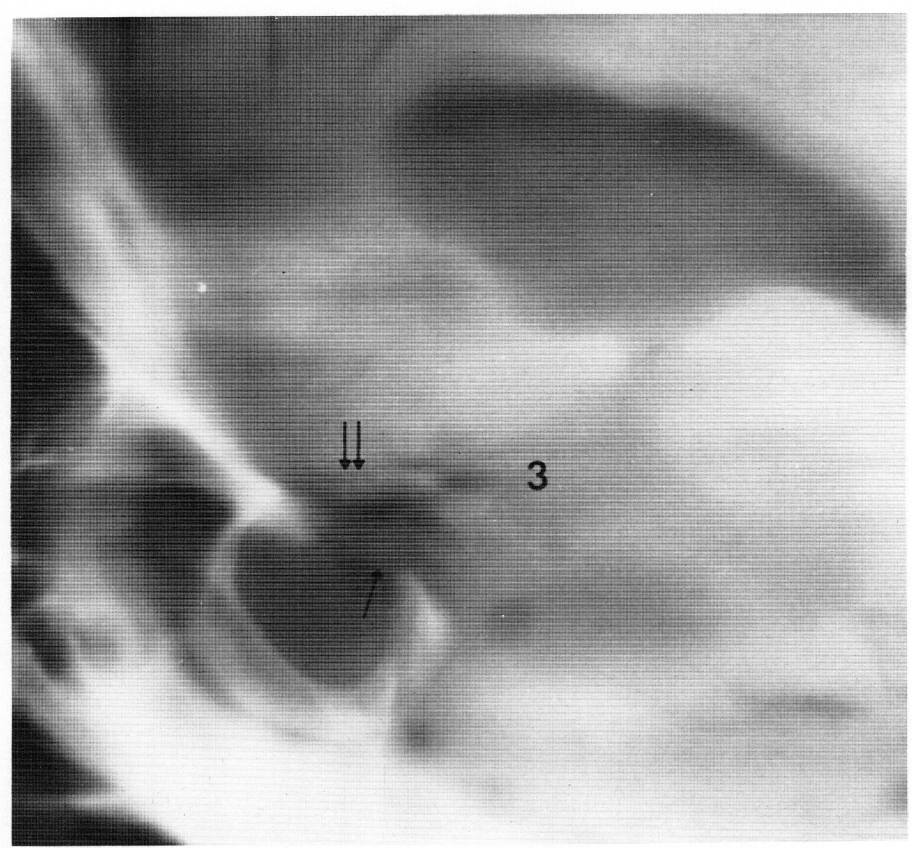

Fig. 20. Pneumoencephalogram, brow-up lateral tomogram. A soft-tissue density (single arrow) is seen immediately above the diaphragma sellae. The density is separate from the optic nerves (double arrows). Detail of this quality is difficult to obtain with thick-section CT. Diagnosis: Suprasellar adenoma.

Craniopharyngiomas in adults may have sellar changes; expansion, widening of the sellar outlet, and shortening of the dorsum are seen in 50% of the cases[24] (see Chapter 10, Figs. 2 and 4). At angiography, there are no specific features distinguishing a craniopharyngioma from an avascular adenoma. Suprasellar calcification, which is seen in 35% of adult and 80% of childhood craniopharyngiomas, can be detected by plain films, tomography, or CT and, if seen, suggests the correct diagnosis (see Chapter 10, Fig. 4). Calcification can also occur with meningiomas, pituitary adenomas (see Chapter 10, Fig. 1), and aneurysms. The incidence of calcification in these conditions is less than with craniopharyngiomas. Abnormal CT scans are not invariably found with craniopharyngiomas, even with large tumors.[25] If the clinical findings suggest progressive optic chiasm dysfunction and the CT scan is normal because the tumor is isodense with the brain and does not enhance after contrast-medium administration, PEG is recommended to define the tumor.

Enlargement of the sella associated with a suprasellar mass as seen on a

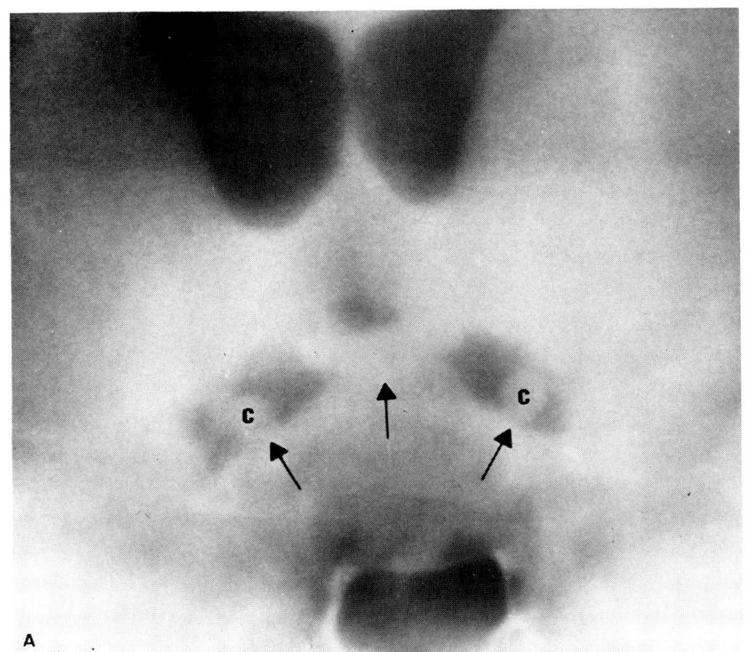

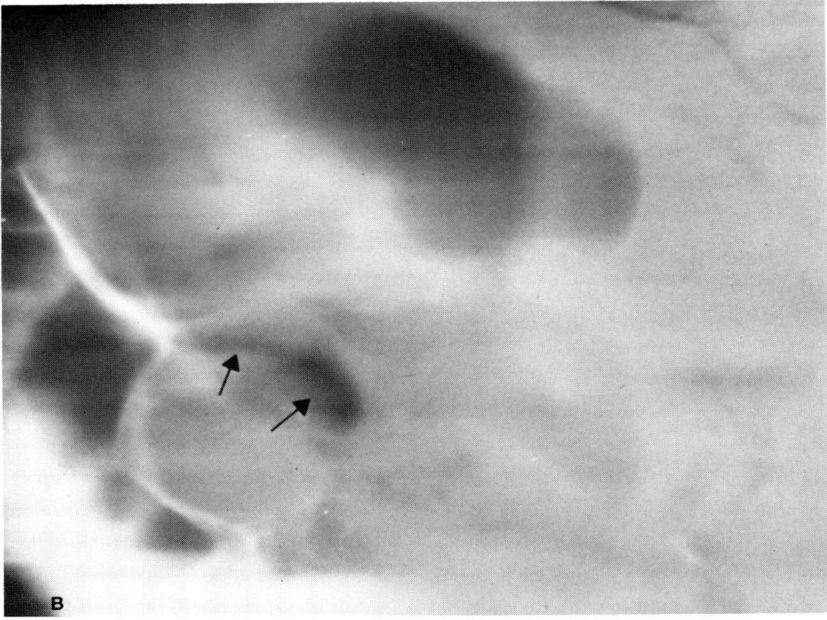

Fig. 21. (A) Pneumoencephalogram, frontal tomogram. A soft-tissue density (arrows) is seen elevating both carotid arteries (c) and the optic chiasm. (B) Lateral tomogram. The sella is enlarged. The soft-tissue density (arrows) is seen elevating the optic nerves. Diagnosis: Pituitary adenoma.

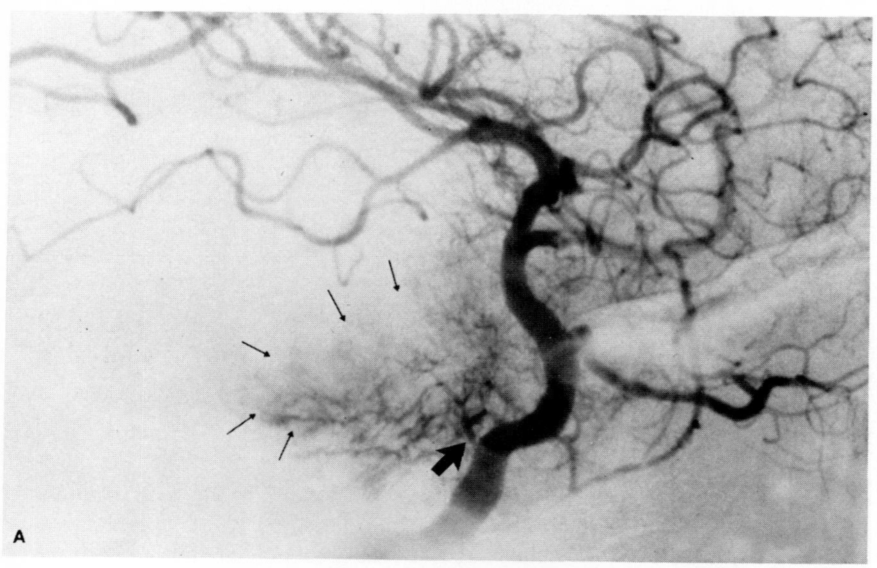

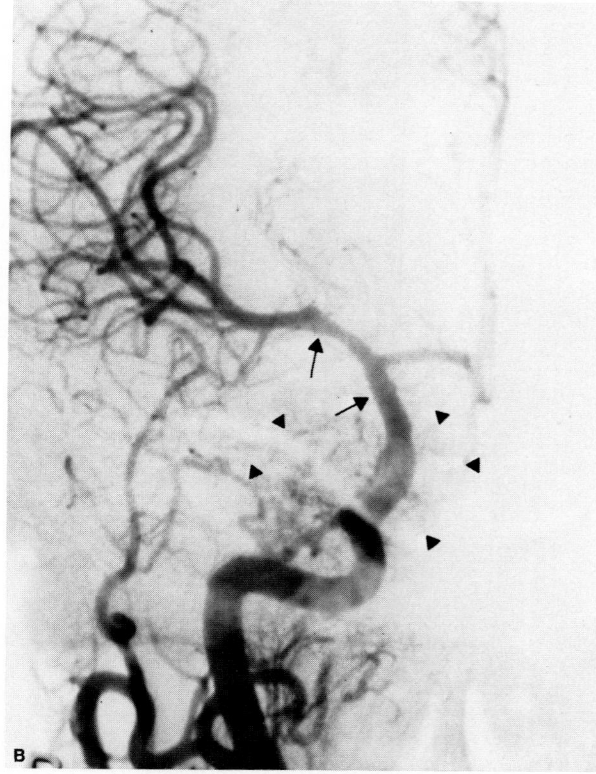

Fig. 22. (A) Right carotid angiogram, lateral projection. A meningohypophyseal artery (large arrow) is seen originating from the cavernous carotid artery and supplying a large vascular tumor (small arrows). The sylvian triangle is also elevated. (B) Frontal projection. Elevation and stretching of the proximal middle cerebral artery and terminal carotid artery (arrows) are seen. Again, note the tumor vascularity (arrowheads). Diagnosis: Vascular adenoma with parasellar and suprasellar extension.

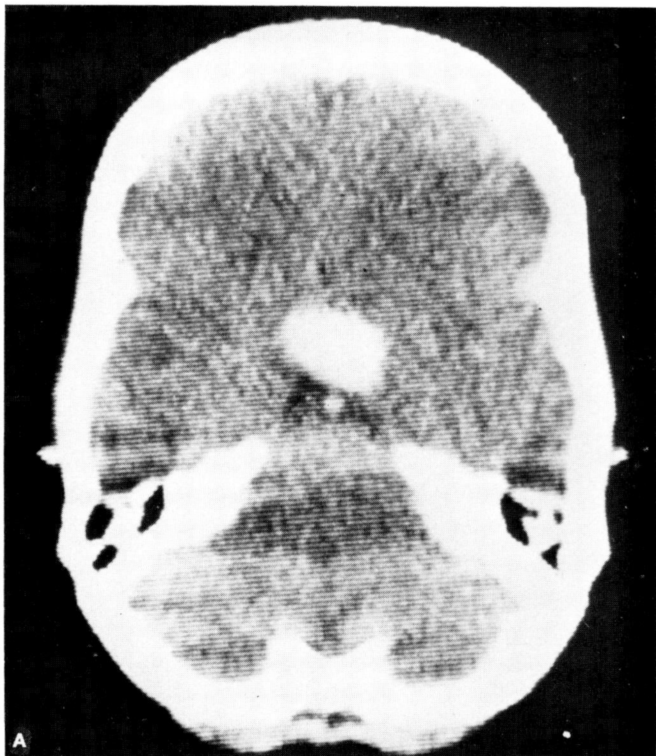

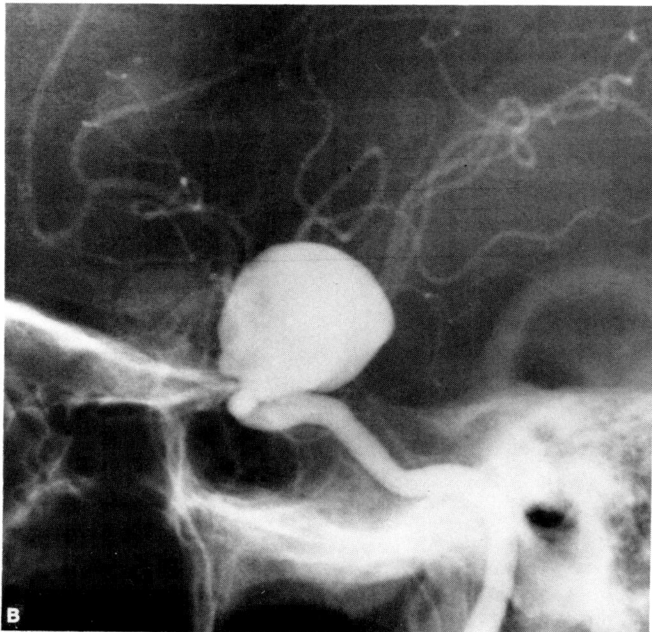

Fig. 23. (A) Contrast-enhanced CT scan demonstrating an enhancing suprasellar mass. (B) Left carotid angiogram demonstrating a large aneurysm originating from the terminal internal carotid artery.

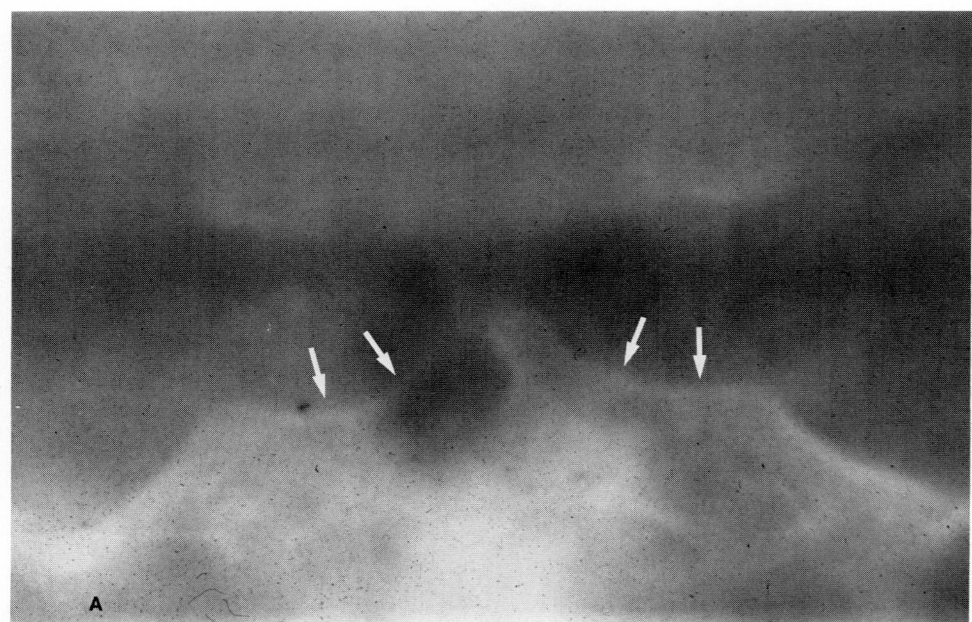

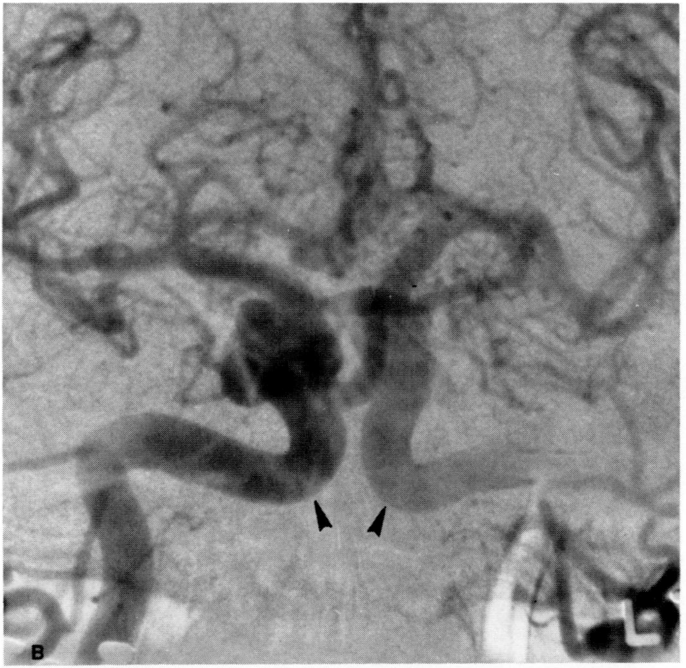

Fig. 24. (A) Tomogram of the sella, anteroposterior projection. Bilateral symmetrical erosions (arrows) of the sella are present. (B) Carotid angiograms, arterial phases, superimposed subtraction prints, demonstrating precavernous carotid arteries (arrowheads) abutting each other. Diagnosis: Ectatic carotid arteries. Reproduced from Wolpert *et al.*,[14] with the permission of *CT: The Journal of Computed Tomography*.

CT scan may also be due to an aneurysm of the carotid or basilar systems (Fig. 23). For this reason, angiography should be carried out in every case of a suprasellar mass diagnosed by CT, whether with or without demonstrable sellar abnormalities, unless the patient has an elevated GH or ACTH level or a significantly elevated serum prolactin level (>200 ng/ml). If there is anything unusual, however, about either the sellar changes (Fig. 24) or the character of the suprasellar CT appearance, particularly if curvilinear calcification is present, angiography should be performed.

References

1. S. Franks, H.S. Jacobs, and J.D.N. Nabarro, Studies of prolactin in pituitary disease, *J. Endocrinol.* **67**:55, 1977.
2. J.L. Antunes, E.M. Housepin, A.G. Frantz, D.A. Holub, R.M. Hui, P.W. Carmel, and D.O. Quest, Prolactin-secreting pituitary tumors, *Ann. Neurol.* **2**:148–153, 1977.
3. K.D. Post, B.J. Biller, L.S. Adelman, M.E. Molitch, S.M. Wolpert, and S. Reichlin, Results of selective transsphenoidal adenomectomy in women with galacterrhea–amenorrhea, *J. Am. Med. Assoc.* **242**:158–162, 1979.
4. P.H. Dubois, D.P. Orr, R.J. Hoy, D.L. Hebert, and E.R. Heinz, Normal sellar variations in frontal tomograms, *Radiology* **131**:105–110, 1979.
5. J.N. Bruneton, J.P. Drouillard, J.C. Sabatier, G.P. Elie, and J.F. Tavernier, Radiologic variants of the normal sella turcica, *Radiology* **131**:99–104, 1979.
6. R.B. Geehr, W.E. Allen, S.L.G. Rothman, and D.D. Spencer, Pluridirectional tomography in the evaluation of pituitary tumors, *Am. J. Roentgenol.* **130**:105–109, 1978.
7. H.A. Swanson and G. du Boulay, Borderline variants of the normal pituitary fossa, *Br. J. Radiol.* **48**:366–369, 1975.
8. J. Hardy, Transsphenoidal surgery of hypersecreting pituitary tumors, in: *Diagnosis and Treatment of Pituitary Tumors* (P.O. Kohler and G.T. Ross. eds.), pp. 183–185, Excerpta Medica, Amsterdam, 1973.
9. W.D. Robertson and T.H. Newton, Radiologic assessment of pituitary microadenomas, *Am. J. Roentgenol.* **131**:389–493, 1978.
10. D.L. Kleinberg, G.L. Noel, and A.G. Frantz, Galactorrhea: A study of 235 cases including 48 with pituitary tumors, *N. Engl. J. Med.* **296**:589–599, 1977.
11. C. Gyldensted and A. Karle, Computed tomography of intra- and justasellar lesions: A radiological study of 108 cases, *Neuroradiology* **14**:5–14, 1977.
12. R. Rozario, S.B. Hammerschlag, K.D. Post, S.M. Wolpert, and I. Jackson, Diagnosis of empty sella with CT scan, *Neuroradiology:* **13**:85–88, 1977.
13. N.E. Leeds and T.P. Naidich, Computerized tomography in the diagnosis of sella and parasellar lesions, *Semin. Roentgenol.* **12**: 121–136, 1977.
14. S.M. Wolpert, Computed tomography of the skull base in the coronal plane, *J. Comput. Tomogr.* **2**:31–37, 1978.
15. S.M. Wolpert, K.D. Post, B.J. Biller, and M.E. Molitch, The value of computed tomography in evaluating patients with prolactinomas, *Radiology* **131**(1):117–119, 1979.
16. A. Syvertsen, V.M. Haughton, A.L. Williams, and J. Cusick, The computed tomographic appearance of the normal pituitary gland and pituitary microadenomas, *Radiology* **133**:385–391, 1979.
17. M.E. Molitch, G.B. Hieshima, S. Marcovitz, I.M.D Jackson, and S.M. Wolpert, Coexisting primary empty sella syndrome and acromegaly, *Clin. Endocrinol.* **7**:261–263, 1977.
18. B.P. Drayer, A.E. Rosenbaum, J.S. Kennerdell, A.G. Robinson, W.O. Bank, and Z.L. Deeb, Computed tomographic diagnosis of suprasellar masses by intrathecal enhancement, *Radiology* **123**:339–344, 1977.
19. J.B. Tyrrell, R.M. Brooks, P.A. Fitzgerald, *et al.*, Cushing's disease: Selective trans-sphenoidal resection of pituitary microadenomas, *N. Engl. J. Med.* **298**:753–758, 1978.

20. J. Danziger, S. Wallace, and S. Handel, The sella tursica in primary end-organ failure, *Radiology* **131:**111–115, 1979.
21. D.F. Powell, H.L. Baker, Jr., and E.R. Laws, The primary angiographic findings in pituitary adenomas, *Radiology* **110:**589–595, 1974.
22. G. Di Chiro, and E. Lindgren, Bone changes in cases of suprasellar meningioma, *Acta Radiol.* **38:**133–138, 1952.
23. L.J. Rubinstein, *Tumors of The Central Nervous System,* Armed Forces Institute of Pathology, Washington, D.C., 1972.
24. M. Banna, Radiology, in: *Pituitary and Parapituitary Tumors* (J. Hankinson and M. Banna, eds.), pp. 135–136, W.B. Saunders, London, 1976.
25. B. Volpe, K.M. Foley, and J. Howieson, Normal CAT scans in craniopharyngioma, *Ann. Neurol.* **3:**87–89, 1978.

IV

Treatment of Pituitary Tumors

15

Medical Therapy of Pituitary Tumors

MARK E. MOLITCH

1. Introduction

Medical therapy of pituitary tumors is directed at decreasing the overall effects of the hormonal oversecretion of these tumors. With the possible exception of prolactinomas and growth-hormone-secreting adenomas, which may show morphological regression after treatment with dopamine agonists, there is no evidence that any form of medical therapy reduces the size of tumors. Therefore, medical therapy should be thought of as adjunctive, rather than definitive, therapy. Accordingly, there is no place for the medical therapy of "functionless" tumors except for the obvious hormonal replacements (hydrocortisone, thyroxine, gonadal steroids, vasopressin) that may be needed if the tumor, by its mass effects, causes hypopituitarism. Detailed testing of both functionless and functioning tumors should always be performed (see Chapter 11), especially after ablative therapy, so that proper hormone replacement can be given (see Chapter 20). This chapter will deal with the specific medical therapies that have been used to treat the hormonal syndromes that result from tumors secreting growth hormone (GH), adrenocroticotropic hormone (ACTH), and prolactin (PRL), i.e., acromegaly, Cushing's disease, and the galactorrhea–amenorrhea–impotence syndromes.

The basic concept underying the medical therapies attempted with these tumors is the fact that most pituitary adenomas (and most endocrine adenomas in general) are not completely autonomous. Many of these tumors respond to some of the same stimuli and suppressive agents to which normal pituitaries respond, although the responses may be quantitatively and even qualitatively different. Such responsiveness has been well shown for acromegaly,[1,2] Cushing's disease (see Chapter 7), and PRL secreting adenomas (see Chapter 4).

MARK E. MOLITCH • Tufts University School of Medicine; Department of Medicine, Division of Endocrinology, Tufts–New England Medical Center Hospital, Boston, Massachusetts 02111.

2. Growth Hormone and Acromegaly

The neurotransmitter and physiological regulation of GH secretion is quite complex and has been reviewed extensively.[3–5] Essentially, α adrenergic, dopaminergic, and serotoninergic pathways are stimulatory to GH secretion in the normal individual, while β-adrenergic stimulation is inhibitory. In acromegalics, however, although the responses to adrenergic and serotininergic stimuli are qualitatively normal,[6–8] the response to dopaminergic stimulation is opposite to that in normals; i.e., it is inhibitory.[9,10] Recent pharmacological approaches to the therapy of acromegaly have been primarily aimed at reducing GH secretion through dopaminergic stimulation.

In addition to trying to decrease GH secretion, other approaches have been to reduce the biological effectiveness of the high GH levels. Most of the actions of GH on the growth of bone cartilage and other tissues appear to be mediated through the GH-mediated generation of 7000-molecular-weight proteins known as somatomedins.[11,12] Reduction of the biological activity of the excessively secreted GH has been achieved with estrogens.

2.1. Dopamine Agonists

Boyd *et al.*[13] were the first to show that administration of L-dopa (a precursor of dopamine) resulted in a rise in GH in normals, but subsequently Liuzzi *et al.*[14] demonstrated that L-dopa had an inhibitory effect on GH secretion in acromegaly. However, in view of its short-lived action, L-dopa is not adequate therapy for this condition.[9] The dopaminergic agonist bromocriptine* was then shown to have a more prolonged action, GH levels remaining suppressed for 6–12 hr after a single dose.[15] The site of action of dopaminergic agonists appears to be at the pituitary and not the hypothalamic level in acromegalics, because dopamine, which does not cross the blood–brain barrier, is as effective as L-dopa in lowering GH levels in acromegalics.[16] Dopamine does not raise GH levels in normals, however,[16] thus indicating that in normals, the site of dopaminergic effects to raise GH is mediated at the hypothalamic level.[17]

Long-term studies have found bromcriptine to be effective in lowering GH levels in about 70–80% of acromegalics. The GH response is clearly dose-dependent, a dose of 7.5 mg/day being effective in only 1 of 8 patients in the series of Summers *et al.*[18] and a dose of 10 mg per day being effective in 7 of 12 patients in the series of Chiodini *et al.*,[19] but doses of up to 5 mg every 6 hr were effective in 58 of 73 patients in the series of Wass *et al.*[20] and in 19 of 21 in the series of Sachdev *et al.*[21] Occasionally, further reductions in GH were seen with doses higher than 20 mg/day.[20] In these last two series, the GH reductions were to less than 50% of basal levels in many patients who responded, the absolute level reached being a function of the basal level in most cases. Normal levels of GH were attained in only about 20% of cases. Al-

* This drug was released by the FDA on August 1, 1978, in the United States and is marketed by Sandoz, Inc., under the name Parlodel. As of this writing (October 1979), this drug has been approved for use only in the treatment of the galactorrhea–amenorrhea syndrome for short periods of time and is not approved for the treatment of acromegaly in this country.

though GH levels decreased immediately, the levels continued to decline over several weeks, with the maximum response seen at 8–12 weeks. Two patients in the series of Sachdev *et al.*[21] "escaped" partially at about 6 months; in one case, GH rose to pretreatment levels. Concomitant with a reduction in GH levels, there was an improvement in glucose tolerance, a reduction in soft-tissue volume including a decreased shoe and ring size, an improvement in facial features, and a decrease in sweating. Three more recent series of smaller numbers of patients also show similar results.[22–24] The only negative report with this drug has come from Dunn *et al.*,[25] who noted that only five of seven patients could tolerate the drug in 10 to 20-mg doses, clinical improvement occurred only in two, and significant GH reduction occurred in only one patient. Side effects of therapy have included nausea, constipation, depression, postural hypotension, and vasospasm. Recently, Wass *et al.*[26] have shown a reduction in tumor size in two patients treated with bromocriptine, suggesting that this drug may have antitumor activity as well.

We have recently had limited quantities of bromocriptine made available to us through the courtesy of Drs. Frank Cuellar and Richard Elton of Sandoz, Inc., for the treatment of acromegalics who still had elevated GH levels after pituitary surgery or irradiation or both. In five of six patients tested so far, a test dose of 2.5 mg bromocriptine resulted in marked falls in GH levels (Fig. 1). In the patient with the highest GH levels, the basal GH levels decreased to about one third of her pretreatment levels (Fig. 2), with no further decrement seen above 20 mg/day. Despite the failure of her GH levels to fall to normal, she has shown considerable clinical improvement with a decrease in appetite, perspiration, hand size, and foot size, and an improvement in facial features. One patient has had a similar clinical improvement on 10 mg/day, although his GH levels did not change on therapy (basal GH levels range between 7 and 15 ng/ml). It is difficult to explain this discrepancy except to hypothesize that in this patient, the radioimmunoassayable GH may not correspond to the bioactive GH. A similar discrepancy has been reported by others.[20] Werner *et al.*[22] have shown that in patients in whom bromocriptine induced a clinical

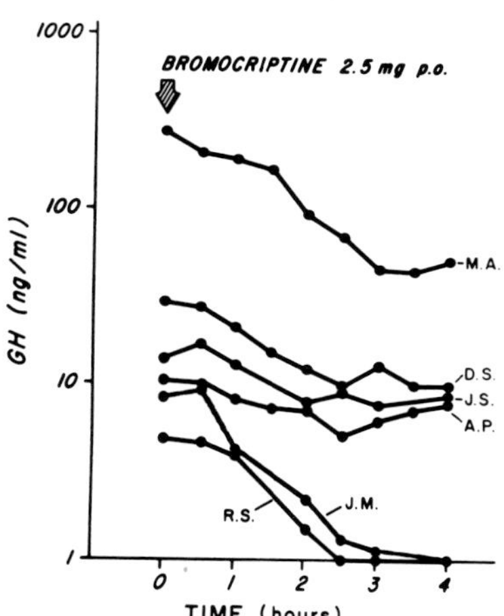

Fig. 1. Bromocriptine tolerance test. The GH response to a test dose of 2.5 mg bromocriptine is shown for six patients with acromegaly.

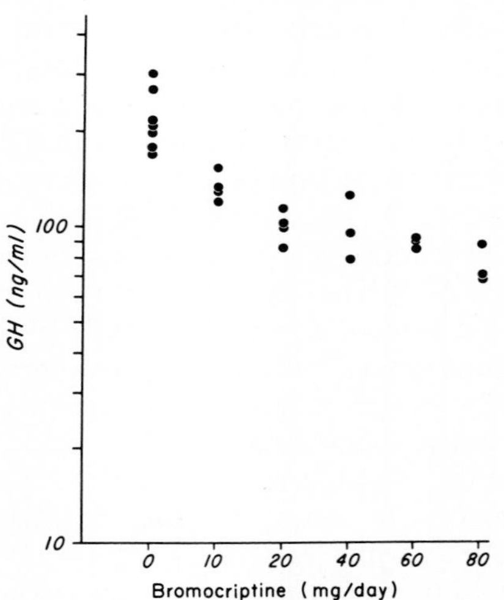

Fig. 2. Basal GH levels in an acromegalic patient being treated with varying doses of bromocriptine.

response but no decrease in plasma GH concentrations, there was significant decrease in somatomedin A as measured by a radioreceptor assay. We have not found a good correlation between somatomedin C levels and clinical response in our patients.[27]

Recently, the ergot lergotrile mesylate, which is also a dopamine agonist, has been found to be effective in six of nine patients with acromegaly.[28] This drug, however, has been withdrawn from further human studies because animal toxicity studies have shown an unacceptable incidence of genital tumors. Lysuride hydrogen maleate, a new ergot derivative, has also been shown to lower GH levels in acromegalics in preliminary studies.[29] In general, this class of drugs appears to be very useful in the treatment of acromegaly and is reasonably well tolerated. It is to be hoped that additional ergot derivatives will be developed that may have even more specific action.

2.2. Serotonin Antagonists

The serotonin antagonists cyproheptadine (Periactin®) and methysergide (Sansert®) have been shown to partially inhibit the normal GH elevation seen with such stimuli as hypoglycemia,[7,30] arginine,[31] and exercise.[30] The effects of serotonin antagonists on the sleep-induced rise in GH are controversial; methysergide has been shown to augment[32] and cyproheptadine has been shown to inhibit[33] the sleep-induced rise in GH. Recently, Feldman *et al.*[8] found that cyproheptadine administered for 2 days lowered plasma GH concentrations in four of six acromegalics and methysergide decreased plasma GH concentrations in one of four patients. Chiodini *et al.*,[34] however, found no effect of cyproheptadine given acutely in four acromegalics. A third drug, metergoline, which has been said to be a serotonin antagonist, has also been found to decrease GH levels in acromegalics.[35] However, Chiodini *et al.*[34] have found that the inhibitory effects of both metergoline and bromocriptine on GH in acromegalics can be blocked with pimozide, a specific dopamine-receptor blocker, suggesting that metergoline probably works through dopaminergic rather than serotonergic pathways. Although long-term data on the usefulness of serotonin antagonists in the therapy of acromegaly are not yet available, this group of agents may be another promising approach to the medical therapy of acromegaly. It is unlikely that cyproheptadine will be used for chronic therapy because the large doses required may cause an undesirable increase in appetite, and nearly all patients gain excessive weight.

2.3. Medroxyprogesterone Acetate

The progestational agent medroxyprogesterone acetate (MPA) (Provera®) was initially found to decrease the GH response to such stimuli as hypoglycemia and arginine in normals.[36] In 1970, Lawrence and Kirsteins[37] reported that oral MPA in a dose of 40 mg daily in divided doses resulted in decreased basal GH levels in 10 of 12 acromegalics and in arginine-stimulated GH levels of 9 of 11 of these acromegalics. Long-term follow-up showed improvement of soft-tissue volume, decreased perspiration, and decreased headaches associated with reduction in GH levels in 7 of 10 patients treated for 1–38 months.[38] Unfortunately, many subsequent studies showed that MPA was useful in only a small number of patients; in six separate series, only 8 of a total of 48 patients responded with sustained decrements of GH.[39–44] At present, it seems reasonable to offer a trial of MPA to patients who have not completely responded to ablative therapy and who do not have access to or do not respond to bromocriptine, although the success rate with this drug is only on the order of 10–20%.

2.4. Estrogens

Estrogen therapy has been known for many years to ameliorate many of the clinical features of acromegaly. Detailed studies by Schwartz *et al.*[45] showed that although estrogen therapy did not affect circulating GH levels, it did result in a reduction in urinary calcium and hydroxyproline and a reduction in serum phosphorous. Subsequent work by these investigators has shown that these apparently beneficial clinical effects are due to interference with GH-mediated somatomedin generation by the liver.[46,47] In current practice, estrogens are used infrequently in the management of acromegaly. They would be used only as a last resort in patients who had received maximal attempts at ablative therapy and who did not respond hormonally and clinically to bromocriptine or even MPA. Caution should be used in their administration because of the many known side effects of estrogens in women,[48] the increased cardiovascular risk associated with estrogens in men,[49] and the possibility that estrogen use may predispose to apolexy of pituitary tumors.

2.5. Other Agents

Chlorpromazine was initially shown by Kolodny *et al.*[44] to be effective in reducing GH levels and improving clinical symptoms in one acromegalic patient. However, in a study of eight patients by Dimond *et al.*,[50] GH decreased only modestly in two patients, and there was no clinical improvement in any of the eight with 3–6 months of therapy with chlorpromazine. Similarly, no effect was seen on GH secretion in five patients with acromegaly treated with chlorpromazine by Alford *et al.*[51] At present, it does not seem to be useful in the therapy of acromegaly.

The hypothalamic hormone somatostatin, which is capable of inhibiting GH, thyroid-stimulating hormone (TSH), and other nonpituitary hormones in normals, is also capable of inhibiting GH secretion in acromegaly.[52–54] Because of these effects on hormones other than GH and because of the very short biological half-life of injected somatostatin, various analogues have been synthesized to provide specificity and longer duration of action. Although some success has been achieved along these lines,[55,56] the use of somatostatin for the treatment of acromegaly is still only a possibility for the future.

3. Cushing's Disease

As in acromegaly, the medical therapy of Cushing's disease should be regarded as second-line therapy compared to ablative therapy of the pituitary or adrenals. Medical therapy is clearly indicated in at least five situations; (1) in the pre-operative period when a decrease in hypercortisolism for a number of weeks to months may enable the patient to tolerate surgery better; (2) in patients too old or ill to undergo surgery; (3) in patients not cured by pituitary ablation and who cannot tolerate adrenalectomy; (4) as an adjunct to pituitary ablative therapy in patients who after adrenalectomy develop increased ACTH secretion and an increase in the size of a pituitary tumor (Nelson's syndrome); and (5) as adjunctive therapy to suppress hormone secretion while awaiting the effects of pituitary irradiation. Obviously, therapy for each patient must be individualized, and there may well be other specific indications for medical therapy, but these are less clearly defined.

The neurotransmitter regulation of corticotropin-releasing factor (CRF)-mediated ACTH secretion is less well understood than that for GH secretion. α-Adrenergic stimulation and β-adrenergic blockade result in a rise in ACTH. Serotonergic and cholinergic pathways also appear to be stimulatory to ACTH secretion.[57] As discussed earlier (see Chapter 7), although the secretion of ACTH is abnormally high in this disease, it is not completely unresponsive to neurotransmitter alteration or exogenous steroids. In recent years, several agents have been employed in Cushing's disease to decrease either ACTH secretion by alteration of this neurotransmitter regulation or corticosteroid secretion by blocking of the synthesis of these steroids within the adrenal cortex.

3.1. Antiserotonin Agents

In normal subjects, the serotonin antagonist cyproheptadine (Periactin®) has been found to block the rise in ACTH induced both by hypoglycemia and by metyrapone, which interferes with cortisol synthesis in the adrenal cortex at the 11-hydroxylation step.[58,59] In 1975, Krieger *et al.*[60] reported the successful use of cyproheptadine in the treatment of three patients with Cushing's disease with normal sella turcicas. A dose of 24 mg/day of this drug resulted in a normalization of cortisol and ACTH levels and clinical remission in all three cases. Discontinuation of the cyproheptadine resulted in the return of cortisol levels to pretreatment levels within 1 month in one case. Subsequently, many letters to the editors of the *New England Journal of Medicine* and *The Lancet* reported both successes and failures of this agent; Dr. Krieger's informal registry of such cases found that as of mid-1978, about 60% of 80 cases of Cushing's disease treated with cyproheptadine responded successfully.[61] Our own experience with the prolonged use of cyproheptadine at a 24 mg/day dosage in a patient with Cushing's disease was unsuccessful. Cyproheptadine has also been found to be successful in lowering ACTH levels in some cases of Nelson's syndrome.[61–63] Unfortunately, relapses occur in all patients when treatment is discontinued.

Metergoline, an ergot derivative with antiserotinergic and antidopaminergic activity, has also been found to lower ACTH levels in normals and patients with Addison's disease.[64] In Cushing's disease, however, it has been successful in lowering ACTH and cortisol levels in only one or two cases reported thus far.[64,65]

3.2. Bromocriptine

Only preliminary studies have been performed with this drug. These have shown an initial decrease in ACTH levels in seven of eight patients with Cushing's disease and in one patient with Nelson's syndrome with a test dose of 2.5 mg.[66,67] A similar test dose of 2.5 mg bromocriptine in one of our patients with Nelson's syndrome resulted in no change in ACTH levels. Longer-term usage of this drug alone in patients with Cushing's disease has given variable results in the few patients so treated thus far.[68,69]

3.3. Adrenolytic Therapy

The drug mitotane (*o,p'*-DDD) (Lysodren®) has been used for over 15 years in the therapy of adrenal carcinoma and appears to cause selective destruction of the zona fasciculata and zona reticularis of the adrenal cortex.[70] Low-dose (3 g/day) therapy with mitotane for Cushing's disease has been used since the 1960's. Four patients were successfully treated by Temple *et al.*[71] with doses of 3 g/day; two of these patients were eventually able to stop the drug. In a recent larger series, Schteingart *et al.*[72] have found that of 18 patients, 14 achieved normal cortisol levels, 3 were improved, and 1 did not improve with a 4 g/day initial dose and 0.5–2.0 g maintenance dose. Six of the 18 patients were maintained in remission off the mitotane. Recently, Luton *et al.*[73] achieved excellent results in 63% of 62 patients with an initial dose of 12 g/day and a maintenance dose of 8 g/day. In all of these series, the dose of mitotane was tolerated quite well with little in the way of side effects. Therefore, this drug would appear to have many advantages in therapy if speed of reduction of hypercortisolism is not an issue, since the response time varied from 2 to 12 months.

Aminoglutethimide is known to interfere with an early step in steroidogenesis, the conversion of cholesterol to pregnenolone.[74] A recent review of

33 cases of Cushing's disease in the literature treated with this drug[75] found that 42% of patients had both biochemical and clinical improvement, 15% had only biochemical improvement, and 42% showed no improvement. Side effects included sedation, rash, nausea, headaches, and malaise, but usually were tolerable.[75] A decrease in aldosterone secretion was also seen in some patients, but it was not of clinical significance.[76]

The 11-hydroxylase inhibitor metyrapone, commonly used as a diagnostic agent in the evaluation of the hypothalamic–pituitary–adrenal axis, has been employed chronically to decrease cortisol levels in Cushing's disease. Jeffcoate *et al.*[77] have treated 13 patients for 2–66 months with 0.5–4.0 g/day of metyrapone with biochemical and clinical success in all patients. Concomitant irradiation to the pituitary was administered to 9 patients, and in the others, 1 had a bilateral adrenalectomy, 1 had a transfrontal hypophysectomy, and 1 had had a partial pituitary infarction prior to starting the drug. Although ACTH levels rose with metyrapone in these patients, none "escaped" clinically or biochemically. Five irradiated patients were subsequently withdrawn from the metyrapone with resulting continued remission. The major side effect of the therapy was hirsutism and acne that was mild in most cases. Thus, metyrapone may also prove to be useful in the adjunctive therapy of Cushing's disease. Finally, combinations of these drugs may prove to be beneficial in certain patients.[78]

4. Prolactin Hypersecretion

PRL secretion is regulated by PRL-inhibitory factor(s) (PIF), one of which is dopamine, and by PRL-releasing factor(s) (PRF), one of which is thyrotropin-releasing hormone (TRH). The inhibitory component for PRL, unlike that for the other pituitary hormones, dominates over the releasing component.[57] Dopaminergic stimulation therefore results in a decrease in PRL secretion, while dopamine-receptor blockers (e.g., phenothiazines, haloperidol, pimozide) result in increased PRL secretion.[79] Serotonergic stimulation results in increased PRL secretion.[80] The roles of adrenergic pathways in the regulation of PRL secretion are not clear.[81]

The state of hyperprolactinemia is usually associated with reproductive dysfunction or galactorrhea or both, and is not potentially life-threatening or disfiguring, as are acromegaly and Cushing's disease. Because of this and because many patients with high PRL have normal sellas by polytomography, the indications for medical therapy are much broader with this syndrome. All patients who have no radiographic evidence of pituitary tumors and are symptomatic from their high PRL levels (i.e., galactorrhea, amenorrhea, impotence) are candidates for medical therapy. Obviously, a number of such patients have microadenomas that many enlarge during the course of medical therapy. When such tumors become apparent by X-ray or visual-field impairment, they can then be resected. Medical therapy has largely been confined to the use of bromergocryptine and has been very successful.

4.1. Bromocriptine

L-Dopa has been found to result in a 1- to 2-hr suppression of PRL levels in hyperprolactinemic patients but does not produce a sustained therapeutic effect.[82,83] The long-acting dopamine-receptor agonist bromocriptine has been highly successful in reducing PRL levels, restoring menses, and stopping galactorrhea with little side effects. In the great number of series that have now been reported,[84–96] bromocriptine was successful in normalizing serum PRL levels in 80–90% of patients, with cessation of galactorrhea in over 90% and restoration of normal menstrual flow in 80–90%. All these patients had normal sella turcicas and visual fields during bromocriptine therapy.

Data from our own series[97] of 17 patients treated with bromocriptine are shown in Fig. 3. PRL levels were reduced to normal in all but 2 patients, and galactorrhea disappeared in all. Menses returned in all but 4; interestingly, 3 of these 4 were later found to have tumors—2 pituitary adenomas (initial PRLs of 432 and 164) and 1 a hypothalamic sarcoma (initial PRL of 13). Two

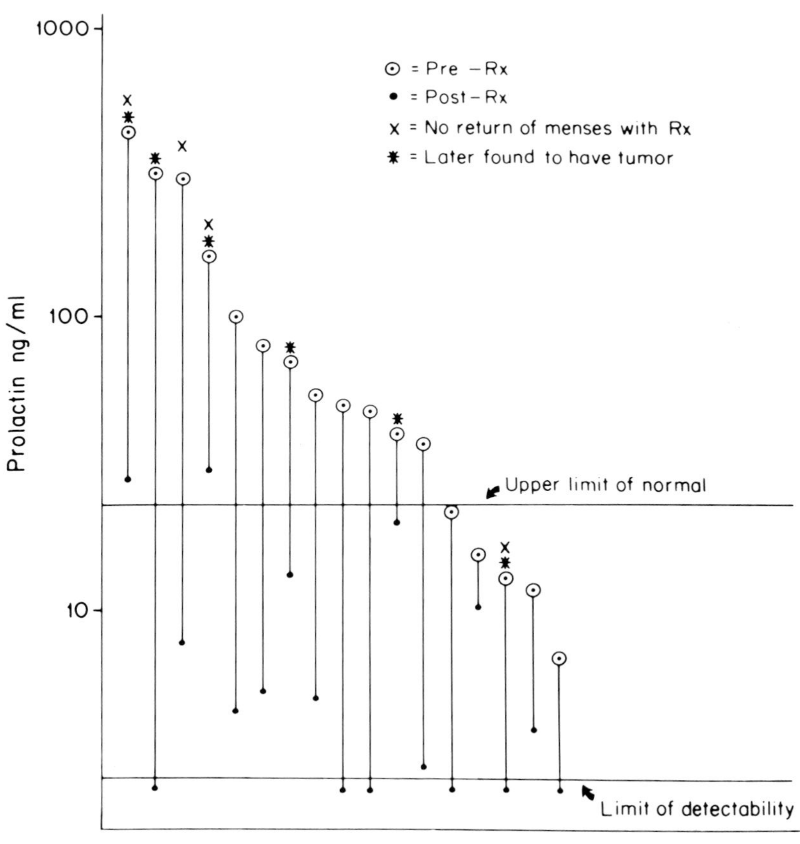

Fig. 3. Effects of bromocriptine therapy on PRL secretion in patients with galactorrhea and amenorrhea.

other patients who had return to menses and normalization of PRL with bromocriptine later developed abnormal sella tomograms and had microadenomas at surgery. Side effects of the therapy noted in our patients included nausea, dyspepsia, headaches, postural hypotension, and rarely depression and anxiety, but therapy was interrupted by these side effects in only 3 cases.

While bromocriptine has been shown to be effective in lowering PRL levels in most patients with and without radiographically demonstrable tumors, there is in addition some *in vitro* evidence that it may have some direct antitumor effects.[98–100] Clinically, reduction in tumor size as evidenced by improvement in visual fields, sella tomography, or computed tomography (CT) has been noted in a modest number of patients.[26,101–107] Unfortunately, we (see below) and others have noted tumor growth in some patients treated with bromocriptine. Bromocriptine has also been useful as adjunctive therapy in patients whose tumors have not been completely cured by surgery or radiotherapy and who were still hyperprolactinemic. We have been able to lower prolactin levels to normal in six such women, and Carter *et al.*[108] were able to lower prolactin levels to normal in seven of ten men who were still hyperprolactinemic following surgery or irradiation.

Although it was initially believed that bromocriptine acted at the hypothalamic level, it is now well established that it acts directly on pituitary dopamine receptors. Diefenbach *et al.*[109] have shown that PRL secretion can be suppressed by L-dopa in monkeys that have been stalk-sectioned, and infusion of dopamine (which does not cross the blood–strain barrier) in humans results in a decrease in PRL secretion,[110] indicating a direct pituitary action.

In summary, bromocriptine appears to be an excellent agent for the therapy of hyperprolactinemic states, including patients who have pituitary tumors. In this latter group, some caution is needed, however. The remission of galactorrhea and amenorrhea may lessen the physician's concern about the presence of a tumor and may lead to decreased vigilance in the follow-up. The eventual demonstration by X-ray of tumors in 5 patients (4 pituitary and 1 hypothalamic) out of 17 in our series of patients initially without sellar enlargement and who were treated with bromocriptine illustrates this point. In addition, patients treated with this drug should use mechanical contraception. We have found that patients can conceive even before their first menses after starting the drug.[97] Since pregnancy can cause a rapid enlargement of PRL-secreting tumors,[103,111–114] these patients must be watched with great care. Finally, although there is no known teratogenicity attributable to this drug so far,[115] the number of pregnant women who have received this drug is still small. Obviously, the drug should be stopped once pregnancy occurs. Because of this enlargement of PRL-secreting tumors during pregnancy, we do not advise administering bromocriptine for the purpose of facilitating pregnancy in women with abnormal sella polytomography.

4.2. Other Drugs

Another ergot derivative, lergotrile mesylate, has been shown to be effective in lowering PRL levels by dopaminergic stimulation,[116] and early clinical trials have shown it to be effective in the treatment of galactorrhea.[117] Our own experience showed this drug to be effective in inducing a cessation of galactorrhea in two patients, with partial reduction of elevated PRL levels in one (130 to 31 ng/ml) and a reduction of PRL from 9.6 to 2.5 ng/ml in the other (B. Biller, M. Molitch, and S. Reichlin, unpublished observations). Unfortunately, all human studies have had to be terminated because long-term studies of this drug in rats showed the development of an excess of gonadal and genital neoplasms. The new ergot derivative lisuride also appears to have PRL-lowering properties in preliminary studies.[118]

Pyridoxine (vitamin B_6), a cofactor in the biosynthesis of dopamine, was reported to decrease PRL levels and suppress galactorrhea in preliminary studies,[119] but subsequent studies with larger numbers of patients have not confirmed these early reports.[120]

Because serotonin is known to be stimulatory to PRL secretion, several studies have attempted to suppress PRL levels using serotonin blocking agents. Cyproheptadine, an antiserotoninergic and antidopaminergic drug, has little short-term effect on PRL levels,[121] but with longer-term therapy it has been shown to lower PRL levels to normal in patients with minimally elevated PRL levels,[122] but not in those with higher levels (over 50 ng/ml).[122,123] Methysergide, another antiserotoninergic agent with mixed dopaminergic agonist antagonist activity, has been shown to decrease PRL levels in short-term studies,[124,125] but long-term therapy with methysergide has been relatively ineffective.[123] Finally, metergoline, an antiserotoninergic agent with dopaminergic properties,[34] was able to reduce PRL level in short-term studies[121,125] and longer-term studies[123] have shown it to be effective in restoring menses and PRL levels to normal in about one-third of women treated.

5. Conclusions

The seven years that have elapsed since the last review of this subject[38] have witnessed a remarkable expansion of information in this area. The medical therapy of the hormonal oversecretion of these tumors represents a direct and rapid application to the clinical management of patients of knowledge obtained from basic science research in the areas of the neurotransmitter and hypophysiotropic hormone regulation of pituitary hormone secretion and neuroendocrine pharmacology.

Although more sophisticated hormonal and radiological diagnostic procedures have resulted in the detection of these tumors at an earlier stage and the newer microneurosurgical and irradiation techniques have resulted in more complete ablation of these tumors with less chance of hypopituitarism, complete cures are still not achieved in some patients with prolactinomas and in many patients with Cushing's disease and acromegaly. Because of this, the expanding armamentarium available for the medical therapy of the hormonal oversecretion of such tumors is of critical importance. Table 1 lists the pharmacological agents that have been discussed.

For acromegaly, bromergocryptine is clearly the drug of choice, but since 10–20% of patients do not respond adequately, it may be necessary to use

TABLE 1. Medical Therapy of Hormone Oversecretion by Pituitary Tumors—1980

Hormone	Therapy	Efficacy[a]
GH	Bromocriptine	+++
	Lergotrile	++[b]
	Cyproheptadine	++[b]
	Metergoline	++[b]
	Lysuride	++[b]
	Medroxyprogesterone acetate	+
	Estrogens	++
	Chlorpromazine	0
	Somatostatin analogues	?
ACTH	Cyproheptadine	++
	Bromergocryptine	+[b]
	Metergoline	++[b]
	Mitotane (*o*, *p*′-DDD)	+++
	Aminoglutethimide	+++
	Metyrapone	++
PRL	Bromocriptine	++++
	Lergotrile	+++[b]
	Lysuride	++[b]
	Pyridoxine	0[b]
	Cyproheptadine	+[b]
	Metergoline	++[b]

[a] Symbols: (++++) excellent; (+++) very good; (++) good; (+) fair; (0) no effect.
[b] Based on preliminary data.

other agents. In Cushing's disease, cyproheptadine may be useful in about 50% of the patients. Adrenolytic therapy with mitotane, metyrapone, or aminoglutethimide may also be quite useful. Finally, for hyperprolactinemic states, bromergocryptine is at present the only effective medical therapy. Clearly, there is a need for more pharmacological agents for the treatment of these syndromes.

References

1. P.E. Cryer and W.H. Daughaday, Regulation of growth hormone secretion in acromegaly, *J. Clin. Endocrinol. Metab.* **29**:386, 1969.
2. A.M. Lawrence, I.D. Goldfine, and L. Kirsteins, Growth hormone dynamics in acromegaly, *J. Clin. Endocrinol. Metab.* **31**:239, 1970.
3. S. Reichlin, Regulation of somatotrophic hormone secretion, in: *Handbook of Physiology–Endocrinology*, Vol. 4, Part 2 (E. Knobil and W.H. Sawyer, eds.), pp. 405–447, Williams and Wilkins, Baltimore, 1974.
4. J.B. Martin, Brain regulation of growth hormone secretion, in: *Frontiers of Neuroendocrinology*, Vol. 4 (L. Martini and W.F. Ganong, eds.), pp. 129–168, Raven Press, New York, 1976.
5. J.B. Martin, P. Brazeau, G.S. Tannenbaum, J.D. Willoughby, J. Epelbaum, L.C. Terry, and D. Durand, Neuroendocrine organization of growth hormone regulation, in: *The Hypothala-*

mus (S. Reichlin, R.J. Baldessarini, and J.B. Martin, eds.), pp. 329–355, Raven Press, New York, 1978.

6. P.E. Cryer and W.H. Daughaday, Adrenergic modulation of growth hormone secretion in acromegaly: Alpha- and beta-adrenergic blockade produce qualitatively normal responses but no effect on L-dopa suppression, *J. Clin. Endocrinol. Metab.* **44**:977, 1977.
7. C.H. Bivens, H.E. Lebovitz, and J.M. Feldman, Inhibition of hypoglycemia-induced growth hormone secretion by the serotonin antagonists cyproheptadine and methysergide, *N. Engl. J. Med.* **278**:236, 1973.
8. J.M. Feldman, J.W. Plonk, and C.H. Bivens, Inhibitory effect of serotonin antagonists on growth hormone release in acromegalic patients, *Clin. Endocrinol.* **5**:71, 1976.
9. P.G. Chiodini, A. Liuzzi, L. Botalla, G. Cremascoli, and F. Silvestrini, Inhibitory effect of dopaminergic stimulation on GH release in acromegaly, *J. Clin. Endocrinol. Metab.* **38**:200, 1974.
10. G.M. Molinatti, F. Camanni, F. Massare, and G.C. Isaia, Dopaminergic control of growth hormone secretion in normal and acromegalic subjects, *Panminerva Med.* **17**:101, 1975.
11. R.H. Chochinov and W.H. Daughaday, Current concepts of somatomedin and other biologically related growth factors, *Diabetes* **25**:994, 1976.
12. W.H. Daughaday, Hormonal regulation of growth by somatomedin and other tissue growth factors, *Clin. Endocrinol. Metab.* **6**:117, 1977.
13. A.E. Boyd, H.E. Lebovitz, and J.B. Pfeiffer, Stimulation of growth hormone secretion by L-dopa, *N. Engl. J. Med.* **283**:1425, 1970.
14. A. Liuzzi, P.G. Chiodini, L. Botalla, G. Cremascoli, and F. Silvestrini, Inhibitory effect of L-dopa on GH secretion in acromegalic patients, *J. Clin. Endocrinol. Metab.* **35**:941, 1972.
15. M.O. Thorner, A. Chait, M. Aitken, G. Benker, S.R. Bloom, C.H. Mortimer, P. Sanders, A.S. Mason, and G.M. Besser, Bromocryptine treatment of acromegaly, *Br. Med. J.* **1**:299, 1975.
16. G. Verde, G. Oppizzi, G. Colussi, G. Cremascoli, L. Botalla, E.E. Müller, F. Silvestrini, P.G. Chiodini, and A. Liuzzi, Effect of dopamine infusion on plasma levels of growth hormone in normal subjects and in acromegalic patients, *Clin. Endocrinol.* **5**:419, 1976.
17. D. Parkes, Bromocriptine, *Adv. Drug. Res.* **12**:247, 1977.
18. V.K. Summers, L.J. Hipkin, M.J. Diver, and J.C. Davis, Treatment of acromegaly with bromocryptine, *J. Clin. Endocrinol. Metab.* **40**:904, 1975.
19. P.G. Chiodini, A. Liuzzi, L. Botalla, G. Oppizzi, E.E. Múller, and F. Silvestrini, Stable reduction of plasma growth hormone (hGH) levels during chronic administration of 2-Br-α-ergocryptine (CB-154) in acromegalic patients, *J. Clin. Endocrinol. Metab.* **40**:705, 1975.
20. J.A.H. Wass, M.O. Thorner, D.V. Morris, L. Rees, A.S. Mason, A.E. Jones, and G.M. Besser, Long-term treatment of acromegaly with bromocriptine, *Br. Med. J.* **1**:875, 1977.
21. Y. Sachdev, A. Gomez-Pan, W.M.G. Tunbridge, A. Duns, D.R. Weightman, R. Hall, and S.K. Goolamali, Bromocriptine therapy in acromegaly, *Lancet* **2**:1164, 1975.
22. S. Werner, K. Hall, and H.E. Sjoberg, Bromocriptine therapy in patients with acromegaly: Effects on growth hormone, somatomedin A and prolactin, *Acta Endocrinol.* **88**(Suppl. 216):199, 1978.
23. L. Lundin, S. Ljunghall, L. Wide, and H. Bostrom, Bromocriptine therapy in 11 patients with acromegaly, *Acta Endocrinol.* **88**(Suppl. 216):207, 1978.
24. A. Nilsson, Experiences with bromocriptine treatment in acromegaly—a preliminary report, *Acta Endocrinol.* **88**(Suppl. 216):217, 1978.
25. P.J. Dunn, R.A. Donald, and E.A. Espiner, Bromocriptine suppression of plasma growth hormone in acromegaly, *Clin. Endocrinol.* **7**:273, 1977.
26. J.A.H. Wass, P.J.A. Moult, M.D. Thorner, J.E. Dacie, M. Charlesworth, A.E. Jones, and G.M. Besser, Reduction of pituitary-tumor size in patients with prolactinomas and acromegaly treated with bromocriptine with and without radiotherapy, *Lancet* **1**:66, 1979.
27. A.C. Moses, M. Molitch, B. Biller, I.M.D. Jackson, C. Sawin, and S. Reichlin, Bromocriptine in treating acromegaly resistant to surgery or radiation therapy, *Clin. Res.* **27**:574A, 1979.
28. D.L. Kleinberg, M. Schaaf, and A.G. Frantz, Studies with lergotrile mesylate in acromegaly, *Fed. Proc. Fed. Am. Soc. Exp. Biol.* **37**:2198, 1978.
29. A. Liuzzi, P.G. Chiodini, G. Oppizzi, L. Botalla, G. Verde, L. DeStefano, G. Colussi, K.J. Graf and R. Horowski, Lisuride hydrogen maleate: Evidence of a long lasting dopaminergic activity in humans, *J. Clin. Endocrinol. Metab.* **46**:196, 1978.
30. G.A. Smythe and L. Lazarus, Suppression of human growth hormone secretion by melatonin and cyproheptadine, *J. Clin. Invest.* **54**:116, 1974.

31. Y. Nakai, H. Imura, H. Sakurai, H. Kurahachi, and T. Yoshimi, Effect of cyproheptadine on human growth hormone secretion, *J. Clin. Endocrinol. Metab.* **38**:446, 1974.
32. W.B. Mendelson, L.S. Jacobs, J.D. Reichman, E. Othmer, P.E. Cryer, B. Trivedi, and W.H. Daughaday, Methysergide: Suppression of sleep-related prolactin secretion and enhancement of sleep-related growth hormone secretion, *J. Clin. Invest.* **56**:690, 1975.
33. K. Chihara, Y. Kato, K. Maeda, S. Matsukura, and H. Imura, Suppression by cyproheptadine of human growth hormone and cortisol secretion during sleep, *J. Clin. Invest.* **57**:1393, 1976.
34. P.G. Chiodini, A. Liuzzi, E.E. Müller, L. Botalla, G. Cremascolli, G. Oppizzi, G. Verde, and F. Silvestrini, Inhibitory effect of an ergoline derivative, metergoline, on growth hormone and prolactin levels in acromegalic patients, *J. Clin. Endocrinol. Metab.* **43**:356, 1976.
35. G. Delitala, A. Masala, S. Alagna, L. Devilla, and G. Lotti, Growth hormone and prolactin release in acromegalic patients following metergoline administration, *J. Clin. Endocrinol. Metab.* **43**:1382, 1976.
36. S. Simon, M. Schiffer, S.M. Glick, and E. Schwartz, Effect of medroxyprogesterone acetate upon stimulated release of growth hormone in men, *J. Clin. Endocrinol. Metab.* **27**:1633, 1967.
37. A.M. Lawrence and L. Kirsteins, Progestins in the medical management of active acromegaly, *J. Clin. Endocrinol. Metab.* **30**:646, 1970.
38. A.M. Lawrence and T.C. Hagen, Alternatives to ablative therapy for pituitary tumors, in: *Diagnosis and Treatment of Pituitary Tumors* (P.O. Kohler and G.T. Ross, eds.), pp. 297–312, American Elsevier, New York, 1973.
39. W.B. Malarkey and W.H. Daughaday, Variable response of plasma GH in acromegalic patients treated with medroxyprogesterone acetate, *J. Clin. Endocrinol. Metab.* **33**:424, 1971.
40. I.M.D. Jackson and B.J. Ormston, Lack of beneficial response of serum GH in acromegalic patients treated with medroxyprogesterone acetate (MPA), *J. Clin. Endocrinol. Metab.* **35**:413, 1972.
41. J.S. Rake, S.A. Hafiz, M.H. Lessof, and G.J.A.I. Snodgrass, A trial of medroxyprogesterone acetate in acromegaly, *Clin. Endocrinol.* **1**:181, 1972.
42. R.L. Atkinson, Jr., R.C. Dimond, W.J. Howard, and J.M. Earll, Unsuccessful treatment of acromegaly with medroxyprogesterone acetate, *Acta Endocrinol.* **77**:19, 1974.
43. Z. Josefsberg, Z. Laron, S. Mathias, and R. Keret, Long-term administration of medroxyprogesterone acetate (MPA) to acromegalic patinets, *Clin. Endocrinol.* **3**:195, 1974.
44. H.D. Kolodny, L. Sherman, A. Singh, S. Kim, and F. Benjamin, Acromegaly treated with chlorpromazine: A case study, *N. Engl. J. Med.* **284**:819, 1971.
45. E. Schwartz, E. Echemendia, M. Schiffer, and V.A. Panarrello, Mechanism of estrogenic action in acromegaly, *J. Clin Invest.* **48**:260, 1969.
46. E. Wiedemann and E. Schwartz, Suppression of growth hormone–dependent human serum sulfaction factor by estrogen, *J. Clin. Endocrinol. Metab.* **34**:51, 1972.
47. E. Wiedemann, E. Schwartz, and A.G. Frantz, Acute and chronic estrogen effects upon serum somatomedin activity, growth hormone and prolactin in man, *J. Clin. Endocrinol. Metab.* **42**:942, 1976.
48. W.D. Odell and M.E. Molitch, The pharmacology of contraceptive agents, *Annu. Rev. Pharmacol.* **14**:413, 1974.
49. Veterans Administration Co-operative Urological Research Group, Treatment and survival of patients with cancer of the prostate, *Surg. Gynecol. Obstet.* **124**:1011, 1967.
50. R.C. Dimond, S.R. Brammer, R.L. Atkinson, Jr., W.J. Howard, and J.M. Earll, Chlorpromazine treatment and growth hormone secretory responses in acromegaly, *J. Clin. Endocrinol. Metab.* **36**:1189, 1973.
51. F.B. Alford, H.W.G. Baker, H.G. Burger, D.P. Cameron, and E.J. Keogh, The secretion rate of human growth hormone. II. Acromegaly: Effect of chlorpromazine treatment, *J. Clin. Endocrinol. Metab.* **38**:309, 1974.
52. R. Hall, G.M. Besser, A.V. Schally, D.H. Coy, D. Evered, D.J. Goldie, A.J. Kastin, A.S. McNeilly, C.H. Mortimer, C. Phenekos, W.M.G. Tunbridge, and D. Weightman, Action of growth-hormone-release inhibitory hormone in healthy men and in acromegaly, *Lancet* **2**:581, 1973.
53. G.M. Besser, C.H. Mortimer, D. Carr, A.V. Schally, D.H. Coy, D. Evered, A.J. Kastin, W.M.G. Tunbridge, M.D. Thorner, and R. Hall, Growth hormone release inhibiting hormone in acromegaly, *Br. Med. J.* **1**:352, 1974.

54. S.S.C. Yen, T.M. Siler, and G.W. DeVane, Effect of somatostatin in patients with acromegaly, *N. Engl. J. Med.* **290:**935, 1974.
55. D. Sarantakis, J. Teichman, E.L. Lien, and R.L. Fenichel, A novel cyclic undecapeptide, WY-40,770, with prolonged growth hormone release inhibiting activity, *Biochem. Biophys. Res. Commun.* **73:**336, 1976.
56. N. Grant, D. Clark, V. Garsky, I. Jaunakais, W. McGregor, and D. Sarantakis, Dissociation of somatostatin effects: Peptides inhibiting the release of growth hormone but not glucagon on insulin in rats, *Life Sci.* **19:**629, 1976.
57. J.B. Martin, S. Reichlin, and G.M. Brown, *Clinical Neuroendocrinology*, F.A. Davis, Philadelphia, 1977.
58. J.W. Plonk, C.H. Bivens, and J.M. Feldman, Inhibition of hypoglycemia-induced cortisol secretion by the serotonin antagonist cyproheptadine, *J. Clin. Endocrinol. Metab.* **38:**836, 1974.
59. J.W. Plonk and J.M. Feldman, Modification of adrenal function by the anti-serotonin agent cyproheptadine, *J. Clin. Endocrinol. Metab.* **42:**291, 1976.
60. D.T. Krieger, L. Amorosa, and F. Linick, Cyproheptadine-induced remission of Cushing's disease, *N. Engl. J. Med.* **293:**893, 1975.
61. D.T. Krieger, Pharmacological therapy of Cushing's disease and Nelson's syndrome, Presented at the International Symposium on Recent Advances in the Diagnosis and Treatment of Pituitary Tumors, San Francisco, California, June 1978.
62. D.T. Krieger and M. Luria, Effectiveness of cyproheptadine in decreasing plasma ACTH concentrations in Nelson's syndrome, *J. Clin. Endocrinol. Metab.* **43:**1179, 1976.
63. J. Cassar, K. Mashiter, G.F. Joplin, L.H. Rees, and J.J.H. Gilkes, Cyproheptadine in Nelson's syndrome, *Lancet* **2:**426, 1976.
64. F. Cavagnini, U. Raggi, P. Micossi, A. DiLandro, and C. Invitti, Effect of an antiserotoninergic drug, metergoline, on the ACTH and cortisol response to insulin hypoglycemia and lysine vasopressin in man, *J. Clin. Endocrinol. Metab.* **43:**306, 1976.
65. C. Ferrari, A. Bertazzoni, and M. Ghezzi, More on cyproheptadine in Cushing's disease, *N. Engl. J. Med.* **296:**576, 1977.
66. G. Benker, K. Hackenberg, B. Hamburger, and D. Reinwein, Effects of growth hormone release inhibiting hormone and bromocryptine (CB-154) in states of abnormal pituitary adrenal function, *Clin. Endocrinol.* **5:**187, 1976.
67. S.W.J. Lamberts and J.C. Birkenhager, Effect of bromocriptine in pituitary-dependent Cushing's syndrome, *J. Endocrinol.* **70:**315, 1976.
68. G.M. Besser, W.J. Jeffcoate, and S. Tomlin, The use of metyrapone and bromocriptine in the control of Cushing's syndrome, Program of the Vth International Congress of Endocrinology, Hamburg, Germany, 1976, Abstract No. 492.
69. A.L. Kennedy and D.A.D. Montgomery, Bromocriptine for Cushing's disease, *Br. Med. J.* **1:**1083, 1977.
70. J.A. Lubitz, L. Freeman, and R. Okun, Mitotane use in inoperable adrenal cortical carcinoma, *J. Am. Med. Assoc.* **223:**1109, 1973.
71. T.E. Temple, Jr., D.J. Jones, Jr., G.W. Liddle, and R.N. Dexter, Treatment of Cushing's disease: Correction of hypercortisolism by *o,p'*DDD without induction of aldosterone deficiency, *N. Engl. J. Med.* **281:**801, 1969.
72. D.E. Schteingart, H.S. Tsao, C.I. Taylor, W.I. Sivitz, and R. Victoria, Chronic suppression of adrenal function with *o,p'*DDD in Cushing's disease, Program of the 57th Annual Session of the American College of Physicians, Philadelphia, 1976, Abstract No. 1.
73. J.P. Louton, J.A. Mahoudeau, P. Bouchard, P. Thieblot, M. Hawte Converture, D. Simon, M.H. Laudat, Y. Touitou, and H. Bricaire, Treatment of Cushing's disease by *o,p'*DDD. Survey of 62 cases, *N. Eng. J. Med.* **300:**459, 1979.
74. R.N. Dexter, L.M. Fishman, R.L. Ney, and G.W. Liddle, Inhibition of adrenal corticosteroid synthesis by aminoglutethimide: Studies of the mechanism of action, *J. Clin. Endocrinol. Metab.* **27:**473, 1967.
75. R.I. Misbin, J. Canary, and D. Willard, Aminoglutethimide in the treatment of Cushing's syndrome, *J. Clin. Pharmacol.* **16:**645, 1976.
76. L.M. Fishman, G.W. Liddle, D.P. Island, N. Fleischer, and D. Kuchel, Effects of amino-glutethimide on adrenal function in man, *J. Clin. Endocrinol. Metab.* **27:**481, 1967.
77. W.J. Jeffcoate, L.H. Rees, S. Tomlin, A.E. Jones, C.R.W. Edwards, and G.M. Besser, Metyrapone in long-term management of Cushing's disease, *Br. Med. J.* **2:**215, 1977.

78. D.F. Child, C.W. Burke, D.M. Burley, L.H. Rees, and T.R. Fraser, Drug control of Cushing's syndrome, *Acta Endocrinol.* **82**:330, 1976.
79. J. Meites, Catecholamines and prolactin secretion, *Adv. Biochem. Psychopharmacol.* **16**:139, 1977.
80. J.A. Clemens, B.D. Sawyer, and B. Cerimele, Further evidence that serotonin is a neurotransmitter involved in the control of prolactin secretion, *Endocrinology,* **100**:692, 1977.
81. J.A. Clemens, Neuropharmacological aspects of the neural control of prolactin secretion, in: *Hypothalamus and Endocrine Functions* (F. Labrie, J. Meites, and G. Pettetier, eds.), pp. 283–301, Plenum Press, New York, 1976.
82. W.B. Malarkey, L.S. Jacobs, and W.H. Daughaday, Levodopa suppression of prolactin in nonpuerperal galactorrhea, *N. Engl. J. Med.* **285**:1160, 1971.
83. M. Edmonds, H. Friesen, and R. Volpe, The effect of levodopa on galactorrhea in the Forbes–Albright syndrome, *Can. Med. Assoc. J.* **107**:534, 1972.
84. E. Del Pozo, L. Varga, H. Wyss, G. Tolis, H. Friesen, R. Wenner, L. Vetter, and A. Uettwiler, Clinical and hormonal responses to bromocriptine (CB-154) in the galactorrhea syndromes, *J. Clin. Endocrinol. Metab.* **39**:18, 1974.
85. R. Rolland, L.A. Schellekens, and R.M. Lequin, Successful treatment of galactorrhea and amenorrhea and subsequent restoration of ovarian function by a new ergot alkaloid 2-brom-α-ergocryptine, *Clin. Endocrinol.* **3**:155, 1974.
86. K. Seki, M. Seki, and T. Okamura, Effect of CB-154 (2-Br-α-ergocryptine) on serum follicle stimulating hormone, luteinizing hormone, and prolactin in women with the amenorrhea–galactorrhea syndrome, *Acta Endocrinol.* **79**:25, 1975.
87. J.E. Tyson, B. Andreassen, J. Huth, B. Smith, and H. Zacur, Neuroendocrine dysfunction in galactorrhea–amenorrhea (after oral contraceptive use), *Obstet. Gynecol.* **46**:1, 1975.
88. R.F. Spark, J. Pallotta, and F. Naftolin, Galactorrhea–amenorrhea syndromes: Etiology and treatment, *Ann. Intern. Med.* **84**:532, 1976.
89. R.P. Dickey and S.C. Stone, Effect of bromo-ergocryptine on serum hPRL, hLH, hFSH, and estradiol 17-β in women with galactorrhea–amenorrhea, *Obstet. Gynecol.* **48**:84, 1976.
90. P. Fossati, G. Strauch, and J. Tourniaire, Étude de l'activité de la bromocriptine dans les états d'hyperprolactinemie: Resultats d'un essai cooperatif chez 135 patients, *Nouv. Presse Med.* **5**:1687, 1976.
91. A.M. Mroueh and T.M. Siler-Khodr, Bromocryptine therapy in cases of amenorrhea–galactorrhea, *Am. J. Obstet. Gynecol.* **127**:291, 1977.
92. Y. Floersheim-Shacar and P.J. Keller, Treatment of hyperprolactinemia–anovulation syndrome, *Fertil. Steril.* **28**:1158, 1977.
93. C.M. March, O.A. Kletzky, and V. Davajan, Clinical response to CB-154 and the pituitary response to thyrotropin-releasing hormone–gonadotropin releasing hormone in patients with galactorrhea–amenorrhea, *Fertil. Steril.* **28**:521, 1977.
94. H.G. Friesen and G. Tolis, The use of bromocriptine in the galactorrhea–amenorrhea syndromes: the Canadian Cooperative Study, *Clin. Endocrinol.* **6**(Suppl.):91s, 1977.
95. M.O. Thorner and G.M. Besser, Bromocriptine treatment of hyperprolactinemic hypogonadism, *Acta Endocrinol.* **88**(Suppl. 216):131, 1978.
96. T. Bergh, S.J. Nillius, and L. Wide, Hyperprolactinaemic amenorrhea—results of treatment with bromocriptine, *Acta Endocrinol.* **88**(Suppl. 216):147, 1978.
97. A.E. Boyd, S. Reichlin, and R.N. Turksoy, Galactorrhea–amenorrhea syndrome: Diagnosis and therapy, *Ann. Intern. Med.* **87**:165, 1977.
98. R.M. MacLeod and J.E. Lehmeyer, Suppression of pituitary tumor growth and function by ergot alkaloids, *Cancer Res.* **33**:849, 1973.
99. H.M. Lloyd, J.D. Meares, and J. Jacobi, Effects of oestrogen and bromocryptine on *in vivo* secretion and mitosis in prolactin cells, *Nature (London)* **255**:497, 1975.
100. K.S. McCarty, Jr., D. Bredesen, R. Schomberg, R. Kramer, and C. Hammond, Effects of 2 bromergocryptine on organ-cultured human prolactin-secreting micro-adenomas, Program of the 27th Annual Meeting of the Congress of Neurological Surgeons, San Francisco, October 1977.
101. B. Corenblum, B.R. Webster, C.B. Mortimer, and C. Ezrin, Possible antitumor effect of 2-bromo-ergocryptin (CB-154 Sandoz) in 2 patients with large prolactin secreting pituitary adenomas, *Clin. Res.* **23**:614A, 1975.
102. B. Corenblum, Bromocriptine in pituitary tumors, *Lancet* **2**:786, 1978.

103. T. Bergh, S.J. Nillius, and L. Wide, Clinical course and outcome of pregnancies in amenorhoeic women with hyperprolactinemia and pituitary tumors, *Br. Med. J.* **1**:875, 1978.
104. L.G. Sobrinho, M.C.P. Nunes, M.A. Santos, and J.C. Mauricio, Radiologic evidence for regression of prolactinoma after treatment with bromocriptine, *Lancet* **2**:257, 1978.
105. S.J. Nillius, T. Bergh, P.O. Lundberg, J. Stahle, and L. Wide, Regression of a prolactin-secreting pituitary tumor during long-term treatment with bromocriptine, *Fertil. Steril.* **30**:710, 1978.
106. R.A. Vaidya, S.D. Aloorkan, N.R. Rege, B.T. Maskati, R.P. Jahangin, A.R. Sheth, and S.K. Pandya, Normalization of visual fields following bromocriptine treatment in hyperprolactinemic patients with visual field constriction, *Fertil. Steril.* **29**:632, 1978.
107. A.M. McGregor, M.F. Scanlon, K. Hall, D.B. Cook, and R. Hall, Reduction in size of a pituitary tumor by bromocriptine therapy, *N. Engl. J. Med.* **300**:291, 1979.
108. J.N. Carter, J.E. Tyson, G. Tolis, S. Van Vliet, C. Faiman, and H.G. Friesen, Prolactin-secreting tumors and hypogonadism in 22 men, *N. Engl. J. Med.* **299**:847, 1978.
109. W.P. Diefenbach, P.W. Carmel, A.G. Frantz, and M. Ferin, Suppression of prolactin secretion by L-dopa in the stalk-sectioned rhesus monkey, *J. Clin. Endocrinol. Metab.* **43**:638, 1976.
110. H. Leblanc, G.C.L. Lachelin, S. Abu-Fadil, and S.S.C. Yen, Effects of dopamine infusion on pituitary hormone secretion in humans, *J. Clin. Endocrinol. Metab.* **43**:668, 1976.
111. D.F. Child, H. Gordon, K. Mashiter, and G.F. Joplin, Pregnancy, prolactin and pituitary tumors, *Br. Med. J.* **4**:87, 1975.
112. N. Husami, R. Jewelewicz, and R.L. Vande Wiele, Pregnancy in patients with pituitary tumors, *Fertil. Steril.* **28**:920, 1977.
113. S.W.J. Lamberts, H.J. Seldenrath, H.G. Kwa, and J.C. Birkenhager, Transient bitemporal hemianopsia during pregnancy after treatment of galactorrhea-amenorrhea syndrome with bromocriptine, *J. Clin. Endocrinol. Metab.* **44**:180, 1977.
114. P.B. Nelson, A.G. Robinson, D.F. Archer, and J.C. Maroon, Symptomatic pituitary tumor enlargement after induced pregnancy, *J. Neurosurg.* **49**:283, 1978.
115. M.O. Thorner, Prolactin, *Clin. Endocrinol. Metab.* **6**:201, 1977.
116. J.A. Clemens, E.B. Smalstig, and C.J. Shaar, Inhibition of prolactin secretion by lergotrile mesylate: Mechanism of action, *Acta Endocrinol.* **79**:230, 1975.
117. R.E. Cleary, R. Crabtree, and L. Lemberger, The effect of lergotrile on galactorrhea and gonadotropin secretion, *J. Clin. Endocrinol. Metab.* **40**:830, 1975.
118. R. Horowski, H. Wendt, and K.J. Graf, Prolactin-lowering effect of low doses of lisuride in man, *Acta Endocrinol.* **87**:234, 1978.
119. E.N. McIntosh, Treatment of women with the galactorrhea-amenorrhea syndrome with pyridoxine (vitamin B_6), *J. Clin. Endocrinol. Metab.* **42**:1192, 1976.
120. G. Tolis, R. Laliberte, H. Guyda and F. Naftolin, Ineffectiveness of pyridoxine (B_6) to alter secretion of growth hormone and prolactin and absence of therapeutic effects on galactorrhea-amenorrhea syndromes, *J. Clin. Endocrinol. Metab.* **44**:1197, 1977.
121. C. Ferrari, A. Paracchi, M. Rondena, R. Beck-Peccoz, and G. Faglia, Effect of two serotonin antagonists on prolactin and thyrotrophin secretion in man, *Clin. Endocrinol.* **5**:575, 1976.
122. J. Wortsman, N.G. Soler, and J. Hirschowitz, Cyproheptadine in the management of the galactorrhea-amenorrhea syndrome, *Ann. Intern. Med.* **90**:923, 1979.
123. P.G. Crosignani, M. Peracchi, G.C. Lombrosco, E. Reschini, A. Mattei, A. Caccamo, and A. D'Alberton, Antiserotonin treatment of hyperprolactinemia amenorrhea: Long-term follow-up with metergoline, methysergide, and cyproheptadine, *Am. J. Obstet. Gynecol.* **132**:307, 1978.
124. R. D. D'Agata, S. Ando, L. Iachello, V. Pezzino, S. Gulizia, and U. Scapagnini, Decrease of prolactin by methysergide in amenorrheic hyperprolactinemic women, *J. Clin. Endocrinol. Metab.* **45**:1116, 1977.
125. C. Ferrari, R. Caldara, P. Rampini, P. Telloli, M. Romussi, A. Bertazzoni, G. Polloni, A. Mattei, and P.G. Crosignani, Inhibition of prolactin release by serotonin antagonists of hyperprolactinemic subjects, *Metabolism* **27**:1499, 1978.

16

General Considerations in the Surgical Treatment of Pituitary Tumors

KALMON D. POST

1. Historical Background

In 1886, Marie[1] suggested a relationship between acromegaly and pituitary tumors. By 1893, Caton and Paul[2] reported an attempt at removal of a growth hormone (GH)-producing tumor via craniotomy and middle fossa approach. In 1905, Krause[3] suggested an approach through the anterior cranial fossa, and in 1906, Sir Victor Horsley[4] reported on 10 cases approached via the middle fossa. The techniques were crude and visibility poor; alternative routes were sought. The first extracranial transsphenoidal procedure was probably that by Schloffer[5] in 1907, although Giordano[6] had suggested a transsinus approach in 1897. Cushing[7] began using a transsphenoidal approach in 1909, and thereafter performed over 200 cases via this route. Until then, the operation involved considerable dissection of the frontal sinus, nose, ethmoids, and sphenoids and was very disfiguring. In 1910, Halstead[8] performed surgery through a transoronasal route with an incision through the mucosa above the upper teeth, utilizing the submucosal techniques of Kocher.[9] In 1910, Oscar Hirsch[10] did the first of 413 transsphenoidal procedures,[11,12] and introduced Harvey Cushing to the procedure. Cushing's reputation attracted many patients, and within several years he had performed over 100 cases.[13] By 1925, he had operated on 231 pituitary tumors through a transsphenoidal route with a 5% mortality in the precortisone, preantibiotic era. Frazier[14] performed both operations, transsphenoidal and transcranial, before 1913, with the modern view of utilizing the transsphenoidal approach to small enclosed tumors and tumors growing downward, while using the transcranial approach to tumors growing upward. The mortality rates differed significantly: 3.4% for the former and 30% for the latter.[15]

KALMON D. POST • Tufts University School of Medicine; Department of Neurosurgery, Tufts–New England Medical Center Hospital, Boston, Massachusetts 02111.

Nevertheless, because of some difficulties with the transsphenoidal approach such as infection and cerebrospinal fluid (CSF) rhinorrhea (which would be overcome later), Cushing returned to the transcranial operation and developed the midline subfrontal approach, which still remains a standard procedure.[7,13,16,17] The decreased recurrence rate with the transcranial operation, less than half that with the transsphenoidal operation, as well as the frequent occurrence of visual compression as an indication for surgery made the transcranial approach the more popular for the next several decades.[18,19] Antibiotics, unavailable to Cushing, reduced the risk of infection, but the most important historical event related to pituitary surgery was undoubtedly the discovery in 1950 of adrenal steroids for pre-,intra-, and postoperative care.[20]

The transsphenoidal approach was resurrected by Guiot and Thipaut,[21] who in 1959 reported on the advantages of the transsphenoidal operation using image-intensified fluoroscopy. Hardy and co-workers further modernized the procedure by introducing the use of the operating microscope, which had the advantage of both magnification and significant improvement in focal illumination.[22,23]

The marked benefits of stereoscopic magnification with intense illumination in delineating the normal tissue from tumor as well as the use of microinstruments were rapidly adapted for both the transsphenoidal and transcranial approaches to pituitary tumors. Other advances, including bipolar coagulation,[24] fixed head-holders, and self-retaining retractors, also aided in reducing morbidity by decreasing brain manipulation and consequent edema. Bipolar coagulation permitted fine dissection without spread of current into adjacent optic nerves or other neural tissue. Microinstruments allowed the dissection of microadenomas with preservation of normal pituitary gland and surrounding nerves.

The specifics of either surgical approach will be discussed in the following two chapters. However, certain considerations must be discussed first: What are the indications for pituitary surgery? What is the goal of surgery for the different tumors that we encounter? What are the advantages and disadvantages of each operation? How do we compare results?

2. Indications

Pituitary tumors can be divided into two broad categories, hypersecreting and nonfunctional. The hypersecreting tumors may produce adrenocorticotropic hormone (ACTH), GH, thyroid-stimulating hormone (TSH), and prolactin, singly or in combination. Because of the effects of the excessive hormones, patients usually present for treatment while the tumors are small, and therefore mass effect with compression of the neural structures is less common as an early manifestation. Nonfunctional tumors, on the other hand, unless noted as incidental findings on skull X-rays or causing headaches or mild endocrinopathies, are usually seen when they are large, producing both mass effect with visual changes and hypopituitarism secondary to compression of the gland.

Formerly, radiation was the treatment of choice in small tumors when diagnosis was reasonably certain on visual, endocrinological, and radiological bases. Primary decompression was reserved for (1) large tumors with vision compromised to 20/200 or worse, (2) cystic adenomas, (3) pituitary apoplexy, or (4) uncertain diagnosis.[25,26]

At present, however, the guidelines discussed below are utilized.

2.1. Nonfunctional Tumors (Table 1)

The size of the nonfunctional tumor may mandate surgical intervention. Progressive visual deficit, of either acuity or fields, has been an implicit surgical indication in our clinic. Similarly, any cranial nerve deficit other than that of the optic nerve demands surgical treatment.

Other mass effects, such as CSF obstruction with hydrocephalus, generalized increased intracranial pressure from the tumor volume in the frontal or middle fossae, and focal neuroendocrine deficits via hypothalamic dysfunction, also mandate surgical removal and decompression. This is true for functional tumors as well.

Both Costello[27] and Kernohan and Sayre[28] demonstrated that in autopsies performed on patients without known evidence of pituitary dysfunction, as many as 23% had pituitary adenomas, presumably nonfunctional and requiring no treatment. (Although they had no signs of Cushing's disease or acromegaly, prolactin secretion could have been present.) Undoubtedly, then, a large proportion of small nonfunctional or prolactin-secreting tumors may have a benign natural history. Therefore, the incidental nonfunctional tumor without neurological or endocrinological deficit can be either followed conservatively with serial sella tomography or computed tomography (CT) scan until evidence of growth is present, or it may be treated with radiation therapy to arrest growth, but surgery is not usually performed. Occasionally, for psychological reasons, a patient will desire even a small tumor removed, and this is done.

Sheline[29] commented on 32 such patients observed conservatively without treatment. Eight were diagnosed at autopsy, and all had large sellas. Their endocrine function was not known, but none had required treatment. Eight were lost to follow-up. Of the remaining 16, half had visual-field defects and half did not. These were then observed conservatively for up to 20 years. Of

TABLE 1. Nonfunctional Tumors: Indications for Surgery

1. Progressive visual loss—acuity or fields
2. Extraocular motor cranial nerve dysfunction (i.e., III, IV, VI)
3. Increased intracranial pressure from local mass effect
4. CSF obstruction and hydrocephalus
5. Pituitary apoplexy
6. Uncertain diagnosis
7. Tumor recurrence after radiation treatment
8. CSF leak

the 16, 14 eventually showed signs of growth and came to treatment: 7 had increased field defects, and 1 had a permanent CSF leak. Sheline concluded, from this limited group, that it might be hazardous to deter treatment. In his opinion, any patient with a visual-field defect, no matter how slight, should be recommended for treatment and not watched conservatively.

2.2. Functional Tumors (Table 2)

2.2.1. Adrenocorticotropic Hormone

Cushing's disease is almost always secondary to a pituitary microadenoma,[30,32] but X-ray studies of the sella are more often normal than abnormal. In a series of 86 patients with Cushing's disease, only 20 were appreciated to have abnormalities on sella tomograms or plain skull X-rays.[33] Tyrrell *et al.*[30] explored the sella in 20 consecutive cases of Cushing's disease, 8 of whom had normal sellae by X-ray study. In 2, there were technical difficulties that precluded intrasellar exploration, but in 17 of the other 18, a microadenoma was found and removed. In the other patient, a hypophysectomy was performed and a 1.5-mm adenoma was seen in the specimen. All but one of these patients had their hypercortisolism corrected. This study and others[30–32] suggest that all, or almost all, Cushing's disease is secondary to a pituitary microadenoma. For this reason, careful evaluation of Cushing's syndrome is mandatory (see Chapter 7). We recommend sellar exploration of all cases with Cushing's disease. The systemic effects of elevated ACTH and cortisol, such as hypertension, diabetes mellitus, osteoporosis, obesity, and myopathy, contribute to the 50% 5-year mortality and are considered significant enough to mandate early surgical intervention with any size tumor (see Chapter 7). The low morbidity of pituitary surgery is an advantage compared with adrenalectomy. Additionally, the risk of Nelson's syndrome, reportedly 0–10%[34,35] after adrenalectomy, is negated. The cure rate and rapidity of response following surgery have made this modality superior to radiation therapy, except perhaps in children, in whom a recent report[36] has shown excellent results with radiation. Jennings *et al.*[36] conceded that only 15% of patients over 20 years of age with Cushing's disease were controlled by pituitary irradiation alone,

TABLE 2. Functional Tumors: Indications for Surgery

1. All indications listed for nonfunctional tumors (Table 1)
2. Cushing's disease in adult—any size tumor
3. Nelson's syndrome
4. Acromegaly—any size tumor
5. Prolactinomas
   a. Macroadenoma with extrasellar extension
   b. Microadenoma if:
      (i) progressive growth demonstrated
      (ii) pregnancy desired
      (iii) refractory to ergocryptine
   c. Radiation failures
6. TSH-producing tumors (rare)

while others report some benefit in approximately half of patients with Cushing's disease.[37,38] Nelson's syndrome, whether it is truly developed after adrenalectomy or represents the further growth of an occult tumor initially responsible for the Cushing syndrome, has also been treated surgically. This tumor tends to have more aggressive growth patterns, and early removal is suggested.

2.2.2. Growth Hormone

Excessive GH has many serious adverse systemic effects such as hypertension, diabetes mellitus, cardiomyopathy, cerebrovascular disease, and chronic pulmonary disease.[39] The death rate is almost twice that expected from the general population, making therapy imperative (see Chapter 6). Surgical removal of a GH-secreting adenoma is absolutely indicated when there are additional mass effects of the tumor. GH-secreting adenomas do not tend to be as large as nonfunctional tumors when first discovered. Irradiation has been widely used. Roth *et al.*[40] reported that 19 of 20 patients with acromegaly had a mean fall in plasma GH of 51% by 1–2 years. In 7 patients studied at 2½–4 years after treatment, the mean decrease was 76% (range 60–89%), but plasma GH was normal in only 3, was modestly elevated in 2, and was considerably elevated in 2. Aloia *et al.*[41] had 6 of 12 patients with normal GH after at least 1 year following irradiation. Overall, there was a 70% mean decrease of GH levels by 6–25 months. There does not appear to be any superior benefit with proton-beam irradiation. Kjellberg *et al.*[42,43] reported a 46% decrease in GH in treated patients. Results with conventional and heavy-particle irradiation are beneficial, yet there is a significant time delay before GH is reduced, and more important, the GH may never be normalized. Even when significant reduction occurs, GH levels may still be elevated above normal levels, a less than ideal result. Similarly, medical treatment, as discussed in Chapter 15,[44] offers some benefits, but does not destroy the tumor. Therefore, we consider surgery to be the primary mode of therapy.

2.2.3. Prolactin

Prolactinomas have become the most common pituitary tumor, making up between 30 and 70% of most series.[45,46] If the tumor is large with neurological deficits, surgery is mandatory, just as in nonfunctional tumors. The issue, however, is more complex for smaller tumors, particularly microadenomas as defined by Hardy.[47,48] Male patients with prolactinomas have generally required surgery because they present late in the course with visual-field defects.[49] Since the standard evaluation of impotent males should now include a prolactin determination, more male patients will be discovered with small tumors. Women with amenorrhea–galactorrhea syndromes often present with infertility and are found to have hyperprolactinemia and asymmetric sellae on tomography.[50,51] The reported results of ergocryptine's lowering prolactin and promoting pregnancy are encouraging,[52–54] but the numerous reports of tumor enlargement during pregnancies induced by the drug[55–59] are a source of concern. Since with microadenomas the cure rate by selective adenomectomy is so high, the morbidity extremely low, and mortality zero, we have favored surgery when pregnancy is desired or when there is evidence of tumor growth.[60]

Although several recent reports[61,62] have shown evidence of tumor shrinkage during treatment with ergocryptine, further studies are required to evaluate such therapy as a means of reducing tumor size. If these are confirmed, then surgery may be indicated only for those patients who are medical–treatment failures. Last, a tumor that has been refractory to radiation therapy is a surgical candidate. There is no evidence to date that radiation therapy is effective enough against prolactin-secreting tumors to consider radiation as the primary form of therapy (see Chapters 21 and 22).

2.3. Pituitary Apoplexy

The sudden enlargement of a pituitary adenoma secondary to either hemorrhage or hemorrhagic infarction associated with acute neurological deficits has been an absolute indication for surgical decompression in our clinic. Although some patients may recover spontaneously from this state, even with the addition of high-dose glucocorticoid therapy, the risks of waiting are large in relation to the risks of decompression even in an acutely ill, elderly patient. The following case history exemplifies the possible benefits:

A 72-year-old woman presented in April 1977 with a history of nausea, vomiting, and diarrhea for 1 week. She had also felt sluggish, both mentally and physically. Neurological and visual examination were normal. Evaluation showed her to be hypothyroid and hyponatremic (Na, 112), probably secondary to inappropriate antidiuretic hormone secretion. She had an enlarged sella, and a suprasellar mass was seen on CT scan. Radiation treatment was given with 5000 rads.

Three months later, she developed severe bifrontal headaches and over a period of 3 days lost vision almost completely. On admission, her pupils were 7 mm and nonreactive. There was no light perception O.D., but finger-counting was present in the nasal field O.S. Extraocular movements were limited solely to trace abduction and depression O.D.; no movement was possible O.S. Severe ptosis was noted.

A CT scan (Fig. 1) demonstrated a dense enhancing pituitary lesion with suprasellar extension up to the inferior portion of the third ventricle. An emergency transsphenoidal operation was performed with the removal of the bulk of a hemorrhagic infarcted pituitary adenoma.

Postoperatively, she regained acuity of 20/20 O.S. with a full field, and 20/20 O.D. with an irregular concentric contraction of the field O.D. A mild right VI nerve paresis remained. She has remained well on replacement therapy.

2.4. Uncertain Diagnosis

If there is doubt as to the clinical diagnosis of sellar lesions, specific tissue diagnosis is mandatory, especially if radiation therapy is considered. Arachnoid cysts, Rathke's cleft cysts, craniopharyngiomas, dermoids, epidermoids, and chordomas may be present and be refractory to radiation treatment.[63]

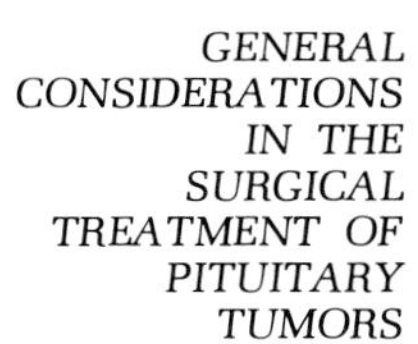

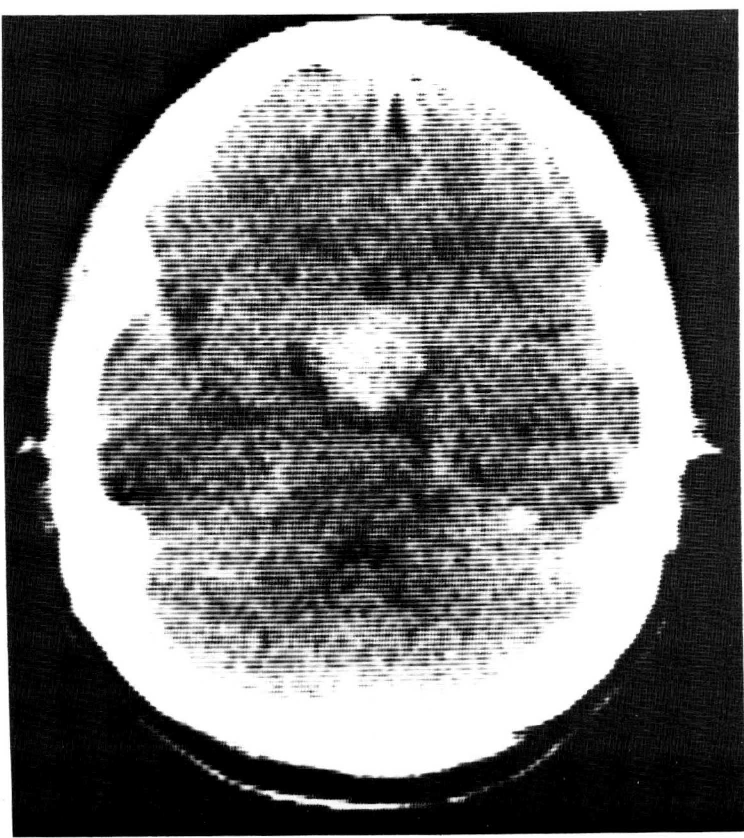

Fig. 1. Nonenhanced CT scan demonstrating a suprasellar lesion with increased density consistent with hemorrhage into a pituitary adenoma.

2.5. Treatment Failures

Patients who have been treated unsuccessfully with other modalities and show evidence of tumor growth or persistence of hypersecretion are operative candidates.

2.6. Cerebrospinal Fluid Leaks

Rarely, patients will present with rhinorrhea secondary to tumor growth or previous radiation therapy. Usually, these tumors are more aggressive with destruction of the floor and dura. Surgery is mandatory to seal the leak and prevent meningitis. Radiotherapy may also be required.

3. Goals of Surgery (Table 3)

To fully appreciate the goals of surgical therapy, we must separate the nonfunctional tumors from the hypersecreting adenomas. The distinction is

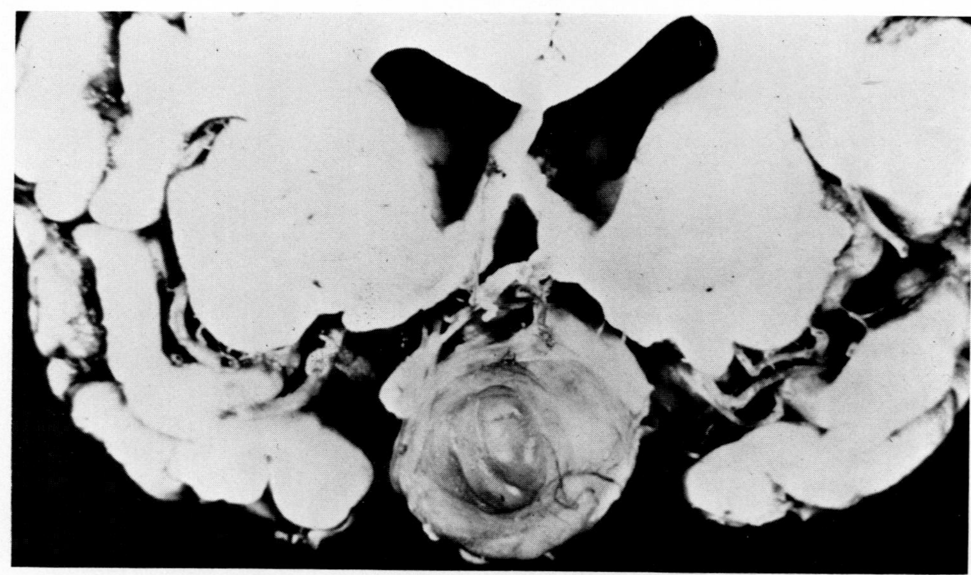

Fig. 2. Photograph of a large nonfunctional tumor compressing the adjacent neural structures.

important on several accounts. First, as discussed previously, the nonfunctional tumors tend to be larger with significant suprasellar expansion when evaluated, while the hypersecreting tumors tend to be smaller. Ideal therapy for all adenomas would be total removal while sparing the normal gland and restoring any lost neurological and pituitary function. This goal is more readily achieved with a small adenoma than with a very large mass. Figures 2 and 3 demonstrate this contrast; one tumor is very large with distortion of the adjacent structures and without identifiable normal gland (Fig. 2), while the other is a microadenoma and can be readily removed from the gland (Fig. 3). The goals of therapy will clearly be different. The risks of manipulating adjacent structures are increased when these tissues are stretched and distorted by a large mass, so that subtotal removal of the tumor, leaving its capsule against the optic nerves and chiasm, may be advisable with a large tumor. The pituitary gland may not be identifiable adjacent to a large mass, or it may be extremely thin and fragile, while this is not the case with a microadenoma.

Second, the effects of hypersecretion may be more devastating than the mass effects, and therefore normalization of the elevated hormone becomes the primary concern. To accomplish this, all tumor tissue must be either removed or destroyed, whereas we need be concerned only with removing the mass effect and preventing future growth in nonfunctional tumors. If pituitary function has been severely or completely lost prior to surgery, it is unusual for it to be regained even after selective total tumor removal.[64] Since nonfunctional tumors generally respond well to radiation therapy, with a recurrence rate in the range of 7%,[18,25] surgery can be more conservative to eliminate the mass lesion, with adjunctive radiation being used to stop further growth. Effectiveness of radiation therapy for hypersecreting tumors depends on the type

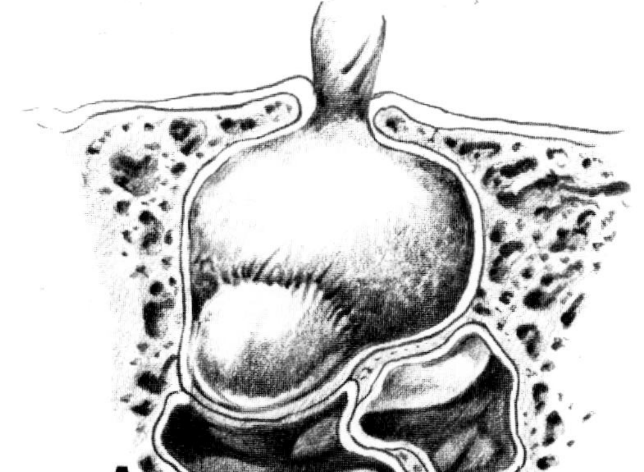

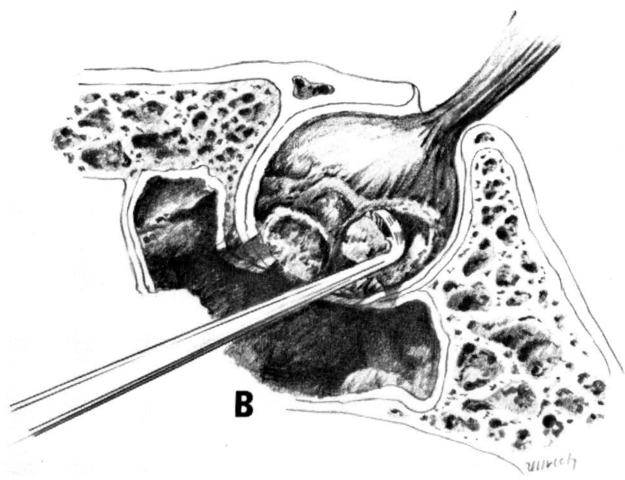

Fig. 3. Diagram of a microadenoma contained within the pituitary gland.

of adenoma, as previously discussed. Cure of a secreting tumor thus requires more radical surgery than is needed for nonfunctional lesions. All tumor tissue must be removed surgically, since even a minute residual fragment may continue to have severe effects. Success is therefore more easily achieved when the tumor is small and readily separable from the normal gland. Realistic goals of adenoma management will depend on the size of the tumor found at surgery. The goal of treatment for a small functioning tumor is to perform a selective total removal without injury to the normal gland. In a moderate-size functional tumor, the goal is still total removal while sparing the normal gland, but the distinction between adenoma and gland is less evident, and intraoperative decisions are more difficult. Leaving questionable tumor (i.e., selective subtotal removal) risks a noncure, while removal of nor-

TABLE 3. Goals of Surgery

A. Nonfunctional tumors
  1. Total removal if capsule separates readily
  2. Selective subtotal removal[a] or nonselective subtotal removal[b]

B. Functional tumors
  1. Cushing's disease
    a. Selective total removal[c] if possible
    b. Nonselective total removal[d] if adenoma not clearly defined from gland
  2. Nelson's disease
    a. Selective total removal[c] if possible
    b. Nonselective total removal[d] if adenoma not clearly defined from gland
  3. Acromegaly
    a. Selective total removal[c] if possible
    b. Nonselective total removal[d] if adenoma not clearly defined from gland in an adult beyond childbearing age
    c. Selective subtotal removal[a] if adenoma not clearly defined from gland in young or child-bearing age
      Possible repeat surgery if not successful
  4. Prolactinoma
    a. Selective total removal[c] if possible
    b. Selective subtotal removal[a] if adenoma not clearly defined from gland
    c. Nonselective subtotal removal[b] in large tumors where gland not identified

[a] Selective subtotal removal is performed when the normal pituitary gland has been identified with a biopsy and remains, but there may be residual pathological tissue. In this case, a second-stage procedure is often preferred to producing panhypopituitarism by the removal of the remnant of the normal gland.
[b] Nonselective subtotal removal consists of partial removal of the sella contents including the normal and pathological tissue, with some residual tissue remaining.
[c] Selective total removal is performed when the normal pituitary has been well identified and biopsied, and all the pathological tissue is removed.[76]
[d] Nonselective total removal consists in radical excision of all the intrasellar contents including the normal and pathological tissue.

mal gland, which appears abnormal only because of the distortion, would lead to hypopituitarism. These risks must be balanced in regard to age, sexual capabilities, and desires for pregnancy, the significance of the clinical disease (i.e., ACTH more significant than prolactin elevation), and the presumed future course of the disease.[65] In large secreting tumors, aggressive removal is required, but some or most pituitary function will, in all probability, be lost. At times, therefore, a nonselective total removal with radical excision of the intrasellar contents is indicated (see Table 3).

Nonfunctional tumors, on the other hand, need only be debulked to remove the compressive component from the surrounding neural structures (nonselective subtotal removal). Adjunctive radiation therapy will then generally prevent recurrence. If, however, the capsule separates readily during dissection, it too is removed.

Functional tumors must be considered individually.

3.1. Cushing's Disease

This is a serious life-threatening illness, and therefore the goal of surgery must be total removal. In the case of microadenomas, the distinction between tumor and normal gland is often possible, and a selective total removal can be performed. However, if a clear distinction cannot be made or if the microadenoma cannot be found, then total hypophysectomy must be considered to achieve cure (i.e., a nonselective total removal where both tumor and gland are removed).

In support of hypophysectomy are the following considerations: A microadenoma not found during the exploration may be present in the resected specimen with a resultant cure. If hyperplasia is the pathology, it will be cured. A second operation, i.e., bilateral adrenalectomy, will be avoided, and possibly Nelson's disease prevented. Hypopituitarism will of course result; however, this may be more benign than the disease, and the use of endocrine-replacement medications can restore hormonal profiles to normal.

Against hypophysectomy are the following considerations: An unnecessary hypophysectomy in the event of mistaken diagnosis such as occult ectopic ACTH production would be avoided. The morbidity of hypophysectomy such as hypopituitarism, including possible diabetes insipidus, is avoided. This is particulary important in patients still in the childbearing age group, in whom fertility may be a serious consideration and long-term gonadotropin replacement necessary.

The final decision must be individualized and be well thought out prior to exploration.

3.2. Nelson's Disease

Considerations similar to those indicated above for Cushing's disease exist for this entity. However, the surgical removal must be as complete as possible, even to the point of total hypophysectomy, because the alternate options of therapy are not as extensive; i.e., adrenalectomy is not an alternate possibility with Nelson's disease.

3.3. Acromegaly

Acromegaly is also a serious illness, but not as damaging as Cushing's disease. A selective total removal is the usual goal and is generally achievable. However, if the tumor is not clearly distinguishable from the gland, then the decisions will differ according to the individual clinical settings. An older patient may be treated most effectively with a nonselective total removal with resultant hypopituitarism. A younger patient still in childbearing years may benefit from a more conservative removal leaving normal tissue. Should the GH remain elevated following this removal, then either a second surgical procedure or another form of treatment such as ergocryptine or radiotherapy might be considered. These approaches must be individualized, but generally the surgeon need not be quite as aggressive as with Cushing's disease.

3.4. Prolactinomas

Elevated prolactin has not thus far been demonstrated to have any systemic effects other than interfering with regulation of gonadotropin secretion and causing galactorrhea. In patients with microadenomas presenting as an infertility problem, we have been attempting selective total removal of the adenoma, sparing the normal gland. As will be seen in Chapter 18, this approach has been reasonably successful. In cases where the distinction between tumor and gland is not completely evident, frozen-section techniques have been a useful adjunct,[66] but if uncertainty persists, a more conservative procedure has been carried out (i.e., selective subtotal removal). This is preferable to a more aggressive removal where hypopituitarism might result in refractory infertility, a situation possibly worse than the initial disease. If prolactin remains elevated after such a subtotal removal, then another modality such as ergocryptine or radiation has been recommended. As the natural history of this disease is observed in the future, the best course of action will become more obvious. In larger prolactin-secreting tumors, an approach similar to that outlined above for nonfunctional tumors is followed.

4. Surgery and Radiation

Radiation therapy is discussed fully in Chapter 21. However, the relationship between surgery and radiation therapy deserves further comment here. Cushing's 338 pituitary tumor cases reviewed by Henderson[18] demonstrated a clearly improved prognosis with postoperative radiation. Tumor recurrence was reduced to 13% in patients operated on subfrontally and then given radiation. Similar techniques utilizing modern equipment have reduced the recurrence rate even further to approximately 7%.[25,67–75] Radiation therapy is therefore given following removal of larger nonsecreting tumors, since the recurrence rate is significantly lowered. Radiation is also used for most large hormone-secreting tumors if total removal is not achieved or if the tumor has produced extensive sellar destruction. Indication for radiation therapy with smaller tumors is less well defined. It is not used following removal of a hypersecreting microadenoma if the elevated hormone returns to normal. It is often given if abnormal hypersecretion persists or if there has been extensive destruction of the sella floor. However, although proliferation may be impeded, excessive secretory ability may remain, and medical therapy may also be needed to control hypersecretion.

Radiation treatment influences subsequent surgical management. Although it may produce some infarction and softening of the tumor, making the central portion readily removable, the distinction between normal gland and tumor is made more difficult. Several years after radiation, marked scarring and fibrotic tissue in the sella with retraction of the diaphragm may produce a secondary empty sella. Selective excisions thereafter are extremely difficult, and radical procedures are necessary.[76]

5. Choice of Surgical Approach

There are advantages and disadvantages to both the transsphenoidal and the transcranial operation. These are summarized in Tables 4 and 5.

For large nonfunctioning tumors, we almost always approach via the

TABLE 4. Transcranial Approach: Advantages and Disadvantages

1. Advantages
   a. Surgery is performed through a sterile field without contamination from the sinuses.
   b. Visibility of the neurological structures offers the ability to protect them during surgical removal of the adenoma.
   c. There is the ability to alter the approach, i.e., subfrontal, lateral, depending on the anatomy and pathology.
   d. The approach is familiar to all neurosurgeons and not unique for this disease.

2. Disadvantages
   a. This is a major operation with significant morbidity and mortality.
   b. The operation is not well tolerated by acutely ill or aged patients.
   c. Significant manipulation of the frontal or temporal lobes is required.
   d. There is often unilateral anosmia.
   e. Even slight trauma to severely stretched optic nerves may worsen vision.
   f. This approach does not readily allow visual differentiation of gland from tumor.
   g. This method does not allow removal of tumor that has extended into the sphenoid sinus.

transsphenoidal route. The size of the tumor makes little difference as long as suprasellar extension, if present, is in the midline and the sella is enlarged. Figure 4 shows an example of an adenoma that reached well into the third ventricle and was removed from below. The suprasellar portion must communicate widely with the intrasellar portion; otherwise, instruments cannot be readily or safely passed into the suprasellar region. Because most adenomas are soft, the suprasellar portion of the tumor usually drops into the sella (see Chapter 18). Of 80 cases of large nonsecreting tumors reported by Hardy and Vezina,[77] 46 had significant suprasellar expansion. In all but 3, the dome collapsed into the sella during surgery. In the other 3, postoperative encephalography showed subsequent collapse. However, if there is extension anteriorly beneath the frontal lobe (Fig. 5), or laterally into the middle fossa, then transcranial surgery is necessary. If the sella is small or if there is a dumbbell-shaped tumor, waisted by a tight diaphragma sella, transcranial surgery will be necessary.

TABLE 5. Transsphenoidal Approach: Advantages and Disadvantages

1. Advantages
   a. Morbidity and mortality are extremely low.
   b. Trauma to the brain is minimized.
   c. The operation is tolerated extremely well by acutely ill and aged patients.
   d. This approach allows visual differentiation of small tumors within the gland.
   e. Anesthetic and convalescent times are short.

2. Disadvantages
   a. The neural structures adjacent to the large tumor cannot be visualized.
   b. The approach is through a nonsterile field (although we have had only one case of meningitis in over 100 cases).
   c. Capabilities are limited if the diagnosis is questionable.
   d. A suprasellar extension into frontal fossa, middle fossa, or retroclival area that is very asymmetric cannot be removed.

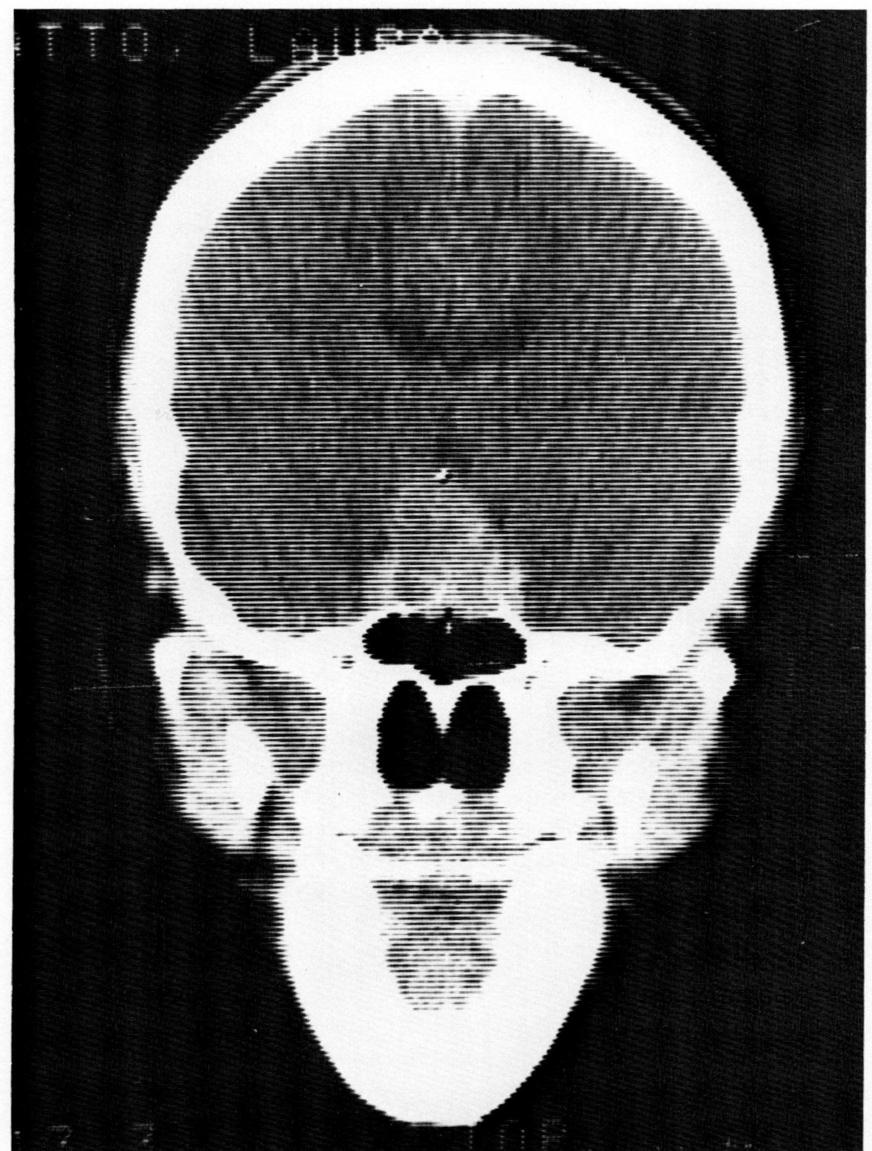

Fig. 4. Enhanced coronal CT scan of 16-year-old female with a midline suprasellar extension into the third ventricle of a prolactin-secreting adenoma that was removed via a transsphenoidal route.

Nonfunctional tumors with multidirectional intracranial extension (Fig. 6) preclude transcranial surgery and are decompressed from below. Likewise, tumors extending predominantly into the sphenoid sinus are best removed transsphenoidally (Fig. 7).

Nonfunctioning tumors in elderly or acutely ill patients, as well as in patients with severe general medical problems, are approached transsphenoi-

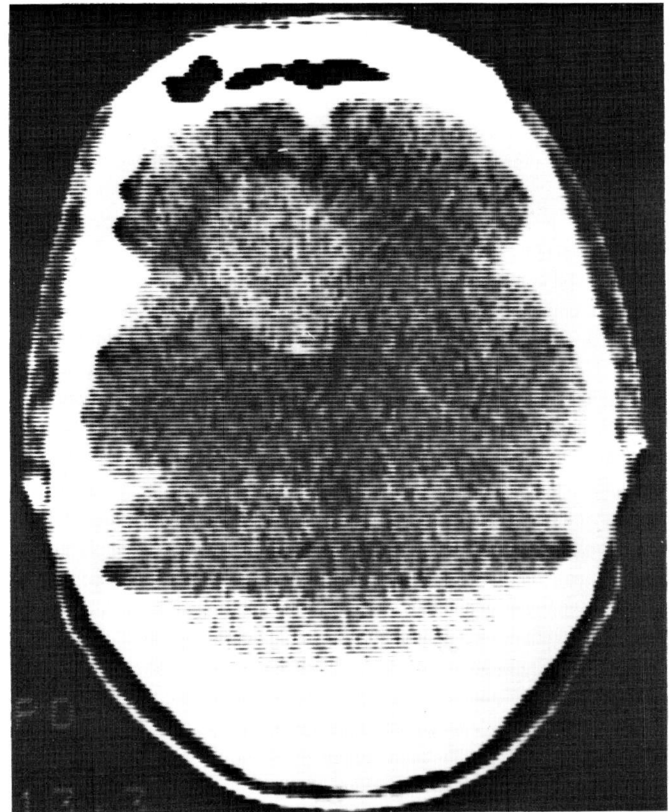

Fig. 5. Enhanced CT scan of an acromegalic patient with an extremely large subfrontal suprasellar tumor extension requiring craniotomy for removal.

dally, since the risks of transcranial surgery would be too great. In situations wherein the vision is severely compromised so that further manipulation would endanger remaining vision, transsphendoidal surgery is considered safer, since there is less trauma to the optic nerves and chiasm. Vision is restored more frequently and rapidly following this type of operation.[78]

Pituitary apoplexy, as in the case summarized previously, is usually seen in acutely ill patients, possibly with associated meningitis. Surgery is better tolerated and more rapidly performed through the sphenoid sinus. I have used the open surgical technique with excellent results. Zervas and Mendelson[79] reported on three cases of apoplexy treated successfully with a stereotaxic transnasal technique. They were able to aspirate 4–6 cc of dark blood and necrotic fragments of adenoma with rapid improvement of the visual deficits.

Functional tumors are graded according to the classification described by Hardy[48] and similarly by Guiot,[65] which is demonstrated in Chapter 14. For lower-grade microadenomas, transsphenoidal surgery is ideal, since the direct exposure of the pituitary gland allows complete differentiation of the tumor

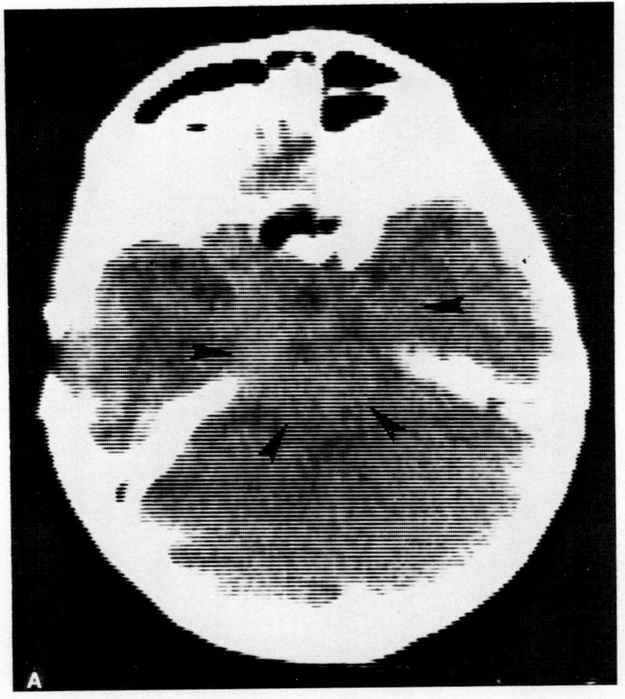

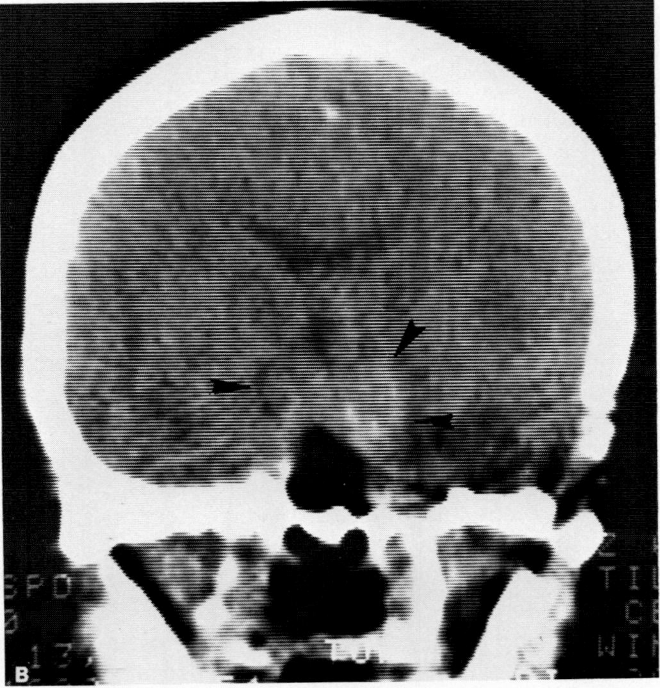

Fig. 6. Enhanced horizontal (A) and coronal (B) CT scans of a patient presenting with a CSF leak and a recurrence of a nonfunctional tumor (arrows) 7 years after resection via craniotomy. Multidirectional intracranial extension as well as the CSF rhinorrhea made the transsphenoidal route indicated.

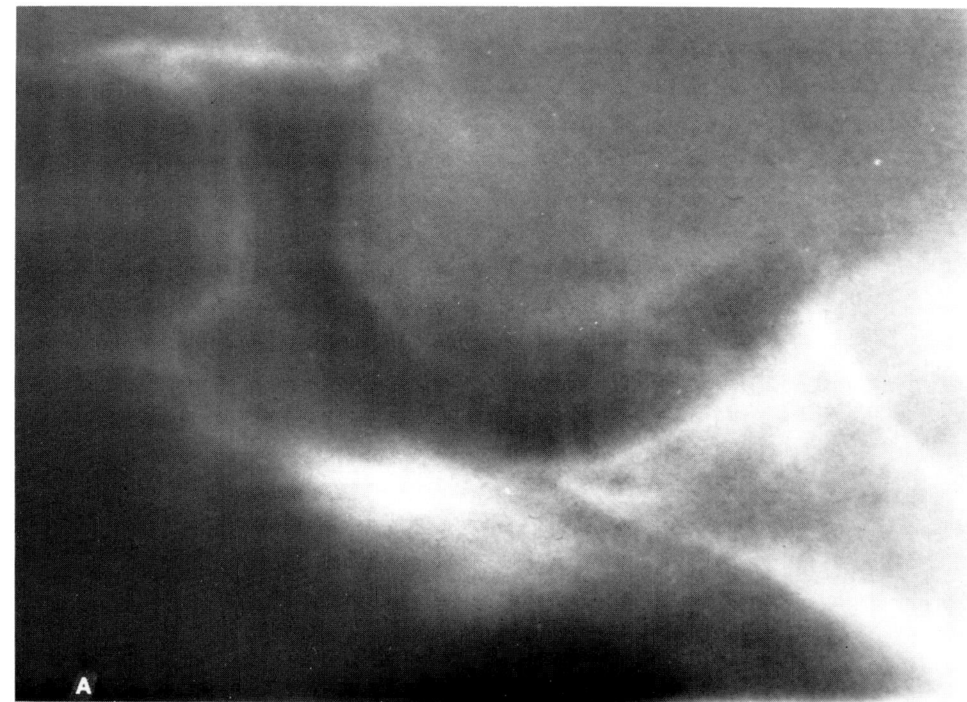

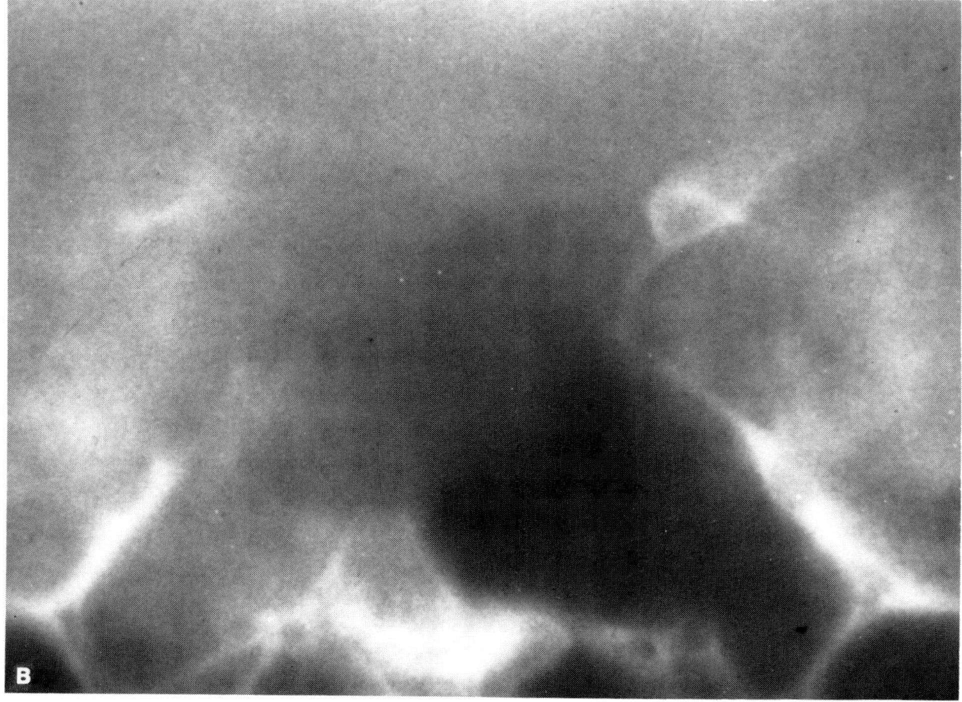

Fig. 7. Lateral (A) and anteroposterior (B) tomograms of a patient with a prolactin-secreting tumor with significant extension into the sphenoid sinus.

from the gland so that a selective total removal is accomplished. Grade II patients also benefit from the direct exposure of the transsphenoidal approach, but differentiation of tumor from gland becomes more difficult. Grades III and IV are generally more resistant to a surgical endocrine cure, and they are treated in a fashion similar to nonfunctional tumors, with perhaps a more aggressive removal. Transsphenoidal surgery is performed with the same restrictions applied to nonfunctional tumors. Attempts at total removal are made with either approach, more so than with the nonfunctional tumors, because of the lower response to adjunctive radiotherapy.

Another contraindication to transsphenoidal surgery is intercurrent nasal or paranasal sinus infection. Most often, surgery can be delayed until this is appropriately treated. However, if the situation is urgent, then the approach would best be performed away from the infected spaces, i.e., via craniotomy.

6. Interpretation of Surgical Results

The various types of pituitary tumors, as well as their various forms of treatment, mandate that the terms used to compare results be standardized. When comparing results from different surgical approaches, modern techniques must be compared to equally modern techniques. It seems inappropriate to me to use 30-year-old surgical statistics for cure rates, recurrences, or complications when one compares the results of more recent modalities such as microsurgery, supervoltage radiation, heavy-particle radiation, or medical therapy. Advances in surgical techniques, particularly the microscope and microdissections, which apply equally to the transsphenoidal operation and the transcranial operation, have made some of the "classic" series archaic.

"Cure" should be defined in the strictest sense, i.e, total tumor removal and total normalization of the elevated hormone in a hypersecreting adenoma. A 90 or 95% reduction of an elevated hormone cannot be considered a cure if the final level remains above the normal range. "Improved" would be a better classification for this situation, or "remission," which implies a reduction of function to normal with the additional implication that some tumor remains and may become active again in the future. In concert with removing the tumor, we must also be concerned with the morbidity of the resection, in particular as regards the other hormonal function. Deficiencies in other hormones may be present preoperatively, and these may not return to normal.[64] During the resection, other hormonal function may be lost, and in certain instances this is acceptable and in others it is not acceptable. With microadenomas, there should be no new deficiencies, while, it is to be hoped, previous deficiencies will resolve. With Cushing's disease or Nelson's syndrome, however, there may be loss of some normal function if a very aggressive procedure is carried out to secure complete elimination of the tumor. This may be considered reasonable, while it would be unacceptable with a prolactin-secreting adenoma. With larger tumors, the accepted morbidity of hormone function loss is greater as the emphasis of treatment shifts toward eliminating the mass effects and neurological compromise. A patient should be considered "worse" if the morbidity of the resection is greater than acceptable for that particular type and size adenoma. Any neurological morbidity is considered worse.

Therefore, when evaluating results of any modality of treatment, it must be clear that similar groups are being compared so that accurate conclusions can be reached. The definitions of "cure," "improved," "remission," and "worse" should be constant, but the accepted endocrine morbidity may vary with the adenoma's secreting characteristics and size.

7. Summary

Considerations for surgery such as indications, goals, and approaches vary in secreting and nonsecreting tumors. Nonfunctional tumors are surgical candidates if there is any type of mass effect noted, visual or other. Incidental nonfunctioning tumors may become surgical candidates if there is evidence of progressive growth. Functional tumors secreting ACTH, GH, or TSH are almost always considered candidates for surgery, while there is still some question regarding prolactin-secreting microadenomas. In the latter situation, if pregnancy is desired or if there is evidence of progressive growth, then surgery is indicated. In large secreting adenomas, surgery is again almost always recommended.

Patients with pituitary apoplexy, CSF leaks, recurrence after radiation treatment, or uncertain diagnoses are almost always surgical candidates.

The goals of surgery differ. In nonfunctional tumors, attempts may be made at total removal, but a subtotal removal followed by radiation therapy is often safer and just as effective. In secreting microadenomas, the goal is a selective total removal sparing the normal gland. A spectrum of aggressiveness exists with ACTH-secreting tumors mandating a complete removal, at times with sacrifice of the normal gland. GH-secreting tumors are also removed aggressively, but the normal gland is usually preserved in questionable situations, while in prolactin-secreting tumors, a more conservative procedure is planned with utmost care for preservation of the normal gland, even at the expense of leaving adenoma tissue *in situ*. For large secreting tumors, goals are similar to those for nonsecreting tumors, but a more aggressive removal is pursued.

The choice of surgical approach depends on the size and location of the tumor. Microadenomas and tumors extending into the sphenoid sinus are always approached via the transsphenoidal route. Large tumors with suprasellar extensions in the midline are also approached transsphenoidally as long as there is a larger sella and open communication between the intrasellar and suprasellar components. Transcranial surgery is performed for asymmetric extension into the frontal or middle fossa, or for tumors with dumbbell shape and limited communication between the intrasellar and suprasellar components.

Preoperative radiation does not preclude surgical intervention, but it makes selective removal of an adenoma more difficult because of the scarring and increased difficulty in distinguishing adenoma from normal gland.

Finally, the terms "cure," "improved," "remission," and "worse" must be well defined so that accurate comparisons of therapy for each type and size of tumor may be made with meaning. Also, modern series must be compared with equally modern series from other forms of therapy for meaningful evaluations.

References

1. P. Marie, Sur deux cas d'acromegalie: Hypertrophie singuliere, non congenitale, des extremities superieures, inferieure et cephalique, *Rev. Med.* (*Paris*) **6**:297–333, 1886.
2. R. Caton and F.T. Paul, Notes of a case of acromegaly treated by operation, *Br. Med. J.* **2**:1421–1432, 1893.
3. F. Krause, Hirnchirurgie, *Dtsch. Klin.* **8**:953–1024, 1905.
4. V. Horsley, On the technique of operation on the central nervous system, *Br. Med. J.* **2**:411, 1906.
5. H. Schloffer, Erfolgreiche Operation eines Hypophysecentumors auf nasalem Wege, *Wien. Klin. Wochenschr.* **20**:621–624, 1907.
6. F. Giordano, *Compendio Chir. Operat. Ital.* **2**:100, 1897 (quoted by G.J. Heuer, The surgical approach and the treatment of tumors and other lesions about the optic chiasm, *Surg. Gynecol. Obstet.* **53**:489–518, 1931).
7. H. Cushing, Partial hypophysectomy for acromegaly with remarks on the function of the hypophysis, *Ann. Surg.* **50**:1002–1017, 1909.
8. A.E. Halstead, Remarks on the operative treatment of tumors of the hypophysis, with the report of two cases operated on by an oro-nasal method, *Surg. Gynecol. Obstet.* **10**:494–502, 1910.
9. T. Kocher, Die Verletzungen der Wirbelsäule zugleich als Beitrag zur Physiologie des menschlichen Ruckenmarks Mitt a.d., *Grenzgeb. Med. Chir.* **1**:415–580, 1896.
10. O. Hirsch, Endonasal method of removal of hypophyseal tumours: With report of two cases, *J. Am. Med. Assoc.* **55**:772, 1910.
11. O. Hirsch, Pituitary tumours: A borderland between cranial and trans-sphenoidal surgery, *N. Eng. J. Med.* **254**:937–939, 1954.
12. O. Hirsch, Life-long cures and improvements after trans-sphenoidal operation of pituitary tumours (thirty-three patients followed for 20–37 years), *Acta Ophthalmol.* (*Copenhagen*) *Suppl.* **56**:60, 1959.
13. H. Cushing, Surgical experiences with pituitary disorders, *J. Am. Med. Assoc.* **63**:1515–1525, 1914.
14. C.H. Frazier, An approach to the hypophysis through the anterior cranial fossa, *Ann. Surg.* **57**:145–150, 1913.
15. C.H. Frazier and F.C. Grant, Pituitary disorder, a digest of 100 cases, with remarks on the surgical treatment, *J. Am. Med. Assoc.* **85**:1103–1106, 1925.
16. H. Cushing, *The Pituitary Body and Its Disorders: Clinical States Produced By Disorders of the Hypophysis Cerebri*, p. 341, J.B. Lippincott, Philadelphia, 1912.
17. H. Cushing, *Intracranial Tumors: Notes upon a Series of Two Thousand Verified Cases with Surgical–Mortality Percentages Pertaining Thereto*, Charles C. Thomas, p. 150, Springfield, Illinois, 1932.
18. W.R. Henderson, The pituitary adenomata: Follow-up study of surgical results in 338 cases (Dr. Harvey Cushing's series), *Br. J. Surg.* **26**:811–921, 1939.
19. H.C. Johnson, Surgery of the hypophysis, in: *A History of Neurological Surgery* (W.E. Walker, ed.), pp. 152–177, Hafner, New York, 1967.
20. E.C. Kendall, Some observations on the hormone of the adrenal cortex designated Compound E, *Mayo Clin. Proc.* **24**:298, 1949.
21. G. Guiot and B. Thibaut, L'extirpation des adenomes hypophysaires par voie transsphenoidale, *Neuro-Chirur.* (*Stuttgart*) **1**:133, 1959.
22. J. Hardy, *Microsurgery Applied to Neurosurgery* (M.G. Yasargil, ed.), pp. 180–193, Academic Press, New York, 1969.
23. J. Hardy, A. Panisset, A. Marchildon, and A. Lanthier, Microsurgical selective anterior pituitary ablation for diabetic retinopathy, *Can. Med. Assoc. J.* **100**:785–792, 1969.

24. L.I. Malis, Bipolar coagulation in microsurgery, in: *Microsurgery Applied to Neurosurgery* (M.G. Yasargil, ed.), pp. 41–45, Academic Press, New York, 1969.
25. C.H. Chang and J.L. Pool, The radiotherapy of pituitary chromophobe adenomas, *Radiology* **89:**1005, 1967.
26. L.M. Davidoff, Symposium on pituitary tumours. IV. Discussion of papers, *J. Neurosurg.* **19:**22, 1962.
27. R.T. Costello, Subclinical adenoma of the pituitary gland, *Am. J. Pathol.* **12:**205–215, 1936.
28. J.W. Kernohan and G.P. Sayre, Tumors of the pituitary gland and infundibulum, in: *Atlas of Tumor Pathology, 1st Series*, Fascicle 36, Armed Forces Institute of Pathology, Washington, D.C., 1956.
29. G.E. Sheline, Comment in discussion, in: *Diagnosis and Treatment of Pituitary Tumors* (P.O. Kohler and G.T. Ross, eds.), pp. 157–158, Excerpta Medica, Amsterdam, 1973.
30. J.B. Tyrrell, R.M. Brooks, P.A. Fitzgerald, P.B. Cofoid, P.H. Forsham, and C.B. Wilson, Cushing's disease: Selective trans-sphenoidal resection of pituitary microadenomas, *N. Engl. J. Med.* **298**(14):753–758, 1978.
31. W.H. Daughaday, Cushing's disease and basophilic microadenomas (editorial), *N. Engl. J. Med.* **298**(14):793, 1978.
32. R.M. Salassa, E.R. Laws, Jr., P.C. Carpenter, and R.C. Northcutt, Transsphenoidal removal of pituitary midroadenoma in Cushing's disease, *Mayo Clin. Proc.* **53:**24–28, 1978.
33. D.P. MacErlean and F.H. Doyle, The pituitary fossa in Cushing's syndrome: A retrospective analysis of 93 patients, *Br. J. Radiol.* **49:**820–826, 1976.
34. R.M. Salassa, T.P. Kearns, J.W. Kernohan, *et al.*, Pituitary tumors in patients with Cushing's syndrome, *J. Clin. Endocrinol. Metab.* **19:**1523–1539, 1959.
35. T.J. Moore, R.G. Dluhy, G.H. Williams, and J.P. Cain, Nelson's syndrome: Frequency, prognosis, and effect of prior pituitary irradiation, *Ann. Intern. Med.* **85**(6):731–734, 1976.
36. A.S. Jennings, G.W. Liddle, and D.N. Orth, Results of treating childhood Cushing's disease with pituitary irradiation, *N. Engl. J. Med.* **297**(18):957–962, 1977.
37. D.N. Orth and G.W. Liddle, Results of treatment in 108 patients with Cushing's syndrome, *N. Engl. J. Med.* **285:**243, 1971.
38. F.C. Dohan, A. Raventos, N. Boucot, and E. Rose, Roentgen therapy in Cushing's syndrome without adrenocortical tumor, *J. Clin. Endocrinol. Metab.* **17:**8, 1957.
39. A.D. Wright, D.M. Hill, C. Lowy, and T.R. Fraser, Mortality in acromegaly, *Q. J. Med.* **39:**1–16, 1970.
40. J. Roth, P. Gorden, and K. Brace, Efficacy of conventional pituitary irradiation in acromegaly, *N. Engl. J. Med.* **282**(25):1385–1391, 1970.
41. J.F. Aloia, M.S. Roginsky, and J.O. Archambeau, Pituitary irradiation in acromegaly, *Am. J. Med. Sci.* **267**(2):81–87, 1974.
42. R.N. Kjellberg, A. Shintani, A.G. Frantz, and B. Kliman, Proton-beam therapy in acromegaly, *N. Engl. J. Med.* **278**(13):690–695, 1968.
43. R.N. Kjellberg and B. Kliman, Radiosurgery therapy for pituitary adenoma, Presented at a Symposium on Pituitary Tumors, Tufts–New England Medical Center, Boston, Massachusetts, April 5, 1978.
44. M.E. Molitch, Medical therapy of pituitary tumors, in: *The Pituitary Adenoma* (K.D. Post, I.M.D. Jackson, and S. Reichlin, eds.), Plenum Press, New York, 1980.
45. S. Franks, H.S. Jacobs, and J.D.N. Nabarro, Studies of prolactin in pituitary disease, *J. Endocrinol.* **67:**55, 1977.
46. J.L. Antunes, E.M. Housepian, A.G. Frantz, D.A. Holub, R.M. Hui, P.W. Carmel, and D.O. Quest, Prolactin-secreting pituitary tumors, *Ann. Neurol.* **2:**148–153, 1977.
47. J. Hardy, *Clinical Neurosurgery* p. 16, Williams and Wilkins, Baltimore, 1969.
48. J. Hardy, Trans-sphenoidal microsurgical removal of pituitary adenoma, in: *Recent Progress in Neurological Surgery*, p. 86, Excerpta Medica, Amsterdam, 1974.
49. J.N. Carter, J.E. Tyson, G. Tolis, S. Van Vliet, C. Faiman, and H.G. Friesen, Prolactin-secreting tumors and hypogonadism in 22 men, *N. Engl. J. Med.* **299**(16):847–852, 1978.
50. S.M. Wolpert, The radiology of pituitary adenomas—an update, in: *The Pituitary Adenoma* (K.D. Post, I.M.D. Jackson, and S. Reichlin, eds.), Plenum Press, New York, 1980.
51. J.L. Vezina and S.J. Tudor, Prolactin-secreting pituitary microadenomas: Roentgenologic diagnosis, *Am. J. Roentgenol. Radium Ther. Nucl. Med.* **120:**46–54, 1974.

52. R.F. Spark, J. Pallotta, F. Naftolin, and R. Clemens, Galactorrhea–amenorrhea syndromes: Etiology and treatment, *Ann. Intern. Med.* **84:**532–537, 1976.

53. M.O. Thorner, A.S. McNeilly, C. Hagan, and G.M. Besser, Long-term treatment of galactorrhea and hypogonadism with bromocriptine, *Br. Med. J.* **2:**419–422, 1974.

54. E. Del Pozo, L. Varga, H. Wyss, G. Tolis, H. Friesen, R. Wenner, L. Vetter, and A. Uettwiler, Clinical and hormonal response to bromocriptine (CB 154) in the galactorrhea syndromes, *J. Clin. Endocrinol. Metab.* **39:**18–26, 1974.

55. M.A. Galconer and M.A. Stafford-Bell, Visual failure from pituitary and parasellar tumours occurring with favourable outcome in pregnant women, *J. Neurol. Neurosurg. Psychiatry* **38:**914–930, 1975.

56. P.B. Nelson, A.G. Robinson, D.F. Archer, and J.C. Maroon, Symptomatic pituitary tumor enlargement after induced pregnancy: Case report, *J. Neurosurg.* **49:**283–287, 1978.

57. M.D. Thorner, G.M. Besser, A. Jones, J. Daice, A.E. Jones, and C.N. Shealy, Bromocriptine treatment of female infertility: Report of 13 pregnancies, *Br. Med. J.* **4:**694–697, 1975.

58. R.H. Wiebe, C.B. Hammond, and S. Handwerger, Treatment of functional amenorrhea–galactorrhea with 2-bromoergocryptine, *Fertil. Steril.* **28:**426–433, 1977.

59. J.T.W. Van Dalen and E.L. Greve, Rapid deterioration of visual fields during bromocriptine-induced pregnancy in a patient with a pituitary adenoma, *Br. J. Ophthalmol.* **61**(2):729–733, 1977.

60. K.D. Post, B.J. Biller, L.S. Adelman, M.E. Molitch, S.M. Wolpert, and S. Reichlin, Results of selective transsphenoidal adenomectomy in women with galactorrhea–amenorrhea, *J. Am. Med. Assoc.* **242**(2):158–162. 1979.

61. B. Corenblum, B.R. Webster, C.B. Mortimer, and C. Ezrin, Possible antitumour effect of bromocriptine in two patients with large prolactin-secreting pituitary adenomas, *Clin. Res.* **34:**614, 1975 (abstract).

62. A.M. McGregor, M.F. Scanlon, and K. Hall, Reduction in size of a pituitary tumor by bromocriptine therapy, *N. Engl. J. Med.* **300:**291–293, 1979.

63. K.D. Post and D.L. Kasdon, Sellar and parasellar lesions mimicking adenoma, in: *The Pituitary Adenoma* (K.D. Post, I.M.D. Jackson, and S. Reichlin, eds.), Plenum Press, New York, 1980.

64. C.S. McLanahan, J.H. Christy, and G.T. Tindall, Anterior pituitary function before and after trans-sphenoidal microsurgical resection of pituitary tumors, *Neurosurgery* **3**(2):142–145, 1978.

65. G. Guiot, Transsphenoidal approach in surgical treatment of pituitary adenomas: General principles and indications in non-functioning adenomas, in: *Diagnosis and Treatment of Pituitary Tumors* (P.O. Kohler and G.T. Ross, eds.), pp. 159–178, Excerpta Medica, Amsterdam, 1973.

66. L.S. Adelman and K.D. Post, Intraoperative frozen section technique for pituitary adenomas, *Am. J. Surg. Pathol.*, February, 1979.

67. B.S. Ray and R.H. Patterson, Symposium on pituitary tumors. 1. Surgical treatment of pituitary adenomas, *J. Neurosurg.* **19:**1, 1962.

68. B.S. Ray and R.H. Patterson, Surgical experience with chromophobe adenomas of the pituitary gland, *J. Neurosurg.* **34:**726, 1971.

69. H.J. Svien and M.Y. Colby, Pituitary chromophobe adenomas: Comparative results of surgical and roentgen treatment, *Behav. Neurol.* **1:**35, 1969.

70. T.P. Hayes, R.A. Davis, and A. Raventos, The treatment of pituitary chromophobe adenomas, *Radiology* **98:**149, 1971.

71. S.G. Elington and W. McKissock, Pituitary adenomata: Results of combined surgery and radiotherapeutic treatment of 260 patients, *Br. Med. J.* **1:**263, 1967.

72. G.E. Sheline, E.B. Boldrey, and T.L. Phillips, Chromophobe adenomas of the pituitary gland, *Am. J. Roentgenol.* **92:**160, 1964.

73. S.B. Heimbach, Étude uivie de 105 cas d'adenomes chromophobes et acidophiles de l'hypophyse, dument verifies apres traitement par operation transfrontale et radiotherapie (Krayenbuhl's series), *Acta Neurochir. (Vienna)* **7:**101, 1959.

74. J.I. Neurnberger and S.R. Korey, *Pituitary Chromophobe Adenomas*, Springer-Verlag, New York, 1953.

75. W. Tonnis, D. Oberdisse, and F. Weber, Bericht über 264 operierte Hypophysenadenome, *Acta Neurochir. (Vienna)* **2**(3):133, 1952.

76. J. Hardy, Transsphenoidal surgery of hypersecreting pituitary tumors, in: *Diagnosis and Treatment of Pituitary Tumors* (P.O. Kohler and G.T. Ross, eds.), pp. 170–194, Excerpta Medica, Amsterdan, 1973.
77. J. Hardy and J.L. vezina, Transsphenoidal neurosurgery of intracranial neoplasm, in: *Advances in Neurology* (R.A. Thompson and J.R. Green, eds.), pp. 261–274, Raven Press, New York, 1976.
78. P. Demailly, G. Guiot, and A. Oproiu, Resultats visuels des exereses d'adenomes hypophysaires par voie transsphenoidale, *Arch. Ophthalmol. (Paris)* **27**:5, 1967.
79. N. Zervas and G. Mendelson, Treatment of acute hemorrhage of pituitary tumors, *Lancet* **1**:604, 1975.

17

Anatomical Aspects of the Transseptal Approach to the Sphenoid Sinus

BRUCE W. PEARSON, EUGENE B. KERN, THOMAS J. McDONALD, and EDWARD R. LAWS, Jr.

1. Introduction

Approximately one quarter of the brain's surface is supported by the frontal, ethmoid, and sphenoid bones. Each of these bones is pneumatized by sinus cavities that in turn derive from the nasal cavity. Not surprisingly, the subject of rhinological anatomy continues to engage the attention of surgeons called on to approach the base of the skull. Transseptal transphenoidal hypophysectomy provides a notable example of the validity of this interest. The first half of the transseptal operation proceeds through normal nasal anatomy.

Since 1973, we have enjoyed the privilege of collaboration in the performance of over 600 transseptal transsphenoidal approaches to the sella.[1] This has prompted reappraisal of the anatomy of the nose and septum by reference to the skull and the cadaver. The purpose of this chapter is not to advance a specific operative technique, but to lay out the anatomical foundation on which the transseptal approach to the sella is based.

2. The External Nose

2.1. Cosmetic Analysis

The shape of the nose reflects the thickness of the skin and the form of the underlying nasal skeleton. Despite wide variations with age, race, sex, culture, and aesthetic persuasion in what might be called the norm, several generalizations can be made.

BRUCE W. PEARSON, EUGENE B. KERN, and THOMAS J. McDONALD • Department of Otolaryngology, Mayo Medical School, Rochester, Minnesota 55901. *EDWARD R. LAWS, Jr.* • Department of Neurological Surgery, Mayo Medical School, Rochester, Minnesota 55901.

Patients examine their own noses from the front (in the mirror). They are sensitive to the reactions of others, who view them mainly from the side. In the frontal view, minimal deviation of the nose to one side or broadening of the base of the nose above the upper lip (both possibilities from septal surgery alone) are poorly tolerated by young and discerning women. An external nasal scar, particularly across the dorsum, a bulbous nasal tip, or any deformation or asymmetry of the nostril rim are so strongly resented that few nasal operations have survived that have risked their production. In the profile view, saddle depressions of the nasal dorsum and retraction of the nasolabial angle to a sharper angle than 90° in a man or 100° in a woman are generally considered deformities. This appearance denotes injury; it is not produced in nature. The structural deficiency responsible for a depressed dorsum and a retracted columella is not nasal but septal in origin.

2.2. Influence of the Septum

The upper third of the external nose is projected by bone. The middle third is borne by the septal cartilage. The profile line is created by the anterosuperior ("dorsal" in surgical parlance) border of the septal cartilage. The lateral walls of the external nose are defined by the upper lateral cartilages, which extend from the dorsal border of the septum like two triangular tabs. Superiorly, they underlap the nasal bones and the frontal processes of the maxilla. Inferiorly, they end in a free margin, curled outward, above the upper margin of the alar cartilage. Medially, they are continuous with the septal cartilage. The lower third of the nose is the tip or lobule (Fig. 1).

The tip is supported by two parallel U-shaped cartilages opening backward. These cartilages (the alar cartilages) consist of a broad, thin lateral crus, an anterior dome, and a curved strutlike medial crus (Fig. 1). The tip is self-supporting and largely independent of the septum, except that the feet of the medial crura rise and flare laterally to lightly embrace the anteroinferior (caudal) border of the septum several millimeters anterior to the apex of the nasal spine. To some extent, the maintenance of tip projection depends on the integrity of this loose synchondrosis.

The nasolabial angle is normally filled out by the soft tissue of the columella and the philtrum. The thickened lower edge of the septum, and its blending with the nasal spine, are responsible for maintaining this shape. By palpating your own nose and feeling the lower (caudal) edge of the septal cartilage through the skin, you can confirm these relationships.

The dorsal and caudal borders of the septum meet at an anterior corner (the anterior–inferior or septal angle). This angle is situated in the slight depression just above the nasal tip (the supratip region). It has nothing to do with the forward projection of the tip! Deviations of the septal angle to the right or left, however, even subtle ones, give the nasal dorsum a peculiar S-shaped twist.

Transseptal surgery risks damage to the septal cartilage. The cosmetic effect of the excessive loss of septal cartilage is flattening or saddling of the nasal dorsum, a mild assymmetric nasal twist, slight loss of tip projection, and conversion of the smooth nasolabial angle into a retracted crevice. In an

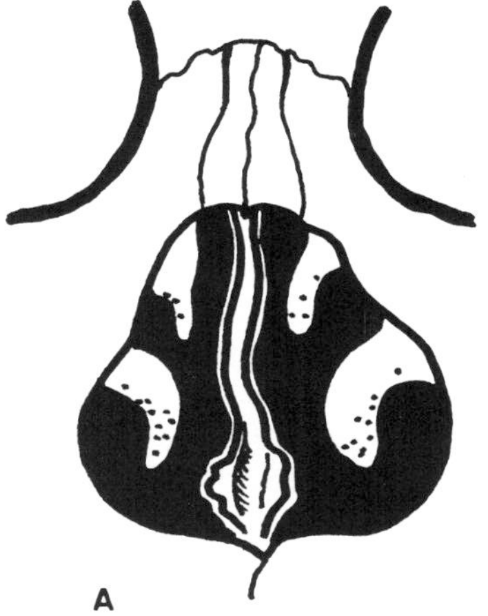

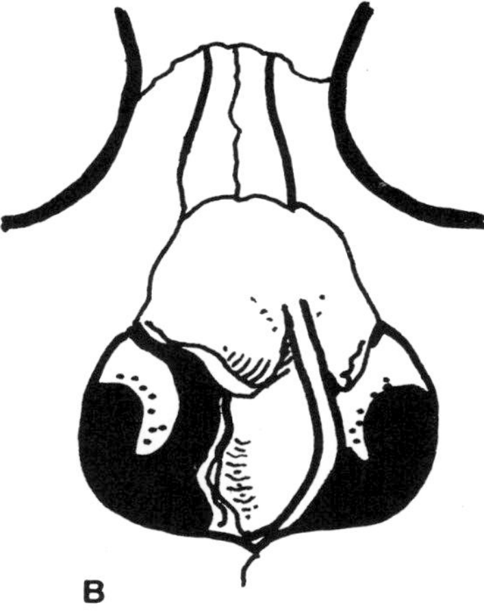

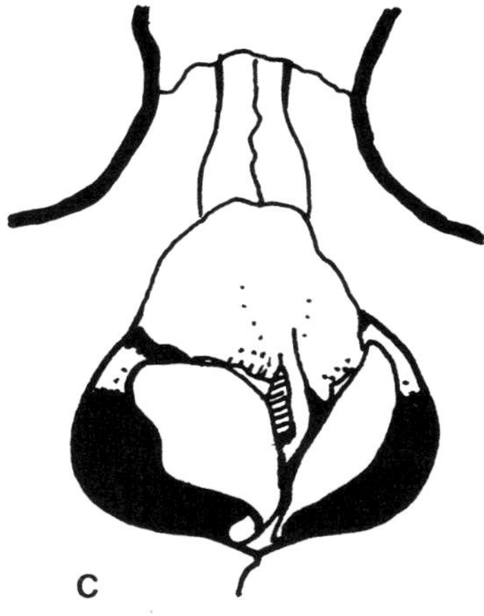

Fig. 1. The cartilaginous skeleton of the external nose from the front is erected on the septum. Consequently, septal surgery risks external cosmetic deformity. (A) The bony septum along with its groove to receive the cartilage and its anterior premaxillary wings can be seen. (B) The septal cartilage and the upper lateral cartilages that support the middle third of the nose are one continuous structure. (C) The alar cartilages that give definition and support to the nasal tip are separate from the skeptal skeleton. Injury is avoided by initiating septal dissections at the caudal edge of the septum.

acromegalic, this merely converts a heavy nose to a pugilistic nose. But in the attractive young prolactin secretor, whose confidence is already shaken by her amenorrhea, this deformity is a significant blow to the self-image.

3. The Nasal Cavity

3.1. Nostril

The nostril is the margin of the nasal vestibule. The vestibule is that part of the nasal cavity lined by skin and bearing sweat glands and hair follicles. On the septal side, the skin blends almost imperceptibly with the mucosa over the septal cartilage, but on the lateral side, the transition to mucosa is sharply demarcated by the nasal valve.

Nostrils in the white-skinned races are oriented longitudinally, while in blacks they are more transverse. The out-turned feet of the medial crura indent the medial border of each nostril and render it kidney-shaped. Anteriorly, a fold of skin and connective tissue unites the lower edges of the crura to form the floor of an anterior vestibular recess.

The lateral rim of the nostril is not supported by cartilage. It gradually expands with fibrofatty tissue as it approaches its junction with the face. The rounded lateral prominence thus formed is called the nasal "ala" ("wing").

The nostril may be considered an incision in the face that exposes but limits access to the nasal cavity. If full advantage of the nasal cavity is to be taken and the space afforded by one side combined with that afforded by the other, the nostril (except in the occasional acromegalic) must be bypassed or enlarged. To preserve midline orientation and avoid deforming the nostril rim in any way, the sublabial approach has been advocated.

3.2. Valve

The lower edge of the upper lateral cartilage raises a fold on the inside of the lateral nasal wall well within view of the examiner. This fold is supported by the thin, outwardly rolled cartilaginous free border of the upper lateral cartilage and is braced by the facial musculature. It must remain stiff enough to resist the negative pressure of strong inspiration; otherwise, it will collapse against the septum and occlude the nose. The nasal valve is the flow-limiting segment of the nasal airway. Small almost minuscule obstructions placed at this site, mucosal crusts, for example, produce major symptoms. Long-standing congenital obstructions are often tolerated without complaint, but acute and acquired obstructions, such as may follow injury or surgery, are not. Although the subjective nature of nasal obstruction is not fully understood, marked increases in nasal resistance and a drop in the critical collapsing pressure of the valve can be demonstrated rhinomanometrically in patients with structural deformity in this area.

3.3. Nasal Atrium

Between the valve area and the beginning of the turbinates on the lateral nasal wall, the nasal cavities are smooth and symmetrical. These areas, the nasal atria, are bounded laterally by the osseous lateral nasal walls (frontal process of the maxilla, not nasal bones), superiorly by the nasal bones, and medially by the thickened junction between the posterosuperior border of the septal cartilage and the anteroinferior border of the ethmoid plate. Septal resection in this area is not attended by cosmetic sequelae.

3.4. Turbinates and Meati

The middle and superior turbinates are critical obstructive elements to transnasal surgery. Fortunately, they consist of cavernous vascular tissue on a very thin bony support. The cavernous tissue can be vasoconstricted with cocaine, and the turbinates can be mobilized and outfractured. Resection is not tolerated; it produces obstruction, due to crusting. The "superior" turbinate is actually posterosuperior, and stands in the way of the sphenoethmoidal recess. Fortunately, its base is the posterior ethmoid air cell complex, and it can easily be fractured aside. In patients with capillary fragility (e.g., Cushing's disease), this act causes early delayed periorbital ecchymosis, of sometimes dramatic appearance but certainly little consequence.

The middle turbinate hoods the middle meatus, which is the recipient site of all the sinus ostia except the posterior ethmoids and sphenoids. Its attachment to the lateral nasal wall (ethmoids again) is oblique, passing from high anterior to low posterior in the nose. On the other hand, the oblique trajectory of the pituitary speculum across the nose passes from low anterior to high posterior. The tips of the speculi almost meet the middle turbinates at right angles. Difficulty inserting the speculum may therefore arise because the tips evaginate the septal mucoperichondrium up into the middle meatus, arresting the instrument and risking a perforation.

The inferior turbinate is a separate bone, shaped like an inverted canoe. Because of its shape and its stronger foundation, it is more resistant to outfracture than the other turbinates. The inferior turbinates lie opposite the lower portion of the septal cartilage. In the act of opening the pituitary speculum, the septal mucosa is strongly compressed against these bony projections. Inspection of the mucosa when the speculum is removed will sometimes reveal that the mucosa has been split by the compression. This should be repaired.

3.5. Choana

The choana is the posterior aperture of the nasal chamber. It is a ring of bone. Starting at the apex of the right choana and working clockwise around its margin, we would encounter in turn the ala of the vomer, the vomer itself, the crest and horizontal process of the palatine bone, the vertical plate of the palatine bone, and the sphenoid process of the palatine bone. Thus, the vomerine ala and the palatine sphenoid process arch from medial and lateral, respectively, to form a strong vault under the floor of the sphenoid sinus. This renders the floor much thicker than the face of the sphenoid, which consists of a thin membrane bone, the sphenoid concha. Sometimes the vomerine ala break away with the rostrum when it is avulsed.

3.6. Physiology of the Normal Nasal Airway

The nose is an extremely sophisticated air conditioner. Assuming the septum remains intact, the nose is actually two air conditioners, in parallel. Clinical observation and nasal resistance experiements have shown that one nasal chamber transmits the bulk of the airflow while the other takes a rest. Every 5 or 6 hr, the decongested or working side responds to the desiccating and irritating effects of the inspired airstream by congesting. At the same time, the turbinates on the opposite side decongest. Thus, the nasal cavities are two parallel resistors, reciprocally varying their resistance in a cyclic manner. This pehnomenon, the nasal cycle, proceeds without symptoms because the total nasal resistance is constant[2] (Fig. 2).

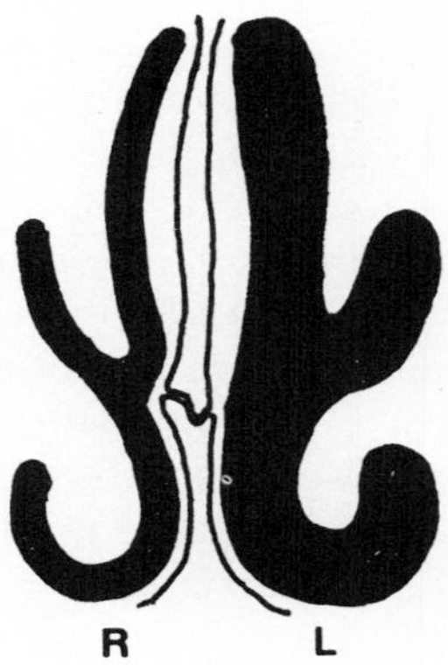

Fig. 2. Cross section of the nasal cavity during the normal nasal cycle. The turbinates on the right are physiologically congested.

It is not hard to appreciate the role of the nasal septum in this physiological sequence. It divides the nose in two. It varies in thickness and plane to mirror the anatomy of the turbinates. As a result, the air passages are approximately 2–3 mm wide throughout the length of each nasal cavity.

The nasal cavity is lined by pseudostratified ciliated columnar epithelium. On this lies the thin watery fluid layer in which the cilia beat. Borne along on the surface of this water and the tips of the cilia is the layer of mucus that contacts the air, captures particulate matter, and eventually carries it to the pharynx for disposal.

If as a result of surgery a close relationship between septal and turbinate mucosa is destroyed, and the turbinates become incapable of maintaining the 2- to 3-mm airway, the inspired airstream desiccates the fluid layer, the mucociliary mechanism is destroyed, and stagnant mucus accumulates to obstruct the nose. Thus, the consequence of septal perforation or septal deviations caused by transseptal surgery is a chronic obstructive rhinitis. Notice that paradoxical as it may seem, the loss of tissue inside the nose leads to obstruction, not patency.

4. The Premaxilla

4.1. Nasal Spine and Premaxilla

The anterior nasal spine is a pyramidal projection of bone based on the lower margin of the pyriform aperture. It has three sides and three margins. The upper side is a horizontal plateau, while the right and left sides curve downward and laterally to blend with the incisive fossae. Sharp median and inferior margins separate the right and left sides like a ship's bowstem. The two lateral margins curl backward and outward to disappear into the pyriform margin. The superior plateau is enclosed by these margins, and is continuous with the floor of the nose, on either side of the maxillary crests.

The right and left sides of the nasal spine are smooth and concave, but the uppermost surface is flat and streaked with fine, bony laminae that flow backward into the nasal chamber. Two of these laminae arise from a paramedian position to dominate the rest. These are called the "maxillary crests." The midline depression embraced by these crests continues backward and upward to meet an identical groove on the superior margin of the vomer.

The size and symmetry of the maxillary crests are quite variable. About 1 cm poterior to the plane of the pyriform aperture, the maxillary crests terminate in a position that overlooks the incisive foramen.

The immediate relationships of the nasal spine are the septal cartilage, the soft tissues of the upper lip, the base of the columella, and the anterior nasal mucoperichondrium and mucoperiosteum. The septal cartilage is borne from before backward by the membranous columella, the flat upper surface of the nasal spine, the midline groove between the maxillary crests, and finally the vomer. Dense fibrous adhesions bind the cartilage and the overlying nasal mucoperichondrium firmly into the maxillary crests and groove. Interwoven horizontal fibers joining the right and left anterior inferior nasal mucoperichondrial membranes pass almost like a sheet between the cartilage and the bone anterior to the maxillary crests. Thus, the septal cartilage lying immediately above the nasal spine is more mobile than that embraced by the maxillary crest. Behind the premaxilla, the junction between the septal cartilage and the vomer is less complex. The mucoperichondrium and mucoperiosteum are much less firmly attached, and surgical submucoperichondrial elevations proceed more easily (Fig. 3).

The soft tissues of the upper lip, which lie immediately anterior to the sharp median inferior margin of the nasal spine, can be stretched over it with a speculum inserted through the lower end of a hemitransfixion incision, and incised. Those attached to the right and left sides of the nasal spine can be scraped aside with a Mackenty elevator. Then the thin Cottle elevator may be passed over the right and left sides of the nasal spine to elevate the densely attached mucosa just below the maxillary crests. The adjacent mucosa on the floor of the nose is less firmly attached and is raised by passing curved elevators over the pyriform margin and along the bony nasal floor.

Such a dissection has been termed by Cottle *et al.*[3] the maxilla–premaxilla approach. Terminological confusion has arisen because the term "premaxilla" (which is the embryological unit of bone anterior to the incisive foramen and bearing all the incisor teeth as well as the nasal spine and maxillary crests) has been used to refer only to the maxillary crests. The submucoperichondrial elevations lying below the maxillary crests have been termed the "inferior tunnels." Similarly, an elevation of mucoperichondrium from the left side of the septal cartilage has been called a "left anterior tunnel" and submucoperiosteal elevations from the ethmoid plate and vomer have been called "posterior tunnels" (Figs. 3 and 4). This terminology proves convenient enough in describing septal procedures that it is widely used among rhinologists. The fact that the sphenopalatine artery bisects the inferior tunnel as it runs from the septal mucosa to the incisive foramen is of little consequence in septal reconstructive surgery and has been largely ignored. It assumes considerable importance in transseptal hypophyseal surgery because

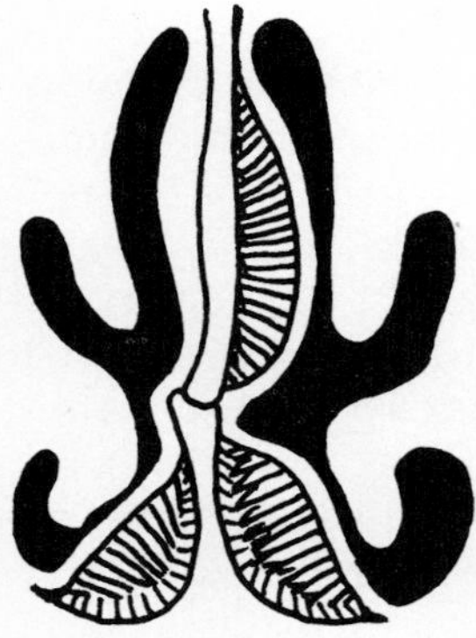

Fig. 3. Cross section of the nose illustrating the location of the left anterior and bilateral inferior submucoperichondrial tunnels. Perforations tend to begin at the site of adherence to the underlying septal skeleton along the osteocartilaginous junction.

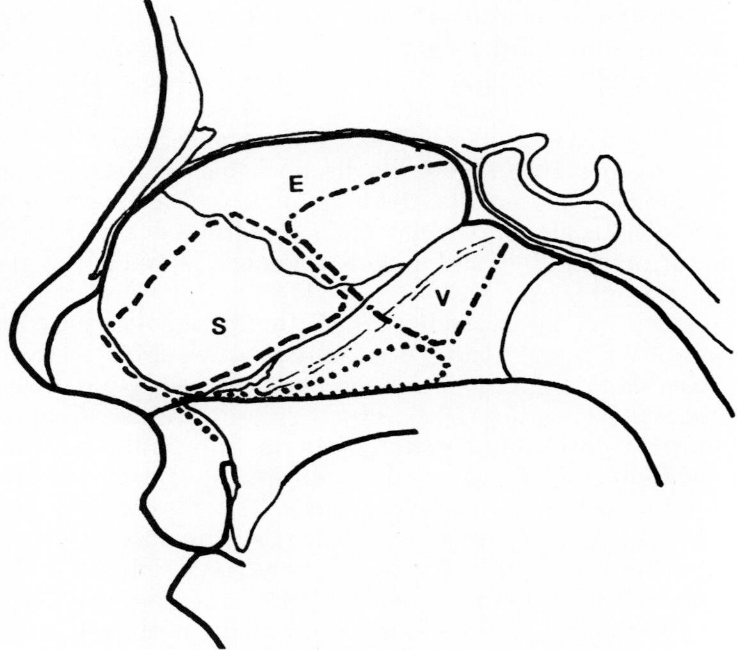

Fig. 4. Septal skeleton and the position of the left submucoperichondrial tunnels. (____) Anterior tunnel; (....) inferior tunnel; (_._._) posterior tunnel; (E) ethmoid plate; (S) septal cartilage; (V) vomer.

of the need to displace mucoperiosteal flaps so widely away from the septum and floor of the nose and the necessity of avoiding excessive hemorrhage when this is done (Fig. 5).

4.2. Soft-Tissue Coverings

The soft tissue covering the premaxilla is much more densely attached than the tissue we find covering the maxilla, the vomer, or the septal carti-

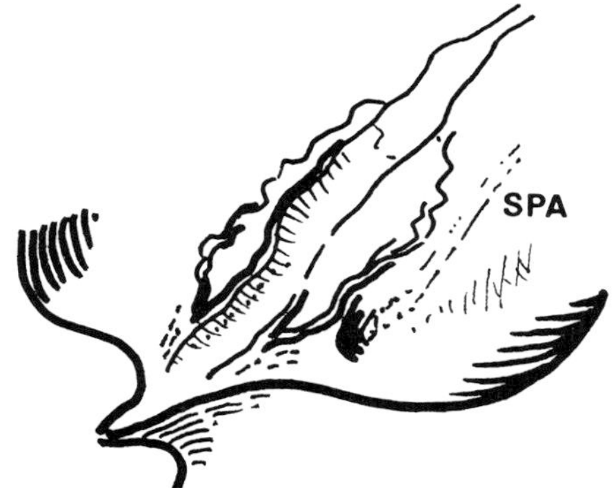

Fig. 5. Anterior nasal spine. The groove for the sphenopalatine artery can be seen angling along the vomer toward the incisive foramen. The premaxillary wings are prominent. (SPA) Sphenopalatine artery.

lage. This fact combined with the variable and often poorly understood anatomy in this region confronts the transseptal pituitary surgeon with the most difficult part of a dissection early in the procedure. To release the mucoperiosteum from the region requires a meticulous sharp dissection. This is accomplished from above through a septal incision. The nasal spine is a guide, and the bony surfaces can be approached directly. If the dissection is attempted from below, the nasal spine is an obstruction, some of the dissection is blind, and mucoperiosteal perforation (and its consequences, intraoperative hemorrhage, loss of flap tension and exposure, and postoperative crusting and perforation) is a greater risk (see Fig. 3).

5. The Nasal Septum

5.1. Supporting Structures

Complications in septal surgery are avoided by preserving chiefly the septal mucosa, secondarily the septal cartilage, and least of all the bony components of the septum. The nasal spine is an exception.

The main components of the skeleton of the nasal septum are the ethmoid plate, the vomer, and the septal cartilage (see Fig. 2).

The ethmoid plate descends from the cribriform above. Its anterior border, which abuts the septal cartilage, is about 3 mm thick, but everywhere else it thins to paper. The vomer (Latin: "ploughshare") is a stronger bony lamina that thrusts forward and downward in the midline from the sphenoid floor to the low bony crest on the palate. Its posterior margin separates the choanae; its anterosuperior margin articulates with the lower edge of the ethmoid plate, then the lower edge of the septal cartilage. The septal cartilage stands like a quadrangular plate the borders of which articulate with the nasal dorsum, the ethmoid plate, the vomer, the premaxilla, the nasal spine, and the columella. The posterior tail of the septal cartilage extends back along the junction of the ethmoid and the vomer as far as the sphenoid rostrum. This junction, and to some extent the septal tail, define the "line of sight" to the sphenoid sinus.

5.2. Mucosa

The mucoperichondrium is firmly adherent to the anterior 1.5 cm of the septal cartilage. It requires careful sharp dissection to remain deep to the perichondrium anteriorly, but care is rewarded by a bloodless submucosal elevation over the rest of the septum. Failure to establish this plane leads to bleeding, tears, and complications.

The septal cartilage is avascular. Its nutrition derives by diffusion from the closely adherent nasal mucoperichondrium. The mucoperichondrium need be elevated over the left side of the septal cartilage only. This leads to the ethmoid plate. If we dislocate this osteocartilaginous junction by displacing the cartilage to the right, the right septal mucoperichondrium remains attached to the cartilage anteriorly, but strips up off the ethmoid plate and posterior vomer posteriorly. This technique preserves the blood supply to the septal cartilage, but yields complete bilateral exposure of the ethmoid plate and upper vomer, which will be resected.

The vomerine and ethmoid plates are bony, rigid, and functionally unnecessary plates in the posterior septum. However, they do serve as a guide to the plane of dissection between the right and left septal mucoperichondrial flaps. The flaps are loosely attached to these bones, so bilateral posterior submucoperichondrial tunnels elevate readily all the way back to the face of the sphenoid. Bony posterior spurs, common along the ethmo–vomerine junction, often thin these flaps at their apices. Visualization can be maximized by resecting bone and especially the spurs as the submucoperichondrial tunneling proceeds. Care is required in extracting bone fragments; the sharp projecting edges can easily lacerate the septal mucosa.

The septal mucoperichondrial flaps derive some blood supply from the ethmoid arteries above, but their major vessel is the sphenopalatine artery. Arising from the maxillary, it enters the nose from the lateral wall through the sphenopalatine foramen behind the middle turbinate. It crosses below the floor of the sphenoid to the septum, then angles downward and forward, parallel to and a few millimeters below, the upper margin of the vomer. At the incisive foramen, the sphenopalatine artery leaves the mucosa and funnels down into the incisive foramen to the palate (see Fig. 5).

5.3. Submucosal Tunnels

At the completion of a transnasal (as opposed to sublabial) submucosal septal dissection, five tunnels need to be connected. These are (1) a left anterior (over the septal cartilage), (2) and (3) bilateral inferior (over the floor and premaxilla), and (4) and (5) bilateral posterior (over the bony septum) (see Figs. 3 and 4).

Before the sublabial incision is made (to introduce a speculum), the adequacy of the elevation should be checked against several criteria. First, have all the densely attached fibers of the nasal spine and maxillary crest been truly detached, or was this area bypassed to get at the easier dissection posteriorly? If the flaps are still tethered in this area, reduced exposure and a difficult speculum insertion are likely. Second, has the inferior tunnel been completed by dividing the sphenopalatine artery, or does this vessel still pin the mucosa down to the incisive foramen at the junction of the floor and the septum? The sphenopalatine artery can be specifically identified, cauterized, and released. Otherwise, when the speculum is introduced and opened, the artery can be stretched and torn. In hypertension and vascular fragility (e.g., Cushing's disease), a torn sphenopalatine artery bleeding vigorously at the front of the nose and flooding the deeper field can greatly impede the surgery.

We prefer to dissect and connect the septal submucosal tunnels and to resect the bony septum via the nasal approach. The sublabial incision is added only to bypass the nostrils, which, except in some acromegalics, are too small to allow the pituitary speculum in. The better angle of visualization in the premaxillary region saves tears. The caudal border of the septal cartilage can be visualized for orientation. The nasal spine is to low to obstruct the view from this angle. The dense mucosal attachments of the premaxilla (the cause of tears) can be attacked from above, in front, and below. A thorough release of tension in the anterior dissection yields good exposure posteriorly. The "feel" of instruments dissecting over the rostrum and face of the sphenoid is unimpeded by anterior elements.

The sublabial incision is used to release the soft tissues of the upper lip from the bony premaxilla and to introduce the sphenoid speculum. The perichondrium has already been released from the premaxilla, and the speculum slides directly into the septal space already created by the nasal dissection between the septal cartilage and the left mucoperichondrial flap. The nasal spine can be preserved for cosmesis and used as a midline anchorage for reconstructing the septum. The speculum blades, and later the optical pathways of the microscope, simply straddle the spine.

6. The Sphenoid Sinus

6.1. Rostrum, Floor, Face, and Ostia

The criteria of adequate exposure posteriorly in the septal space are these: Are the sphenoid rostrum (Floor and face) so widely uncovered that the medial edges of the sphenoid ostia can be visualized or palated by the dissector? If they cannot, chances are the superior turbinate has been inadequately outfractured. Can the floor of the sphenoid sinus and the rostrum, a large mass of heavy bone, be distinguished from the anterior face of the sphenoid, which is small and thin?

The floor of the sphenoid sinus is a laminate of bony components. The sphenoid body, the ala of the vomer, the vaginal processes of the pterygoid plates, and the sphenoid processes of the vertical plates of the palatine bones form a formidable barrier to sinusotomy through the sphenoid floor. The anterior face of the sphenoid is smaller and more delicate. The sphenoid concha, a membranous bony remnant of the embryological cartilaginous nasal capsule, forms this surface. Each concha is thinned in its center to nothingness, forming ostia of variable size. The right and left concha are separated in the midline by a vertical bar of heavy bone from the roof to the rostrum. The bar defines the true midline; the intrasinus septum does not. To enter the sphenoid sinus, the rostrum is simply avulsed. By transecting the vertical bar above the rostrum and the bony floor it with a chisel, the lines of avulsion can be controlled.

6.2. The Interior of the Sphenoid Sinus

The view of the sphenoid sinus interior permitted by the transseptal approach points one directly at the midline. There is safety in this. The vulnerable relationships (e.g., optic nerve, carotid artery, cavernous sinus, oculomotor nerve) are laterally situated. The intrasinus septa are usually not midline. Often, they are multiple. Vertical secondary septi occur laterally and transverse secondary septi superiorly, which splits the sinus asymmetrically into a right and left, upper and lower, or right, middle, and left set of subdivisions. Preoperative anteroposterior tomograms aid in recognizing the individual peculiarities of each case.

The normal sphenoid sinus mucosa is extremely thin and weak. Its consistency is poorly compatible with total stripping. Surgical avulsion of mucosa is generally complete.

The manner in which the sella meets the roof of the sphenoid is sometimes quite variable. This angle is acute and sharply defined. Every variation between this and a smooth blending between the roof and the sella is possible. Inferiorly, the anatomy is also quite variable. The floor of the normal sella may be clearly defined in a well-pneumatized sinus that reaches back toward the clivus, or it may be undefinable in the so-called "presellar" pattern of pneumatization. In the latter instance, the region between the floor of the sella and the floor of the sphenoid is filled with cancellous bone. An image intensifier demonstrating the lateral view intraoperatively is helpful to ensure that the surgical opening into the sella is on target, especially when the upper and lower angles are poorly defined.

6.3. Variations in Pneumatization

The lateral recesses of a well-pneumatized sphenoid are out of view. It is worth studying a sagitally sectioned skull to appreciate the important relationships of a well-pneumatized lateral wall. High and anteriorly, the optic nerves indent the hollowed root of the lesser sphenoid wing. The internal carotid artery rims the floor of the sella laterally just below and in front of the junction between the sella and the lateral sinus wall. Inferiorly, pneumatization can extend out into the greater wing of the sphenoid and down to the pterygoid process. In doing so, it throws into relief the bony walls of the maxillary nerve (foraman rotundum) and vidian nerve (pterygoid canal).

Approximately 2% percent of our cases have nonpneumatized sphenoid sinus. Some have regarded this as an impediment to transsphenoidal surgery. Cancellous bone fills the sphenoid and the face of the sella. Nevertheless, this bone readily hollows out with a curette. The cancellous trabeculae are gritty but weak, and the limits imposed by the compact bony envelope enclosing the sphenoid are easily recognized. Thus, the sphenoid sinus can be surgically pneumatized and enlarged to sufficient dimensions to permit transsphenoidal hypophysectomy.

7. Conclusions

In this chapter, we have attempted to focus on some of the less obvious anatomical features of the nasal septum and sphenoid that have proven to be of importance during the performance of slightly more than 600 transseptal transsphenoidal hypophysectomies. Through the recognition of these details, it is hoped that the surgical principles of the transseptal operation may be more clearly understood and widely applied. It would appear that sophistication in carrying out the rhinological aspects of the transseptal transphenoidal approach to the hypophysis is largely a matter of understanding the septal anatomy and appreciating its role in nasal function. Transnasal instruments and techniques developed for the correction of nasal septal deviation greatly simplify the transseptal approach to the sphenoid. The time is probably at hand when no patient with a pituitary tumor need fear nasal mutilation or postoperative nasal dysfunction.

References

1. E.B. Kern, B.W. Pearson, T.J. McDonald, and E.R. Laws, Jr., The trans-septal approach to lesions of the pituitary and parasellar regions, *Laryngoscope* **89,** Suppl. 15, May 1979.
2. M. Hasegawa, E.B. Kern, and P.C. O'Brien, Dynamic changes of nasal resistance, *Ann. Otol. Rhinol. Laryngol.* **88:**66–71, 1979.
3. M.H. Cottle, R.M. Loring, G.G. Fischer, and I.E. Gaynon, The "maxilla premaxilla" approach to extensive nasal septum surgery, *Arch. Otolaryngol.* **68:**301, 1958.

18

Transsphenoidal Surgery for Pituitary Tumors

KALMON D. POST

1. Introduction

The transsphenoidal approach to the sella dates back to Schloffer,[1] who in 1907 reported the decompression of a growth hormone (GH)-producing tumor via this route. He had modified the operation of Giordano[2] by not resecting the frontal sinus or floor of the anterior fossa. Further modifications ensued, including a submucosal dissection,[3] a sublabial incision,[4] the use of a headlight,[5] and image-intensified fluoroscopy.[6] Hardy[7–10] added the operating microscope and microsurgical techniques to the procedure, so that with minimal morbidity and mortality, both microadenomas and large tumors could be safely removed or decompressed while sparing the pituitary gland.

Other methods including stereotaxic techniques were developed, such as ultrasonic irradiation, cryosurgery, gold and yttrium implants, and thermal radiofrequency lesions. Arslan[11] utilized ultrasonic irradiation via a midline transphenoidal route on 41 acromegalic patients. However, this method was not very accurate. Cross *et al.*,[12] Richards *et al.*,[13] and DiTullio and Rand[14] reported on cryosurgical techniques. The mortality and morbidity were high, with meningitis, cerebrospinal fluid (CSF) leaks, and ocular nerve palsies being all to common. Two limitations for tumors were encountered: (1) tumors were not usually centrally placed in the sella; and (2) there was a lack of differentiation between tumor and normal gland.[15] Yttrium-90 implants were initially used for hypophysectomy for cancer.[16] However, the complications were significant because of anatomical variations in sella and gland size and shape, as well as in the position of the chiasm. Conway *et al.*[17] reported on 8 acromegalic patients treated with yttrium-90. All had effective control of their acromegaly, although significant late complications such as CSF leaks

KALMON D. POST • Tufts University School of Medicine; Department of Neurosurgery, Tufts–New England Medical Center Hospital, Boston, Massachusetts 02111.

and optic nerve and carotid artery damage were seen in over 50%.[18] Zervas and Hamlin[19] used radiofrequency lesions with similar limitations as for cryosurgical techniques, particularly a high incidence of CSF leaks.

2. Technique

The orbitoethmoidal approach, to expose the sella, is used by some surgeons with the claim that it offers a shorter distance to the sella, a higher and therefore less obstructed view of the stalk, no devitalization of the incisor teeth, fewer operative manipulations of the teeth, and no nasal packing. However, it requires a facial incision (lateral rhinotomy), and the midline landmarks cannot be utilized. More important, it approaches the sella obliquely, leaving an entirely blind quadrant.

I have preferred the sublabial midline ororhinoseptal transsphenoidal approach because it respects the desire to reach the sella squarely, allows symmetric visualization for safe dissection avoiding the risk of trauma to the more laterally placed neurovascular structures, allows visualization of the diaphragma area with easy manipulation of instruments in the suprasellar area, and is performed through a concealed incision.

The following technique is basically that described by Hardy,[9,10] with some modifications from Wilson,[20] Tindall *et al.*,[21] Collins,[18,22] and our own experience.

The patient is given cortisone acetate, 50 mg, the night before surgery, and an additional 100 mg hydrocortisone via intravenous drip just prior to and again during surgery. General anesthesia is used with an orotracheal tube. The mouth and throat are packed with moist sponges to prevent aspiration. After the anesthesiologist has completed the intubation, the patient is turned into a lateral position, and a subarachnoid catheter is placed percutaneously in the lumbar area for instillation of air or drainage of CSF during the surgery.[23] The patient is then returned to the supine position with the head flexed 15° and tilted toward the left shoulder so that the surgeon may assume a direct, comfortable position looking straight into the surgical field without strain (see Fig. 1). The head is secured either with tape or with a three-pin head-holder. The operating table is moved into position so that the patient's head will be in line with a portable image-intensified fluoroscope with the horizontal beam centered on the sella. Radiofluoroscopic control is used intermittently during the procedure as a guide in the early dissection toward the sella, and later to help visualize the instruments during the suprasellar dissection. Lead shielding is attached to the fluoroscope, and radiation readings on several occasions have shown a maximum radiation rate of 10 mrem/h at approximately 8 inches. Outside the 8-inch area, the radiation rate is 1 mrem/h. For a cumulative 10 min of total radiation on-time (an extremely high estimate), the exposure would be 1.6 mrem, well within safe levels.

Cocaine (4%) in solution is applied to the nasal mucosa with applicator sticks to decongest the mucosa (100 mg maximal dosage). The face, nasal mucosa, gingiva, and the right lateral thigh are prepped with an antiseptic solution. The sublabial mucosa, anterior nasal spine, and membranous system

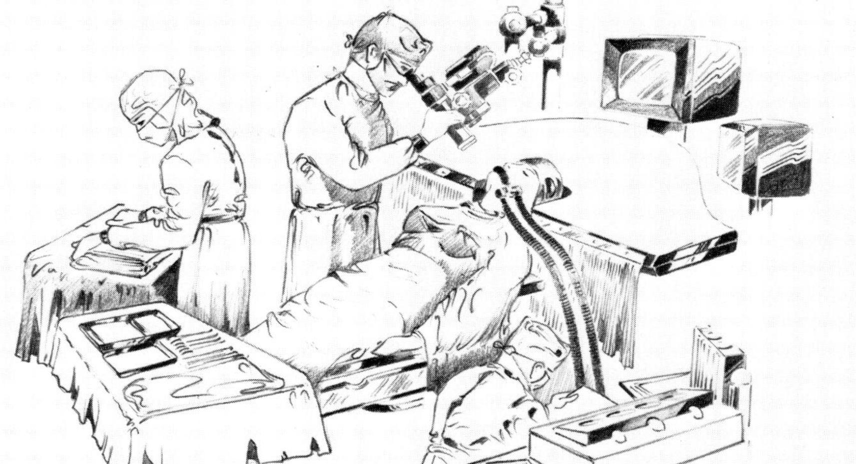

Fig. 1. Diagramatic representation of operative setup for transsphenoidal approach to the sella. Note the position of the patient's head, surgeon's position, lead-shielded fluoroscope with televised image, and operative microscope.

are infiltrated with 10 cc ½% xylocaine with epinepherine 1:200,000 U, so that the mucosa is lifted off the cartilaginous septum. An adhesive plastic drape is applied to cover the exposed face. The field is completely draped, and sterile sponges placed in the mouth, leaving only the gingiva exposed.

A 3- to 4-cm incision is made in the gingiva just above the gingivo–labial fold and is carried through the periosteum (Fig. 2). The periosteum is elevated superiorly, exposing the pyriform aperture in the maxilla.

The lateral and inferior edges of the maxilla are removed using a Kerrison rongeur to expand the opening for later insertion of the nasal speculum. It is important that the lateral ascending edges be removed, because these will be limiting factors to opening the speculum. Hemostasis is obtained with bone wax.

Beginning laterally, the nasal mucosa is elevated from the floor bilaterally, creating inferior tunnels along the nasal septum. This plane is carried medially, separating the mucosa from the cartilaginous septum as well. A good initial infiltration aids greatly. At times, it is difficult to turn the corner from the inferior tunnel along the septum, and a No. 15 blade is used to cut medially into the cartilaginous septum at the superior point of the anterior nasal spine. This maneuver will initiate a subchondral separation of the mucosa from the septum and establish the medial plane. A blunt dissector, such as a Penfield No. 2, may be used to complete the elevation. As the elevation proceeds deep along the septum toward the vomer, fluoroscopy is used to assure the correct direction. I have used both a bilateral approach as performed

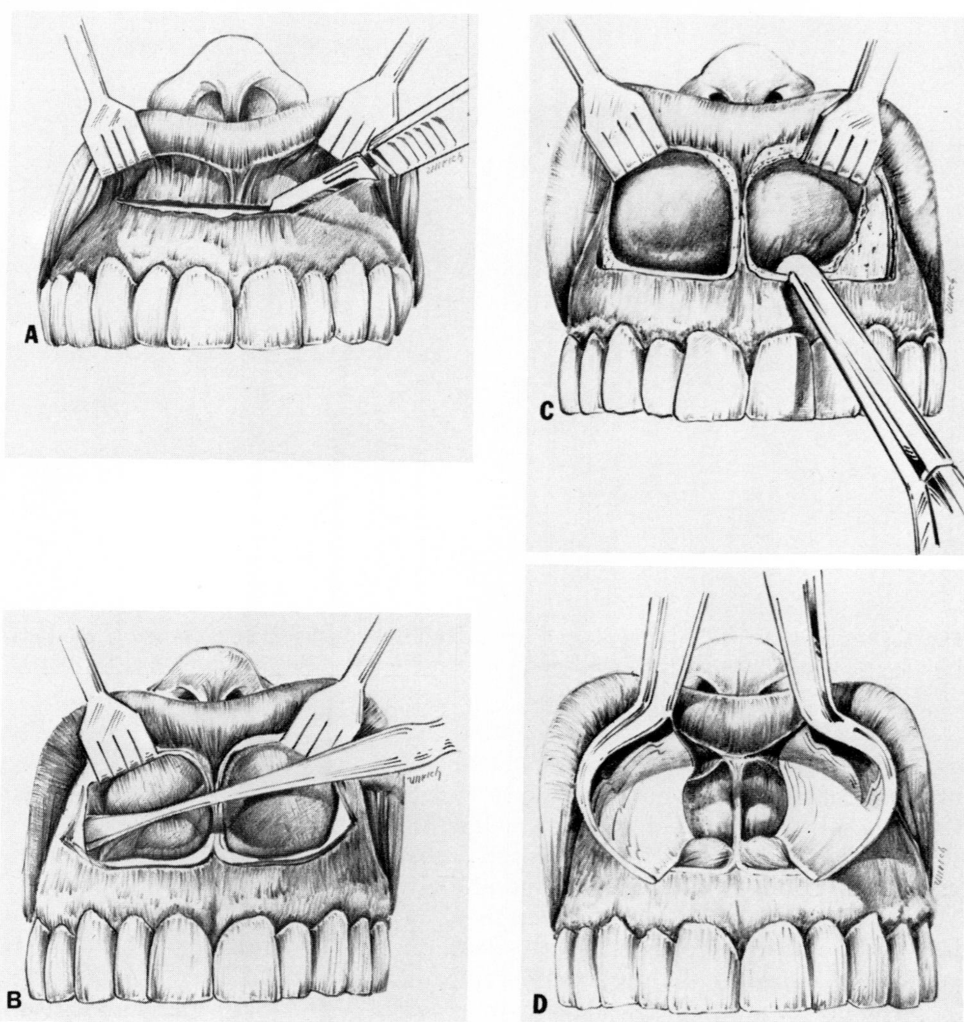

Fig. 2. (A) Diagram of position of gingival incision. (B) Submucosal dissection beginning inferolaterally. (C) Enlargement of the pyriform aperture in the maxilla. Note particularly the enlargement laterally to allow opening of the speculum. (D) Insertion of the bivalve speculum during a bilateral approach. Septum remains in midline.

by Hardy[8] and Wilson[20] and a unilateral approach as described by Tindall *et al.*,[21] and now prefer the latter to assure the health of the septum. The anterior nasal spine is removed flush with the floor, and the base of the septum is disarticulated from its attachment to the vomer and the ethmoid plate, but left attached superiorly. It is then retracted to the side with the intact mucosa, exposing the anterior edge (keel) of the vomer and anterior wall of the sphenoid sinus. The mucosal elevations are completed before the cartilage is disarticulated to allow stability during elevation. The nasopalatine artery, which is anteromedial, may at times cause bleeding and must be coagulated. A Hardy bivalve nasal speculum of appropriate length is inserted, a blade on each side of the vomer, and opened. While opening the speculum, a mallet is occasionally used to seat the tip of the retractor against the anterior wall of the sphenoid sinus, which is curving away from the surgeon. The amount of pressure needed to open the speculum is usually not great, and a speculum spreader is not required. However, the turbinates may occasionally be hypertrophied, as in acromegaly, and the spreader is used. The force applied by nasal speculums during transsphenoidal operations has recently been reported by Hardy *et al.*[24] with the conclusion that if there is adequate removal of the ascending edges of the maxillae, there will not be an excessive pressure exerted on the tissues.

Through this early portion of the operation, a headlight is sufficient. At this point, however, the operating microscope with 12.5× straight eyepieces and a 300-mm lens is brought into use. A binocular sidearm is available on the left for the assistant, and a television camera and 16-mm movie camera are mounted on the right side. Initially, 10-power magnification is sufficient, but once the sella is exposed, 16-power is used. At times during the intrasellar dissection, 25-power will be necessary.

The vomer is removed by grasping it as close to the sphenoid sinus wall as possible and twisting rather than biting, so that a large piece can be removed intact for use during the sella closure if cartilage has not been obtained for this purpose. The opening in the anterior sphenoid sinus wall is enlarged so that the lateral portions of the sella as well as the upper and lower edges as seen with fluoroscopy are readily visualized. The speculum is not advanced into the sphenoid sinus because this maneuver can cause a basal skull fracture as well as damage to the optic nerves or carotid arteries. The sinus mucosa is completely exenterated to prevent a future mucocele, and a piece is sent for culture.

The septations of the sphenoid sinus are correlated with the anteroposterior (AP) tomograms for correct sella orientation, and then removed. The sella floor is now in full view, and any asymmetries can be appreciated. Usually, the floor is readily opened with a blunt dissector in the thinned area. Occasionally, a small osteotome or air drill is necessary to make the initial opening. It is then enlarged laterally until the medial edges of the cavernous sinus become apparent. The opening is carried superiorly to several millimeters below the tuberculum and inferiorly to the horizontal sella floor.

If an anterior transverse dural sinus is present, it is coagulated with bipolar cautery. A rectangular window in the dura is removed, presenting an opening almost equal to that of bone. Troublesome bleeding from the dura or epidural space is controlled with bipolar cautery or with small pieces of Surgicel (Johnson & Johnson) tucked along the edge. Hemostasis should be complete before entering the gland; otherwise, vision will be constantly hampered and differentiation of adenoma from gland made difficult. Once the gland is exposed, the adenoma will often begin to extrude as a soft, purplish-gray suctionable tissue (Fig. 3).

With macroadenomas, ring currettes and suction are utilized to remove the bulk of the tumor. The tumor is usually very soft and readily suctionable, making removal easy. However, the mass will occasionally be very fibrous

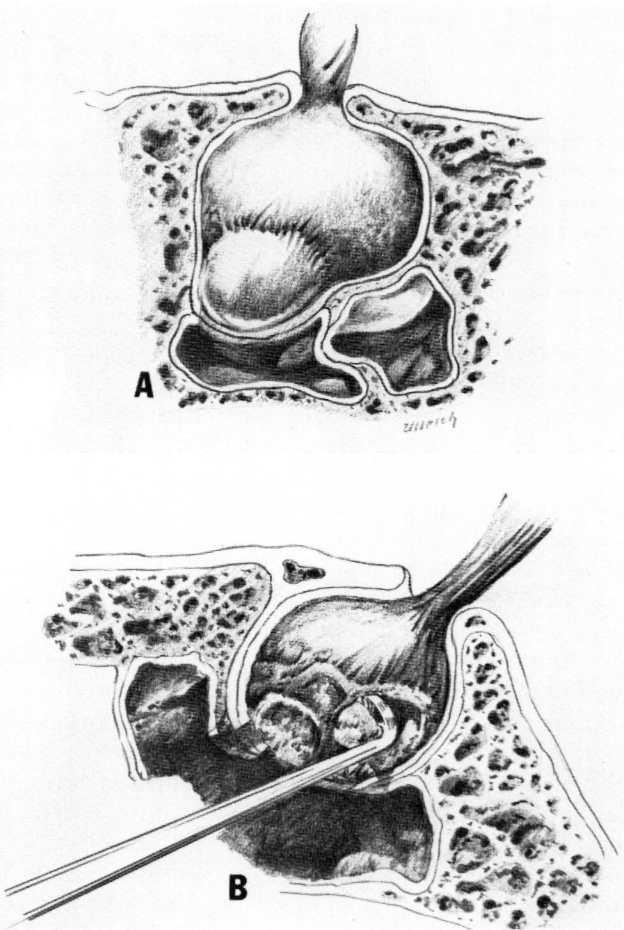

Fig. 3. (A) Diagram of microadenoma in inferolateral position of the gland. It is immediately evident on opening the sella. (B) Microdissectors and currettes are used to selectively remove the tumor.

and nonsuctionable, requiring the use of sharp dissection. This occurred in 5% of Hardy's cases[25] and in 6% of Guiot's cases.[26] Instillation of air through the subarachnoid catheter will help by both outlining the superior pole of the tumor and forcing the suprasellar extension of the tumor down into the sella for removal. Televised fluoroscopy is used to guide the placement of instruments during the suprasellar dissection (Fig. 4). As the tumor descends, the air above the capsule will be seen to descend as well. A Valsalva maneuver performed by the anesthesiologist will also help force the tumor down into the sella. The capsule, which is the diaphragma sella, should never be pulled down, since this will lead to tears and CSF leaks, as well as possible optic nerve injury. Lateral extension is removed with care to prevent injury to the cavernous sinus. Bleeding may occur while stroking the lateral walls, but this is readily controlled with tamponade. Care must be taken with all size tumors to ensure that the diaphragma and arachnoid are not torn, thus minimizing the risk of postoperative CSF leak. A dental mirror may be used to inspect the obscured portions of the operative field for residual tumor.

With microdenomas, the tumor may not be immediately evident on opening the dura, and the gland must be incised. There is often an asymmetry of appearance or texture that will suggest the correct location to be incised. After explanation laterally and inferiorly outside the gland, if the gland appears totally normal, a vertical incision is made into the gland on the side with the tomographic abnormality. If the tumor is not seen, slight pressure on the gland will often cause the tumor to extrude. I have also used a horizontal incision into the lower third of the anterior gland if laterality cannot be determined. Again, slight pressure on the gland will help identify the adenoma as a softer, purplish tissue, as opposed to the firm, yellow, nonsuctionable gland. Two areas where tumor can be missed are high and anterior to the stalk and very posterolateral. Once the tumor is located, microdissection techniques are used to separate the tumor from the gland and remove it either in one piece or

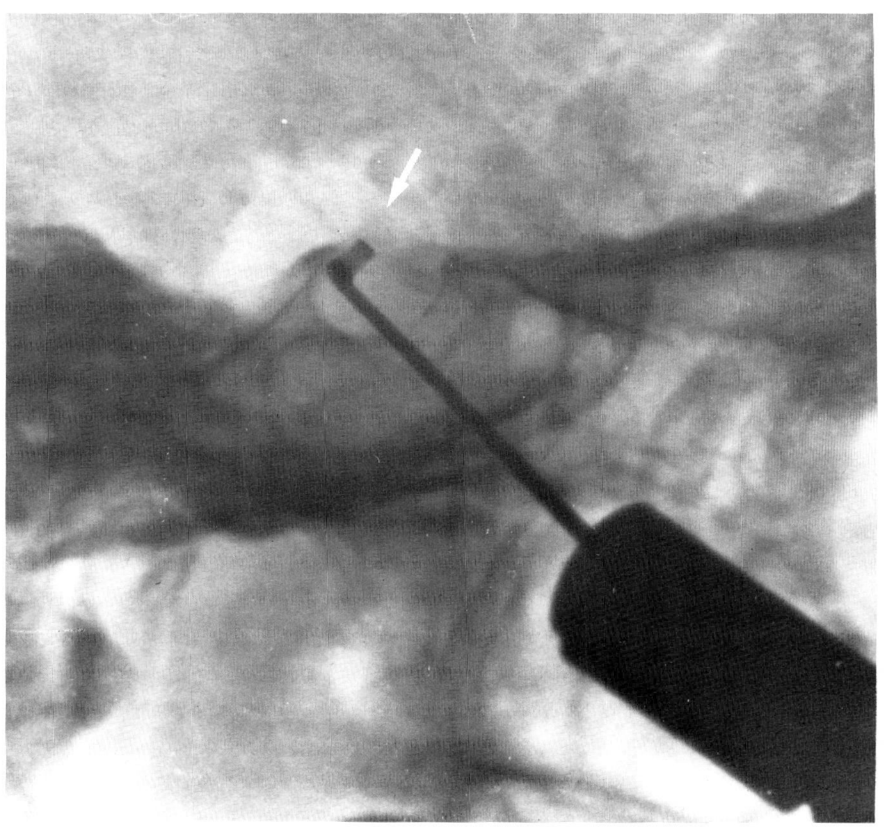

Fig. 4. Lateral X-ray of sella during surgery. Note air above the sella outlining the upper margin of the tumor (arrow).

piecemeal. It may be difficult to differentiate the exact border between tumor and normal gland, and we have utilized a technique of frozen-section stains[27] to help in this distinction. Multiple microbiopsies are taken from the tumor bed, and if any evidence of tumor is seen, another arc of tissue is removed. Only a small percentage of the normal gland is removed in this manner, and since it is well established that only 15–20% of the normal gland is needed for normal function, a wide safety range exists.[28,29] A common mistake is removing just the necrotic portion and leaving the active tumor, thinking it is normal gland. Experience in visualizing the difference between tumor and gland is vital to avoid this error. The nonnecrotic tumor is often gray, soft, mealy and easily suctionable, as opposed to the normal gland, which is not.

With smaller tumors, the arachnoid may herniate into the sella during the dissection, obstructing the view and obscuring segments of tumor in superior recesses. CSF can be removed via the lumbar catheter, decompressing this pouch and exposing the residual tumor.

When tumor removal is complete, the bed is irrigated with absolute alcohol to destroy any residual tumor cells. With moderate or large tumors, a piece of fat is taken from the thigh and placed in the sella with care that the normal gland not be compressed. In microadenomas, this step is often omitted. With large tumors, a clip is often placed on the diaghragma to judge radiographically the amount of packing necessary and to evaluate recurrence postoperatively. The sella is then closed with a piece of the vomer or nasal cartilage in the manner described by Hardy (Fig. 5). If CSF is exposed during

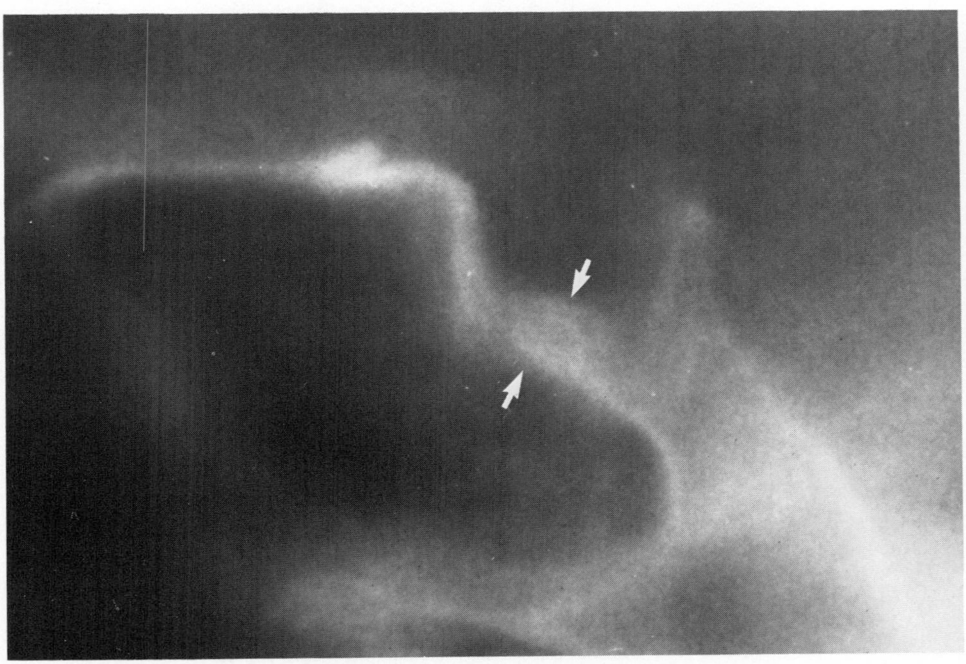

Fig. 5. Postoperative lateral tomogram showing the sella defect closed with a bone (arrows) from the vomer.

the dissection, a piece of fascia lata is also placed within the sella adjacent to the exposed arachnoid and a second piece is placed in the sphenoid sinus against the anterior sella wall. The speculum is removed, the gingiva sutured with chromic catgut, and the nasal mucosa reapproximated to the septum with intranasal Vaseline gauze impregnated with bacitracin ointment. This is removed on the third or fourth postoperative day.

Intraoperative antibiotics (usually Oxacillin) are given and continued postoperatively for 48 hr. If copious CSF was evident during the dissection, the spinal drainage catheter is left in place for 48–72 hr postoperatively to divert the CSF and allow the sella to seal.

3. Anatomical Pitfalls

The foregoing description is general and does not discuss some of the dangers and variations necessitated by anatomical variance. The following sections will review some of these problems.

3.1. Sphenoid Sinus

The sphenoid sinus has considerable variation in size, shape, symmetry, and pneumatization. On the basis of pneumatization, three general types are seen: conchal, presellar, and sellar[30] (see Fig. 6). The conchal type is more

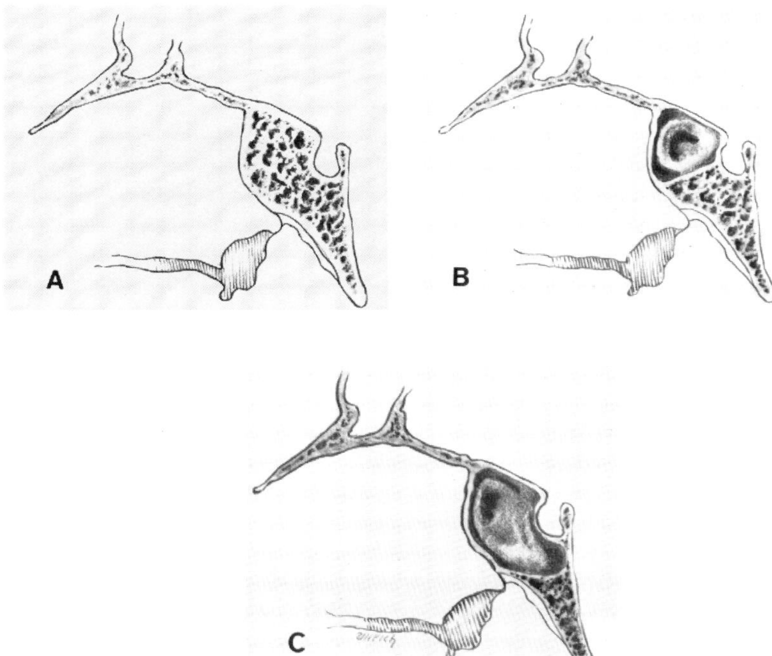

Fig. 6. Diagrams of variations in the sphenoid sinus: (A) conchal, 3% in adults; (B) presellar, 11%; (C) sellar, 86%.

common in children, but accounts for only 3% in adults, while the presellar is seen in 11% and the sellar type in 86%. The sellar type is completely pneumatized and extends well under the sella toward the clivus. The presellar type is pneumatized only in the portion of the sinus anterior to the sella. The conchal type is not pneumatized, and the sphenoid bone beneath the sella is made of dense bone up to 2 cm thick. The latter type is not a contraindication to transsphenoidal surgery, but does make it necessary to use an air drill to reach the sella. Televised fluoroscopy is mandatory here, because visual landmarks are not available.

There is usually one major vertical septum oriented in the sagittal plane, but it is often deflected to one side, inserting on the wall over the carotid canal. Preoperative AP tomography helps identify these septa for orientation in this plane during surgery, especially since the fluoroscopy is only in the lateral plane. Following a deviating septum as though it were midline can lead the surgeon directly into the carotid artery. Renn and Rhoton[31] found a single major septum in 68%, and it was off midline in 46%. No major septum existed in 28% and no minor septum in 18%. Hammer and Radberg[32] found the major septum midline in 25%, while Kinnman[33] noted this in 41.9%. A total of 35% deviated right and 22% deviated left. Multiple irregular minor septations are also seen (see Fig. 7), and these can be easily removed during the approach.

The carotid arteries may bulge into the inferolateral wall of the posterior portion of the sphenoid sinus (see Fig. 8), this occurring 71% of the time in the study of Renn and Rhoton.[31] This bulge was usually covered by bone, but 4% were covered only by mucosa and 66% had less than 1-mm-thick bone protecting the artery.

The optic canals protruded into the superolateral part of the sphenoid

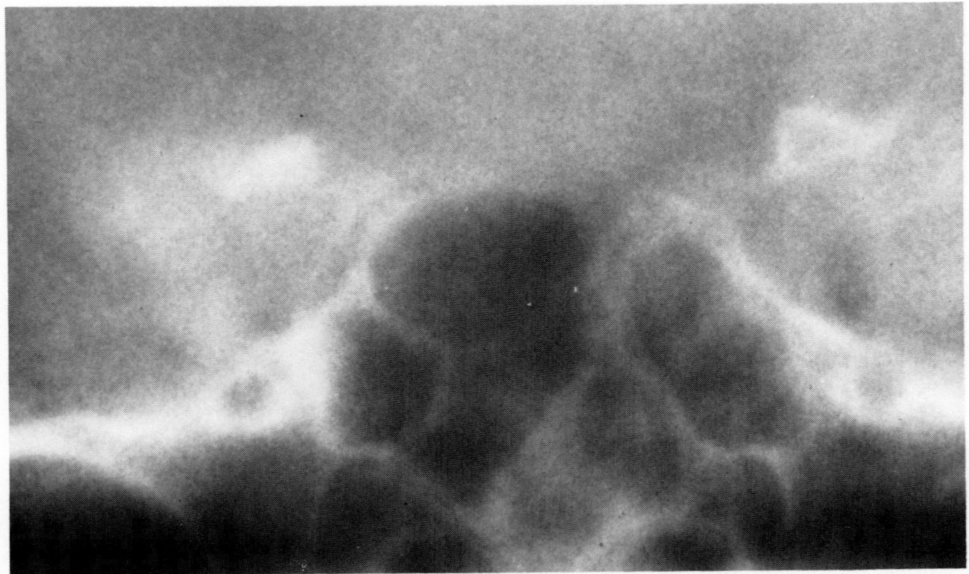

Fig. 7. AP tomogram demonstrating a sphenoidal sinus with multiple septa.

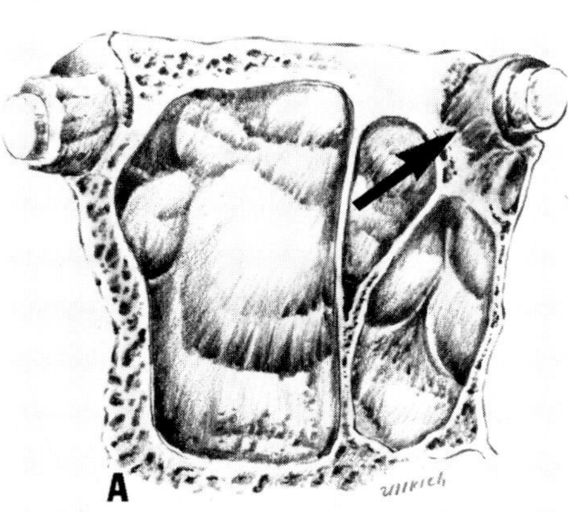

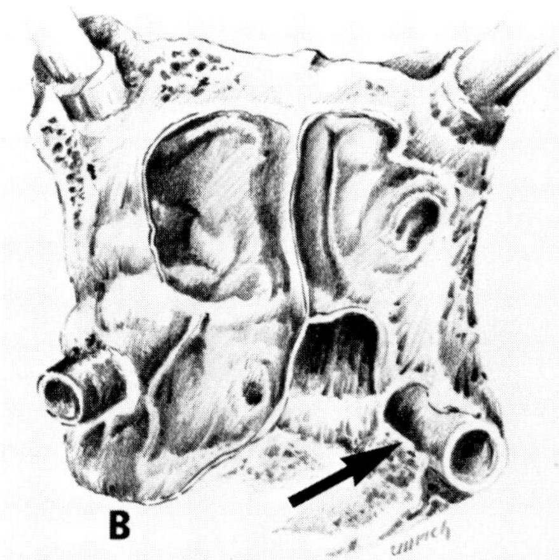

Fig. 8. (A) Diagram of central portion of sphenoid sinus. Note the optic nerve (arrow) covered only by optic sheath and sinus mucosa, unprotected by bone. (B) Diagram of central portion of sphenoid sinus. Note the carotid artery (arrow) covered only by sinus mucosa, unprotected by bone and subject to injury.

sinus as well (see Fig. 8), and in 4%, the nerves were covered only by optic sheath and sinus mucosa, requiring particular care to avoid injuring them.[31]

Because of potential injury to the carotid arteries and optic nerves, the lateral walls of the sphenoid sinus must be respected. Insertion of the speculum within the sinus could injure these structures as well as cause a basal skull fracture when opened.

3.2. Sella Turcica

A thin sella floor (1 mm or less) was found in 72% by Bergland *et al.*[34] and in 82% by Renn and Rhoton.[31] Generally, with tumors, the floor is even thinner and possibly totally eroded. In a child, however, the floor may be much thicker,[34] requiring an air drill or osteotome for opening.

The anterior intercavernous sinus (circular sinus) is variable in size and position. It was present in 76% of specimens studied,[31] but not wholly within the diaphragma sella, extending in front of the gland in 10%. In 4.9% of Hardy's cases operated on for hypophysectomy,[8] there was medial displacement or expansion of the cavernous sinus that was seen as a bluish tinge in the anterior dura. Bergland *et al.*[34] found that 85% of specimens had an anterior intercavernous sinus as well. These variations may complicate the dural opening and require that the opening be eccentric at times, with considerable effort required for hemostasis utilizing bipolar coagulation and tamponade. The venous sinuses, however, occasionally have to be crossed for adequate exposure and differentiation of tumor from gland.

3.3. Intrasellar Contents

The normal shape of the pituitary gland is somewhat variable, with certain variations caused by the position of the carotid arteries. Of the group studied by Renn and Rhoton,[31] 28% showed evidence of the carotid artery protruding through the medial wall of the cavernous sinus, indenting the gland. This occurred in 22% with Bergland *et al.*[34] and in 6% with Hardy.[8] The mean distance between artery and the lateral surface of the gland in nontumor subjects was 2.3 mm,[31] and the average separation of the two carotid siphons is 12 mm. However, with tortuous arteriosclerotic arteries, kissing vessels may occur, indenting and distorting the gland. Care must be taken to identify such vessels during surgery, particularly if arteriography has not been done preoperatively.

The diaphragma sella was found to be as thick as one layer of dura in 38% of cases, while extremely thin over some portion of the pituitary gland in the other 62%. In 28–56% of patients, the opening in the diaphragm was 5 mm or greater.[8,31,34] In situations where the dura is thin, or the opening large, particular care is needed during transsphenoidal surgery, so that this barrier is not violated. An arachnoid pouch within the sella was present in 20% of Bergland's cases and in 15.4% of Hardy's with a 2:1 female/male predominance. The frequency of an arachnoidal diverticulum increases with advancing age in females (below 40: 6%; above 40: 19.6%).[8]

It is usual that the diaphragma sella extends from the superior aspects of the posterior clinoid process to the superior margin of the tuberculum sellae. However, the attachment is often found several millimeters below this point,[34] and care must be taken when opening the dura, lest the opening be extended supradiaphragmatic, leading to CSF leakage.

3.4. Discussion

From the preceding discussion, it is apparent that certain variants of anatomy are considered disadvantageous to transsphenoidal surgery, but not contraindications:

1. A markedly deviated nasal septum or other nasal pathology.
2. A conchal or presellar type of sphenoid sinus without a sellar floor bulge into the sinus.
3. Carotid arteries that are not covered by bone in the sphenoid sinus.
4. Optic canals with bony defects in the sphenoid sinus.
5. A sphenoid sinus without a major septum to aid in orientation.
6. An overly thick sella floor.
7. A large anterior intercavernous sinus.
8. Carotid arteries that approach the midline within the sella.
9. A thin or deficient diaphragma sella.
10. A large intrasellar arachnoid pouch.

4. Results

As discussed in Chapter 16, the objectives are different for large nonfunctional tumors and small functional tumors. The surgical goal for large nonfunctional adenomas is to eliminate the mass effects without risk to neurological function or to life. A total surgical removal is usually not achievable, and postoperative conventional irradiation is given. With functional microadenomas, the objective is a total tumor removal, sparing the normal gland and either maintaining or restoring normal endocrine function. With Grades III and IV functional adenomas,[8] this is not always technically feasible; tumor tissue may remain and normal gland may not be identified. With invasive tumors, an endocrine cure is not usually possible.

4.1. Nonfunctional Tumors

Nonfunctional tumors are usually seen when presenting as mass lesions with visual impairment from suprasellar extension. The results are comparable to those reported below for large functional tumors. A subtotal removal is usually performed, followed by radiation therapy. Since there is no tumor marker such as an excessive hormone level, a total resection cannot be confirmed. Therefore, radiation therapy has been given following surgical removal of all nonfunctional tumors. The recurrence rate is clearly lowered with this combined therapy (see Chapters 16 and 21).

In a report on the results of transsphenoidal decompression of the optic nerves and chiasm in 62 patients for lesions in and about the sella, 45 of which were pituitary adenomas, 81% were improved, 11% unchanged, and 5% worse.[35]

4.2. Prolactin-Secreting Tumors

A series of 43 women with amenorrhea–galactorrhea–hyperprolactinemia syndromes were found to have prolactin-secreting adenomas on the basis of radiologic and endocrine studies outlined in Chapter 4, and were operated on via the transsphenoidal route.[36] All but one of the patients had galactorrhea, abnormal sella polytomes and/or visual fields, amenorrhea with low basal serum gonadotropins [luteinizing hormone (LH)/follicle-stimulating hormone (FSH)] despite decreased serum estradiol, and elevated basal serum prolactins. The indications for surgery were: (1) desire for pregnancy; (2) enlargement of tumor while under observation; (3) failure of medical treatment; (4) suprasellar tumor with mass effect; and (5) profuse galactorrhea or debilitating headache. All patients were restudied endocrinologically 6–8 weeks following surgery with the following tests: (1) TRH stimulation test with bloods for TSH and prolactin; (2) GnRH stimulation with bloods for LH and FSH; (3) insulin hypoglycemia stimulation with bloods for glucose, prolactin, GH, and cortisol; (4) 14-hr dehydration test; (5) basal T_4, T_3, progesterone, and estradiol; and (6) Goldmann visual fields. The follow-up period for the entire group ranged from 5 to 10 months, with an average of 18.6 months.

Follow-up of patients after the 8-week postoperative endocrine profile occurred at intervals of 3 months, and included yearly sella polytomography and hormonal reevaluation.

At surgery, pituitary adenomas were found in all patients. Thirty-three of 43 had eosinophilic granules on light microscopy.

The endocrine results are summarized in Table 1. "Cure" was defined in the strictest sense, i.e., complete normalization of prolactin (<25 ng/ml), normal menses, cessation of galactorrhea, and either resolution of or no additional hormone deficiencies. "Improved" meant considerable reduction of prolactin levels without significant other hormone deficiencies. "Unchanged" indicated no significant difference in any parameter, while "worse" indicated significant postoperative hormonal deficiencies.

In the Grade I group, 23 of 27 patients had normal prolactin levels after surgery, 22 of 27 had return of menses, 5 patients desiring pregnancy conceived, and 24 of 27 had resolution of galactorrhea. Of the 27, 4 developed partial hormonal deficiencies postoperatively. A 43-year-old woman who specifically requested an aggressive sella exenteration "to be certain that tumor would never recur" had panhypopituitarism. Of the other three, ACTH-, LH-, and antidiuretic hormone (ADH)-reserve deficiency occurred, respectively.

In the Grade II group, 3 of 6 patients had normalization of prolactin, 3 of 6 had return of menses (1 subsequent pregnancy), and 3 of 6 had resolution of galactorrhea. Postoperatively, one patient had GH-reserve deficiency, and one patient had GH-, ACTH-, and LH-reserve deficiency. Another had resolution of secondary hypothyroidism.

Of the Grade III patients, 4 of 8 had normalization of prolactin, 3 of 8 had return of menses (all having subsequent pregnancies), and 5 of 8 had resolution of galactorrhea. Two patients had new pituitary deficiencies postoperatively. One Grade IV C patient with marked elevation of prolactin (1017.8 ng/ml preoperatively) had significant improvement of prolactin (29.9 ng/ml postoperatively) with resolution of galactorrhea, but no return of menses, although there has been only 18 months of follow-up since postoperative radiation therapy. The other Grade IV C patient had an exenteration of her sella with panhypopituitarism and resolution of visual-field defects postoperatively.

Of Grade I patients, 85.2% were cured and 14.8% were improved. None was unchanged or worse. Of 6 Grade II patients, 2 were cured, 2 were significantly improved, and 2 were unchanged. Of 8 patients in Grade III, 4 were cured and 2 were improved, while 2 with suprasellar extension (SSE) were either unchanged or worse. One Grade IV patient with marked SSE had significant improvement, while the other was considered cured of tumor even in the

TABLE 1. Summary of Endocrine Results (Prolactinomas)

Grade	Number of patients	Cured	Improved	Unchanged	Worse
I	27	23 (85.2%)	4 (14.8%)	—	—
II	6	2 (33.3%)	2 (33.3%)	2 (33.3%)	—
III No SSE[a]	2	1 (50%)	1 (50%)	—	—
SSE	6	3 (50%)	1 (16.7%)	1 (16.7%)	1 (16.7%)
IV SSE	2	1 (50%)	1 (50%)	—	—
TOTALS	43	30 (69.8%)	9 (20.9%)	3 (7.0%)	1 (2.3%)

[a] (SSE) Suprasellar extension.

face of intentional panhypopituitarism. Overall, 69.8% were cured, 20.9% improved, 7.0% unchanged, and 2.3% worse.

Eighty percent of patients had complained of headache preoperatively, and all had total resolution of this symptom postoperatively. Five patients had visual-field defects (bitemporal hemianopsia) preoperatively, which completely resolved following surgery. There were no other preoperative neurological signs. Mortality is zero.

Complications are listed in Table 2. One patient had unexplained unilateral proptosis for 6 days postoperatively, which resolved spontaneously. CT scan failed to show a blood clot or other abnormality such as engorged ophthalmic veins. Two patients operated on early in the series had CSF leakage postoperatively, one of whom required reoperation and packing to seal the leak.

Four patients had nasal septal perforation, one of whom is symptomatic with crusting. One patient had a minor fracture of the maxilla requiring no treatment, assumed to be from opening the nasal speculum.

We have not had any other complications involving visual acuity, visual fields, or extraocular movements.

4.2.1. Discussion

An important consideration in the management of prolactinoma patients is that infertility is often an important problem and normal gonadotropin function must be retained. The benign nature of the tumor cannot be disregarded, and the therapy must not be worse than the disease. The ideal treatment is total removal of the tumor while maintaining normal pituitary function so that menses are restored and pregnancy may occur.

The success rates of normalizing prolactin levels in hyperprolactinemic patients utilizing bromergocryptine range from 85 to 100%.[36–38] Because of the high rate of pregnancy achieved with this drug, and the significant risk of pituitary tumor enlargement during pregnancy with potential neurological impairment,[39,40] bromocriptine usage should be limited to patients without any radiographic evidence for tumor.[40] Therefore, I believe that hyperprolactinemic patients who are demonstrated to have a tumor should first be treated with ablative therapy. Since, in our own and other experienced

TABLE 2. Complications: Prolactinomas

Complications	Occurrence
Mortality	0/43
Morbidity	
CSF leak	2/43 (1 re-op)
Perforated nasal septum	4/43
Fracture of maxilla	1
Transient proptosis	1 (1 week duration, ? etiology)
Infection (meningitis)	0
Persistent partial ADH insufficiency	3

hands,[41–43] the therapeutic success of transsphenoidal surgery in Grade I adenomas approaches the efficacy of bromergocryptine, we feel that surgery should be the treatment of choice in such patients.

The size of the tumor is a limiting factor in the success of treatment. The excellent results realized in a patient with a prolactin-secreting microadenoma, unaccompanied by abnormalities in secretion of other hormones, cannot be expected in a patient with a large tumor compromising normal pituitary function, or with a tumor having significant SSE. In the latter situations, a nonselective total removal or a subtotal removal followed by radiation therapy may be more advisable. In the localized microadenomas, a selective adenomectomy, sparing the normal gland, should be attempted.[25]

I agree with Collins[44] and Wilson *et al.*[45] that many patients with normal sella radiography do harbor adenomas, and that before abnormal polytomes are seen, approximately 25% of the sella will be filled with tumor. I initiated surgical exploration in selected patients with suggestive endocrine history and abnormal endocrine studies, yet normal polytomes. The first such patient was found to have a 5-mm adenoma and is included in this series. However, in the second patient, a tumor was not found, and at present I elect to operate only when radiographic studies are abnormal.

Three patients were reexplored transsphenoidally after initial failure to normalize prolactin. In two patients, further intrasellar tumor tissue could not be found and hyperprolactinemia persisted. In a patient reoperated on because of visual-field defects in association with a postoperative empty sella, residual tumor was removed with normalization of prolactin, the arachnoid pouch was elevated, and the sella packed. Postoperatively, her visual-field defect resolved and prolactin was normal. On the basis of this experience, I have decided not to reexplore the sella if the primary procedure has failed to effect a cure. Rather, other modes of therapy, including irradiation and/or bromocriptine, are used to arrest residual tumor growth and/or normalize prolactin.

Postoperatively, patients who had macroadenomas, with or without SSE, have been given conventional radiation therapy with the Betatron if serum prolactin remains elevated. Patients who had microadenomas and postoperative elevation of prolactin have been offered either radiation therapy or bromergocryptine.

Although the average follow-up of 18.6 months is somewhat short, we have seen only one patient with normal prolactin levels postoperatively develop hyperprolactinemia and galactorrhea unassociated with menstrual abnormalities 28 months after surgery.

4.3. ACTH-Secreting Tumors

Several series have recently been reported on the results of selective transsphenoidal removal of ACTH-producing microadenomas in Cushing's disease.[46–49] The diagnosis of Cushing's disease was made generally by the clinical syndrome associated with hypercortisolism, nonsuppressibility of plasma or urinary corticosteroid levels with overnight or low-dose dexamethasone, and suppression of adrenocortical steroid levels to less than 50%

of baseline levels with high-dose dexamethasone.[47] Combining these series (Table 3) shows that 19 of 63 patients (30%) had normal sellas seen on pleuridirectional tomography. Of the 63, 57 (90%) were considered Grade I microadenomas, and 56 of the 57 were found at surgery. One tumor measuring 1.5 mm was found in the pituitary gland during pathological study after a total hypophysectomy was performed.[47]

The results are summarized in Table 3. Of Grade I adenomas, 93%, or 84% of the total group of 63 patients, were cured of their hypercortisolism with no mortality and minimal morbidity. One patient became panhypopituitary after total hypophysectomy was performed when the adenoma could not be found during exploration. Five patients developed transient diabetes insipidus.[47] Two patients thought to be cured developed evidence of continued tumor growth and were treated further, one with total hypophysectomy and the other with radiation, with excellent results.[49]

A period of hypocortisolism requiring hydrocortisone replacement therapy occurred after tumor removal in most patients experiencing a remission.[47,50] In one series, the shortest duration of postoperative steroid replacement was 3 months and the longest 24 months, with the average being 9 months.[50] Generalized hypopituitarism was not seen in any patient other than those subjected to intentional hypophysectomy. Exemplary data from one study[47] of 17 patients in whom preoperative and postoperative data were available show comparison mean values: morning plasma ACTH levels of 116 pg/ml fell to 27 pg/ml; morning plasma cortisol of 29 μg/100 ml fell to 5μg/100 ml; baseline urinary 17-hydroxycorticosteroid level of 23 mg/24 hr fell to 4 mg/24 hr; and urinary free cortisol fell from 509 μg/24 hrs to 34 μg/24 hr.[47]

In general, the results also show a return to normal feedback regulatory

TABLE 3. Cushing's Disease Results

Authors	Number of patients	Grade	Tumor found	Total hypophysectomy	Number cured	Complications
Tyrell *et al.*[47]	20 (8 normal sella)	20 Grade I	17 (2 unsuccessful)	1	17 (1 total hypophysectomy; 16 selective removal)	1 panhypopituitarism (hypophysectomy) 5 transient diabetes insipidus
Hardy[49]	25 (11 normal sella)	19 Grade I 3 Grade II 3 Grades III and IV	19 3 0	— — —	17 3 0	2 recurred, requiring total hypophysectomy, 1 raidcal 3 with abnormal X-rays; no tumor found
Salassa *et al.*[48]	18 (all abnormal X-rays	18 Grade I	17	—	16	1 patient—no tumor found at surgery or autopsy after unrelated death
TOTALS:	63	57 Grade I	56		53 93% of Grade I 84% of total	

control with a return of normal responsiveness to feedback inhibition by the "low-dose" dexamethasone test, and normal response to metyrapone.[46,48] Circadian rhythms also returned.

Nelson's disease has been far more difficult to treat. Hardy[49] reported 9 cases, 3 with normal sella, 3 Grade I, and 3 Grade II. Five patients were cured and 4 were improved. One patient with abnormal X-rays was explored, but no tumor was seen. Salassa *et al.*[50] reported on 14 patients, with 30% showing a pronounced decrease in hyperpigmentation. Seventy percent had continued elevation of plasma ACTH despite adequate replacement treatment with both glucocorticoid and mineralocorticoid steroids. In our clinic, two patients with Nelson's syndrome, both Grade IV, were explored. One patient, age 16, was cured and now has normal plasma ACTH values while on replacement glucocorticoid and mineralocorticoid, and has normal pituitary function. The other patient was improved, but not cured. Wilson and Dempsey[45] report poor results as well. Only 2 of 18 patients achieved normal postoperative values of plasma ACTH.

4.4. Growth-Hormone-Secreting Tumors

More data are available on the results of transsphenoidal surgery for acromegaly than for any of the other pituitary tumors. Several larger series have been well studied and were recently reported.[46,49,51–54]

Overall, these studies show that for a Grade I microadenoma secreting GH, a biological cure can be expected in more than 90%, with GH levels reduced to below 10 ng/ml. With prior treatment, the results are not as good. Prior surgery tends to distort the anatomy more than radiation therapy does and therefore is associated with the least successful results.

With diffuse adenomas not previously treated, the cure rate is closer to 75%, while with invasive adenomas, the cure rate falls to approximately 50%. The results parallel rather closely those seen with prolactin-secreting adenomas when grouped according to size and extension.

Complications are also similar, with transient diabetes insipidus seen in about 10%, and other anterior pituitary dysfunction increasing in frequency with tumor size and the radical nature of removal necessitated by the larger tumors. Hardy[49] reported that 14% had improvement of preoperative anterior pituitary hormone deficiencies, while 11% had new deficiencies postoperatively, 77% of which were intentional with radical removal. Laws[54] reported 6% partial anterior pituitary deficiency with microadenomas, 32% partial or complete deficiencies with diffuse adenomas, and 54% partial or complete deficiencies with invasive adenomas.

Patients with visual loss preoperatively improved in a manner similar to that noted previously for nonfunctional tumors.

Wilson and Dempsey[45] reported that patients initially cured and followed for up to 6 years have not shown recurrence of the adenoma. If a cure has not been achieved with residual elevation of GH or obvious tumor remaining, then postoperative radiation therapy is given.[45,52–55]

5. Complications

Cushing's mortality rate in 1932 was 5.2%.[56] Hirsch[57] reported a preantibiotic mortality rate of 5.4% and a postantibiotic rate of 1.5%. Guiot,[26] in 582 cases, noted a rate of 1.3%, and Hardy,[49] in over 500 cases, reported a rate of about 2%. Both Guiot and Hardy had the advantage of steroids and antibiotics as well as the modern advances of image-intensified fluoroscopy and the operating microscope. Other recent series of transsphenoidal tumor removals report mortalities from 0 to 2%.[46,49,54] Our mortality has been zero through the first 100 tumor patients.

Specific complications of transsphenoidal surgery have been extensively reviewed.[58] Intracranial complications are the most severe and include hypothalamic and optic nerve and chiasm injury, by either direct or secondary vascular effects, hemorrhages, meningitis, and major arterial damage. Hematomas occur in about 1%.[26,36,46]

Visual impairment is more likely if the tumor capsule is transversed or if it is adherent to the visual apparatus. Interference with small vessels to the chiasm can cause ischemic changes. Overpacking of the sella after tumor removal can compress the optic system, and, likewise, underpacking can lead to a secondary empty sella syndrome with eventual herniation of the optic nerves and chiasm causing visual defects.

With tumors wholly contained within the sella, it is unusual to see visual changes; however, in our clinic, there has been one patient who had previously undergone transsphenoidal surgery for a prolactin microadenoma and presented with visual loss from a secondary empty sella (see Chapter 10, Fig. 17). Guiot[26] reported 5 of 475 patients who developed postoperative empty sella syndromes with visual deterioration requiring reoperation. Two had significant improvement, one had slight improvement, and two were failures.[26]

The incidence of visual complications, however, is low. Of 129 patients with normal vision preoperatively, none developed visual impairment postoperatively, while 2 of 45 patients with preoperative visual loss had transient increase of visual impairment after transsphenoidal surgery for pituitary tumor.[35] In our series of 100 consecutive tumor patients undergoing transsphenoidal surgery, one patient has had significant visual loss. This was a 67-year-old woman with normal vision and a very large tumor extending 2 cm above the sella. At 48 hr postoperatively, she developed monocular blindness secondary to a hematoma. Permanent visual worsening or loss occurs in 1–4%.[46,49,54] Extracular motor palsies may occur from manipulation of the cavernous sinus or overpacking of the sella, but are usually transient.

Major arterial injury can occur during the initial exposure in the cavernous sinus or with medially displaced arteries in the sella. This may lead to major vessel occlusion, spasm, or false aneurysm formation. Overpacking of the sella can cause carotid compression.

Meningitis is usually secondary to postoperative CSF leak, but may occur from organisms introduced during surgery. The incidence of CSF leak and meningitis is low, 1.3–4%.[26,58] Our incidence is 3%. Leaks occur more frequently when the diaphragma sella is torn during surgery or when an intrasellar arachnoid diverticulum or enlarged opening in the diaphragma exists.

Sphenoid sinus and nasofacial complications include diastasis or fracture of the hard palate, fracture of the skull base or maxilla secondary to excessive opening of the nasal speculum, delayed mucocele formation, sinusitis, nasoseptal perforation, and external nasal deformity.

Endocrinological complications include partial or complete hypopituitarism and diabetes insipidus. Persistent partial or total ADH insufficiency is seen in approximately 4–5% of patients.[36,46,54] In a study by McLanahan *et al.*,[59] anterior pituitary hormones were measured pre- and postoperatively in 40 patients with pituitary adenomas treated via transsphenoidal surgery. Of 23 patients with normal anterior-lobe function preoperatively, 91% were normal postoperatively as well. Of 17 patients with impaired function preoperatively, 40% regained normal function, 18% improved, 24% remained the same, and 18% were further impaired by the procedure. The conclusion was that the likelihood of recovery of pituitary function varied inversely with the degree of preoperative impairment and the size of the tumor. This corroborated the approach of a more aggressive surgical procedure for small, minimally symptomatic pituitary tumors.[59]

6. Summary

The transsphenoidal operation with the use of the operating microscope allows the selective removal of hyperfunctioning pituitary adenomas while sparing the normal gland. Approximately 85% of patients with microadenomas can achieve an endocrine cure. Large tumors may be adequately decompressed with excellent visual results, at least comparable to, and perhaps better than, those achieved with any other modality. Postoperative radiation therapy is used in conjunction to lessen the recurrence rate. The morbidity and mortality are minimal, offering a new dimension in safety for treatment of pituitary adenomas.

References

1. H. Schloffer, Erfolgreiche Operation eines Hypophysecentumors auf nasalem Wege, *Wien. Clin. Wochenschr.* **20:**621–624, 1907.
2. G. Giordano, *Compendio Chir. Operat. Ital.* **2:**100, 1897 (quoted by G.J. Heuer, The surgical approach and the treatment of tumors and other lesions about the optic chiasm, Surg. *Gynecol. Obstat.* **53:**489–518, 1931).
3. T. Kocher, Die Verletzungen der Wirbelsäule zugleich als Beitrag zur Physiologie des menschlichen Ruckenmarks Mitt a.d., *Grenzgeb. Med. Chir.* **1:**415–580, 1896.
4. A.E. Halstead, Remarks on the operative treatment of tumors of the hypophysis, Surg. *Gynecol. Obstet.* **10:**494–502, 1910.
5. A.B. Kanavel, The removal of tumors of the pituitary body by an infranasal route: A proposed operation with a description of the technique, *J. Am. Med. Assoc.* **53:**1704–1707, 1909.
6. G. Guiot and B. Thibaut, L'extirpation des adenomes hypophysaires par voie transsphenoidale, *Neuro-Chirur.* (*Stuttgart*) **1:**133, 1959.
7. J. Hardy, *Microsurgery Applied to Neurosurgery* (M.D. Yasargil, ed.), pp. 180–193, Academic Press, New York, 1969.

8. J. Hardy, Transsphenoidal microsurgery of the normal and pathological pituitary, *Clin. Neurosurg.* **16:**185–217, 1969.
9. J. Hardy, Trans-sphenoidal hypophysectomy, *J. Neurosurg.* **34:**581, 1971.
10. J. Hardy, Trans-sphenoidal microsurgical removal of pituitary adenoma, in: *Recent Progress in Neurological Surgery,* p. 86, Excerpta Medica, Amsterdam, 1974.
11. M. Arslan, Ultrasonic hypophysectomy in acromegaly: Report of 41 cases, *Otol. Rhinol. Laryngol.* **35:**134–140, 1973.
12. J.N. Cross, K.W.M. Grossart, R.J. Kellett, J.A. Thomson, A. Glynn, W.B. Jannett, J.H. Lazarus, and M.H.C. Webster, Treatment of acromegaly by cryosurgery, *Lancet* **1:**215–216, 1972.
13. S.J. Richards, J.P. Thomas, and D. Kilby, Transethmoidal hypophysectomy for pituitary tumours, *Proc. R. Soc. Med.* **67:**889–892, 1974.
14. M.V. DiTullio, Jr., and R.W. Rand, Efficacy of cryohypophysectomy in the treatment of acromegaly, *J. Neurosurg.* **46**(1):1–11, 1977.
15. W.F. Collins, Jr., Transsphenoidal surgery of pituitary adenomas, in: *The Pituitary: A Current Review* (M.B. Allen, Jr., and V.B. Mahesh, eds.), pp. 431–442, Academic Press, New York, San Francisco, and London, 1977.
16. G.H. Bateman, Transsphenoidal hypophysectomy: A review of 70 cases treated in the past two years, *Trans. Am. Acad. Ophthalmol. Otolaryngol.* **63:**103–110, 1962.
17. L.W. Conway, F.T. O'Fogludha, and W.F. Collins, Stereotactic treatment of acromegaly, *J. Neurol. Neurosurg. Psychiatry* **32:**48–59, 1969.
18. W.F. Collins, Hypophysectomy: Historical and personal perspective, in: *Clinical Neurosurgery: Proceedings of the Congress of Neurological Surgeons* (R.H. Wilkins, ed.), pp. 68–78, Williams & Wilkins, Baltimore, 1974.
19. N.T. Zervas and H. Hamlin. Stereotaxic thermal pituitary ablation, *Acta Neurochir.* **21**(Suppl.):165–168, 1974.
20. C.B. Wilson, Personal communication.
21. G.T. Tindall, W.F. Collins, and J.A. Kirchner, Unilateral septal technique for transsphenoidal microsurgical approach to the sella turcica: Technical note, *J. Neurosurg.* **49:**138, 1978.
22. W.F. Collins, Personal communication.
23. K.D. Post and B.M. Stein, Spinal drainage catheter: Technical note, *Neurosurgery* **4**(3):255, 1979.
24. J. Hardy, P.R. Townsend, and D.G. Cerundolo, Forces applied by nasal speculums during transsphenoidal operations, *Surg. Neurol.* **10:**361, 1978.
25. J. Hardy, Transsphenoidal surgery of hypersecreting pituitary tumors, in: *Diagnosis and Treatment of Pituitary Tumore* (P.O. Kohler and G.T. Ross, eds.), pp. 179–194, Excerpta Medica, Amsterdam, 1973.
26. G. Guiot, Transsphenoidal approach in surgical treatment of pituitary adenomas: General principles and indications in non-functioning adenomas, in: *Diagnosis and Treatment of Pituitary Tumors* (P.O. Kohler and G.T. Ross, eds.), pp. 159–178, Excerpta Medica, Amsterdam, 1973.
27. L.S. Adelman and K.D. Post, Intraoperative frozen section technique for pituitary adenomas, *Am. J. Surg. Pathol.* **3**(2):173–175, 1979.
28. S. Saglam, C.L. Kragt, C.B. Wilson, S.L. Kaplan, and M. Barker, Graded cryohypophysectomy in the rhesus monkey: Histopathology and endocrine function, *J. Neurosurg.* **36:**169–177, 1972.
29. J.M. Van Buren and D.M. Bergenstal, An evaluation of graded hypophysectomy in man, *Cancer* **13:**155–171, 1960.
30. C.A. Hamberger, G. Hammer, G. Norlen, *et al.*, Transantrosphenoidal hypophysectomy, *Arch. Otolaryngol.* **74:**2–8, 1961.
31. W.H. Renn, and A.L. Rhoton, Jr., Microsurgical anatomy of the sellar region, *J. Neurosurg.* **43:**288–298, 1975.
32. G. Hammer and C. Radberg, The sphenoidal sinus: An anatomical and roentgenologic study with reference to transsphenoidal hypophysectomy, *Acta Radiol.* **56:**401–422, 1961.
33. J. Kinnman, Surgical aspects of the anatomy of the sphenoidal sinuses and the sella turcica, *J. Anat.* **124**(3):541–553, 1977.
34. R.M. Bergland, B.S. Ray, and M. Torack, Anatomical variations in the pituitary gland and adjacent structures in 225 human autopsy cases, *J. Neurosurg.* **28:**93–99, 1968.
35. E.R. Laws, J.C. Trautman, and R.W. Hollenhorst, Transsphenoidal decompression of the optic nerve and chiasm: Visual results in 62 patients, *J. Neurosurg.* **46:**717–722, 1977.

36. K.D. Post, B.J. Biller, L.S. Adelman, M.E. Molitch, S.M. Wolpert, and S. Reichlin, Results of selective transsphenoidal adenomectomy in women with galactorrhea–amenorrhea, *J. Am. Med. Assoc.* **242**(2):158–162.
37. M.O. Thorner, A.S. McNeilly, C. Hagan, and G.M. Besser, Long-term treatment of galactorrhea and hypogonadism with bromocriptine, *Br. Med. J.* **2**:419–422, 1974.
38. E. Del Pozo, L. Varga, H. Wyss, G. Tolis, H. Friesen, R. Wenner, L. Vetter, and A. Euttwiler, Clinical and hormonal response to bromocriptine (CB-154) in the galactorrhea syndromes, *J. Clin. Endocrinol. Metab.* **39**:18–26, 1974.
39. Editorial, Pituitary tumors and pregnancy, *Lancet* **1**:404, 1976.
40. P.B. Nelson, A.G. Robinson, D.F. Archer, and J.C. Maroon, Symptomatic pituitary tumor enlargement after induced pregnancy, Presented at the American Association of Neurological Surgeons Annual Meeting, New Orleans, Louisiana, April 1978.
41. R.J. Chang, W.R. Keye, Jr., J.R. Young, C.B. Wilson, and R.B. Jaffe, Detection, evaluation, and treatment of pituitary microadenomas in patients with galactorrhea and amenorrhea, *Am. J. Obstet. Gynecol.* **128**:356–4363, 1977.
42. J. Hardy, Transsphenoidal microsurgical treatment of hypersecreting pituitary adenomas, Presented at the American College of Physicians, Neuroendocrine Course, Montreal, Canada, March 1978.
43. G.T. Tindall, C. Scott, C.S. McLanahan, and J.H. Christy, Transsphenoidal microsurgery for pituitary tumors associated with hyperprolactinemia, *J. Neurosurg.* **48**:849–860, 1978.
44. W.F. Collins, Jr., Transsphenoidal surgery of pituitary adenomas, in: *The Pituitary* (M.B. Allen, Jr., and V.B. Mahesh, eds.), pp. 431–442, Academic Press, New York, 1977.
45. C.B. Wilson and L.C. Dempsey, Transsphenoidal microsurgical removal of 250 pituitary adenomas, *J. Neurosurg.* **48**:13–22, 1978.
46. A.M. Schnall, J.S. Brodkey, B. Kaufman, and O.H. Pearson, Pituitary function after removal of pituitary microadenomas in Cushing's disease, *J. Clin. Endocrinol. Metab.* **47**(2):410–417, 1978.
47. J.B. Tyrell, R.M. Brooks, P.A. Fitzgerald, P.B. Cofoid, P.H. Forsham, and C.B. Wilson, Cushing's disease: Selective trans-sphenoidal resection of pituitary microadenomas, *N. Engl. J. Med.* **298**(14):753–758, 1978.
48. R.M. Salassa, E.R. Laws, Jr., P.C. Carpenter, and R.C. Northcutt, Transsphenoidal removal of pituitary microadenoma in Cushing's disease, *Mayo Clin. Proc.* **53**:24–28, 1978.
49. J. Hardy, Recent advances in the diagnosis and treatment of pituitary tumors, International Symposium held in San Francisco, California, May 31–June 4, 1978.
50. R.M. Salassa, T.P. Kearns, J.W. Kernohan, R.G. Sprague, and C.S. MacCarty, Pituitary tumors in patients with Cushing's syndrome, *J. Clin. Endocrinol. Metab.* **19**:1523–1539, 1959.
51. J. Garcia-Uria, J.M. del Pozo, and G. Bravo, Functional treatment of acromegaly by transsphenoidal microsurgery, *J. Neurosurg.* **49**:36–40, 1978.
52. M.A. Giovanelli, E.D.F. Motti, A. Paracchi, P. Beck-Peccoz, B. Ambrosi, and G. Faglia, Treatment of acromegaly by transsphenoidal microsurgery, *J. Neurosurg.* **44**:677–686, 1976.
53. H. Sang U, C.B. Wilson, and J.B. Tyrrell, Transsphenoidal microhypophysectomy in acromegaly, *J. Neurosurg.* **47**:840, 1977.
54. E.R. Laws, Jr., The neurosurgical management of acromegaly: Results in 82 patients treated between 1972 and 1977, Presented at the AANS Annual Meeting in April 1978 (Paper No. 33).
55. J. Hardy, M. Somma, and J.L. Vezina, Treatment of acromegaly: Radiation or surgery?, in: *Current Controversies in Neurosurgery* (T.P. Morley, ed.), pp. 377–391, W.B. Saunders, Philadelphia, 1976.
56. H. Cushing, Intracranial tumors, in: *Notes upon a Series of Two Thousand Verified Cases with Surgical–Mortality Percentages Pertaining Thereto,* p. 150, Charles C. Thomas, Springfield, Illinois, 1932.
57. O. Hirsch, Pituitary tumours: A borderland between cranial and trans-sphenoidal surgery, *N. Engl. J. Med.* **254**:937–939, 1954.
58. E.R. Laws, Jr., and E.B. Kern, Complications of trans-sphenoidal surgery, *Clin. Neurosurg.* **23**(Chapt. 29):401–416, 1975.
59. C.S. McLanahan, J.H. Christy, and G.T. Tindall, Anterior pituitary function before and after trans-sphenoidal microsurgical resection of pituitary tumors, *Neurosurgery* **3**(2):142–145, 1978.

19

Transfrontal Surgery for Pituitary Tumors

KALMON D. POST

1. Introduction

The advantages and disadvantages of the transcranial route were outlined in the chapter on general considerations (Chapter 16). The primary disadvantages are the greater morbidity and mortality, the greater threat to vision, and the particular inability to adequately differentiate a microadenoma from the normal gland because direct visualization is not readily achieved. The mortality rates are generally higher than with the transsphenoidal procedures, with some reports ranging between 4.5 and 35%.[1–10] The morbidity is also higher than with the transsphenoidal procedure and will be discussed under complications (Section 4).

Nevertheless, even with widespread experience with the transsphenoidal operation, there are specific indications for a transcranial approach to pituitary adenomas. A tumor with suprasellar extension but without an enlarged sella, or an hourglass-shaped tumor, must be removed from above. Similarly, very asymmetric lateral extension beneath the temporal lobe or anterior extension to the subfrontal area requires removal from above (Fig. 1). Invasive tumors tend to grow into the cavernous sinus[11] and have been considered unresectable and therefore decompressed from below. MacKay and Hosobuchi[12] reported on two cases with cavernous sinus invasion approached by craniotomy and direct opening of the sinus with total tumor removal. If this group of adenomas can be identified preoperatively as invasive, they may be a further indication for craniotomy or a bidirectional removal with two operations. Transcranial surgery is definitely more advantageous when additional pathology, such as an aneurysm, is also present (Fig. 2).

KALMON D. POST • Tufts University School of Medicine; Department of Neurosurgery, Tufts–New England Medical Center Hospital, Boston, Massachusetts 02111.

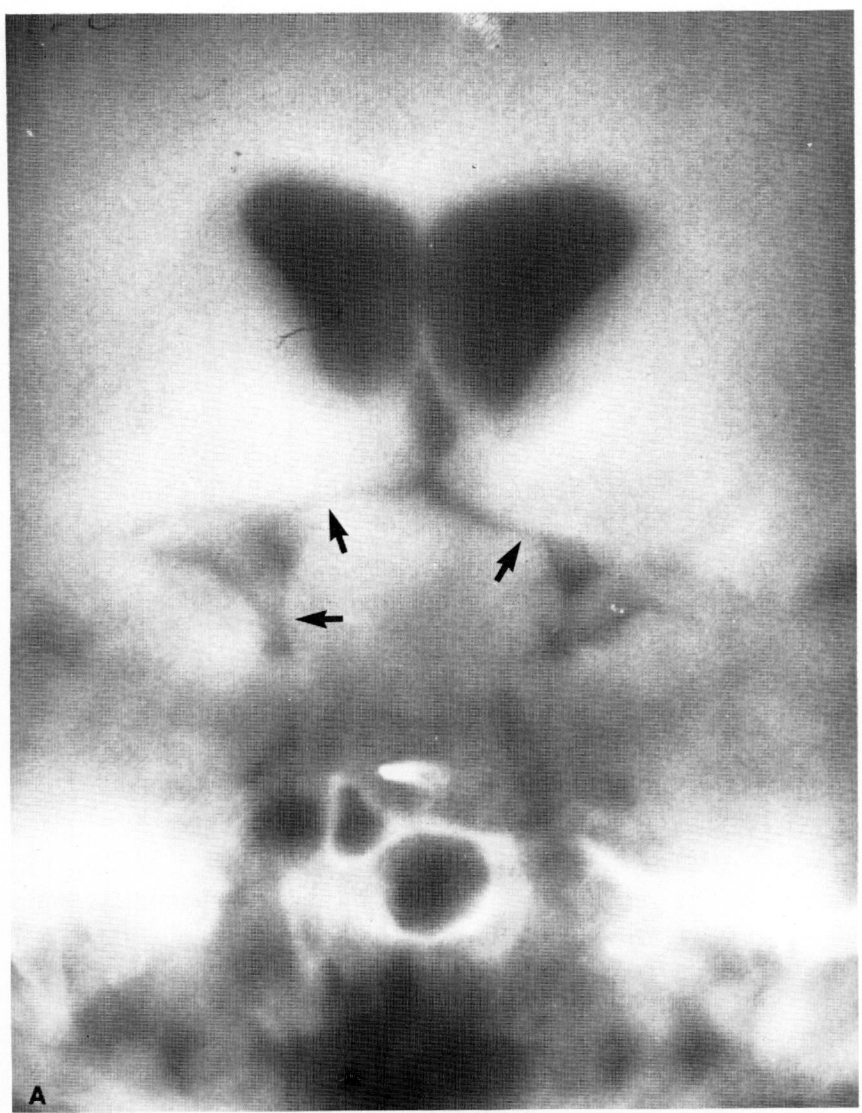

Fig. 1. (A) Anteroposterior (AP) tomogram during pneumoencephalogram demonstrating large suprasellar extension of a recurrent pituitary adenoma (arrows). (B) Computed tomography (CT) scan with contrast enhancement demonstrating lesion extending from the suprasellar cistern forward beneath the right frontal lobe. (C) Intraoperative photograph of the same patient demonstrating the anterior extension of the tumor along the planum sphenoidale.

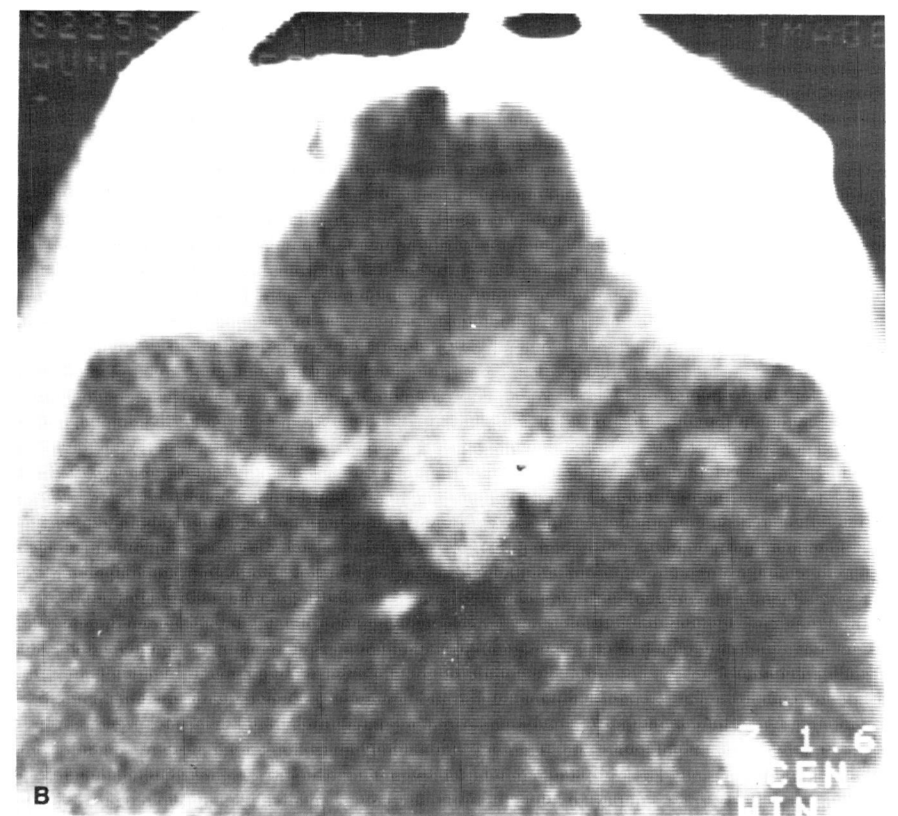
B

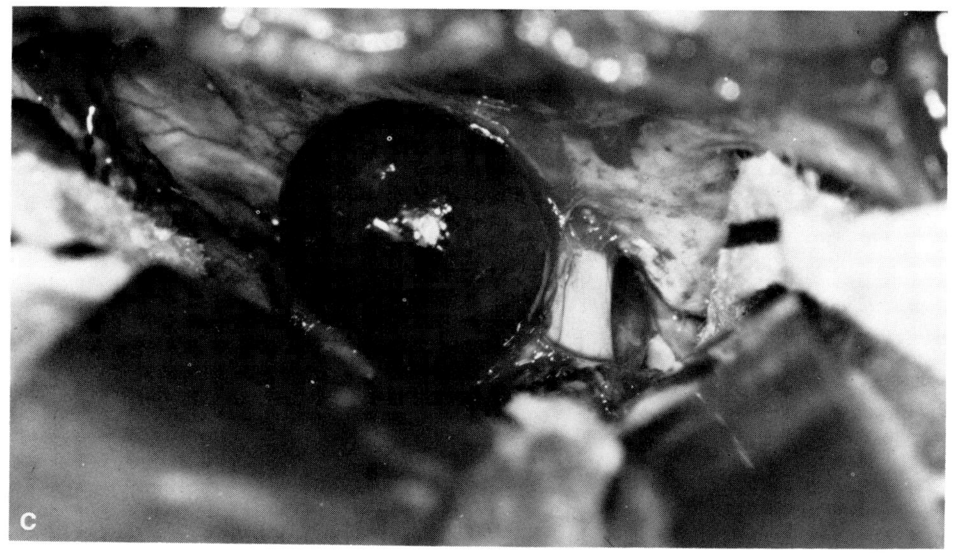
C

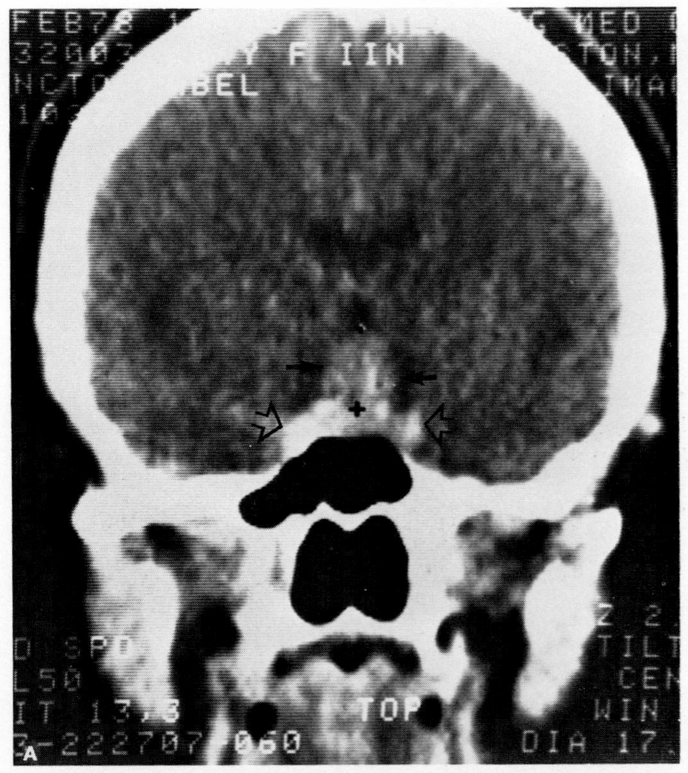

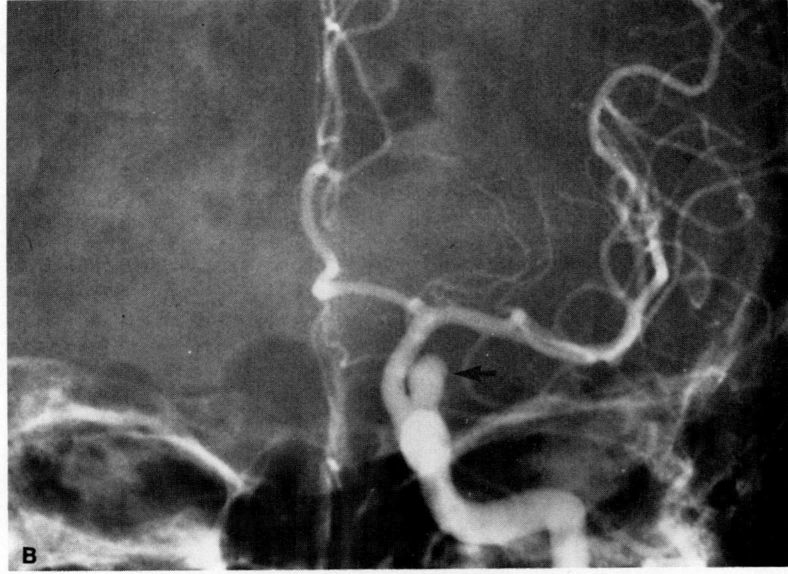

Fig. 2. (A) Coronal CT scan with enhancement demonstrating suprasellar lesion (solid arrows) as well as enhancing parasellar lesions (open arrows). (B) AP left carotid arteriogram of same patient demonstrating slight elevation of A-1 segment of the left anterior cerebral artery. Additionally, an aneurysm on the supracavernous portion of the internal carotid artery is demonstrated (arrow).

2. Anatomical Considerations

Using a transcranial approach, the optic nerves, chiasm, and major arteries present a barrier to exposure of the tumor. Anatomical variation of the location of these structures necessitates the direction of the approach: (1) between the optic nerves and below the chiasm (interneural–subchiasmatic) (see Fig. 4); (2) between the carotid artery and the optic nerve (optico–carotid) (see Fig. 5); or (3) transfrontal–transsphenoidal as described by Rand.[13]

In normal position, the chiasm overlies the diaphragma sella and pituitary gland. A prefixed chiasm overlies the tuberculum sellae, and a postfixed chiasm overlies the dorsum sellae (Fig. 3). There is some variation, with an incidence of 80% normal, 9% prefixed, and 11% postfixed in the series of Bergland *et al.*[14] and 75% normal, 10% prefixed, and 15% postfixed in the study of Renn and Rhoton.[15] In the presence of a prefixed chiasm, the tuberculum sellae may project as much as 2 mm behind the anterior margin of the chiasm. In normal position, the distance between the tuberculum and the anterior margin of the chiasm averaged 4 mm, while with a postfixed chiasm, the average distance was 7 mm.[15] Additionally, the tuberculum may project above the superior surface of the optic nerves as they enter the optic canals as described in 44% of cases studied by Renn and Rhoton. These variations may indicate the direction of growth of the suprasellar component of the adenoma,

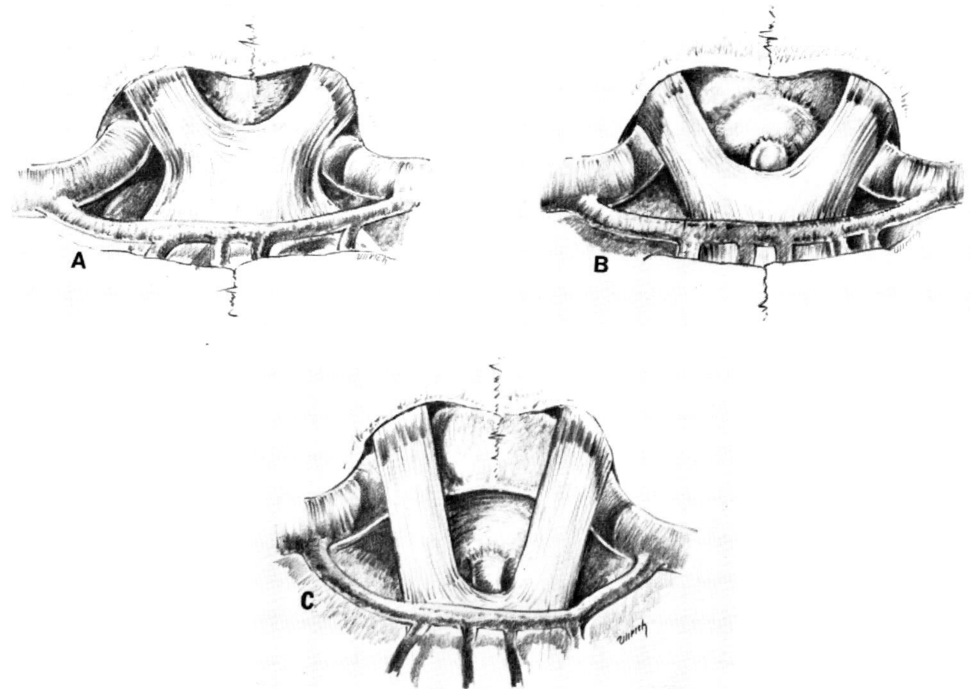

Fig. 3. Diagrams demonstrating variations in the position of the optic nerves and chiasm: (A) prefixed chiasm; (B) normal position of chiasm; (C) postfixed chiasm (see the text).

as well as dictate the surgical approach for its removal. If the procedure is hampered by a prefixed chiasm or a protruding tuberculum, it may be necessary to remove the tuberculum.[13]

Another surgical hazard concerns the relationship of the posterior margin of the optic canals and the optic nerves. There may be an absence of bone over the nerves for a distance varying from 0.5 to 8.0 mm, the average being 3 mm, so that they are covered only by dura.[15] Coagulation on the dura may be hazardous[16] and should be performed as though the nerves were immediately adjacent to the dura.

The position of the carotid and anterior cerebral arteries is also variable. The internal carotid arteries are most closely approximated in the supraclinoid area in 82% of cases, in the cavernous sinus–sella level in 14%, and in the sphenoid sinus in 4%.[15] The junction of the anterior communicating artery with the anterior cerebral arteries is usually above the chiasm (70%), but occasionally above the optic nerves (30%). When anteriorly placed, the arteries are frequently tortuous and elongated, in some instances even touching the tuberculum sellae or planum sphenoidale.

The vascular anatomy has been eloquently illustrated by Rhoton and coworkers.[15,17–19] The supraclinoid internal carotid gives off perforating branches including the superior hypophyseal artery that runs to the optic nerves, chiasm, anterior hypothalamus, and anterior perforating substance. The anterior cerebral and anterior communicating arteries provide multiple small branches to the superior surface of the optic chiasm, the anterior hypothalamus, the anterior perforating substance, and the region of the optic tract. The upper centimeter of the basilar artery provides an average of eight branches from its posterior and lateral surfaces to the diencephalon and midbrain. The posterior cerebral artery proximal to the posterior communicating artery as well as the posterior communicating artery give rise to multiple perforating branches, including the thalamoperforating and medial posterior choroidal arteries. These branches might be stretched over the top of suprasellar tumors. Care must be taken to preserve these vessels. This can be accomplished only with microscopic techniques.

Considerable anatomical variations of the osseous structures in this region occur. These include ligamentous connections between the clinoid processes, bone continuity between the anterior and posterior clinoid processes, and complete absence of the clinoid processes.[20] These variations must be appreciated to protect the vital neural and vascular structures during dissection.

The variants that are considered most disadvantageous to the transfrontal approach are[16]:

1. A prefixed or normal positional chiasm with 2 mm or less between the chiasm and tuberculum sellae.
2. A prominent tuberculum sellae.
3. Carotid arteries that approach the midline within or above the sella turcica.
4. Anterior cerebral arteries that have a prefixed course above the optic nerves.

3. Surgical Techniques

Mannitol, hyperventilation, and spinal drainage are all used to minimize the amount of brain retraction that will be necessary.

With the patient in the supine position under general anesthesia, the head is fixed in a Mayfield head-holder and turned 15° to the opposite side. Dandy[21] devised a small frontotemporal craniotomy flap through which he removed both large and small pituitary tumors. This flap is still commonly used, as is the bicoronal and classic unilateral frontal incision. All are effective in exposing the frontal bone as low as the supraorbital ridge and frontal floor. The bicoronal flap may be more cosmetic, since it is completely concealed behind the hairline. The choice of side for the bone flap is dictated by the side of lateral extension. If the tumor is midline, then the nondominant side is chosen, although some surgeons prefer to enter on the side with the more affected optic nerve. Others prefer the side with the less affected optic nerve so that it may be immediately identified and protected.

The frontal sinus may have to be traversed to accomplish this, but the frontal floor must be reached to minimize the retraction of the frontal lobe. A flap of periosteum is turned down over the sinus and sutured to the dura to seal the opening. With lateral extension, a more lateral approach is used with a pterional bone flap. The bone is removed flush with the temporal floor, and the sphenoid ridge is rongeured away. The lateral transcranial route has the advantages of not sacrificing the olfactory nerve and of allowing removal of tumor from the middle fossa, third ventricle, interpeduncular cistern, and suprasellar region with a prefixed chiasm.[22,23]

The dura is opened along the base, and the frontal lobe is elevated. With the frontal approach, the optic nerve is found by following the olfactory nerve, and with the lateral approach, the sphenoid ridge is followed.

Veins bridging the temporal lobe to the dura are coagulated and divided to prevent bothersome bleeding while retracting the lobe. Self-retaining retractors are placed on the frontal and temporal lobes to maintain the exposure of the optic nerve and suprasellar region.

The use of the operating microscope has refined transcranial surgery for pituitary adenomas. Instrumentation, including microdissectors with 1 to 2-mm tips, bipolar coagulation,[24] self-retaining retractors, and fixed head-holders, also offers an advantage to the surgeon. Bipolar coagulation allows fine coagulation while minimizing the dangerous spread of current into the adjacent optic nerves and other neural structures. Saline irrigation during the coagulation reduces heating even further and prevents tissue sticking to the instruments. Self-retaining retractors allow gentle, constant retraction on the brain for long periods of time.

If spinal drainage was not used, the arachnoid of the chiasmatic cistern is opened and cerebrospinal fluid (CSF) removed with suction. The optic nerve and carotid artery are dissected free from the arachnoid, and the arachnoid over the frontal lobe is opened to allow further retraction exposing the tumor, chiasm, and arteries. The tumor is preferably approached between the optic nerves and below the chiasm (interneural–subchiasmatic approach) (Fig. 4).

However, an approach between the carotid artery and optic nerve (optico–carotid approach) (Fig. 5) may be necessary if: (1) there is a prefixed chiasm; (2) there is asymmetric extension of the tumor that widens the space between the optic nerve and carotid artery; or (3) there are no major perforating branches from the carotid artery passing across this area to the optic nerves, chiasm, or hypothalamus.[16] With a prefixed chiasm, another choice is the subfrontal transsphenoidal approach described by Rand.[13]

The tumor capsule is coagulated with bipolar cautery and punctured with

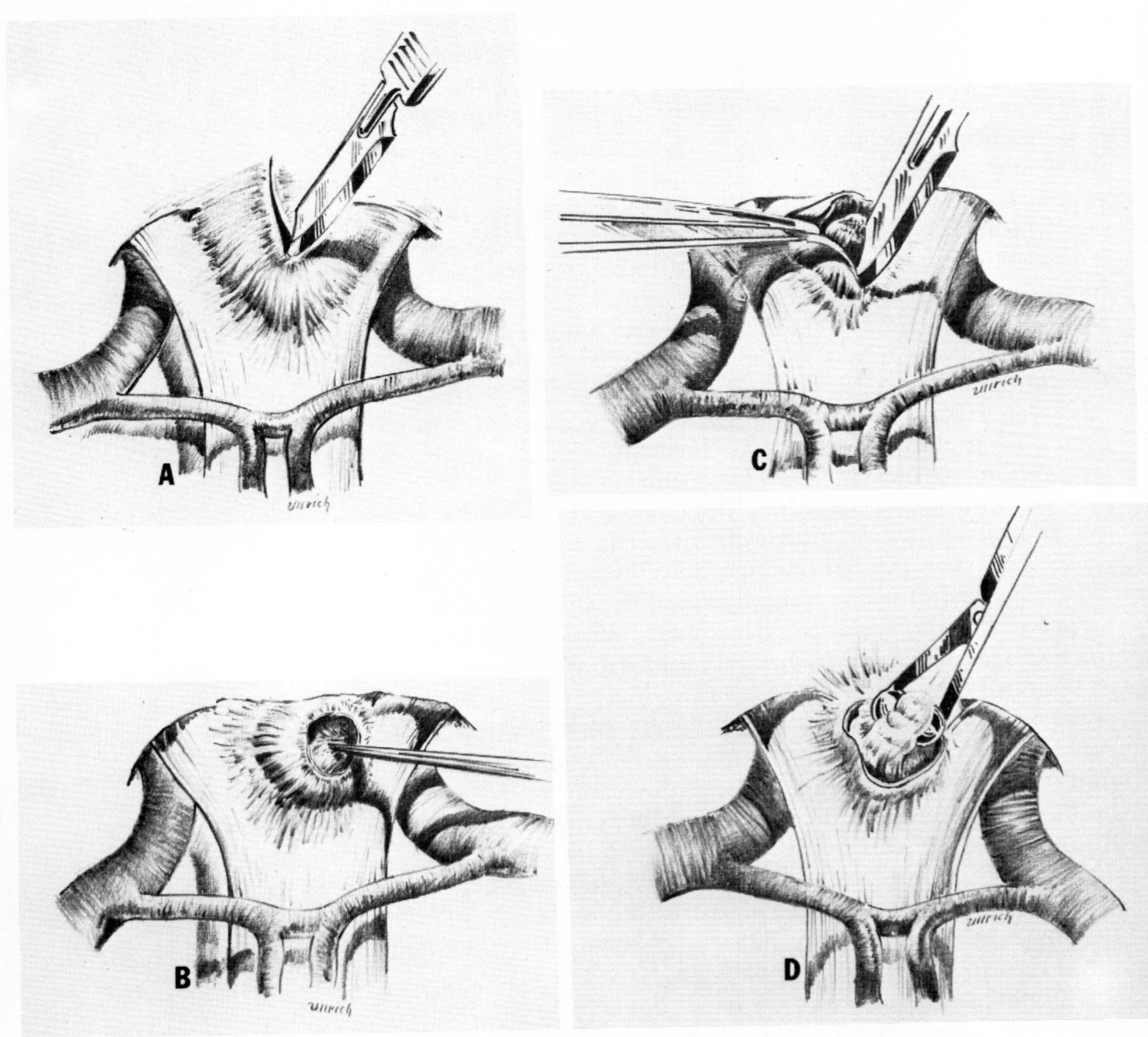

Fig. 4. Diagrammatic demonstration of an interneural–subchiasmatic tumor removal (see the text): (A) opening of arachnoid over tumor and nerves; (B) needling tumor for cystic component; (C) opening tumor sharply; (D) intracapsular piecemeal removal of tumor; (E) dissection of capsule if it separates readily; (F) piecemeal removal of capsule; (G) microdissection of vessels from capsule; (H) sella packed with muscle after removal.

a needle to see whether there is a cystic component and to ensure that an aneurysm is not present. The capsule is opened widely between the optic nerves or between the optic nerve and carotid artery. An intracapsular piecemeal removal is then carried out using suction, ring currettes, and tumor forceps. No attempt is made to remove the capsule until it has collapsed. If it fails to collapse, it is usually because of remaining pieces of tumor within the capsule. Dandy,[21] Ray and Patterson,[25] Stern and Batzdorf,[6] Kempe,[23] and Rhoton and Maniscalco[26] all note that it is not necessary, and in fact may be dangerous, to remove the entire tumor capsule. The portion of the capsule that can be readily dissected away from the optic nerves, chiasm, and arteries is then removed piecemeal. Particular attention must be paid to the perfora-

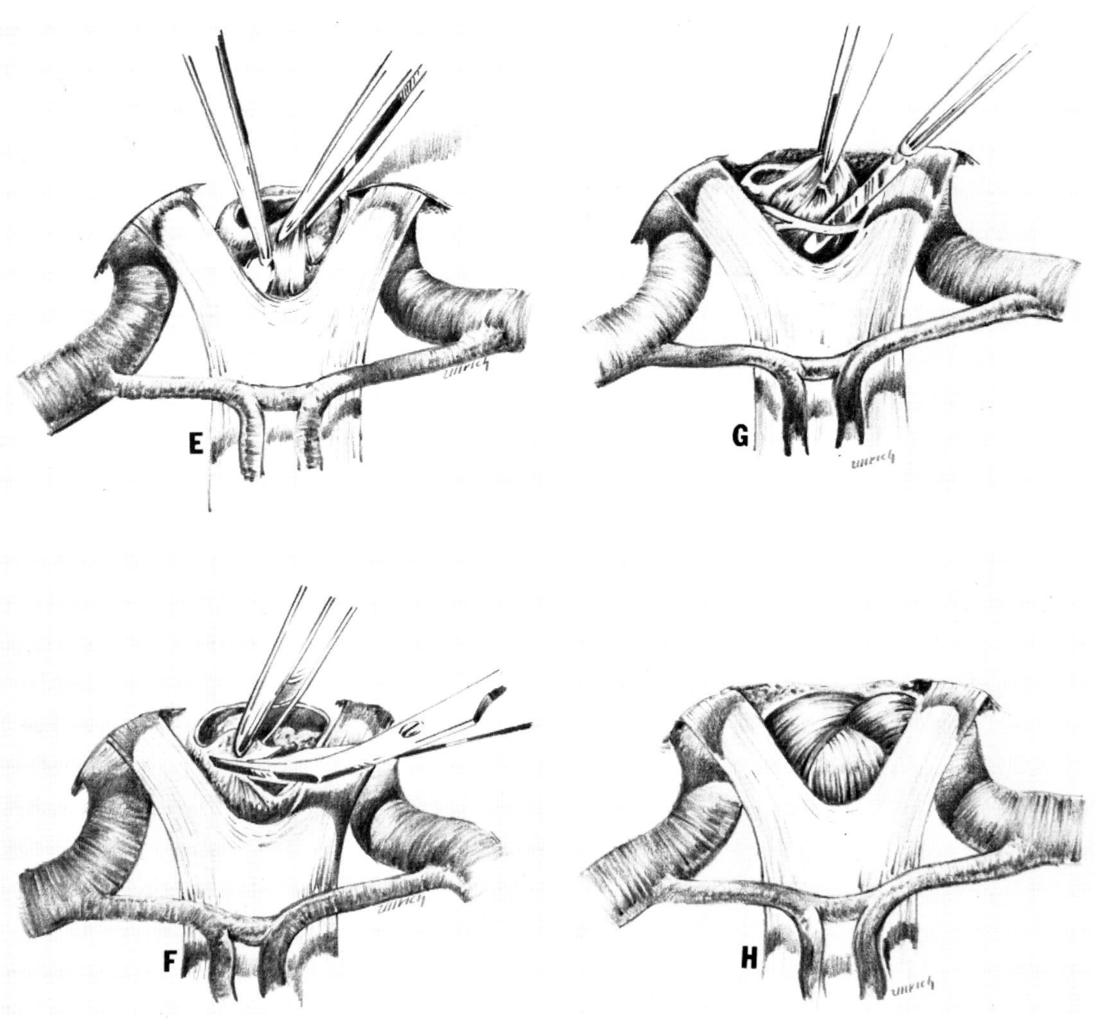

Fig. 4. *(continued)*

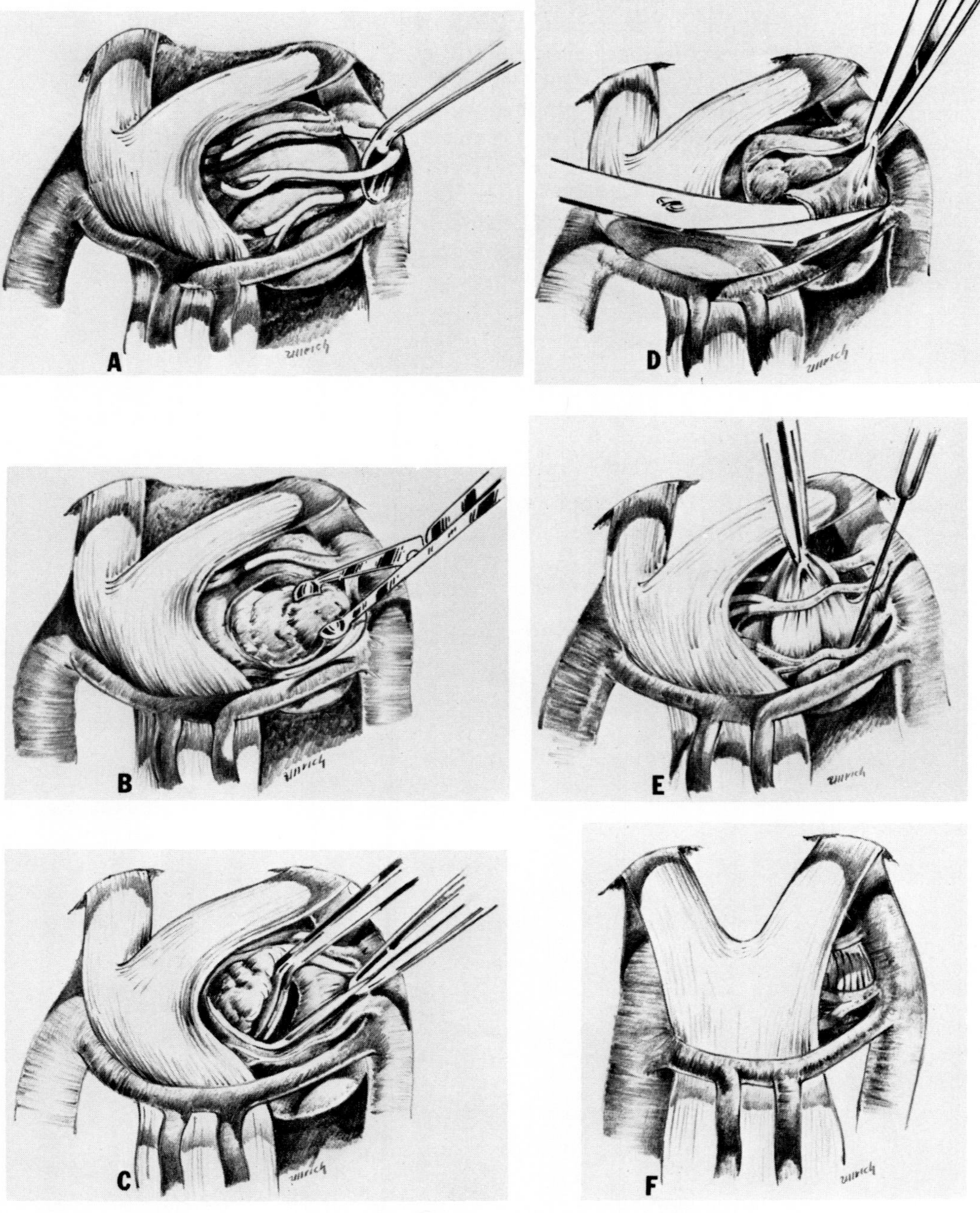

Fig. 5. Diagrammatic demonstration of an optico–carotid tumor removal (see the text): (A) microdissection separating arachnoid and vessels from tumor surface; (B) intracapsular piecemeal removal of tumor after needling; (C) intracapsular dissection of tumor to facilitate piecemeal removal; (D) piecemeal removal of tumor capsule; (E) microdissection to further separate tumor capsule from vessels; (F) resection completed, sella packed with muscle.

ting arteries that pass over the tumor capsule to supply the nerves, chiasm, and hypothalamus. Injury to these vessels may have severe consequences with hypothalamic syndromes, visual loss, and affective disorders. It is usual that the entire capsule cannot be removed. Total radical intracapsular removal followed by radiation, however, is necessary to significantly reduce the recurrence rate.[6,27]

After tumor and partial capsular removal, hemostasis is obtained. A dental mirror is often useful to inspect for further bits of tumor before packing the sella. Packing is done with muscle to prevent herniation of the optic nerves and chiasm into the empty sella postoperatively. The craniotomy is then closed in the usual fashion.

4. Results

Factors that play a role in mortality of pituitary surgery include tumor size, patient age, and concomitant medical problems.

Operative mortality is variable. In one series[25] of 146 patients with chromophobe adenomas, 2 (both of whom were seriously ill with recurrent tumor following previous surgery and radiation therapy) died within 1 month of surgery, a mortality of 1.4%. No deaths occurred in 138 patients operated on for the first time. Other large series have a mortality range of 3–14%,[1,5,27–35] with the majority in the 6–8% range (Table 1). A higher mortality rate (25–33%) is seen generally in large tumors with massive suprasellar extension,[2,6,7,29,32,35–37] or in operations for recurrence. In large tumors, a mortality rate of 18%, and in small tumors a rate of 3.1%, were reported by Wirth *et al.*[27]

TABLE 1. Mortality Rates from Major Published Series

Authors	Number of patients	Mortality rate (%)				
		Large tumor	Small tumor	Primary operation	Secondary operation	Overall
Cushing[1]	205	—	—	—	—	2.4
Bakay[2]	232	35	6.4	—	—	11.3
Tonnis[8]	240	—	—	—	—	11.2
Horrax *et al.*[7]	125	34.5	3.9	—	—	14.1
Rand[9]	67	—	—	—	—	8.9
Martins *et al.*[32]	54	—	—	—	—	5.0
Svien and Colby[36]	117	16.7	2.5	—	—	6.8
Elkington and McKissock[29]	260	33	5.0	—	55	10.0
Jefferson[37]	110	36	2.0	—	—	5.4
Stern and Batzdorf[6]	64	—	—	7	—	5.9
Ray and Patterson[25]	146	—	—	0	25	1.2
MacCarty *et al.*[31]	100	—	—	—	—	3.0
Fager *et al.*[30]	197	—	—	—	—	(2% after 1950)
Wirth *et al.*[27]	157	18	3.1	8	33	8.9
Hankinson and Banna[34]	120					6.66

Mortality rate correlates with the age of the patient, being 3.2% under 50 years of age compared with a rate of 17.2% in patients over 50 years.[27]

In terms of morbidity, seizures are seen as a postoperative complication in 3–4% of cases operated on by a subfrontal route.[38] Postoperative blood clots, infection, and CSF fistulas are uncommon.

Transient diabetes insipidus (DI) was reported following 21% of primary transfrontal operations,[27] persisting beyond 2 weeks in only 12%. Permanent DI is unusual.

Endocrine function is usually deficient in adenoma patients submitted to craniotomy, and it is usually anticipated that recovery will not occur. Occasionally it may, but replacement therapy is most often required (see Chapter 20).

Visual loss has been one of the major indications for transcranial surgery. Of 106 patients reported by Ray and Patterson,[25] 38% of patients had visual symptoms as an initial complaint, and by the time of treatment, 93% had visual disturbances. Following surgery, significant improvement occurred in 80%, and normal vision was achieved in approximately 50%. There was no change in 18%, and 2% were worse. Patients with either previous surgery or radiation did not fare as well. Sheline *et al.*[39] showed that recovery of vision was dependent on the duration of visual impairment. Patients with compression for less than 6 months had a 54% improvement rate. With symptoms for longer than 6 months, the improvement rate was only 15%.

In a series of 120 surgical procedures,[34] patients with normal acuity and only a field defect made full recoveries. The less extensive and more recent acuity impairments made better improvements. Overall, 53.8% made full recoveries, while 86.3% had some improvement with recovery spreading over several months up to 2 years. With microsurgical techniques, results may be even better, with improvement reaching the 90% level.[33]

The visual improvement may be better with radical tumor removal as opposed to subtotal and intracapsular removals. Wirth *et al.*[27] reported 81% improvement in patients treated by radical removal with or without radiation, while only 67% with subtotal removal and radiation improved.

There is a definite risk ranging from 7.5 to 2% that vision will be made worse by transcranial surgery.[25,27,30]

Visual evoked potentials (VEPs) have been measured in patients undergoing adenoma removal, with demonstration that there is immediate improvement in the VEPs during decompression.[40]

Contrasting these results with those achieved via a transsphenoidal removal shows some advantage to the latter approach. In the Mayo series reported by Laws *et al.*,[41] of 42 adenoma patients with visual impairment undergoing transsphenoidal removal, 36 (85.7%) had improvement, while 6 were unchanged. Two patients experienced transient increase in visual impairment following the transsphenoidal procedure. Before surgery, there was a median visual impairment of 17%, while after transsphenoidal surgery, it was only 3%. A comparable Mayo Clinic series of 71 patients who underwent intracranial surgery was reported by Svien *et al.*[42] The median improvement in this series was 18%, but only 10% of the craniotomy series returned to normal vision, while 17% of the transsphenoidal series did. However, the pa-

TABLE 2. Recurrence Rates from Major Published Series

Authors	Number of patients	Recurrence rate (%) Without radiation	With radiation	Average follow-up (yr)
Cushing [1]	205	56	13	5
Bakay [2]	232	—	10–15	5
Martins *et al.* [32]	54	—	6	—
Stern and Batzdorf [6]	64	9.4	—	5.5
Ray and Patterson [25]	146	22	8	—
MacCarty *et al.* [31]	96	31.8	3.0	>5
Van Der Zwan [44]			6	
Wirth *et al.* [27]	157	25.8	11.7	5.3

tients in the transsphenoidal series had less severe visual impairment prior to surgery than did patients in the craniotomy series.[41]

Recurrence rates following surgical removal of adenomas are unquestionably reduced with postoperative radiation (Table 2). With a radical removal plus postoperative radiation, the recurrence rate was lowered to 6.7% in the series of Wirth *et al.*,[27] with an average 5.8-year follow-up. Most recurrences will occur within the first 5 years following treatment,[2,25,27] as shown by Cushing's series,[43] in which 95% of recurrences were within the first 5 years and the latest known recurrence occurred 8 years after surgery. In another report,[27] 8 of 24 recurrences occurred after 5 years (at 6, 8, 10, 11, 11, 12, and 13 years). Therefore, follow-up must extend beyond 5 years.

5. Summary

The transcranial removal of pituitary adenomas is an effective means of therapy; however, the morbidity and mortality are higher than in transsphenoidal surgery even though results are similar. There are situations such as asymmetric suprasellar extension wherein the transcranial procedure is preferred. With microsurgical techniques, the risks can be significantly reduced.

The improvement in visual deficits is comparable to that achieved by the transsphenoidal route; however, there is some risk that as many as 7.5% will have worse vision following manipulation of the optic nerves.

Recurrence rates are clearly related to tumor size and are significantly reduced with postoperative radiation therapy. Follow-up is mandatory beyond 5 years despite the occurrence of most recurrences within that period.

References

1. W.R. Henderson, The pituitary adenomata: Follow-up study of surgical results in 338 cases (Dr. Harvey Cushing's series), *Br. J. Surg.* **26**:811–921, 1939.
2. I. Bakay, the results of 300 pituitary adenoma operations (Olivecrona's series), *J. Neurosurg.* **7**:240, 1950.

3. J.I. Nurnberger and S.R. Korey, *Pituitary Chromophobe Adenomas*, Springer-Verlag, New York, 1953.
4. G. Horrax, M.I. Smedal, J.G. Trump, R.C. Granke, and K.A. Wright, Present-day treatment of pituitary adenomas: Surgery versus X-ray therapy, *N. Engl. J. Med.* **252:**524, 1955.
5. H. Krayenbuhl, Hypophyseal adenomas and craniopharyngioma, in: *Abstracts: II International Congress of Neurological Surgery*, Washington, D.C., *Excerpta Med. Int. Congr. Ser.* **36:**E10–E12, Excerpta Medica, Amsterdam, 1961.
6. W.E. Stern and U. Batzdorf, Intracranial removal of pituitary adenomas: An evaluation of varying degrees of excision from partial to total, *J. Neurosurg.* **33:**564–573, 1970.
7. G. Horrax, J.F. Hare, J.L. Poppen, I.M. Hurxthal, and O.Z. Younghusband, Chromophobe pituitary tumors. II. Treatment, *J. Clin. Endocrinol. Metab.* **12:**631–641, 1952.
8. W. Tonnis, Report of 240 adenomata of the hypophysis, *Zentralbl. Chir.* **77:**2103–2105, 1952.
9. C.W. rand, Notes on pituitary tumors including suggestions of others and personal experiences in 100 cases, *Clin. Neurosurg.* **3:**1–58, 1957.
10. A.S. Obrador, Adenomas of the pituitary based on a neurosurgical experience of 65 operated patients, *Rev. Clin.* **81:**396–440, 1961.
11. Sir Geoffrey Jefferson, *The Invasive Adenomas of the Anterior Pituitary*, pp. 1–63, University of Liverpool Press, Liverpool, England, 1955.
12. A. MacKay and Y. Hosobuchi, Treatment of intracavernous extensions of pituitary adenomas, *Surg. Neurol.* **10:**377–383, 1978.
13. R.W. Rand, Transfrontal transsphenoidal craniotomy in pituitary and related tumors using microsurgical techniques, in: *Microneurosurgery* (R.W. Rand, ed.), pp. 74–86, C.V. Mosby, St. Louis, 1969.
14. R.M. Bergland, B.S. Ray, and M. Torack, Anatomical variations in the pituitary gland and adjacent structures in 225 human autopsy cases, *J. Neurosurg.* **28:**93–99, 1968.
15. W.H. Renn and A.L. Rhoton, Jr., Microsurgical anatomy of the sellar region, *J. Neurosurg.* **43:**288–298, 1975.
16. A.L. Rhoton, Jr., F.S. Harris, and W.H. Renn, Microsurgical anatomy of the sellar region and cavernous sinus, in: *Neuro-ophthalmology: Symposium of the University of Miami and the Bascom Palmer Eye Institute* (J.S. Glaser, ed.), pp. 75–105, C.V. Mosby, St. Louis, 1977.
17. F.S. Harris and A.L. Rhoton, Jr., Microsurgical anatomy of the cavernous sinus, *J. Neurosurg.* **45:**169–180, 1976.
18. D. Perlmutter and A.L. Rhoton, Jr., Microsurgical anatomy of the anterior cerebral–anterior communicating–recurrent artery complex, *J. Neurosurg.* **45:**259–271, 1976.
19. N. Saeki and A.L. Rhoton, Jr., Microsurgical anatomy of the upper basilar artery and the posterior circle of Willis, *J. Neurosurg.* **46:**563–578, 1977.
20. Captain Martin Plaut, Anatomic variations of the sella turcica, *Surg. Neurol.* **10:**259, 1978.
21. W.E. Dandy, The brain, in: *Walter's Practice of Surgery* (D. Lewis, ed.), pp. 1–671, W.F. Prior, Maryland, 1963.
22. J.L. Poppen, The temporal approach to tumors of the sella turcica in the presence of a prefixed chiasma, *J. Neurol. Neurosurg. Psychiatry* **22:**79, 1959.
23. L.G. Kempe, Transcranial approach in pituitary surgery, in: *The Pituitary: A Current Review* (M.B. Allen and V.B. Mahesh, eds.), pp. 421–430, Academic Press, New York, 1977.
24. L.I. Malis, Bipolar coagulation in microsurgery, in: *Microsurgery Applied to Neurosurgery* (M.G. Yasargil, ed.), pp. 41–45, Academic Press, New York, 1969.
25. B.S. Ray and R.H. Patterson, Jr., Surgical experience with chromophobe adenomas of the pituitary gland, *J. Neurosurg.* **34:**726–729, 1971.
26. A.L. Rhoton, Jr., and J.E. Maniscalco, Microsurgery of the sellar region, in: *Neuro-ophthalmology: Symposium of the University of Miami and the Bascom Palmer Eye Institute* (J.S. Glaser, ed.), pp. 106–127, C.V. Mosby, St. Louis, 1977.
27. F.P. Wirth, H.G. Schwartz, and P.R. Schwetschenau, Pituitary adenomas: Factors in treatment, in: *Clinical Neurosurgery*, Vol. 21 (R.H. Wilkins, ed.), pp. 8–25, Williams & Wilkins, Baltimore, 1974.
28. F.C. Grant, Surgical experience with tumors of the pituitary gland, *J. Am. Med. Assoc.* **136:**668–671, 1948.
29. S.G. Elkington and W. McKissock, Pituitary adenomata: Results of combined surgery and radiotherapeutic treatment of 260 patients, *Br. Med. J.* **1:**263, 1967.

30. C.A. Fager, J.L. Poppen, and Y. Takaoka, Indications for and results of surgical treatment of pituitary tumors by the intracranial approach, in: *Diagnosis and Treatment of Pituitary Tumors* (P.O. Kohler and G.T. Ross, eds.), pp. 146–155, Excerpta Medica, Amsterdam, 1973.
31. C.S. MacCarty, E.J. Hanson, R.V. Randall, and P.W. Scanlon, Indications for and results of surgical treatment of pituitary tumors by the transfrontal approach, in: *Diagnosis and Treatment of Pituitary Tumors* (P.O. Kohler and G.T. Ross, eds.), pp. 139–145, Excerpta Medica, Amsterdam, 1973.
32. A.M. Martins, L.G. Kempe, and G.J. Hayes, Pituitary adenomas: Concepts based on twelve years' experience at Walter Reed General Hospital, *Acta Neurochir.* **13:**469–471, 1965.
33. H.A.M. van Alphen, Microsurgical fronto-temporal approach to pituitary adenomas with extrasellar extension, *Clin. Neurol. Neurosurg.* **78**(4):246–256, 1974–1975.
34. J. Hankinson and M. Banna, *Pituitary and Parapituitary Tumours,* W.B. Saunders, London, Philadelphia, and Toronto, 1976.
35. H.J. Svien, W.C. Kennedy, and T.P. Kearns, Results of surgical treatment of pituitary adenoma: the factor of the excessively enlarged sella, *J. Neurosurg.* **20:**669, 1963.
36. H.J. Svien and M.Y. Colby, Jr., *Treatment of Chromophobe Adenomas,* p. 17, Charles C. Thomas, Springfield, Illinois, 1967.
37. A.A. Jefferson, Chromophobe pituitary adenomata: The size of the suprasellar portion in relation to the safety of operation, *J. Neurol. Neurosurg. Psychiatry* **32:**633, 1969.
38. H.J. Svien and M.Y. Colby, Jr., Pituitary chromophobe adenomas: Comparative results of surgical and roentgen treatment, *Behav. Neurol.* **1:**35, 1969.
39. G.E. Sheline, E.B. Boldrey, and T.L. Phillips, Chromophobe adenomas of the pituitary gland, *Am. J. Roentgenol.* **92:**160, 1964.
40. M. Feinsod, J.B. Selhorst, W.F. Hoyt, and C.B. Wilson, Monitoring optic nerve function during craniotomy, *J. Neurosurg.* **44:**29–31, 1976.
41. E.R. Laws, J.C. Trautman, and R.W. Hollenhorst, Transsphenoidal decompression of the optic nerve and chiasm: Visual results in 62 patients, *J. Neurosurg.* **46:**717–722, 1977.
42. H.J. Svien, J.G. Love. W.C. Kennedy, M.Y. Colby, Jr., and T.P. Kearns, Status of vision following surgical treatment for pituitary chromophobe adenoma, *J. Neurosurg.* **22:**47–52, 1965.
43. W.J. German and S. Flanigan, Pituitary adenomas: A follow-up study of the Cushing series, *Clin. Neurosurg.* **10:**72, 1964.
44. A. Van Der Zwan, *Pituitary Tumors,* Thesis, Leiden (De. Kempenaer, Oegstgeest).

20

Endocrine Management after Pituitary Surgery

WILLIAM E. COBB

1. Introduction

The detection and treatment of pituitary-hormone deficiencies constitutes a major part of patient management following surgery for pituitary and hypothalamic tumors. In the immediate postoperative period, the appearance of adrenocorticotropic hormone (ACTH) and/or thyroid-stimulating hormone (TSH) deficiency may be of little importance due to the routine use of corticosteroids and to the long plasma half-life of thyroxine, whereas acute deficiency of the posterior pituitary octapeptide, vasopressin, may result in a life-threatening disturbance of water balance. The management of ACTH, TSH, gonadotropin, and growth-hormone (GH) deficiencies assumes a greater significance in the long-term follow-up of patients beyond the immediate postoperative period. This chapter will review some basic concepts and recent developments in the perioperative use of corticosteroids and in the postoperative detection and treatment of pituitary-hormone deficiencies.

2. Pituitary–Adrenal Function

Glucocorticoids are routinely administered to all patients undergoing surgery for pituitary or hypothalamic tumors regardless of preoperative hypothalamic–pituitary–adrenal (HPA) axis testing. Our goal is to ensure adequate tissue levels of a corticosteroid in patients with normal results on preoperative HPA axis tests who develop ACTH deficiency intraoperatively due to stalk section or hypophysectomy as well as in those with documented preoperative ACTH deficiency. High doses of glucocorticoids may have an addi-

WILLIAM E. COBB • Department of Medicine, Division of Endocrinology, Tufts–New England Medical Center Hospital, Boston, Massachusetts 02111; Quincy City Hospital, Quincy, Massachusetts 02169.

tional beneficial effect by reducing local brain swelling that occurs in response to the trauma of surgery. This widely held but unproven view is derived from the well-known reduction of intracranial pressure effected by pharmacological doses of corticosteroids in patients with cerebral edema from a variety of causes other than hypothalamic–pituitary surgery. High-dose steroids may therefore enhance preservation of postoperative hypothalamic–pituitary function by minimizing the pressure necrosis and impaired blood flow that accompany cerebral edema.

Patients with deficient HPA function should receive on the first day an amount of steroid that matches or exceeds the 24-hr adrenal-steroid output under conditions of maximum stress (≈ 200–400 mg hydrocortisone or its equivalent). Steroids are then tapered to a basal replacement level over a period of 1 week as shown in the following suggested protocol:

Preoperative: Dexamethasone 4 mg (or an equivalent amount of a related corticosteroid) i.m. or i.v. on the morning of surgery
Day 1 (day of surgery): Dexamethasone (or equivalent) 2 mg i.v. every 6 hr beginning with surgery
Day 2: Dexamethasone 2 mg i.v. or p.o.* every 8 hr
Day 3: Dexamethasone 1.5 mg i.v. or p.o.* every 8 hr
Day 4: Dexamethasone 1.0 mg i.v. or p.o.* every 8 hr
Day 5: Dexamethasone 0.5 mg i.v. or p.o.* every 8 hr
Day 6: Dexamethasone 0.5 mg i.v. or p.o.* every 12 hr
Day 7: Dexamethasone 0.75 mg i.v. or p.o.* daily (in divided doses)

The benefit of supplemental steroids in patients with normal HPA function preoperatively, particularly when high doses are used in patients undergoing adenomectomy, is not established. We, and others, however, routinely administer supplemental steroids preoperatively (50–100 mg cortisone acetate p.o. or hydrocortisone parenterally or p.o. the evening prior to surgery) and during surgery (100 mg hydrocortisone i.v.) to patients with microadenomas.[1,2] This approach, although probably not necessary in most instances, provides steroid coverage to patients who may develop partial or complete ACTH deficiency during surgery.

2.1. Postoperative Testing of the Hypothalamic–Pituitary–Adrenal Axis

All patients are discharged from the hospital on a physiological dose of prednisone (5–7.5 mg in a single or in divided doses daily) and rescheduled for further testing of the HPA axis in 6–8 weeks. Significant drug-related HPA-axis suppression has not occurred in our patients receiving prednisone for this short time, a finding consistent with the observation that patients receiving physiological amounts of steroids for up to 72 months tolerate a variety of stressful diagnostic and surgical procedures without supplemental steroid.[3] However, the possible occurrence of a subnormal rise in plasma cortisol during an insulin hypoglycemia test, as has been reported in patients

* When changing over to oral administration, we frequently switch to the equivalent amount of prednisone.

receiving physiological doses of prednisone for over 18 months,[4] cannot be totally excluded. Replacement steroids are discontinued for 48 hr' and the need for continued steroid supplement is based on results of tests of the HPA axis. If adrenal gland unresponsiveness is even remotely suspected, the serum cortisol response to ACTH 1–24 (Cortrosyn®) should first be assessed (see Chapter 11). An impaired cortisol response may be due not only to primary insufficiency of the adrenal but also to chronic hyposecretion of ACTH resulting in adrenal gland atrophy (secondary adrenal insufficiency), as might occur in association with pituitary or hypothalamic disease. Patients who respond poorly to Cortrosyn are excluded from further testing of the HPA axis and maintained on replacement steroids. There is now evidence suggesting that the Cortrosyn test may be all that is required to assess the integrity of the entire HPA axis. Lindholm *et al.*[5] have recently shown a very strong correlation of peak cortisol responses 30 min after Cortrosyn with those obtained during insulin-induced hypoglycemia in patients with hypothalamic or pituitary disease; further study of the usefulness of Cortrosyn in the evaluation of postoperative HPA function is needed. Patients either not tested with Cortrosyn or those who show a normal cortisol response to Cortrosyn may demonstrate a normal or impaired cortisol response to insulin hypoglycemia or metyrapone. Patients with an impaired response but normal basal cortisol levels are at risk of developing acute ACTH deficiency under stress, are instructed only in the use of supplemental steroids (see below), and are routinely retested at 12 to 24-month intervals. Patients with low basal levels and impaired HPA responsiveness are placed on daily physiological steroid replacement.

Exceptions to this plan of steroid management and postoperative testing include patients deficient in HPA function preoperatively or those who had such extensive tumor resection that the probability of permanent hypopituitarism is high. These patients are maintained on replacement steroids for life. Patients undergoing radiotherapy after incomplete removal of a large pituitary adenoma (see Chapters 16 and 21) are maintained on twice the usual physiological replacement dose of corticosteroid (e.g., prednisone 10–15 mg daily in divided doses) throughout the course and for 1 week after completion of radiotherapy; this approach is based on our belief that radiotherapy is sufficiently stressful to require the use of supplemental steroid in patients who may have underlying ACTH deficiency. Dosage is then tapered to physiological levels over 1–2 weeks. Minor physical changes resulting from glucocorticoid excess may occur during the period of radiotherapy, but our overall impression is that the improved energy level and sense of well-being seen with this regimen outweigh the transient side effects of steroid excess. The prolonged use of supraphysiological doses of prednisone increases the likelihood of drug-induced HPA-axis suppression.[6] Therefore, we delay postoperative HPA-axis testing for 6 months or more in this group of patients.

2.2. Management of Chronic Secondary Adrenocortical Insufficiency

Prednisone 5 mg daily in single or divided doses is adequate maintenance therapy for most patients with secondary adrenocortical insufficiency.

Some may require slightly greater or lesser amounts because the normal requirement for glucocorticoid is a function of body size and because bioavailability of prednisone may differ among brands. Slow dissolution and poor absorption of some prednisone tablets have been observed; the *Medical Letter*[7] has reported that Meticortin® (Schering) and Deltasone® (Upjohn and Co.) may be more reliable than other formulations of prednisone. Hydrocortisone 20 mg and cortisone 25 mg daily are considerably more expensive than prednisone (2–3 times the cost of prednisone, on the average), but are of particular value in situations where careful clinical monitoring of dose is desired. In contrast to prednisone and other corticosteroids, the plasma level and 24-hr urinary excretion of these drugs can be measured by a standard radioimmunoassay or competitive protein-binding assay for cortisol[8]; these measurements may allow for more precise adjustment of glucocorticoid dose in children where it is desirable to avoid the adverse effect on growth of excessive glucocorticoids. 11-β-Hydroxyglucocorticoids such as prednisolone (5 mg daily) or the much more expensive methylprednisolone (4 mg daily) are preferred replacement medication in patients with cirrhosis because, unlike prednisone, hepatic 11-keto reduction is not required for biological activity.[6] Dexamethasone (0.75 mg daily) or related glucocorticoids have essentially zero mineralocorticoid activity and thus may be preferred over other glucocorticoids in patients with coexisting salt-retaining disorders or hypertension.

All patients with ACTH deficiency, including those with normal basal cortisol levels but impaired ACTH reserve (and not receiving daily replacement steroids), require an increase in steroid dosage under stress. We advise patients to increase prednisone to 10–15 mg daily for minor stress (e.g., an upper respiratory infection) and to 15–25 mg daily for intermediate stress (e.g., an infectious illness with fever or a dental or minor surgical procedure). A major stress (e.g., major trauma or surgery) usually requires parenteral steroids: 100 mg hydrocortisone 3 or 4 times daily, or its equivalent intravenously. All patients should be provided with Medicalert® identification (necklace or bracelet) that indicates that they are deficient in adrenocortical function and should be instructed in the use of an injectable corticosteroid (e.g., 4 mg dexamethasone phosphate) should the ingestion of an oral preparation be impossible due to vomiting. A relative or friend may administer the intramuscular dose of dexamethasone if the patient is unconscious, prior to seeking medical care. We advise patients not to travel great distances from convenient access to health care facilities unless accompanied by an individual knowledgeable in the parenteral administration of glucocorticoids.

3. Disorders of Antidiuretic Hormone (ADH) Secretion

Deficiency [diabetes insipidus (DI)] or inappropriate secretion of antidiuretic hormone [syndrome of inappropriate ADH (SIADH)] after surgery for hypothalamic or pituitary tumors is often transient and may simply reflect the extreme sensitivity of the hypothalamic–neurohypophyseal unit to local alterations in blood flow, edema, and traction on the pituitary stalk. Permanent disturbance of hormone secretion, especially DI, requires direct damage to the neurohypophyseal unit and is much more dependent on the original size and location of tumor and the extent of surgical resection. Prompt, accurate diagnosis and aggressive treatment are essential for prevention of extreme alterations in solute and water balance that may accompany these syndromes.

3.1. Diabetes Insipidus

In 1938, Fisher *et al.*[9] described a triphasic pattern of development of DI following acute destruction of hypothalamic cell bodies that synthesize ADH. Modern immunohistochemical techniques using antibodies to ADH and its carrier protein, neurophysin, have confirmed that these cell bodies lie predominantly in the supraoptic nucleus, but have also shown that lesser amounts of ADH may be synthesized in the paraventricular nucleus and other hypothalamic sites.[10] The first, or "transient," phase of DI, lasting 1–7 days, represents abrupt cessation of ADH synthesis (in the hypothalamus) and secretion (from the median eminence and posterior pituitary). Direct damage to hypothalamic nuclei or high pituitary stalk section, in which there is 90% or more interruption of axoplasmic flow in the median eminence and below, may elicit this response. The second phase (latent phase or interphase) is characterized by a temporary restoration of ADH secretion. Inappropriate retention of water and hyponatremia (SIADH) may occur during the interphase. Prior removal of the posterior pituitary followed by hypothalamic destruction results in permanent DI without an interphase, suggesting that release of previously stored ADH from the posterior pituitary accounts for the temporary return of function. The third component of this classic response is the permanent development of DI representing irreversible death of cell bodies in the supraoptic nucleus and exhaustion of ADH stores in axon terminals of the median eminence and posterior pituitary. Clinically, two additional patterns of DI are seen[11]: Transient DI, followed by a return to normal function, is the most common type, particularly with less extensive pituitary surgery, as in the transsphenoidal removal of a microadenoma. Permanent DI with no interphase is somewhat less predictable, but, as one might expect, seems to be associated most often with extensive resection of large pituitary or hypothalamic tumors. (Occasional patients with apparent "permanent" DI may, after months or even years, recover adequate posterior pituitary function, as discussed below.)

3.1.1. Management of Diabetes Insipidus in the Immediate Postoperative Period

The management of DI in neurosurgical patients at our institution has recently been reviewed by Shucart and Jackson[12] and will be briefly summaried here.

Most patients demonstrate a relatively concentrated, low-volume urine in the first few hours postoperatively, due at least in part to stimulation of ADH release.[13] Preoperative narcotics[14,15] and barbiturates[16] and surgical stress may cause central stimulation of ADH secretion. Anesthetic agents,[17] through inhibition of cardiovascular reflexes, may potentiate the enhancing effect of volume reduction on ADH secretion. Polyuria, particularly when it occurs in this very early postoperative period, should suggest the diagnosis of DI.

The diagnosis of DI is confirmed by demonstrating an abnormally high serum osmolality (>295 mosmol/kg) and an inappropriately dilute urine (<300 mosmol/kg). If the serum osmolality is normal, we allow the diuresis to continue until a state of mild serum hyperosmolality is achieved, thus avoiding an erroneous diagnosis of DI in a patient undergoing a water diuresis due to overhydration during surgery and the early postoperative period. A normal or high serum and high urine osmolality suggest an osmotic diuresis, most often due to osmotic agents such as mannitol (used to reduce brain swelling), or to glycosuria in a diabetic patient. The latter situation may be easily missed in the mild diet-controlled diabetic who manifests glycosuria only on exposure to high-dose steroids and the stress of surgery. Serum sodium concentration is of particular value in the setting of an osmotic diuresis because dilution of extracellular fluid by the osmotically active agent may result in hyponatremia. Osmotic diuresis may also occur in chronic renal failure.

Corticosteroids and diphenylhydantoin, drugs that have a minor inhibitory effect on ADH release in normals,[18] may aggravate the manifestations of DI in patients with compromised ADH reserve. Aubry *et al.*[19] reported that pretreatment of human subjects with hydrocortisone could raise the osmotic threshold for ADH release during normal saline infusion. Streeten *et al.*[20] have provided more direct support for an effect of steroids on osmoreceptor function by demonstrating that cortisol injected directly into the supraoptic nucleus of the rat results in the excretion of a more dilute urine and that a greater increase in plasma osmolality is needed to stimulate ADH secretion.

Meticulous intake and output records, once- or twice-daily weight, measurement of serum electrolytes and serum and urine osmolalities, and replacement of fluid loss as free water (5% dextrose in water if given intravenously) are basic requirements of successful management.[12] Specific drug therapy is usually withheld in the early postoperative period until urinary output exceeds 250 ml/hr for 2 consecutive hours or unless adequate fluid intake cannot be maintained due to lethargy or an impaired thirst mechanism.[12] The rationale for this approach is that DI may be transient or progress rapidly to the interphase of endogeneous ADH secretion. However, the need to consume large quantities of fluid may be poorly tolerated and interfere significantly with sleep. Under these circumstances, hormonal-substitution therapy may be indicated, regardless of the urinary volume.

Aqueous vasopressin (20 U/ml), because of its brief duration of action, is the preferred agent for acute postoperative DI. The usual dose is 0.1–0.3 ml every 4–6 hr. However, it is at present in short supply and may not be readily available for use in this setting. The longer-acting vasopressin tannate in oil (5 U/ml) is the preparation most often used in the treatment of acute postoperative DI. We have achieved good results with a starting dose of 0.25–0.5 ml i.m. (1.25–2.5 U). The use of the lowest dose may result in a less than maximally concentrated urine and its effect is dissipated more rapidly, thus minimizing the potentially dangerous complication of water intoxication and the less dangerous, but at times disturbing, problem of rapid shifts in serum sodium concentration. As the effect wears off, we allow a water diuresis to persist up to several hours in anticipation of a return of endogenous ADH secre-

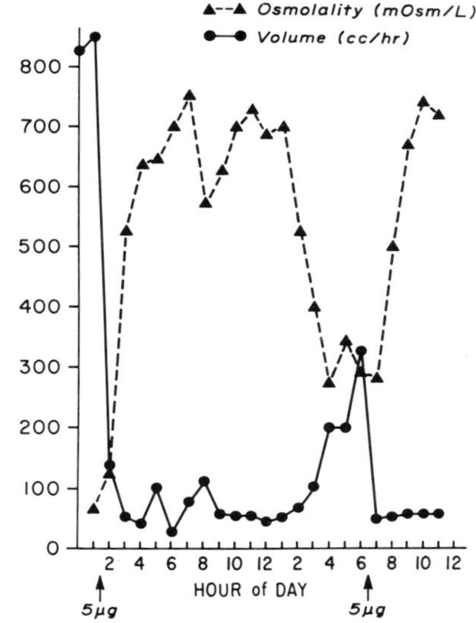

Fig. 1. Effect of 5 μg intranasal dDAVP on volume and osmolality of hourly urine collections in a patient who developed DI after removal of a craniopharyngioma. Reproduced from Cobb *et al.*,[23] with the permission of the *Annals of Internal Medicine*.

tion. Vasopressin tannate is present as a precipitate in oil, so the small particles in the bottom of the vial should be completely dissolved by warming and shaking prior to administration.

1-Deamino-8-D-arginine vasopressin (desmopressin; dDAVP), the recently released vasopressin analogue, has replaced other hormonal preparations in the chronic management of DI (see Section 3.1.2.).[21–24] Administered intranasally through a calibrated plastic catheter (Rhinyle®), it is of limited usefulness in the setting of acute DI following transsphenoidal surgery due to the potential risk of irritating acutely injured nasal mucosa. Very early postoperatively, the nasal passages are occluded with packing, further preventing its effective use. However, following transfrontal craniotomy for hypothalamic or large pituitary tumors with suprasellar extension, dDAVP may be readily administered, even in an unconscious patient[23] (Fig. 1). Compliant patients self-administer dDAVP by gently blowing a measured amount of liquid through the Rhinyle. In the unconscious patient, the calibrated quantity of dDAVP can be safely administered by a nurse or physician after attaching the oral end of the Rhinyle to an air-filled syringe that is gently compressed to expel the liquid high into the nasal passage. We recommend a starting dose of 2.5–5 μg. Repeat doses in the acute setting are determined in much the same way as discussed above for vasopressin tannate in oil. Intravenous dDAVP, available in Europe but not in this country, will most likely render obsolete the use of vasopressin tannate in oil after transsphenoidal surgery. The intravenous dose of dDAVP is approximately one tenth the intranasal dose.

3.1.2. Management of Chronic Diabetes Insipidus

Persistence of DI beyond the immediate postoperative period implies a poor long-term outlook for recovery, particularly after transfrontal surgery. However, an early prognosis regarding long-term disability should be avoided (especially in the setting of transsphenoidal adenomectomy) because many patients have now been observed, after weeks or even years, to recover ADH secretory function. In a few such patients, we have observed the transient reappearance of DI during ethanol ingestion or following an abrupt increase in corticosteroid dosage, implying residual impairment of ADH reserve. (Ethanol, like corticosteroids, effects a central inhibition of release; the mechanism of ethanol's action is unknown.[25])

a. Dehydration Test. Some patients complain of mild polyuria and polydipsia postoperatively, and the question of partial central DI is raised. We use a modification of the dehydration test proposed by Miller *et al.*[26] in 1970 to evaluate such complaints. Patients are deprived of all fluids until the specific gravity of three consecutive hourly urine collections remain constant, usually 6–15 hr after the start of the test in patients with partial DI (in more severe DI, this end point may be attained very quickly; it is important to measure body weight before and during the test—dehydration should be terminated when 3–5% of body weight has been lost). Serum and urine osmolality are measured simultaneously, and dDAVP, 10 μg intranasally, is given. Serum and urine osmolality are measured for an additional 2–4 hr. Patients with central or nephrogenic DI show an abnormally high serum osmolality ($>$ 295 mosmol/kg) and inappropriately low urine osmolality ($<$600 mosmol/kg; often much lower) prior to dDAVP. After dDAVP, a 10% or greater increment in urine osmolality occurs with central but not with nephrogenic DI.

b. Pharmacological Agents Used to Treat Chronic Diabetes Insipidus. 1-Deamino-8-D-argine vasopressin (dDAVP) is the preferred agent for long-term management of central DI.[21–24] Modification of the parent compound, arginine vasopressin, by deamination of position 1 and D-arginine substitution at position 8 has resulted in a compound with high antidiuretic to pressor potency (AD:P = 2000:1) and prolonged duration of action (6–20 hr).[27,28] Control of symptoms by dDAVP is equal to that obtained with chlorpropamide, lysine vasopressin nasal spray, or hydrochlorothiazide. dDAVP is virtually free of side effects, except that headache may occur in some patients, and in the doses usually prescribed does not raise blood pressure and pulse rate or cause abdominal pain. Twice-daily doses of 2.5–20 μg usually result in good control, although once-daily may suffice and occasionally three-times-daily dosage may be needed (Fig. 2). Therapy is best initiated at night. When an evening dose that controls nocturia has been established, a second daily dose, usually in the morning, is added.

The older hormonal preparation, vasopressin tannate in oil, provides good control of DI at a dose of 2.5–5 U (0.5–1.0 ml) every 24–48 hr. Its major disadvantage is the requirement that it be administered intramuscularly. Sterile abscess formation and painful injection sites are common problems, particularly in children. Side effects due to the action of vasopressin on smooth muscle (such as abdominal pain in children or aggravation of coronary artery disease in adults) and allergic reactions due to animal-protein contamination of vasopressin preparations are common problems associated with the chronic use of vasopressin tannate in oil. A short-acting (2–4 hr) nasal spray of synthetic lysine vasopressin (Diapid) (50 U/ml) may be used to treat very mild DI or as an adjunct to vasopressin tannate in oil or nonhormonal preparations (see below). Although the drug is usually well tolerated, local

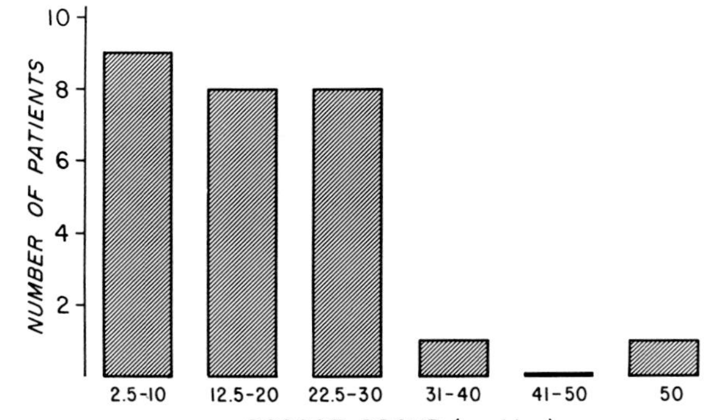

Fig. 2. Frequency distribution of total daily dDAVP dosage in 27 patients with central DI. All except one patient take dDAVP in divided doses 2 or 3 times daily.

and systemic pressor effects may occur, necessitating a change in therapy.[29]

Chlorpropamide, an oral sulfonylurea used to treat DI, clofibrate, an agent used to treat hyperlipidemia, and carbamazepine, an anticonvulsant drug useful in the management of tic douloreux, have been shown to have an antidiuretic effect that is useful in the treatment of patients with chronic DI.[30–33] The mechanism of action of these drugs is complex.[33] Chlorpropamide[34] and clofibrate[30] increase the urinary excretion of ADH, and carbamazepine[35] raises plasma levels of bioassayable ADH, suggesting a direct enhancing effect on ADH secretion. However, newer radioimmunoassays have actually shown no change or a fall in plasma vasopressin level after their use.[36,37] Although these results do not rule out direct stimulation of ADH release, they suggest that all three drugs may act primarily by a different mechanism, perhaps by enhancing ADH action at the renal tubule. The demonstration that chlorpropamide enhances the effect of small amounts of vasopressin on water transport *in vitro* in the toad bladder[38,39] and that clofibrate potentiates the antidiuretic effect of small doses of dDAVP[40] support this concept.

Chlorpropamide (50–500 mg daily) alone is effective in mild degrees of DI, but life-threatening hypoglycemic reactions, particularly in patients with panhypopituitarism, and overhydration resulting in symptomatic hyponatremia, have limited its use.[41] Patients should be forewarned not only of fasting hypoglycemia but also of an "Antabuse-like" reaction that may occur during concurrent ingestion of alcohol. The usual dose of clofibrate is 500 mg 2–4 times daily and of carbamazepine, 400–600 mg daily.

Several reports have suggested that chlorpropamide is of particular value in the syndrome of DI associated with absent or markedly diminished thirst.[42–44] These patients demonstrate hypernatremia with minimal or no fluid deficiency, intact renal tubular response to ADH, and impaired ADH response to osmotic but normal ADH response to volume stimuli.[45] They behave as though osmoreceptor control of thirst and ADH secretion has been "reset" to a higher threshold. Many such patients treated with chlorpropamide have shown a reduction in plasma osmolality and urine volume and a rise in urine osmolality, suggesting that chlorpropamide in this setting may enhance the ability of an osmotic stimulus to activate osmoreceptors in the hypothalamus.

Hydrochlorothiazide (50–100 mg daily) or related thiazide diuretics are effective in nephrogenic as well as in central DI by a mechanism unrelated to ADH action on the kidney. This effect of thiazides is mediated by depletion of total body sodium leading to enhanced proximal tubular reabsorption of salt and water and also by inhibition of free water generation in the diluting segment of the early distal tubule.[46]

3.2. Syndrome of Inappropriate ADH (SIADH)

Preoperative medications (narcotics and barbiturates), anesthetic agents, and surgical stress stimulate ADH secretion and may cause hyponatremia and low urinary volume in the early postoperative period. Untreated hypothyroidism, by a poorly understood defect in urinary dilution,[47,48] coexisting disorders in which there is a reduction in effective circulating plasma volume (such as cirrhosis, nephrotic syndrome, and congestive heart failure) and the perioperative administration of osmotic diuretics such as mannitol may contribute to the development of hyponatremia. In the absence of an identifiable explanation for hyponatremia, inappropriate secretion of ADH resulting from surgical damage to the hypothalamic neurohypophyseal unit must be considered. The diagnosis is supported by the demonstration of low serum osmolality, inappropriately high urine osmolality, and urinary sodium concentration above 20 meq/liter.

SIADH is usually transient, occurs independent of or during the interphase of DI, and may persist for months or years following surgery. Appropriate management requires frequent measurement of body weight, urine and serum osmolality, and serum sodium concentration, and accurate intake and output records in much the same manner as for DI. Fluid intake should be restricted to maintain serum sodium in the normal range (usually 0.5–1.5 liters/day). Severe hyponatremia (115–120 meq/liter or less) or abrupt changes in extracellular sodium concentration may produce central nervous system damage.[49] The degree of CNS disturbance determines the need for more vigorous therapy. The concurrent use of hypertonic saline (3× normal) and furosemide has been proposed as a way to raise serum osmolality without the risk of a large fluid accumulation.[50] Furosemide (Lasix®), because it acts by blocking active sodium transport in the ascending limb of Henle's loop (the concentrating segment) and early distal tubule (diluting segment), results in a urine of high volume with an osmolality that approximates that of plasma. The combined effect of a hypertonic solute load and high volume isosthenuric urine leads to a rapid rise in serum osmolality.

3.2.1. Chronic SIADH

Until recently, fluid restriction was the only effective means for maintaining serum sodium concentration in the normal range. However, the observation that lithium carbonate, used in the treatment of manic–depressive psychosis, and demeclocycline, an antibiotic, could result in nephrogenic DI has prompted their use in SIADH.[51–53] Both drugs act on the renal tubule by a complex mechanism that includes inhibition of adenylate cyclase and a cyclic-AMP-dependent protein kinase.[18] Forrest *et al.*[54] have recently reported that demeclocycline is superior to lithium carbonate in the treatment of SIADH. Of their patients, 30% did not respond to lithium, and of these, two thirds showed potentiation of the CNS effects of hyponatremia. By comparison, serum sodium was restored to normal in all patients receiving demeclocycline. The onset (5–14 days) and cessation (about 5 days) of demeclocycline effect are slow, and the dose must be carefully adjusted because nephrogenic diabetes may occur with excessively high doses.[53] Azotemia has occurred in some patients with coexisting liver or cardiac failure. Photosensitization and opportunistic infection are other potential complications of demeclocycline therapy. The therapeutic dose for demeclocycline is 600–1200 mg daily (in divided doses) and for lithium carbonate 600–900 mg/day. Patients receiving lithium should have frequent determinations of serum levels and the dose adjusted to maintain a therapeutic range.

Miller and Moses[44] have recently shown that the narcotic antagonists oxilorphan and butorphanol are effective in the treatment of neurogenic SIADH, an observation consistent with the known stimulation of ADH release by narcotic agonists. They propose that the osmotic threshold for ADH was raised by these agents. Several patients with the ectopic ADH syndrome did not respond, providing further support for a central mechanism of action.

4. Hypothyroidism

The patient who is euthyroid preoperatively may become deficient in thyroid-stimulating hormone (TSH) or thyrotropin-releasing hormone (TRH) following surgery for a pituitary or hypothalamic tumor, but this is of no consequence in the immediate postoperative period because thyroxine, the thyroidal secretion of which is dependent on TSH stimulation, circulates in plasma with a half-life of 7 days. In contrast, patients with long-standing secondary or tertiary hypothyroidism preoperatively who have received no or inadequate replacement thyroid medication may, on occasion, develop complications in the immediate postoperative period that are due to or aggravated by thyroid deficiency.

Impaired consciousness, ranging from mild lethargy to coma, may occur in the hypothyroid patient following surgery, due to a variety of effects of thyroid deficiency on drug metabolism, respiratory function, fluid and electrolyte balance, and cardiac output. Hypothyroidism may reduce drug metabolism,[55] thus potentiating the effects of sedative, analgesic, and anesthetic medications; reduces the ventilatory drive to a hypoxic and in the severely hypothyroid state, to a hypercapneic stimulus[56]; impairs urinary dilution and sodium excretion, an effect that may result in hyponatremia[47,48]; and causes a reduction in myocardial contractility,[57,58] which may bring about a decrease in cardiac output and cerebral perfusion. Hypothyroidism may also contribute to the development of postoperative ileus and urinary retention. We prefer to treat hypothyroid patients with sodium L-thyroxine for a minimum to 4–8 weeks preoperatively to avoid postoperative complications associated with hypothyroidism. When this is not possible, thyroxine is started in the immediate postoperative period at a dose of 0.025–0.1 mg daily, by mouth. The exact starting dose depends on the age of the patient, duration of hypothyroidism, and whether there is evidence of coexisting coronary artery disease.[59] Intravenous sodium L-thyroxine may be administered when the patient is unable to take medication orally. The dose is one half to three fourths the oral dose based on the demonstration that sodium L-thyroxine tablets are only 60–80% absorbed from the gastrointestinal tract.[60] The best results in the management of myxedema coma have been obtained when up to 0.5 mg of intravenous sodium L-thyroxine has been given to first replete the total body thyroxine pool.[61,62]

4.1. Management of Chronic Central Hypothyroidism

Several groups have now reported that the optimum replacement dose of sodium L-thyroxine is 0.1–0.2 mg daily, the variability being due in part to the dependence of dose on body size.[63,64] We prefer the use of a synthetic thyroxine preparation over crude (desiccated thyroid, thyroglobulin) or synthetic thyroxine–triodothyronine (T_4–T_3) combinations and over synthetic L-triiodothyronine because thyroxine, administered once daily, results in constant levels of T_4 and T_3 in blood.[65] Preparations containing triiodothyronine result in fluctuating serum T_3 levels due to the shorter half-life of T_3 (24 hr) as compared to T_4 and, because these preparations contain lesser amounts of T_4 (none in the case of synthetic L-triiodothyronine), result in low normal or abnormally low serum levels of T_4.[66] Thus, serum levels of T_4 and T_3 obtained with thyroxine can be used, but those obtained with preparations containing triiodothyroine cannot be used, to adequately assess thyroid-hormone dosage.[66] The use of thyroid-hormone levels to properly assess dose is particularly important because serum TSH, a useful measure to follow in primary hypothyroidism, is usually normal or low in central hypothyroidism prior to treatment; the return to normal of an elevated TSH therefore cannot be used to determine the adequacy of thyroid replacement.

5. Hypogonadism

In the management of gonadal insufficiency due to hypothalamic or pituitary tumors, several important points should be kept in mind. Libido in either sex is partly a function of androgen concentration. Patients who are chronically androgen-deficient not only may suffer from a decreased libido (and, in men, signs of hypogonadism), but also often show little interest in beginning treatment to restore sexual feeling. Hypopituitary women usually do not achieve normal libido after estrogen replacement alone because ACTH deficiency results in a loss of adrenal androgens; testosterone [or an equivalent androgen (see below)] at approximately one fourth the dose (or less) of that given to men is usually required to compensate for this loss. It may be necessary to inquire specifically about sex drive because many patients, believing that this is an effect of their illness for which there is no treatment, are reluctant to offer decreased libido as a complaint.

Gonadotropin deficiency does not require treatment in the immediate postoperative period. Chronic gonadal-steroid-replacement therapy in men is carried out with 200–300 mg testosterone enanthate or propionate intramuscularly every 2–4 weeks and in women with ethinyl estradiol 20–50 μg or conjugated estrogens (Premarin®) 0.625–2.5 mg daily. Estrogen treatment is administered to women for 25 days each month; on days 20–25, oral medroxyprogesterone, 5–10 mg daily, is added. This results in the induction of menstrual flow and reverses endometrial hyperplasia, which may occur when estrogens are administered alone. All women require a yearly gynecological examination and Pap smear. Alternative treatments include buccal testosterone propionate (Oreton® propionate), 5–20 mg sublingual daily, in men, or one of the combination oral contraceptives in women.[67] Fluoxymesterone (Halotestin®), 2–10 mg daily by mouth, is a synthetic methyltestosterone derivative that has been used to treat male hypogonadism. It may cause obstructive jaundice in some patients and is therefore less desirable than parenteral or buccal testosterone. Doses of parenteral, buccal, or oral androgens in women are about one fourth the dose given to men. Excessive dosage in women is easily recognized by the appearance of a mild degree of hirsutism.

Successful treatment of infertility using sequential combinations of human menopausal gonadotropin (hMG) and human chorionic gonadotropin (hCG) in patients who have undergone hypophysectomy is now well established,[68,69] so that hypophyseal deficiency need not exclude the possibility of parenthood. Because of its great expense and the occurrence, in some women, of ovarian hyperstimulation, this form of therapy should be administered only by physicians who are familiar with its application.[69] Males may achieve successful impregnation of their spouses after treatment even when sperm concentration does not exceed 10×10^6/ml.[70] Clomiphene citrate, which enhances gonadotropin secretion by blocking estrogen receptors and therefore the negative feedback of estrogen, is of no value in many patients who are infertile after hypophysectomy because gonadotropin reserve is often reduced or absent.

Luteinizing-hormone-releasing hormone (LH-RH) or one of its analogues may prove to be of value in the treatment of infertility due to LH-RH deficiency in the presence of intact pituitary gonadotropins. Mortimer *et al.*[71] reported a rise in plasma androgen levels and improved spermatogenesis in 12 males who were treated with subcutaneous LH-RH for up to 1 year. However, Rabin[72] failed to see an improvement in serum testosterone level in 3 patients with hypogonadotropic hypogonadism treated for 3 months with twice-daily LH-RH even though a plasma LH response occurred with each dose of LH-RH and 1 patient showed a rise in serum testosterone after intramuscular hCG. The potential value of LH-RH and analogues in the treatment of infertility has been further questioned due to the recent demonstration that an LH-RH agonist caused a marked reduction in LH receptors in the testes of male rats and in LH and follicle-stimulating hormone (FSH) receptors in the ovaries of female rats.[73] The decline in receptors was accompanied by a decreased prostatic and testicular weight and serum testosterone concentration in male and by lowered progesterone levels and disrupted corpora lutea in female rats.[73] The status of LH-RH in the treatment of human infertility is currently unresolved.

6. Growth-Hormone Deficiency

Advances in the treatment of GH deficiency have been hampered over the years because of a short supply of human growth hormone (hGH) available only from autopsied human pituitary glands. The yield of GH from a single pituitary gland provides only about 2 weeks of treatment for one child with GH deficiency. Raben,[86] in 1958, was the first to demonstrate the successful treatment of GH-deficient children with extracts of GH from preserved human pituitary glands; numerous clinical trials have since confirmed and extended his initial studies, but until recently, the extraction and preparation of hGH remained essentially unchanged from Raben's initial technique. The preparation currently supplied by the National Pituitary Agency consists of over 95% monomeric GH and is essentially devoid of GH aggregates present in the Raben preparation. The aggregates are themselves biologically inactive and probably contribute in part to the development of GH antibodies in hGH recipients.[74] Moore[74] has recently suggested that the clinical response to monomeric GH may be superior to the older "clinical-grade" GH; in three patients treated with the new preparation, growth velocity was 27% greater in the first year of treatment. Although the use of monomeric GH may prove to be an important advance in the management of GH deficiency, there continues to be a lack of agreement worldwide on the optimal dosage, frequency of administration, and duration of treatment.

In the United States, hGH replacement therapy is offered at many major medical centers under protocols sponsored by the National Pituitary Agency.* To be eligible, patients must generally be less than 60 inches tall and have a growth rate of less than 1.5 inches (4 cm) per year, a bone age of 2 years or more below chronological age, and a diagnosis of GH deficiency confirmed by results of at least two standard tests of GH stimulation. Treatment in most protocols is continued until the child is 5 feet 6 inches (168 cm) tall or until full growth protential has been realized.

A wide range of hGH doses and intervals between injections have been used successfully in the management of GH deficiency. A starting dose of 2–5 IU hGH 3 times weekly is most often used in this country and may be expected to result in a growth increment of 5–15 cm in the first year. The maximum effect is generally seen in the first 3 months, representing a period of so-called "catch-up growth"; growth velocities usually decrease after the first and each subsequent year of treatment. Older children and adolescents, patients with organic disease of the hypothalamus and pituitary, and patients with multiple anterior pituitary hormone deficiencies have been reported to respond less well to hGH treatment. Some reports have emphasized that failure to calculate dosage based on body weight may account for the "blunted" response that occurs in older (and bigger) patients.[75,76] Frasier *et al.*[76] demonstrated that 0.01 IU hGH/kg is not likely to have a beneficial effect and recom-

* For additional information contact: Salvatore Raiti, M.D., Director of the National Pituitary Agency, University of Maryland School of Medicine, 210 W. Fayette St., Baltimore, Maryland 21201; or: Human Growth Foundation, Maryland Academy of Science, 601 Light St., Baltimore, Maryland 21230.

mend that 0.06 IU/kg body weight be used. Higher doses may result in even greater increments in growth velocity; Preece *et al.*[77] have shown that 20 IU per week results in a growth velocity 1.3 times as great as 10 IU weekly without causing a greater advancement in bone age. Although these results indicate that higher-dosage regimens may benefit many patients, the short supply of human pituitaries dictates that consideration be given to the marginal benefit derived from increasing dosage in the patient who is responding well to treatment. Guyda *et al.*[75] have emphasized the importance of improper regulation of other hormone replacement as a possible factor accounting for the poorer responses seen in patients with multiple hormone deficiencies. This is particularly true for corticosteroid replacement; excessive glucocorticoids have been demonstrated to antagonize the action of somatomedin,[78] and Kaplan[79] has even suggested that cortisone replacement be withheld from patients with partial ACTH deficiency while they are undergoing treatment with hGH. Thyroid hormone must be given to achieve the maximum benefit from hGH.[79] It should be recognized that central hypothyroidism has occurred in some patients with idiopathic GH deficiency after beginning hGH treatment[80]; although it is not known whether euthyroid subjects with hypothalamic or pituitary tumors will respond to hGH in a similar manner, the possible development of hypothyroidism in patients who do not require thyroid medication at the outset of treatment should be sought particularly if the growth response during treatment becomes poor.

A highly controversial issue in the treatment of GH deficiency is the concurrent use of gonadal steroids in children beyond the age of puberty who have shown little or no sexual development. Male and female sex steroids, by themselves or in synergism with GH, increase the velocity of linear bone growth, but do so at the expense of a disproportionate increase in bone maturation. The injudicious use of sex steroids could therefore impair the final height achieved. The result from several recent studies indicate that the joint use of GH and sex steroids may benefit certain patients, particularly those at or beyond the age of puberty whose bone maturation assessed by X-ray is far below chronological age.[75,81–85] The reader may wish to refer to the publications cited before initiating such treatment.

References

1. K.D. Post, B.J. Biller, L.S. Adelman, M.E. Molitch, S.M. Wolpert, and S. Reichlin, Results of selective transsphenoidal adenomectomy in women with galactorrhea–amenorrhea, *J. Am. Med. Assoc.* **242:**158, 1979.
2. C.B. Wilson, and L.C. Dempsey, Transsphenoidal removal of 250 pituitary adenomas, *J. Neurosurg.* **48:**13, 1978.
3. T.S. Danowski, J.V. Bonessi, G. Sabeh, R.D. Sutton, M.W. Webster, Jr., and M.E. Sarver, Probabilities of pituitary–adrenal responsiveness after steroid therapy, *Ann. Intern. Med.* **61:**11, 1964.
4. T. Livanou, D. Ferriman, and V.H.Y. James, Recovery of hypothalamo–pituitary–adrenal function after corticosteroid therapy, *Lancet* **2:**856, 1967.
5. J. Lindholm, H. Kehlet, M. Blichert-Toft, B. Dinesen, and J. Riishede, Reliability of the 30 minute ACTH test in assessing hypothalamic–pituitary–adrenal function, *J. Clin. Endocrinol. Metab.* **47:**272, 1978.

6. L. Axelrod, Glucocorticoid therapy, *Medicine* **55:**39, 1976.
7. Oral corticosteroids, *Med. Lett.* **17:**99, 1975.
8. H. Kehlet, C. Binder, and M. Blichert-Toft, Glucocorticoid maintenance therapy following adrenalectomy: Assessment of dosage and preparation, *Clin. Endocrinol.* **5:**37, 1976.
9. C. Fisher, W.R. Ingram, and S.W. Ranson, *Diabetes Insipidus and the Neuro-Hormonal Control of Water Balance: A Contribution to the Structure and Function of the Hypothalamio–hypophysial System*, Edwards Bros., Ann Arbor, Michigan, 1938.
10. E.A. Zimmerman and A.G. Robinson, Hypothalamic neurons secreting vasopressin and neurophysin, *Kidney Int.* **10:**12, 1976.
11. R.V. Randall, E.C. Clark, H.W. Dodge, Jr., and J.G. Love, Polyuria after operation for tumors in the region of the hypophysis and hypothalamus, *J. Clin. Endocrinol.* **120:**1614, 1960.
12. W.A. Shucart and I. Jackson, Management of diabetes insipidus in neurosurgical patients, *J. Neurosurg.* **44:**65, 1976.
13. S. Deutsch, M. Goldberg, and R.D. Dripps, Post-operative hyponatremia with the inappropriate release of antidiuretic hormone, *Anesthesiology* **27:**250, 1966.
14. R.C. DeBods, The antidiuretic action of morphine and its mechanism, *J. Pharmacol. Exp. Ther.* **82:**74, 1944.
15. H. Schneider and E.K. Blackmore, The effect of nalorphine on the antidiuretic action of morphine in rats and man, *Br. J. Pharmacol.* **10:**45, 1955.
16. R.C. DeBoda and K.F. Prescott, The antidiuretic action of barbiturates (phenobarbital, amytal, pentobarbital) and the mechanism involved in this action, *J. Pharmacol. Exp. Ther.* **85:**222, 1945.
17. L. Share, Extracellular fluid volume and vasopressin secretion, in: *Frontiers in Neuroendocrinology* (W.F. Ganong and L. Martini, eds.), pp. 183–210, Oxford University Press, New York, 1969.
18. A.M. Moses, J. Miller, and D.H.P. Streeten, Pathophysiologic and pharmacologic alterations in the release and action of ADH, *Metabolism* **25:**697, 1976.
19. R.H. Aubry, H.R. Nankin, A.M. Moses, and D.H.P. Streeten, Measurement of the osmotic threshold for vasopressin release in human subjects, and its modification by cortisol, *J. Clin. Endocrinol. Metab.* **25:**1481, 1965.
20. D.H.P. Streeten, G.S. Ross, and M. Souma, Osmotic threshold for ADH release: Effects of cortisol introduced into supraoptic nuclei, Presented at the 5th Meeting of the Endocrine Society, Chicago, Illinois, June 20–22, 1973.
21. C.R.W. Edwards, M.J. Kitan, T. Chard, and G.M. Besser, Vasopressin analogue dDAVP in diabetes insipidus: Clinical and laboratory studies, *Br. Med. J.* **3:**375, 1973.
22. A.G. Robinson, dDAVP in the treatment of central diabetes insipidus, *N. Engl. J. Med.* **294:**507, 1976.
23. W.E. Cobb, S. Spare, and S. Reichlin, Neurogenic diabetes insipidus: Management with dDAVP (1-desamino-8-D-arginine vasopressin), *Ann. Intern. Med.* **11:**183, 1978.
24. D.J. Becker and T.P. Foley, 1-Desamino-8-D arginine vasopressin in the treatment of central diabetes insipidus in childhood, *J. Pediatr.* **92:**1011, 1978.
25. J. Wright, Endocrine effects of alcohol, *Clin. Endocrinol. Metab.* **7:**351, 1978.
26. M. Miller, T. Dalakos, A.M. Moses, H. Fellerman, and D.H.P. Streeten, Recognition of partial defects in antidiuretic hormone secretion, *Ann. Intern. Med.* **73:**721, 1970.
27. W.H. Sawyer, M. Acosta, L. Balaspiri, J. Judd, and M. Manning, Structural changes in the arginine vasopressin molecule that enhance antidiuretic activity and specifity, *Endocrinology* **94:**1106, 1974.
28. W.H. Sawyer, M. Acosta, and M. Manning, Structural changes in the arginine vasopressin molecule that prolong its antidiuretic action, *Endocrinology* **95:**140, 1974.
29. J.B. Martin, S. Reichlin, and G.M. Brown, *Clinical Neuroendocrinology*, pp. 83–84, F.A. Davis, Philadelphia, 1977.
30. F. Arduino, F.P.J. Ferray, and J. Rodrigues, Antidiuretic action of chlorpropamide in idiopathic diabetes insipidus, *J. Clin. Endocrinol. Metab.* **26:**1325, 1966.
31. A.E. Meinders, J.L. Touber, and L.A. deUries, Chlorpropamide treatment in diabetes insipidus, *Lancet* **2:**544, 1967.
32. A.M. Moses, J. Howantiz, M. vanGemert, and M. Miller, Clofibrate induced antidiuretics, *J. Clin. Invest.* **52:**535, 1973.
33. M. Miller and A.M. Moses, Drug-induced states of impaired water excretion, *Kidney Int.* **10:**96, 1976.

34. A.M. Moses, P. Numan, and M. Miller, Mechanism of chlorpropamide-induced antidiuresis in man: Evidence for release of ADH and enhancement of peripheral action, *Metabolism* **22:**59, 1973.
35. T. Kimura, K. Matsui, T. Sato, and K. Yoshinaga, Mechanism of carbamazepine (Tegretol)-induced antidiuresis: Evidence for release of antidiuretic hormone and impaired excretion of water load, *J. Clin. Endocrinol. Metab.* **38:**356, 1974.
36. G.L. Robertson and E. Mahr, The mechanism of chlorpropamide antidiuresis in diabetes insipidus: Studies with a new radioimmunoassay for plasma vasopressin, *Endocrinology* **88:**125, 1971.
37. A.E. Meinders, V. Cejka, and G.L. Robertson, The antidiuretic action of carbamazepine in man, *Clin. Soc. Mol. Med.* **47:**289, 1974.
38. S. Mendoze, Effect of chlorpropamide on the permeability of urinary bladder of the toad and the response to vasopressin, adenosine 3′,5′-monophosphate and theophylline, *Endocrinology* **86:**1028, 1970.
39. M. Miller and A.M. Moses, Potentiation of vasopressin action by chlorpropamide *in vivo*, *Endocrinology* **86:**1024, 1970.
40. J.P. Rado and J. Marosi, Prolongation of duration of action of 1-deamino-8-D-arginine vasopressin (dDAVP) by ineffective doses of clofibrate in diabetes insipidus, *Horm. Metab.* **7:**527, 1975.
41. B. Webster and J. Bain, Antidiuretic effect and complications of chlorpropamide therapy in diabetes insipidus, *J. Clin. Endocrinol. Metab.* **30:**215, 1970.
42. J.H. Mahoney and A.D. Goodman, Hypernatremia due to hypodipsia and elevated threshold for vasopressin release: Effects of treatment with hydrochlorothiazide, chlorpropamide and tolbutamide, *N. Engl. J. Med.* **279:**1191, 1968.
43. H.N. Bode, D.M. Harey, and J.D. Crawford, Restoration of normal drinking behavior by chlorpropamide in patients with hypodipsia and diabetes insipidus, *Am. J. Med.* **51:**304, 1971.
44. M. Miller and A.M. Moses, Clinical states due to alteration of ADH release and action, in: *Neurohypophysis: International Conference*, Key Biscayne, Florida, 1976, pp. 153–166, S. Karger, Basel, 1977.
45. F. Plum and R.V. Vitert, Nonendocrine diseases and disorders of the hypothalamus, in: *The Hypothalamus* (S. Reichlin, R.J. Baldessarini, and J.B. Martin, eds.), pp. 415–473, Raven Press, New York, 1978.
46. J.T. Harrington and J.J. Cohen, Clinical disorders of urine concentration and dilution, *Arch. Intern. Med.* **131:**810, 1973.
47. K.M. McDonald, P.D. Miller, R.J. Anderson, R. Berl, and R.W. Schrier, Hormonal control of renal water excretion, *Kidney Int.* **10:**38, 1976.
48. C. Macaron and O. Famuyiwa, Hyponatremia of hypothyroidism: Appropriate suppression of antidiuretic hormone levels, *Arch. Intern. Med.* **138:**820, 1978.
49. A.I. Arieff and R. Guisado, Effects on the central nervous system of hypernatremic and hyponatremic states, *Kidney Int.* **10:**104, 1976.
50. O. Hantman, B. Rossier, R. Zohlman, and R.W. Schrier, Rapid correction of hyponatremia in the syndrome of inappropriate secretion of antidiuretic hormone, *Ann. Intern. Med.* **78:**870, 1973.
51. M.G. White and C.D. Fetner, Treatment of the syndrome of inappropriate secretion of antidiuretic hormone with lithium carbonate, *N. Engl. J. Med.* **292:**390, 1975.
52. A. DeTroyer and J.C. Demanet, Correction of antidiuresis by demeclocycline, *Ann. Intern. Med.* **85:**336, 1975.
53. K. Graze, M. Molitch, and K. Post, Chronic demeclocycline therapy in the syndrome of inappropriate ADH secretion due to brain tumor, *J. Neurosurg.* **47:**933, 1977.
54. J.N. Forrest, M. Cox, C. Hong, G. Morrison, M. Bia, and I. Singer, Superiority of demeclocycline over lithium in the treatment of chronic syndrome of inappropriate secretion of antidiuretic hormone, *N. Engl. J. Med* **298:**173, 1978.
55. M. Eichelbaum, G. Bodem, R. Gugler, C. Schneider-Deters, and H.J. Dengler, Influence of thyroid status on plasma half-life of antipyrine in man, *N. Engl. J. Med.* **290:**1040, 1974.
56. C.W. Zwillich, D.J. Pierson, F.D. Hofeldt, E.G. Lufkin, and J.V. Weil, Ventilatory control in myxedema and hypothyroidism, *N. Engl. J. Med.* **292:**662, 1975
57. W.F. Crowley, Jr., E.C. Ridgway, E.W. Bough, G.S. Francis, G.H. Daniels, I.A. Kourides, G.S. Meyers, and F. Maloof, Noninvasive evaluation of cardiac function in hypothyroidism, *N. Engl. J. Med.* **296:**1, 1977.

58. E.W. Bough, W.F. Crowley, E.C. Ridgway, H. Walker, F. Maloof, G.S. Myers, and G.H. Daniels, Myocardial function in hypothyroidism, *Arch. Intern. Med.* **138:**1476, 1978.
59. W.E. Cobb and I.M.D. Jackson, Management of hypothyroidism, *Am. J. Hosp. Pharm.* **35:**51, 1978.
60. K.W. Wenzel and H.E. Kirschsieper, Aspects of the absorption of oral L-thyroxine in normal man, *Metabolism* **26:**1, 1977.
61. C.E. Menendez and R.S. Rivlin, Thyrotoxic crisis and myxedema coma, *Med. Clin. N. Am.* **57:**1463, 1973.
62. S.C. Werner, Myxedema coma, in: *The Thyroid* (S.C. Werner and S.H. Ingbar, eds.), pp. 971–973, Harper and Row, Hagerstown, Maryland, 1978.
63. D. Evered, E.T. Young, B.J. Ormston, R. Menzies, P.A. Smith, and R. Hall, Treatment of hypothyroidism: A reappraisal of thyroxine therapy, *Br. Med. J.* **3:**131, 1973.
64. J.M. Stock, M.I. Surks, and J.H. Oppenheimer, Replacement dosage of L-thyroxine in hypothyroidism, *N. Engl. J. Med.* **290:**529, 1974.
65. M.I. Surks, A.R. Schadlow, and J.H. Opperheimer, A new radioimmunoassay for plasma L-triiodothyronine: Measurement in thyroid disease and in patients maintained on hormonal replacement, *J. Clin. Invest.* **51:**3104, 1972.
66. I.M.D. Jackson and W.E. Cobb, Why does anyone still use desiccated thyroid USP?, *Am. J. Med.* **64:**284, 1978.
67. J.B. Martin, S. Reichlin, and G.M. Brown, *Clinical Neuroendocrinology*, pp. 370–372, F.A. Davis, Philadelphia, 1977.
68. E. Rosembeg, Medical treatment of male infertility, *Andrologia* **8:**(Suppl. 1):95, 1976.
69. R.H. Glass, Infertility, in: *Reproductive Endocrinology* (S.S.C. Yen and R.B. Jaffe, eds.), pp. 413–417, W.D. Saunders, Philadelphia, 1978.
70. R.J. Sherins, D. Brightwell, and P.M. Sternthal, Longitudinal analysis of semen of fertile and infertile men, in: *New Concepts of the Testis in Normal and Infertile Men: Morphology, Physiology and Pathology* (P. Troen and H.R. Nankin, eds.), pp. 473–488, Raven Press, New York, 1977.
71. C.H. Mortimer, A.S. McNeilly, R.A. Fisher, M.A.F. Murray, and G.M. Besser, Gonadotrophin-releasing hormone therapy in hypogonadal males with hypothalamic or pituitary dysfunction, *Br. Med. J.* **4:**617, 1974.
72. D. Rabin, Diagnosis and preliminary therapeutic use of LH-RH in isolated gonadotropin deficiency, Presented at Workshop on LH-RH Testing, Memphis, Tennessee, December 8–10, 1977.
73. P.A. Kelly, A. deLean, C. Auclair, L. Cusan, G.S. Kledzik, and F. Labrie, Regulation of polypeptide hormone receptors, Presented at Recent Advances in Neuroendocrinology sponsored by the American College of Physicians, Montreal, Quebec, March 6–8, 1978.
74. W.V. Moore, The role of aggravated HGH in the therapy of HGH-deficient children, *J. Clin. Endocrinol. Metab.* **46:**20, 1978.
75. H. Guyda, H. Friesen, J.D. Bailey, G. LeBoeuf, and J.C. Beck, Medical Research Council of Canada therapeutic trial of human growth hormone: First five years of therapy, *Can. Med. Assoc. J.* **112:**1301, 1975.
76. S.D. Frasier, T. Aceto, Jr., A.B. Hayles, and V.C. Mikity, Collaborative study of the effects of human growth hormone in growth hormone deficiency. IV. Treatment with low doses of human growth hormone based on body weight, *J. Clin. Endocrinol. Metab.* **44:**22, 1977.
77. M.A. Preece, J.M. Tanner, R.H. Whitehouse, and N. Cameron, Dose dependence of growth response to human growth hormone in growth hormone deficiency, *J. Clin. Endocrinol. Metab.* **42:**477, 1966.
78. W.H. Daughaday, Hormonal regulation of growth by somatomedin and other tissue growth factors, *Clin. Endocrinol. Metab.* **6:**117, 1977.
79. S.A. Kaplan, Hypopituitarism, in: *Endocrine and Genetic Diseases of Childhood and Adolescence* (L.I. Gardner, ed.), pp. 121–125, W.D. Saunders, Philadelphia, 1975.
80. B.M. Lippe, A.J. VanHerle, S.H. LaFranchi, R.P. Uller, N. Lavin, and S.A. Kaplan, Reversible hypothyroidism in growth hormone–deficient children treated with human growth hormone, *J. Clin. Endocrinol. Metab.* **40:**612, 1975.
81. S. Raiti, E. Trias, L. Levitsky, and M.S. Grossman, Oxandrolone and human growth hormone, *Am. J. Dis. Child.* **126:**597, 1973.
82. M.H. MacGillivray, M. Kolotkin, and R.W. Munschauer, Enhanced linear growth responses in

hypopituitary dwarfs treated with growth hormone plus androgen versus growth hormone alone, *Pediatr. Res.* **8:**103, 1974.

83. A. Aynsley-Green, M. Zachman, and A. Prader, Interrelation of the therapeutic effects of growth hormone and testosterone on growth in hypopituitarism, *J. Pediatr.* **89:**992, 1976.
84. J.M. Tanner, R.H. Whitehouse, P.C.R. Hughes, and B.S. Carter, Relative importance of growth hormone and sex steroids for the growth at puberty of trunk length, limb length, and muscle width in growth hormone deficient children, *J. Pediatr.* **89:**1000, 1976.
85. A. Pertzelan, I. Blum, M. Grunebaum, and A. Laron, The combined effect of growth hormone and methandrostenolone on the linear growth of patients with multiple pituitary hormone deficiencies, *Clin. Endocrinol.* **6:**271, 1977.
86. M.S. Raben, Treatment of pituitary dwarf with human growth hormone, *J. Clin. Endocrinol. Metab.* **18:**901, 1958.

21

Conventional Radiotherapy and Pituitary Tumors

BAHMAN EMAMI

1. Introduction

Most of the tumors that originate in the hypophyseal region are histologically benign, but because of the effects they exert on endocrine function and surrounding structures, they present particular therapeutic challenges. Both surgical and radiotherapeutic approaches date back to the beginning of this century. Schloffer[1] performed the first transsphenoidal procedure in 1906, and in the same year Horsley[2] reported on the intracranial approach to this tumor. Radiotherapy of pituitary tumors was pioneered in 1907 by Gramegna,[3] who treated a 45-year-old acromegalic female, utilizing an intraoral glass applicator and an early Crooks tube with voltage in the range of 80 kV. Temporary improvement of visual fields was achieved with disappearance of headaches. In the same year, Béclère[4] reported the successful radiotherapeutic management of a 16-year-old female with gigantism. He used 100 kV, delivered via a five-treatment-field technique, a technique that is still being used in modified form by many radiotherapists. His patient was alive and well 15 years later.[5] Subsequent reports by Williams,[6] Calamet,[7] Loeb,[8] and others established the role of radiotherapy in the treatment of pituitary tumors. In pioneering studies, Quick[9] and Hirsch[10] implanted radon capsules into the sphenoid via the transnasal route for the treatment of pituitary tumors by brachytherapy (the introduction of radioactive sources directly within and around the tumor).

In the 1930's, considerable controversy existed between neurosurgeons and radiotherapists as to which treatment modality was superior. Cushing[11] believed that radiotherapy would eventually be abandoned in the treatment of pituitary tumors; ironically, the resolution of this issue emerged from sub-

BAHMAN EMAMI • Tufts University School of Medicine; Department of Therapeutic Radiology, Tufts–New England Medical Center Hospital, Boston, Massachusetts 02111.

sequent review of Cushing's own patients.[12] In a follow-up study of Cushing's 338 surgically treated pituitary adenomas, Henderson[12] reported that the 5-year recurrence-free rate of 42% resulting from surgery alone was raised to 74% when postoperative radiotherapy was employed. Although postoperative radiotherapy had been advocated previously,[13] Henderson's study can be considered the basis for combined surgical and radiotherapeutic approach to these tumors.

In the late 1940s, radiotherapy of pituitary tumors consisted of repeated courses of low-dose exposure over a prolonged period of time. Utilization of single intensive courses of irradiation has had its advocates since the report in 1949 of Kerr[14] who demonstrated the superiority of the latter over the prolonged low-dose technique. Ellis[15] subsequently suggested a dose level of at least 4000 rads in 4 weeks, which is currently considered the minimum required dose for many pituitary adenomas.

The utilization of heavy particles in the treatment of these tumors was first proposed by Tobias *et al.*[16] on theoretical grounds. The results of their preliminary studies with rats and mice were included in their first report and in a subsequent communication.[17] Finally, McCombs[18] in 1957 reported the use of this modality in the therapy of pituitary disorders

2. Effects of Irradiation on Normal Hypothalamic–Pituitary Function

The normal adult pituitary has been considered to be relatively radioresistant and hypopituitarism as a result of external radiation to be quite rare. On the one hand, Lawrence *et al.*[19] reported that the pituitaries of young animals are susceptible to irradiation and that hypopituitarism can occur even with modest doses. Large doses of X-ray to the pituitary region have been followed by pituitary insufficiency. Pituitary dwarfism developed in a 12-year-old girl treated for nasopharyngeal carcinoma by a treatment technique that delivered about 9300 rads to the pituitary area,[20] and a 4½-year-old girl with sarcoma of the nasopharynx who received 7500 rads to the pituitary gland showed isolated growth hormone (GH) insufficiency.[21] The cases of three other children with nonpituitary tumors who had pituitary irradiation to doses of 4000–5000 rads and later showed similar suppression of GH were also cited.[21]

Samaan *et al.*[22] studied the function of the hypothalamic–pituitary axis in 15 patients who had radiotherapy for nasopharyngeal cancer. The estimated dose to the pituitary area had been 5000–8305 rads. Of these 15 patients, 14 showed endocrine deficiency (12 hypothalamic dysfunction and 7 pituitary-hormone deficiencies). Functional studies of children with leukemia who have had prophylactic radiotherapy to the brain showed that the suppressive effects on pituitary function could be demonstrated with doses as low as 2400 rads,[23,24] although this effect appeared to be reversible at these low doses.[23] On the other hand, DeSchryver *et al.*[25] performed detailed endocrinological studies in 26 patients with nasopharyngeal carcinoma at least 10 years after irradiation doses of 1700–6800 rads. All patients appeared clinically normal, and only 3 patients had abnormal laboratory findings suggestive of disturbed hypothalamic–pituitary function. Studies by Lederman[26] demonstrated no evidence of hypopituitarism in 241 patients with cancer of the nasopharynx followed for 2–20 years after therapy.

The studies cited above are suggestive of a relative radioresistance of the adult pituitary gland and a greater sensitivity in children. However, this cannot be conclusively stated because the number of patients with long-term endocrinological follow-up examinations is small, and the complete scale of pituitary function tests by current standards has not been performed in any of the reported studies. With recent technical advances in endocrinology, it is possible to detect minor hormonal suppressions in irradiated patients; however, the question of whether these minor changes are of any clinical value remains to be answered.

Susceptibility of neighboring brain tissue to radiation damage precludes delivery of doses in excess of 10,000 rads to the pituitary region by means of external-beam therapy. By utilizing radioactive implants or heavy particles, however, it is possible to deliver higher doses; information about the pituitary-gland tolerance to irradiation is derived from such modalities. McCombs[18] found that with doses under 20,000 rads, there was rarely histological evidence of necrosis, whereas doses above 20,000 rads produced some degree of damage in all patients, and doses above 30,000 rads caused complete necrosis of the gland. Estimated doses to the pituitary by interstitial implant vary between 55,000 and 120,000 rads.[27–29] Because the hypothalamus is relatively radiosensitive,[30] pituitary-function changes after irradiation of the sellar region may be due in part to hypothalamic injury.

3. Pituitary Adenomas

Pituitary adenomas have classically been divided into three types—chromophobe, acidophilic, and basophilic—according to their affinity for specific dyes. Chromophobe adenomas were believed to be nonsecretory; acidophilic and basophilic tumors were responsible for acromegaly and Cushing's disease, respectively. However, recent advances in the fields of radioimmunoassay, immunohistology, and electron microscopy have entirely changed the concepts in regard to these tumors. It is now known that hormone secretion does not necessarily correlate with routine histological characteristics.[31] It is also known that "chromophobe adenomas" may be functional. Indeed, hormone secretion has been demonstrated by many of these tumors.[32–35] Recent classifications such as the one proposed by Kovacs *et al.*[36] have more applicability in differentiating these tumors. These issues, as well as the clinical presentations, morphological and functional characteristics, and diagnostic procedures involved with pituitary tumors, are dealt with in other chapters of this volume; radiotherapeutic approaches to this disease will be reviewed here. It should be emphasized that there is no clear information on differential radiosensitivities of various cell types of pituitary tumors.

3.1. Management of Treatment

As in many areas of cancer therapy, the key to successful management of pituitary tumors is the *multidisciplinary approach*. The essential team of neurosurgeon, radiotherapist, and endocrinologist collaborates with the neuropathologist, neuroradiologist, and neuroophthalmologist for the optimal treatment of these tumors.

3.2. Radiotherapy

After nearly 70 years of experience, there is no longer any doubt that radiotherapy has a major role in the management of pituitary adenomas. Its therapeutic value alone or postoperatively has been well established.[37,38] As mentioned previously, postoperative radiotherapy has improved the recurrence-free rate in one series from 42 to 74%. As part of the multidisciplinary approach, radiotherapy is currently an essential modality in the management of these tumors. This will be discussed with regard to therapeutic doses employed, technique of delivery, and results achieved.

3.2.1. Dose

Recommended doses for treatment of pituitary adenomas were originally based on clinical criteria, i.e., growth of tumor, headache, and visual-field changes. Only recently have new data based on endocrinological responses been integrated into clinical management. The currently recommended conventional dose is between 4000 and 5000 rads administered at the rate of 900–1000 rads/week. Sheline and Wara[39] established a dose response based on clinical grounds with the finding that at 3000 rads, 5 of 9 adenomas recurred; at 3000–4000 rads, 1 of 9; and at 4000 rads, only 5 of 85 showed evidence of recurrence. The data have been confirmed by subsequent published series.[37,40,41]

3.2.2. Technique

Supervoltage equipment is necessary for delivery of the desired dose to the pituitary region with a minimum dose to the normal surrounding tissue. Cobalt-60 teletherapy units, linear accelerators, and betatrons have been used with beam energies ranging from 1.2 to 45 MeV.

Pituitary tumors should be irradiated with the smallest field size that can be obtained with presently available supervoltage therapy units. The central location of pituitary neoplasms within the cranial cavity necessitates careful treatment planning to avoid high doses to the surrounding normal structures and brain.

Various treatment techniques have been utilized for irradiation of these tumors:

1. Parallel opposed-field technique: A pair of temporal fields are treated to a prescribed central axis depth dose at the midline (Fig. 1).
2. Multiple fixed-fields technique: The three-field technique is the most

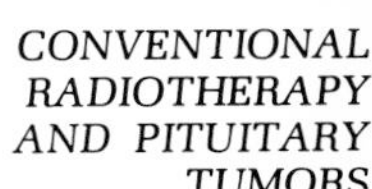

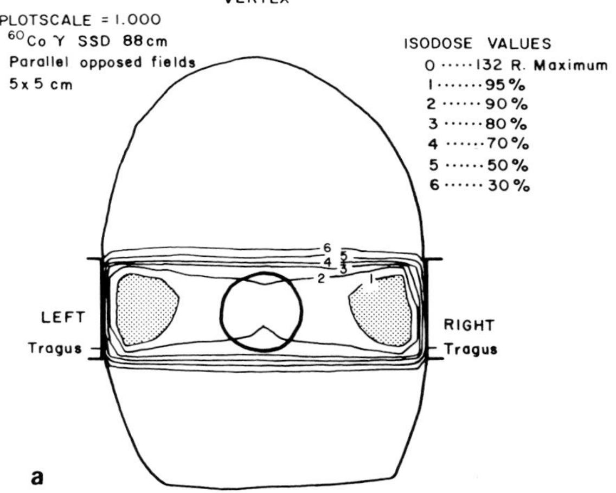

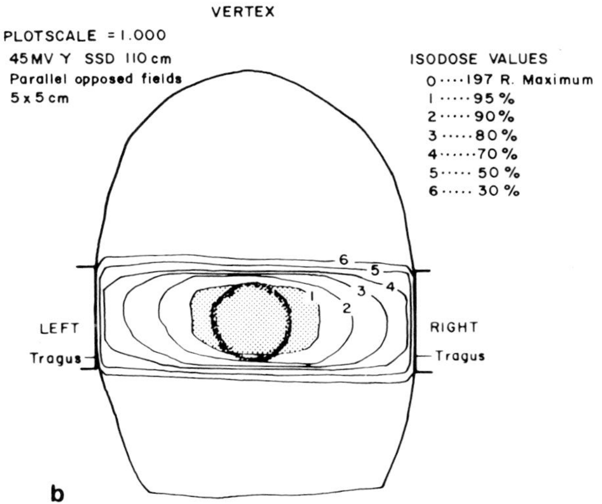

Fig. 1. Dose distribution for parallel opposed-field technique: (A) ^{60}Co; (B) 45 MeV X-rays. The shaded region corresponds to 95–100% of the maximum dose. As seen, for ^{60}Co, the area of maximum dose is outside the tumor volume.

favored of this type, in which a combination of bitemporal fields, which are wedged if low-energy photons are used, and one open vertex field is used (Fig. 2).

3. Rotational techniques:
   a. Coronal arc rotation technique: This is the most frequently utilized form of the rotational techniques, in which arc angles vary from 120° to 180° for the 45 MeV betatron unit and from 80° to 220° for the ^{60}Co units and linear accelerators (Fig. 3).
   b. Wedged double-arc rotation technique: This is for ^{60}Co teletherapy units and is designed along the coronal plane.

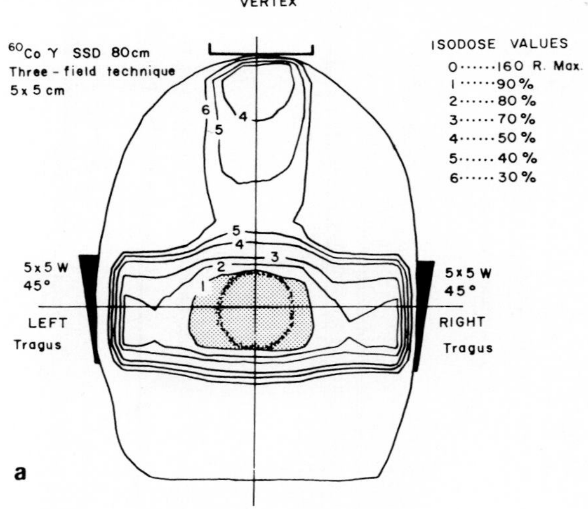

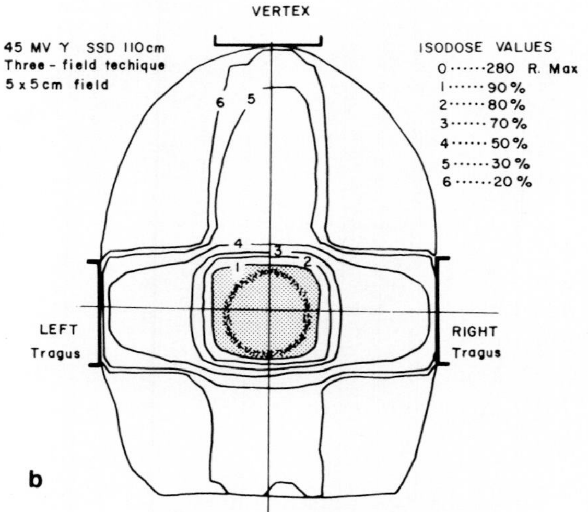

Fig. 2. Dose distribution for three-field technique: (a) ^{60}Co (lateral fields with 45° wedges); (b) 45 MeV X-rays (no wedges for lateral fields). The shaded area corresponds to 95–100% of the maximum dose.

In any technique chosen for treatment, reproducible positioning and immobilization of the patient are of utmost importance.

The selection of a specific technique depends on the availability of equipment and the patient's condition; criteria may thus vary. However, there are a few requirements that are widely recognized:

1. The total target volume should be clearly defined.
2. Dose should be delivered with the highest possible degree of accuracy, and dose distribution throughout the irradiated volume should be known.

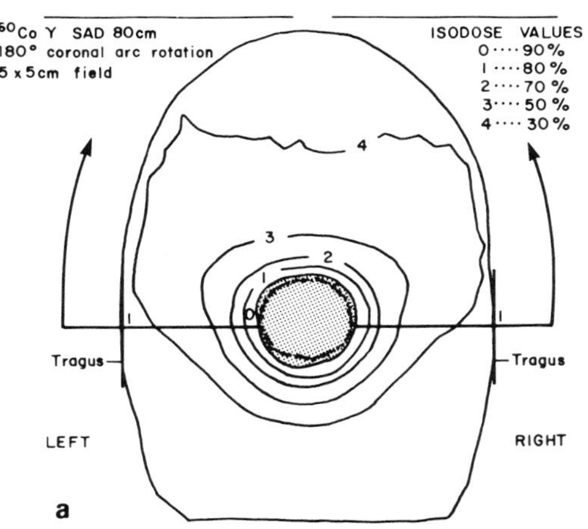

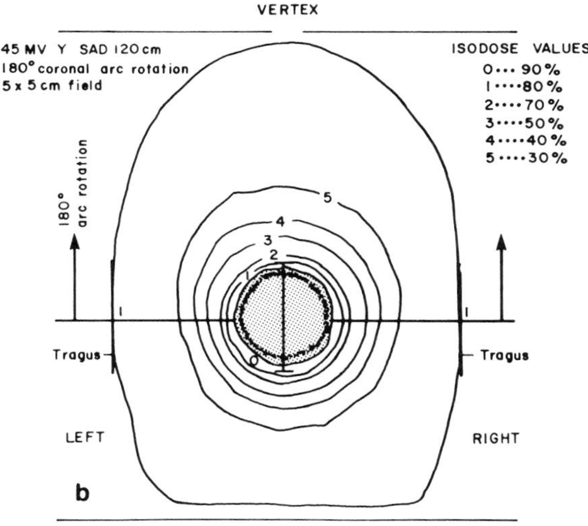

Fig. 3. Dose distribution for 180° coronal arc rotation: (a) ^{60}Co; (b) 45 MeV X-rays. The shaded area corresponds to 95–100% of the maximum dose.

3. Normal tissue within the irradiated volume should receive a minimal dose, with the dose delivered to the target being maximal.
4. The dose delivered to the target volume should be as homogeneous as possible.

Our own group[42] calculated the dose distribution of radiation energies to which the pituitary and surrounding tissue are exposed when a variety of standard radiotherapy techniques are used (Table 1). We concluded that for each treatment plan, 45 MeV X-rays are superior to ^{60}Co. This is manifested by: (1) the maximum dose within the tumor volume; (2) less dose to nonin-

TABLE 1. **Calculated Dose Characteristics for Two Different X-Irradiation Treatment Modalities**[a]

Treatment modality	Maximum dose (rads)	Inhomogeneity (%)
^{60}Cobalt		
Parallel opposed fields	6575[b]	19
Three fields	5555	11
180° Arc	5880	18
90° Wedged arcs	5555	11
45 MeV photons		
Parallel opposed fields	5375	7.5
Three fields	5555	11
180° Arc	5435	8.5

[a] Modified from Ucmakli *et al.*[42]
[b] Not within the tumor volume.

volved regions; (3) less dose inhomogeneity within the tumor volume; and (4) lower integral dose. Parallel opposed ^{60}Co fields are the least desirable plan because of the high dose to noninvolved regions in the temporal lobes. In this calculation, the minimum dose to the tumor volume has been taken as the tumor dose. Thus, the values must be scaled accordingly. The inhomogeneity within the tumor indicates the percentage difference between the maximum tumor dose and the minimum tumor dose. Therefore, an inhomogeneity of 20% indicates that some point within the tumor received a dose 20% higher than the minimum tumor dose.

Another factor that should be considered in selecting a specific plan to fit the therapeutic needs of an individual patient is the position of tumor and its extention. For example, if the tumor has more lateral extension, the three fixed fields of ^{60}Co beams [two wedged lateral and one vertex beam (Fig. 2)] may be more suitable, or if there is extensive extension of tumor toward the frontal lobe, the third field in the three-field fixed technique can be directed through the forehead to ensure adequate coverage of tumor.

3.3. Results of Radiotherapy

The results of radiotherapy of pituitary adenomas have usually been reported separately for the three classically divided subgroups—chromophobe, eosinophilic (acromegaly), and basophilic (Cushing's disease) adenomas—and have generally been analyzed according to (1) tumor control and survival, (2) symptomatic improvement, and (3) improvement in laboratory findings.

3.3.1. Efficacy of Tumor Control

A summary of a review of the literature on the success rate of radiotherapy for so-called "chromophobe adenomas" is presented in Table 2. These results are based primarily on clinical grounds. The table implies that there is no significant difference between the results of radiotherapy alone and those of surgery plus postoperative radiotherapy. However, important points to note are:

1. Because of these patients' longevity, a significant number die of intercurrent disease. Thus, the control rate data in some series are determinate; e.g., in the series of Kramer,[38] absolute and determinate survival rates for radiotherapy (RT) and surgery and radiotherapy (S&RT) were 62 and 82% and 72 and 90%, respectively.
2. Control rates noted for RT alone are for patients in whom radiotherapy has been used as the primary modality. In some series, a subgroup of patients failed initial therapy, and surgery had been utilized for salvage. For example, in the series of Pistenma *et al.*,[40] the recurrence-free rate after initial radiotherapy is 58.6% in 29 patients. Surgery was performed for salvage in 12 patients with additional control in 9, resulting in a final control rate of 89.6%. In the series of Urdaneta *et al.*,[37] of 32 patients primarily treated with radiotherapy, 12 subsequently underwent surgery because of failure to control the disease. The final control figure reported was 86%.
3. In all series cited, both initial radiotherapy and surgery for salvage and surgery plus postoperative radiotherapy demonstrated control rates significantly superior to those for surgery alone.[47,50]

Radiotherapy has also been used in the treatment of recurrent pituitary tumors, which may be the result of surgical or radiotherapy failure. A summary of some reports is presented in Table 3.

TABLE 2. Summary Review of the Literature on Treatment of "Chromophobe Adenomas"

Authors	Year reported	Percentage of control rate[a]			Duration of follow-up (yr)
		RT[b]	S&RT	S	
Horrax *et al.*[43]	1955	88	72	—	1–6
Correa and Lampe[44]	1962	79	76	—	1–5
Emmanuel[45]	1966	75	92	—	4+
Bouchard[46]	1966	71	82	—	5–20
Hayes *et al.*[47]	1971	78	74	45	2–16
Bloom[48]	1973	92.6	91.6	—	5+
Sheline and Wara[39]	1973	93	96	36	5+
Kramer[38]	1973	82	90	—	1–6
Pistenma *et al.*[40]	1975	89.6	84.9	—	5+
Urdaneta *et al.*[37]	1976	86	86	—	5+
Sheline[49]	1978	100	95	43	5+
	MEANS OF TOTALS	85	85	41	

[a] Abbreviations: (RT) radiotherapy alone; (S&RT) surgery and postoperative radiotherapy; (S) surgery alone.
[b] In some series, surgery has been used for salvage of radiotherapy failures and the overall result listed is from combined modalities (see the text).

TABLE 3. Results of Treatment of Recurrences with Radiotherapy

Authors	Year reported	Number of patients: Surgical failure	Radiotherapy failure	Controlled	Follow-up (yr)
Hayes *et al.*[47]	1971	12	—	8	2–16
Kramer[38]	1973		2	1	1–16
		13		6[a]	
Urdaneta *et al.*[37]	1976		5	2	15

[a]Including two patients NED (no evidence of disease) at 5 years, then lost to follow-up. Two patients LFU (lost to follow-up) in less than 1 year counted as failures.

3.3.2. Effect on Visual Symptoms

Improvement of ocular symptoms and the restoration of vision have been judged by many authors to be among the best objective tests of pituitary tumor response to treatment. Initial radiotherapy has been used in treatment of pituitary tumors in the presence of visual symptoms, especially in patients with long-standing visual impairment and in patients who are at high risks for surgery. Because of the various doses and radiotherapeutic techniques used, analysis of the reported literature is complicated. Dyke and Hare[51] classified the response of visual symptoms and signs to radiotherapy into four groups: (1) marked improvement; (2) moderate improvement; (3) condition unchanged; and (4) condition worse. Chang and Pool[52] modified Dyke and Hare's classification and regarded the combination of groups 1 and 2 as being successful response. On the basis of these criteria, they developed a dose–response curve for various radiotherapy treatment programs (Fig. 4). It is generally agreed that with adequate irradiation, satisfactory treatment results

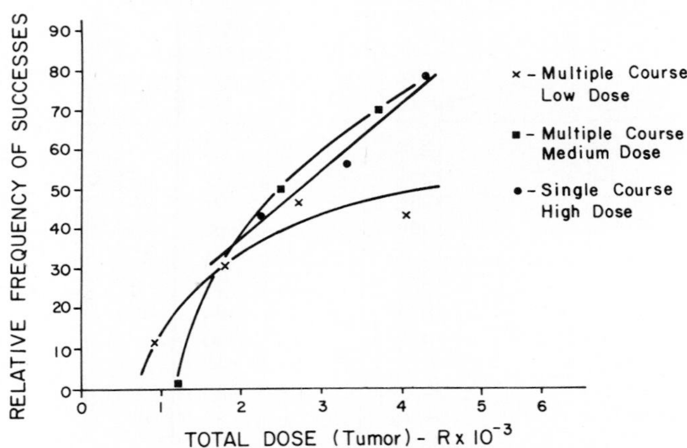

Fig. 4. Effect of different radiation techniques and dosages on successful visual response in patients with pituitary chromophobe adenomas. The curves depict the different responses that are apparently dose-dependent within the dose range used. Reproduced from Chang and Pool [52] with permission from *Radiology*.

(groups 1 and 2 of Dyke and Hare's classification) can be achieved in 70–80% of patients having visual symptoms.[37–40,47]

However, loss of vision during radiation therapy has been reported[41,59] with a relatively high incidence of visual complications (5%) in patients with Cushing's disease.[41] It is unclear whether further visual decline is related to the matured disease, is a direct effect of radiation, or is secondary to tumor swelling induced by the treatment. Because of these complications, at New England Medical Center, if the visual system is comprised, we prefer initial surgical decompression of the tumor followed by radiation therapy.

3.3.3. Effects on Hormonal Hypersecretion

a. Acromegaly. Before the availability of GH assays, the efficacy of treatment for acromegaly was usually judged by clinical evidence. Significant clinical improvement has been reported in 30–80% of patients treated with conventional radiotherapy (supervoltage radiotherapy, total dose of 4000–5000 rads, at a rate of 900–1000 rads/week).[38,44,53,54] Introduction of the GH assay afforded a new means by which the efficacy of therapy could be evaluated. Since then, there has been some criticism of the use of radiotherapy to lower GH levels because of the extended period (6 months to 4 years) after treatment before levels within normal range are attained (Table 4). Considering the long natural history of this disease, there is controversy over whether this delay is a sufficient disadvantage to warrant utilization of more aggressive forms of therapies. A summary of reported series is shown in Table 4.

Most authors agree that when GH levels are lowered to about 10 ng/ml, a satisfactory clinical remission is obtained, but there is serious question of the acceptability of this residual elevation. It is desirable to lower the GH levels to normal range (<5 ng/ml), but this is not reported frequently with radiation therapy alone. In the series reported by Eastman *et al.*,[56] 69% of patients achieved this level at 10 years, and in the series of Lamberg *et al.*,[55] this was achieved in 39% of the patients. It should be noted that in the latter series, fewer than half the patients were adequately treated by current standards and their follow-up was short (1–20 years).

TABLE 4. Response of Elevated Growth Hormone Levels to Conventional Radiotherapy

Authors	Year reported	Patients with GH returned to ≤ 10 ng/ml			
		1 yr	2 yr	5 yr	10 yr
Roth *et al.*[54]	1970	51%[a]	76%[a]	—	—
Lawrence *et al.*[53]	1971	—	77%	—	—
Sheline and Wara[39]	1973	41%	78%	—	—
Kramer[38]	1973	—	75%	—	—
Lamberg *et al.*[55]	1976	53%	—	—	—
Eastman *et al.*[56]	1979	—	—	73%	81%

[a] Mean fall reported in these series.

The level of GH and acromegalic symptomatology are not correlated closely.[40,49,54,56] Nevertheless, the efficacy of radiotherapy has also been analyzed in regard to these symptoms. The results on visual-field abnormalities are similar to what has been indicated before. Regression of soft-tissue abnormalities in 35%[40,53] and improvement of skin thickness in 50% of patients has been achieved.[55]

It is now clear that conventional radiotherapy is an effective modality in reducing GH concentration in acromegalic patients,[38,39,53–55] with few complications.[46,54,56] As shown in Table 4, approximately three fourths of these patients, if appropriately treated, will have GH levels in the normal or near-normal range, the only disadvantage being the slow response. It is an appropriate and effective therapy for acromegaly if the disease is mild and the slow response is not of major clinical concern. It is also the treatment of choice for patients in whom surgery has failed to adequately reduce the GH level.

b. Cushing's Disease. The available data show that approximately 50–60% of patients with Cushing's disease can be treated satisfactorily with pituitary irradiation as the primary modality of therapy.[60, 83–85] In patients treated with adequate doses (4500–5000 rads), control rates of 70% have been achieved.[60] The control rate is greater for children than for adults with Cushing's disease.[86] The average time for clinical and/or biochemical remission is shorter than for acromegaly. Pituitary irradiation has also been used in association with bilateral adrenalectomy in the treatment of Cushing's disease. This is based on the assumption that prior irradiation may prevent Nelson's syndrome. This assumption has not been confirmed, and the development of Nelson's syndrome in adrenalectomized patients has been reported,[85,87] despite pituitary irradiation.

c. Prolactin. Abnormal prolactin secretion by pituitary tumors has been detected more frequently by recently introduced radioimmunoassay techniques,[33–35,71] but reports of X-ray therapy are based on relatively few studies with small numbers of patients. Consequently, the effect of radiotherapy on prolactin secretion is not well known. Malarkey and Johnson[57] had only one patient in their series who was studied both before and after radiotherapy. Comparing this case with a surgically treated patient, they noted a more grad-

TABLE 5. Response of Elevated Prolactin Level to Conventional Radiotherapy[a]

		Posttherapy results	
Treatment[b]	Number of patients	Mean reduction (% of pretherapy value)	Return to normal prolactin level
RT	6	12	0/6[c]
S	16	20	7/16
S&RT	8	15	2/8

[a] From Antunes *et al.*[58] Mean follow-up: 26 months.
[b] Abbreviations: (RT) radiotherapy; (S) surgery; (S&RT) surgery and radiotherapy.
[c] All reduced to near normal.

TABLE 6. Results of Treatment of Prolactin-Secreting Pituitary Tumors

Authors	Therapy[a]		Number of patients responding/treated: Galactorrhea	Amenorrhea	Pregnancy occurred later
Antunes et al.[58]	S		6/13	4/15	2
	RT		4/5	2/5	—
	S&RT		1/3	0/4	—
Gomez et al.[34]	S		6/10	4/8	—
	RT		2/8	4/8	—
	Grade[b]:				
Post (Chapter 18)	S	I	24/27	22/27	5
		II	3/6	3/6	1
		III	5/8	3/8	3
		IV	2/2	0/2	—

[a] Abbreviations: (S) surgery; (RT) radiotherapy; (S&RT) surgery and radiotherapy.
[b] Grade I: the sella turcica is normal in size, with tomography revealing an asymmetry of the floor of the sella; Grade II: the sella turcica is enlarged to various degrees, but the floor is always intact; Grade III: erosion is well localized to one area of the floor of the sella; Grade IV: the entire floor of the sella is diffusely eroded or destroyed.[72]

ual decrease of prolactin level in the patient after treatment with radiotherapy. Antunes *et al.*[58] evaluated the prolactin level pre- and post-therapy in patients with pituitary tumors. Their results are summarized in Table 5.

It is important to note that almost all surgically treated patients had very early disease and almost all patients with very advanced disease were treated with radiotherapy alone or in combination with surgery. The results of surgery for prolactin-secreting microadenomas thus far seem to surpass those of radiation therapy[77] (see also Chapter 18).

The decline in prolactin level was rapid (hours) for surgical cases and more gradual (months) for radiotherapy patients. Gomez *et al.*[34] observed similar results in 19 patients, 8 treated with radiotherapy and 11 with surgery. In the 8 radiotherapy patients, prolactin levels gradually declined to almost normal, with 1 achieving actual normal range. The number of patients studied is small and follow-up is short.

The data in regard to efficacy of radiotherapy on clinical symptoms of prolactin-secreting pituitary adenomas are even more fragmentary. A summary of three recently reported series is presented in Table 6.

3.4. Complications of Radiotherapy

The normal adult pituitary gland appears to be relatively radioresistant. Nevertheless, an incidence of 15–20% hypopituitarism is reported following radiation.[56] Eastman *et al.*[56] have studied 16 patients with acromegaly 10 years after pituitary irradiation and have found the incidence of secondary hypopituitarism to be 19%, of secondary adrenal insufficiency to be 38%, and of secondary gonadal insufficiency to be 58% in men and 50% in women.

The normal tissue effects of areas other than the pituitary are also of major concern. As greater dosages have come into more frequent use, reports of radiation-induced morbidity have appeared in the literature. Brain necrosis, radiation damage to the skin and bone, visual impairment secondary to radiation injury to optic pathways, and hypothalamic dysfunction are among the observed complications.

Two factors appear to have a major influence in these complications: (1) fraction size or the size of daily radiation dose and (2) total dose. The effect of fraction size on the incidence of these complications is shown in Table 7. The total tumor dose is also a contributing factor to the majority of complications that occur following doses in excess of 5000 rads.[61,62] Aristizabal *et al.*[60] reported complications in 1 of 32 cases (3%) with doses below 5000 rads and in 2 of 7 (28%) with doses above. Kramer and Lee[67] reported no major complication in their series of patients with pituitary tumors treated with irradiation. It appears that if daily dose increments are kept to 200 rads or less and the total dose does not exceed the recommended 4400–4600 rads, the complication rate should be minimal. Similarly, it is obvious that if a special condition requires higher doses, as in those being considered for retreatment, higher complication rates should be expected.

Pituitary apoplexy[63] is another complication in which irradiation has been implicated as a contributing factor. Its reported incidence varies from 0%[64] (117 patients) to 4.6%[65] (14/300 patients) and to 7%[66] (155/2205 patients). Although pituitary apoplexy usually occurs spontaneously without any known precipitating factor, it has been reported to occur in association with conditions such as head trauma, estrogen and anticoagulant therapy, and radiotherapy.[63] Because of its infrequent association with irradiation, a direct relationship has not been established. The empty sella syndrome has also been reported after radiotherapy, but many reported cases occur spontaneously. Kramer and Lee[67] have postulated that following irradiation, shrinkage of the adenoma was associated with fibrosis that progressively drew the optic chiasm down into the pituitary fossa and caused symptomatology. Malignant tumors, usually fibrosarcomas, have been reported to occur in the sellar region or other irradiated areas of the brain from 5 to 20 years after treatment

TABLE 7. Effect of Fraction Size on the Incidence of Complications

Authors	Year reported	Fraction size: <200 rads	Fraction size: >200 rads
		Incidence of complications	
Harris and Levene[59]	1975	0/27 (0%)	5/28 (18%)
Aristizabal *et al.*[60]	1977	2/35 (6%)	1/4 (25%)
Aristizabal *et al.*[41]	1977	3/106 (3%)	2/16 (12%)

of pituitary tumors.[68–70] Fortunately, this serious complication is quite rare. Powell *et al.*[68] could find only 15 sarcomas reported in the literature up to 1977, and they added one case of their own. It appears that the risk of malignant transformation is far outweighed by the overall benefit of radiotherapy in the treatment of pituitary tumors.

4. Discussion

It appears that neither surgery nor radiotherapy should be used as the sole therapeutic modality. There was a high recurrence rate after surgery alone, and the addition of postoperative radiotherapy improved the overall results. Conversely, because of a high recurrence rate after initial radiotherapy alone, surgical salvage is necessary in many cases. From the data reviewed above, it is safe to say that a combination of both is the best approach in the treatment of pituitary tumors; however, it is important to note that from reported series it is often difficult to comment on how best to combine the two modalities in any given clinical situation. Recently recognized factors further complicate the issue: (1) The high mortality and morbidity associated with the transfrontal neurosurgical approach has long been a point of contention for radiotherapists. However, recent advances in transsphenoidal microsurgery have enabled neurosurgeons to approach the pituitary with less formidable complications. This approach also has its own limitations, as will be briefly discussed below. (2) In most reports, there is no mention of medical management of these tumors, especially in the early stages of functioning tumors. (3) Only in a few of the recently reported series has the effect of extent of disease on the choice of therapy modality and on the prognosis been thoroughly discussed.

These problems are not easy to solve and have been further complicated by the new functional classifications. Using these functional classifications, it is difficult to decide on the sequence of surgery or radiotherapy, type of surgery, and type and dose of radiotherapy. This disparity in various classifications and their influence on the management decision is not uncommon in oncology. In the majority of neoplastic disorders, such as gynecological oncology, lymphoreticular disorders, and many others, two systems of classification exist: (1) *histopathological and functional classification* and (2) *classification based on anatomical extent of disease or staging.* Although the former are of great help in managing these diseases, the therapeutic decision is generally based on staging. The latter is also of immense prognostic value. To date, there is no formal staging for pituitary tumors that is acceptable to all. With the introduction of new pathological–functional classifications that are gaining more and more acceptance, the need for a formal staging system based on anatomical extent of disease is evident. Herein is proposed a staging system for pituitary tumors based on clinical and radiographic information, *which should be considered as complementary to the functional classification system.* This proposal is based on criteria utilized by Hardy[72] for radiological and by Antunes *et al.*[58] for endocrinological evaluation of these tu-

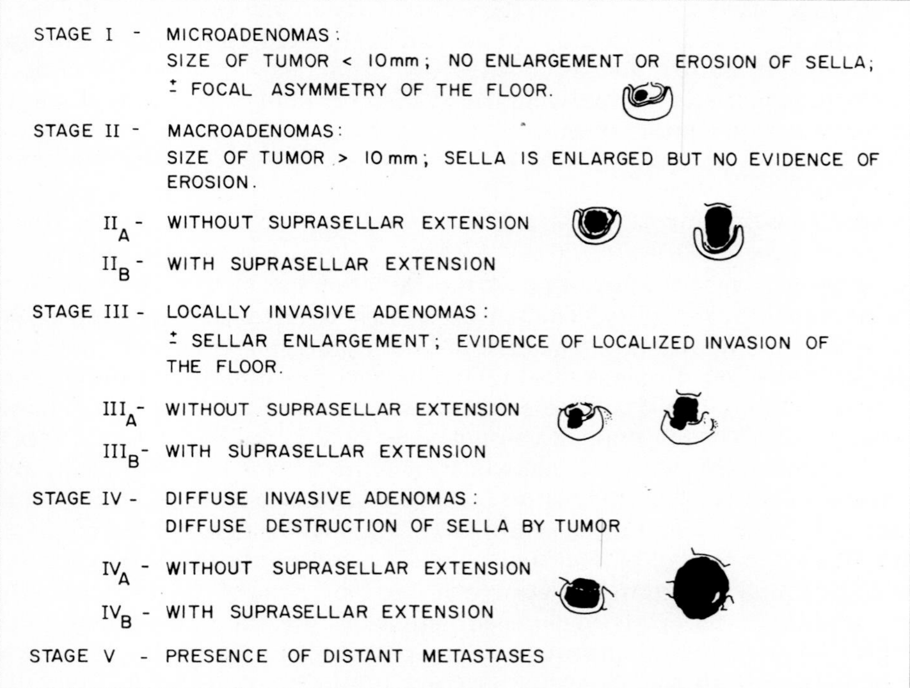

Fig. 5. Proposed staging system.

mors. Hardy's term "grade" is replaced by "stage" because the former term is generally used by oncologists for degree of histological differentiation of tumors, not extent of disease. Using further major modifications, the staging system outlined in Fig. 5 is proposed.

At this point, a few comments are warranted.

1. The clinical presentation of visual symptoms correlates with stage. It is very unlikely to be present in early stages, but more likely to appear in later stages, especially in B categories.

2. There is relatively good correlation between size and extent of tumor and endocrinological activity,[57,58,73–75] although some exceptions can be found.[57]

3. The extent of disease (the basis for the proposed staging) correlates with results.[75,76] For example, suprasellar extension is associated with a lower cure rate than microadenomas.[72,77] Analysis of our own material is indicative of this correlation between tumor extent and results.[77]

4. Pituitary tumors that have previously been reported under the headings "invasive pituitary adenomas,"[75,76,78] "malignant chromophobe adenomas,"[79] and "primary carcinomas of the pituitary"[80,81] can be categorized in an organized and systematic fashion.

5. This system can be useful in evaluating the results of various modes of therapy and follow-ups.[72,82]

4.1. Comments on the Therapeutic Approach Based on the Proposed Staging System.

Within each anatomical stage, functional classification has an important influence on choice of therapy and on the evaluation of clinical response:

In Stage I (microadenomas), if the tumor is nonsecreting, the patient may be totally asymptomatic and usually is not diagnosed unless tomograms are done for other reasons or if headaches are prominent. If such patients have no endocrine abnormalities, as is usually the case, only periodic roentgenographic and endocrinological evaluation is recommended. This is particularly true because of the high prevalence of asymptomatic adenomas and because the natural history of such tumors is not well understood. If the tumor shows signs of growth while under observation, either X-ray therapy or microadenomectomy should be carried out, but there is insufficient data available to make a final judgment as to the relative value of one approach over the other.

If a Stage I patient has significant hypersecretion of ACTH or GH, local therapy is obligatory even though the tumor may be quite small. The proper choice of therapy, i.e., surgery vs. radiotherapy, is reviewed above. The need for treatment of Stage I prolactin-secreting tumors is subject to greater debate, but at New England Medical Center, we favor early treatment.

Stage II tumors, having already revealed their propensity to growth, should have definitive treatment. The relative value of radiotherapy as compared with transsphenoidal adenomectomy for the asymptomatic macroadenoma, assumed to be a chromophobe adenoma, has yet to be determined. It must be emphasized that before initiation of any therapy, examination of the enlarged fossa should include studies to exclude causes of enlarged pituitary fossa including the empty sella syndrome, aneurysms, and craniopharyngiomas.

Stage II nonfunctional tumors are often appreciated as incidental findings on skull X-rays or tomograms taken for other reasons, i.e., head trauma. If there is no compromise of the visual system, then radiation therapy is often the treatment of choice. With significant suprasellar extension, surgical decompression followed by radiation therapy is chosen. Surgery alone may have a significant recurrence rate, since there is no tumor marker to ensure that the tumor has been totally removed surgically. Surgery is more conservative so that the optic nerves and chiasm are not challenged.

Stage II functional tumors are usually treated by transsphenoidal surgery as the first modality at New England Medical Center. If a complete removal is achieved and documented by serial normal hormone levels, then radiation therapy is not offered. However, if the hormone remains abnormally elevated, even minimally so, then postoperative radiation therapy is given immediately in an attempt to completely control the disease.

Patients with tumors of Stage III or IV, regardless of functional state, usually require aggressive combined surgical and irradiation treatment. It is conceivable that the total tumor dose will be slightly higher than what is usually recommended, but no confirming data are available to substantiate this practice. All Stage III and IV nonfunctioning tumors that are treated surgically are also given postoperative irradiation unless they have been previously irradiated. Secreting tumors are treated with postoperative radiation if the elevated hormone is not totally normalized or if there is evidence of recurrence.

ACKNOWLEDGMENTS. The author wishes to express gratitude to Dr. Anthony J. Piro and Dr. Alptekin Ucmakli for their critical and scientific advice and to Ms. Ann Gilboy for her assistance in the preparation and typing of this manuscript.

References

1. J. Schloffer, Zur Frage der Operationen an der Hypophyse, *Beitr. Klin. Chir.* **50**:767, 1906.
2. V. Horsley, Disease of the pituitary gland, *Br. Med. J.* **1**:323, 1906.
3. A. Gramegna, Un cas d'acromegalie traité par la radiothérapie, *Rev. Neurol.* **17**:15, 1909.
4. A. Béclère, The radiotherapeutic treatment of tumors of the hypophysis, gigantism and acromegaly, *Arch. Roentgenol. Rad.* **14**:142, 1909.
5. M.B. Levene, Pituitary radiotherapy, *Radiol. Clin. North Am.* **5**:333, 1967.
6. T.A. Williams, Case of subsidence through radiotherapy of a neoplasm in the region of the hypophysis cerebri, *Wash. Med. Ann.* **15**:103, 1916.
7. C.F. Calamet, Sur un cas d'hemianopsie bitemporale par tumeur de l'hypophyse, *Arch. Ophthalmol.* **35**:103, 1916–1917.
8. C. Loeb, Deep roentgen-ray therapy in the treatment of tumors of the hypophysis, *Trans. Am. Acad. Ophthalmol. Otolaryngol.*, pp. 58–71, 1917–1918.
9. D. Quick, Radium and X-rays in tumors of hypophysis, *Arch. Ophthalmol.* **49**:256, 1920.
10. O. Hirsch, Ueber Radium Behandlung der hypophysen Tumoren, *Arch. Laryngol. Rhinol.* **21**:133, 1921.
11. H. Cushing, *Intracranial Tumors,* Charles C. Thomas, Springfield, Illinois, 1932.
12. W.R. Henderson, Pituitary adenomata: A follow-up study of the surgical results of 338 cases, *Br. J. Surg.* **26**:811, 1939.
13. G.E. Pfahler and E.W. Spachman, Further observations on the roentgen treatment of pituitary tumors, *Am. J. Roentgenol.* **33**:214–226, 1935.
14. H.D. Kerr, Irradiation of pituitary tumors, *Am. J. Roentgenol.* **60**:348, 1949.
15. F. Ellis, Radiotherapy in the treatment of pituitary basophilism and eosinophilism, *Proc. R. Soc. Med.* **42**:853, 1949.
16. C.A. Tobias, H.O. Anger, and J.H. Lawrence, Radiological use of high energy deutrons and alpha particles, *Am. J. Roentgenol.* **67**:1, 1952.
17. C.A. Tobias, D.C. VanDyke, M.E. Simpson, H.O. Anger, R.L. Huff, and A.A. Koneff, Irradiation of the pituitary of the rat with high energy deutrons, *Am. J. Roentgenol.* **72**:1–21, 1954.
18. R.K. McCombs, Proton irradiation of the pituitary and its metabolic effects, *Radiology* **68**:797, 1957.
19. J.H. Lawrence, W.O. Nelson, and H. Wilson, Roentgen irradiation of the hypophysis, *Radiology* **29**:446, 1957.
20. B.C. Tan and N. Kunaratnum, Hypopituitary dwarfism following radiotherapy for nasopharyngeal carcinoma, *Clin. Radiol.* **17**:302, 1966.
21. Z. Fuks, E. Glatstein, G.W. Marsa, M.A. Bagshaw, and H.S. Kaplan, Long term effects of external radiation on the pituitary and thyroid glands, *Cancer* **37**:1152, 1976.
22. N.A. Samaan, M.M. Bakdash, J.B. Caderao, A. Cangir, R.H. Jesse, and A.J. Ballantyne, Hypopituitarism after external irradiation: Evidence for both hypothalamic and pituitary origin, *Ann. Intern. Med.* **83**:771–777, 1975.
23. C. Dacou-Voutetekis, S. Haidas, and L. Zannos-Mariolea, Radiation and pituitary function in children, *Lancet* **2**(7946):1206–1207, 1975.
24. S.M. Shalet, C.G. Beardwell, P.H. Morrisjone, and D. Pearson, Pituitary function after treatment of intracranial tumors in children, *Lancet* **2**(7925):104, 1975.

25. J. DeSchryver, G. Lyunggren, and I. Baryd, Pituitary function in long-term survival after radiation therapy of nasopharyngeal tumors, *Acta Radiol. Ther. Phys. Biol.* **12:**497, 1973.
26. M. Lederman, *Cancer of the Nasopharynx, Its Natural History and Treatment*, Charles C. Thomas, Springfield, Illinois, 1961.
27. S. Young, Pituitary necrosis due to implants of radioactive gold and yttrium, *Lancet* **1:**548, 1957.
28. T. Rasmussen, P.V. Harper, and T. Kennedy, Use of a beta ray point source for destruction of the hypophysis, *Surg. Forum* **4:**681, 1953.
29. G. Notter, A technique for destruction of the hypophysis using Y^{90}-spheres, *Acta Radiol.*, Suppl. 184, 1959.
30. A. Arnold, P. Bailey, and R.A. Harvey, Intolerance of the primate brainstem and hypothalamus to conventional and high energy radiations, *Neurology* **4:**575–585, 1954.
31. R.L. Blaylock and L.G. Kempe, Pituitary adenomas—a re-appraisal of their pathology and treatment, *Neuro-Chir.* **20:**63, 1977.
32. A.M. Landolt, Ultrastructure of human sella tumors: Correlations of clinical findings and morphology, *Acta Neurochir. (Suppl.)* **22:**8, 1975.
33. D.R. Child, S. Nader, K. Mashiter, M. Kigeld, L. Banks, and T.R. Fraser, Prolactin studies in "functionless" pituitary tumors, *Br. Med. J.* **1:**604, 1975.
34. F. Gomez, F.I. Reyes, and C. Faiman, Nonpuerperal galactorrhea and hyperprolactinemia, *Am. J. Med.* **62:**648, 1977.
35. S. Franks, J.D. Nabarro, and H.S. Jacobs, Prevalence and presentation of hyperprolactinemia in patients with "functionless" pituitary tumors, *Lancet* **1:**778, 1977.
36. K. Kovacs, E. Horvath, and C. Ezrin, Pituitary adenomas, *Pathobiol. Annu.* **12:**341, 1977.
37. N. Urdaneta, H. Chessin, and J.J. Fischer, Pituitary adenomas and craniopharyngiomas: Analysis of 99 cases treated with radiation therapy, *Int. J. Radiat. Oncol. Biol. Phys.* **1:**895, 1976.
38. S. Kramer, Treatment of pituitary tumors by radiation therapy, in: *Tumors of the Nervous System* (H.G. Seydel, ed.), p. 91, John Wiley, New York, London, Sydney, and Toronto, Wiley, 1973.
39. G.E. Sheline and W.M. Wara, Radiation therapy of acromegaly and nonsecretory chromophobe adenomas of the pituitary, in: *Tumors of the Nervous System* (H.G. Seydel, ed.), pp. 117–131, John Wiley, New York, London, Sydney, and Toronto, 1975.
40. D. Pistenma, D.R. Goffinet, M.A. Bagshaw, J.W. Hanbery, and J.R. Eltringham, Treatment of chromophobe adenomas with megavoltage irradiation, *Cancer* **35:**1574, 1975.
41. S. Aristizabal, W.L. Caldwell, and J. Avila, The relationship of time–dose fractionation factors to complications in the treatment of pituitary tumors by irradiation, *Int. J. Radiat. Oncol. Biol. Phys.* **2:**667, 1977.
42. A. Ucmakli, H.W. Mower, and B. Emami, Critical analysis of supervoltage photon modalities in the treatment of pituitary neoplasms and craniopharyngiomas, *Int. J. Radiat. Oncol. Biol. Phys.* **2**(Suppl. 2):66–67, 1977.
43. G. Horrax, M.I. Smedal, and J.G. Trump, Present day treatment of pituitary adenomas; Surgery versus X-ray therapy, *N. Engl. J. Med.* **252:**254, 1955.
44. J.N. Correa and I. Lampe, The radiation treatment of pituitary adenomas, *J. Neurosurg.* **19:**626, 1962.
45. I.G. Emmanuel, Symposium on pituitary tumors. Ill. Historical aspects of radiotherapy, present treatment technique and results, *Clin. Radiol.* **17:**154, 1966.
46. J. Bouchard, *Radiation Therapy of Tumors and Diseases of the Nervous System*, p. 181, Lea & Febiger, Philadelphia, 1966.
47. T.P. Hayes, R.A. Davis, and A. Raventos, The treatment of pituitary chromophobe adenomas, *Radiology* **98:**149, 1971.
48. H.J.G. Bloom, Radiotherapy of pituitary tumors, in: *Pituitary Tumors* (J.S. Jenkins, ed.), p. 165, Butterworths, London, 1973.
49. G.E. Sheline, Treatment of chromophobe adenomas of the pituitary gland and acromegaly, in: *Diagnosis and Treatment of Pituitary Tumors* (P.O. Kohler and G.T. Ross, eds.), pp. 201–216, Excerpta Medica, Amsterdam, and American Elsevier, New York, 1978.
50. H.J.G. Bloom, The role of radiotherapy in the management of chiasmal compression, *Proc. R. Soc. Med.* **70:**319, 1977.
51. C.G. Dyke and C.C. Hare, Roentgen therapy of pituitary tumors: A report of 63 cases, *A. Res. Nerv. Ment. Dis. Proc.* **17:**651, 1938.

52. C.H. Chang and J.L. Pool, The radiotherapy of pituitary chromophobe adenomas, *Radiology* **89:**1005–1016, 1967.
53. A.M. Lawrence, S.M. Pinsky, and I.D. Goldfine, Conventional radiation therapy in acromegaly, *Arch. Intern. Med.* **128:**369, 1971.
54. J. Roth, P. Gordon, and K. Brace, Efficacy of conventional pituitary irradiation in acromegaly, *N. Engl. J. Med.* **282:**1385, 1970.
55. B.A. Lamberg, V. Kivikangas, J. Vartianen, C. Raitta, and R. Pelkonen, Conventional pituitary irradiation in acromegaly, *Acta Endocrinol.* **82:**267, 1976.
56. R.C. Eastman and J. Roth, Conventional supervoltage irradiation is an effective treatment for acromegaly, *J. Clin. Endocrinol. Metab.* **48:**931–940, 1979.
57. W.B. Malarkey and C.J. Johnson, Pituitary tumors and hyperprolactinemia, *Arch. Intern. Med.* **136:**40, 1976.
58. J.L. Antunes, E.M. Housepian, A.G. Frantz, D.A. Holub, R.M. Hui, P.W. Carmel, and D.O. Quest, Prolactin-secreting pituitary tumors, *Ann. Neurol.* **2:**148, 1977.
59. J.R. Harris and M.B. Levene, Visual complications following irradiation for pituitary adenomas and craniopharyngiomas, *Radiology* **120:**167, 1976.
60. S. Aristizabal, W.L. Caldwell, J. Avila, and E.G. Mayer, Relationship of time dose factors to tumor control and complications in the treatment of Cushing's disease by irradiation, *Int. J. Radiat. Oncol. Biol. Phys.* **2:**47, 1977.
61. A.N. Martins, J.S. Henry, J.S. Johnson, T.J. Stoffel, and D. Giovanni, Delayed radiation necrosis of the brain, *J. Neurosurg.* **47:**336, 1977.
62. Y. Numaguchi, J.C. Hoffman, Jr., and P.J. Stons, Jr., Basal ganglia calcification as a late radiation effect, *Am. J. Roentgenol.* **123:**27, 1975.
63. J.D. Jacobi, L.M. Fishman, and R.B. Daroff, Pituitary apoplexy in acromegaly followed by partial pituitary insufficiency, *Arch. Intern. Med.* **134:**559, 1974.
64. J.I. Nurnberger and S.R. Korey, *Pituitary Chromophobe Adenomas*, p. 66, Springer, New York, 1953.
65. L.H. Weisberg, Pituitary apoplexy, *Am. J. Med.* **63:**109, 1977.
66. J.A. Lopez, Pituitary apoplexy, *J. Oslo City Hosp.* **20:**17, 1970.
67. S. Kramer and K.F. Lee, Complications of radiation therapy: The central nervous system, *Semin. Roentgenol.* **9:**75, 1974.
68. H.C. Powell, L.F. Marshall, and R.J. Ignelzi, Post-irradiation pituitary sarcoma, *Acta Neuropathol. (Berlin)* **39:**165, 1977.
69. R.L. Sogg, S.S. Donaldson, and C.H. Yorke, Malignant astrocytoma following radiotherapy of a craniopharyngioma, *J. Neurosurg.* **48:**622, 1978.
70. J.C. Gonzalez-Vitale, R.F. Salvin, and J.D. McQueen, Radiation-induced intracranial malignant fibrous histiocytoma, *Cancer* **37:**2960, 1976.
71. S. Nader, K. Mashiter, F. Doyle, and G.F. Joplin, Galactorrhea, hyperprolactinemia and pituitary tumors in the female, *Clin. Endocrinol.* **5:**245, 1976.
72. J. Hardy, Transsphenoidal surgery of hypersecreting pituitary tumors, in: *Diagnosis and Treatment of Pituitary Tumors* (P.O. Kohler and G.T. Ross, eds.), p. 185, Excerpta Medica, Amsterdam, 1973.
73. A.D. Wright, M.S.F. McLachlan, F.H. Doyle, and T.R. Fraser, Serum growth hormone levels and size of pituitary tumor in untreated acromegaly, *Br. Med. J.* **4:**582, 1969.
74. P.H. Sonksen, F.C. Greenwood, J.P. Ellis, C. Lowy, A. Rutherford, and J.D.N. Nabarro, Changes of carbohydrate tolerance in acromegaly with progress of the disease and in response to treatment, *J. Clin. Endocrinol.* **27:**1418, 1967.
75. D. Ludecke, R. Kautsky, W. Saeger, and D. Schrader, Selective removal of hypersecreting pituitary adenomas, *Acta Neurochirurg.* **35:**27, 1976.
76. P.O. Lundberg, B. Drettner, A. Hemmingsson, G. Stenkvist, and L. Wide, The invasive pituitary adenoma, *Arch. Neurol.* **34:**742, 1977.
77. K.D. Post, B.J. Biller, L.S. Adelman, M.E. Molitch, S.M. Wolpert, and S. Reichlin, Results of selective transsphenoidal adenomectomy in women with galactorrhea–amenorrhea, *J. Am. Med. Assoc.* **242**(2):158–162, 1979.
78. A.N. Martins, G.J. Hayes, and L.G. Kempe, Invasive pituitary adenomas, *J. Neurosurg.* **22:**268, 1965.
79. P.W. Rowe and T.K. Jones, Malignant chromophobe adenoma with extensive skull destruction, *Radiology* **86:**532, 1966.

80. E.H. Feiring, L.M. Davidoff, and H.M. Zimmerman, Primary carcinoma of the pituitary, *J. Neuropathol. Exp. Neurol.* **12:**205, 1953.
81. A.S. Fleischer, T. Reagan, and J. Ransohoff, Primary carcinoma of the pituitary with metastasis to the brain stem, *J. Neurosurg.* **36:**781, 1972.
82. I. St. Mileu, Decrease of the sella turcica to normal size, a major sign of the effectiveness of pituitary tumor irradiation, *Strahlentherapie* **152:**410, 1976.
83. S.W.J. Lamberts, F.H. deJong, and J.C. Birkenhager, Evaluation of a therapeutic regimen in Cushing's disease: The predictability of the result of unilateral adrenalectomy followed by external pituitary irradiation, *Acta Endocrinol.* **86:**146–155, 1977.
84. P.R. Hunter, W. Ross, R. Hall, D.B. Cook, D.C. Evered, and J.A. Fleetwood, Treatment of Cushing's disease with adrenal blocking drugs and megavoltage therapy to the pituitary, *Proc. R. Soc. Med.* **67:**35–36, 1974.
85. W. Wild, G.L. Nicolis, and J.L. Galrilone, Appearance of Nelson's syndrome despite pituitary irradiation prior to bilateral adrenalectomy for Cushing's syndrome, *Mt. Sinai J. Med.* **40:**68–71, 1973.
86. A.S. Jennings, G.W. Liddle, and D.N. Orth, Results of treating childhood Cushing's disease with pituitary irradiation, *N. Engl. J. Med.* **297:**957–962, 1977.
87. T.J. Moore, R.G. Dluhy, G.H. Williams, and J.P. Cain, Nelson's syndrome: Frequency, prognosis, and effect of prior pituitary irradiation, *Ann. Intern. Med.* **85:**731–734, 1976.

22

Radiosurgery Therapy for Pituitary Adenoma

RAYMOND N. KJELLBERG and BERNARD KLIMAN

1. Introduction

The dramatic advances of the past two decades afford patients with pituitary adenomas unprecedented prospects of recognition, therapy, and "living happily ever after."

Radioimmunoassay has provided a generation of sophisticated endocrinologists to confirm early pituitary hyperfunction. Neuroradiological computed tomography (CT) scanning and polytomography exquisitely define anatomical disease. Microsurgical excision and particle-beam therapies provide unprecedented safety and effectiveness. Medicinal therapies are showing gratifying promise for some situations.

For our humanitarian and social goals, we can appreciate the value of restoring a relatively youthful and productive population to normal lives and life expectancies. In the framework of "informed consent," we can provide optimistic alternative options to thoughtful, understanding consumer-patients. Short hospitalizations and low complication rates are "cost-effective." We can, nevertheless, amplify our existing capabilities by identifying and solving existing deficiences, as, for example, gaps in our knowledge of epidemiology of pituitary adenomas and long-term, lifetime, follow-up of treated patients.

2. Epidemiology

Available information on the epidemiological factors comes largely from two sources: the analysis by Kurland[1] of the Rochester, Minnesota, region from the 1960s in which the incidence of various cerebral neoplasms was com-

RAYMOND N. KJELLBERG and BERNARD KLIMAN • Harvard Medical School; Massachusetts General Hospital, Boston, Massachusetts 02114.

puted, and Federal government statistics from the U.S. National Center for Health Statistics.[2] Kurland's figures give 1.5 pituitary tumor patients per 100,000 population per year or about 3000 per year in the U.S. Government figures indicate that about 10% of 8000–10,000 brain tumors per year are adenomas, giving perhaps 1000 pituitary tumors per year.

It is not likely that these figures could have anticipated or that they reflect the role that radioimmunoassay has played in the detection of pituitary hyperfunction patients. This advance almost certainly increases the detection rate and does so at an earlier age. Further, it is doubtful that Kurland's or H.E.W. figures include patients with pituitary-dependent Cushing's disease or most of the patients with prolactinomas.

Because many of these patients appear to have the prospect of 25–50 years of productive life, it should be socially "cost-effective" to invest our limited medical resources in such patients.

3. Patients and Indications

Although proton hypophysectomy is usually preferred by the authors, there are specific indications for other methods. These indications can be considered in reference to the total experience of the authors with surgical procedures on the pituitary shown in Table 1. If a patient has suprasellar extension of an adenoma, particularly if visual-field defects exist, open microsurgical transsphenoidal hypophysectomy is normally performed. A patient in whom a full course of prior radiation has been given will usually be treated by transsphenoidal operation. Craniotomy is avoided because of the higher risks associated with this procedure. Transsphenoidal radiofrequency hypophysectomy has not been done by the author (R.N.K.) in recent years.

Two broad indications for therapy of pituitary adenomas exist—hyperfunction and mass. The majority of our adenoma patients have been treated for hyperfunction as follows.

TABLE 1. Surgical Procedures on the Pituitary[a]

Tumor	Open		Stereotactic		Total
	Frontal craniotomy	Transsphenoidal	Transsphenoidal radiofrequency	Bragg peak proton beam	
Functioning					
Acromegaly	3	32	—	431	466
Cushing's disease	3	4	—	113	120
Nelson's syndrome	—	2	—	23	25
Prolactinoma	—	17	—	64	81
Thyrotropinoma	—	1	—	1	2
Nonfunctioning	12	40	1	117	170
TOTALS	18	96	1	749	864

[a] The figures in this table may vary somewhat from those indicated elsewhere in this chapter, depending on the time at which the other figures were prepared.

1. Acromegaly: 466 procedures for patients identified by characteristic clinical findings; nearly always elevated human growth hormone (hGH); hGH always refractive to glucose suppression; and usually, but not always, enlargement of the sella turcica.

2. Cushing's disease: 120 procedures in patients with clinically active Cushing's disease; elevated urinary, or more currently, plasma steroids; and most frequently with a radiographically normal sella.

3. Nelson's syndrome: 25 procedures in totally adrenalectomized Cushing's disease patients; with hyperpigmentation of the skin; elevated plasma ACTH; with or without sellar enlargement.

4. Hyperprolactinemia: 81 procedures in patients with amenorrhea and galactorrhea; elevated prolactin; with or without evidence of enlargement of the sella turcica.

5. Hyperthyrotropinemia: a rare condition. We have treated two such patients, previously thyroidectomized, with elevated TSH and irregular enlargement of the sella turcica.

Patients treated for nonfunctioning pituitary tumors often come to medical attention by virtue of a mass producing visual-field defects. Thus, a relatively large proportion of our procedures in these patients are performed by the open microsurgical transsphenoidal method (40 procedures). Proton hypophysectomy may be performed following open excision hypophysectomy to control proven or suspected recurrence or residual tumor.

Fairly large nonfunctioning pituitary adenomas may be uncovered during the radiographic screening of patients with head injuries, troublesome headache, or for other reasons. Such patients may be followed periodically without therapy and reconsidered if progress of tumor is detected. Others are treated with proton therapy because other involved physicians or the patients themselves are reluctant to allow harboring an untreated proven tumor.

Proton hypophysectomy has been invoked in several instances in patients with proven suprasellar extension, with or without field defects, considering the special circumstances of particular patients. Older, surgically unfit patients may be proton-treated to avoid the risks of general anesthesia and a surgical convalescence. Younger patients, unwilling to risk hypopituitarism, particularly compromise of fertility, may be proton-treated. In any case, the choice of alternative methods of pituitary adenoma patients is guided by consideration of the particular needs of the individual patient. We seek to minimize risk and maximize achievement of therapeutic goals, at minimal cost, and have thus invoked proton hypophysectomy in 117 instances for nonfunctioning adenomas.

4. "Informed Consent"

An important factor influencing a patient's choice of a procedure is the risk, particularly the procedure-related mortality risk. Table 2 illustrates our experience and reported experience of several reputable series. In general, craniotomy is associated with the highest mortality risk and is not commonly employed these days. Transsphenoidal hypophysectomy is quite safe, compa-

TABLE 2. Operative Mortality in Pituitary Tumors

Series	Frontal craniotomy	Transsphenoidal microsurgical	Proton-beam stereotactic	"System"[a]
Author (R.N.K.)	5%	0	0	0.12%
Reported	1–13%[b–e]	1.5–2.5%[f–h]	—	—

[a] Kjellberg's mortality rate for the "system" reflects the fact that we try to elect the lowest-risk procedure consistent with goals of "lifetime-effective" therapy for pituitary adenoma, but that the overall "system" shares the risk of employment of higher-risk procedures when these are indicated as described in the text. The reported operative mortality of the several series cited from past publications probably does not reflect current mortality rates, which are undoubtedly lower.
[b–h] Sources: [b]Ray and Patterson[8]; [c]Mayo Clinic MacCarty *et al.*)[7]; [d]Schwartz (Wirth *et al.*)[9]; [e]Lahey Clinic (Fager *et al.*)[3]; [f]Hirsch[6]; [g]Guiot[4]; [h]Hardy.[5]

rable to appendectomy or cholecystectomy, and experienced operators have mortality rates of 1% or less. Kjellberg's mortality rate for the transsphenoidal procedure is perhaps lucky. Nevertheless, in the process of securing "informed consent," patients are told that the risk is in the range of 0.5–1.0%. Patients given a mortality risk of 1 vs. 0% will often choose 0%, the mortality risk of proton hypophysectomy.

By selecting the lowest mortality-risk alternative appropriate to the needs of the particular patients, our total experience reflects a "system" mortality risk of 0.12% (Table 2). This mortality is that of a single death, 16 years ago, in a craniotomy patient, due to pulmonary embolus.

The other prominent feature of "informed consent" provided to adenoma patients is the prospect of recurrence. Interestingly, it is also important in "cost-effective" considerations. To appreciate an overview of recurrence rates, several series of treated patients were examined. Those shown in Table 3 were

TABLE 3. Pituitary Adenoma: Recurrence Rates[a]

Treatment[b]	Ref. No.	Annual rate (%)	Cumulative (%) 25-Year	Cumulative (%) 50-Year
Craniotomy	10	7.5	100.0	100.0
	7	1.0	25.0	50.0
Craniotomy and Fractionated X-ray therapy	10	1.2	30.0	60.0
	7	2.0	50.0	100.0
Hirsch (TR-SP and radiation)		0.6	15.0	30.0
Transsphenoidal		1.5	38.0	75.0
Proton beam		0.15	3.8	7.5

[a] The craniotomy alone and craniotomy plus fractionated X-ray therapy are present because they provided examples of series with sufficiently long intervals of follow-up (20 years) to justify the computations of annual recurrence rates and to justify the assumption that annual recurrence rates are relatively stable over such long intervals of time. Although Hirsch's interval of follow-up is the longest of any (37 years), it is uncertain as to the extent to which his transsphenoidal operation plus serial radium applications can be applied to contemporary surgical or radiation techniques. The transsphenoidal and proton-beam recurrence rates are the authors' (see the text).

selected because the data allowed computation of annual recurrence rates, and thus the variation in interval of follow-up did not seriously compromise comparison.[3–9]

In fact, several problems compromise the possibility of critical comparisons. To secure 25- or 50-year follow-up, one must deal with procedures performed 25–50 years ago. Only one series, that of Hirsch,[6] falls in this range, a 37-year follow-up with an annual recurrence rate of 0.6%. Hirsch's method is not currently used. Beginning in 1910, he combined transsphenoidal evacuation of tumor with serial applications of a radium pallet. Nevertheless, the length of this follow-up and the low annual rate of recurrence of adenoma have almost not been equaled to this day.

Open excision by craniotomy (FC) with a 20-year follow-up is reported in two series of patients treated by cranitomy.[7,10] These report 7.5% per year and 1% per year recurrence, respectively.

The supplementation of surgical excision by craniotomy with fractionated X-ray therapy (FC+FXR) improved the long-term prospects in one group[10] and impaired the long-term prospects in the other.[7] It is likely that selection of patients in both these groups influenced the outcome.

It has been difficult to secure recurrence rates for microsurgical transsphenoidal hypophysectomy. Kjellberg reviewed his own cases of transsphenoidal hypophysectomized patients, admittedly a selected, nonrandom population. We defined recurrence as indicated in Table 4. Recurrence occurs when symptoms or abnormal laboratory values become abnormal following a remission. It differs from failure, an instance in which remission did not occur. The recurrence rate was 1.5–2% per year, depending on which of certain assumptions are made. The 2% rate, extrapolated to the 50-year interval, leads to recurrence in 100% of patients.

TABLE 4. Pituitary Adenoma Therapy: Proposed Terms and Definitions[a]

Term	Definition
Procedure mortality	Dead due to procedure
Failure	No better or worse
Effective	1. Cured or remission
	2. Improved
	3. Without symptoms
Ineffective	1. Procedure mortality
	2. Failure
Recurrence	1. Endocrine remission followed by hyperfunction
	2. Stable fields or findings followed by worsening, due to solid mass

[a]The definitions are proposed to attempt to construct categories for comparison of results, especially when the indications vary (e.g., hyperfunction, mass, prevent recurrence). The "effective" category includes cases not in "remission" but improved to the extent that no further therapy is immediately contemplated, especially when the prospect exists that "remission" may be forthcoming. We regard the concept and definition of recurrence to be of major importance in assessing "lifetime effectiveness" (see the text).

TABLE 5. Recurrent Pituitary Adenomas[a]

Tumors	Open excision			Proton		
	Number of patients	Recurrences		Number of patients	Recurrences	
		Number	%		Number	%
All adenomas	99	7	7	678	5	0.7
Nonfunctional	45	5	11	114	1	0.9
Acromegaly	33	0	0	396	4	1.0
Cushing's disease	8	0	0	124	0	0
Prolactinoma	13	2	15	44	0	0

[a]The recurrence rates shown are those of R.N.K. It should be appreciated that selection into categories exists by intended and sometimes unintended methods.

In our proton-treated patients, recurrence occurred infrequently. Table 5 shows that one nonfunctioning adenoma recurred, but this patient was inadequately treated by a proton dose excessively low by our present standards. No patients with Cushing's disease or prolactinoma have had recurrence. Of four patients with recurrent acromegaly, three were operated on by R.N.K., and all three showed tissue culture features characteristic of "malignancy" (see below). Thus, we are led to the impression that recurrence is very infrequent in proton-treated patients with typical benign adenomas.

This observation, if confirmed by longer detailed follow-up, is of paramount importance. Figure 1 shows the published and extrapolated cumulative recurrence prospects of therapy by various therapeutic alternatives. It

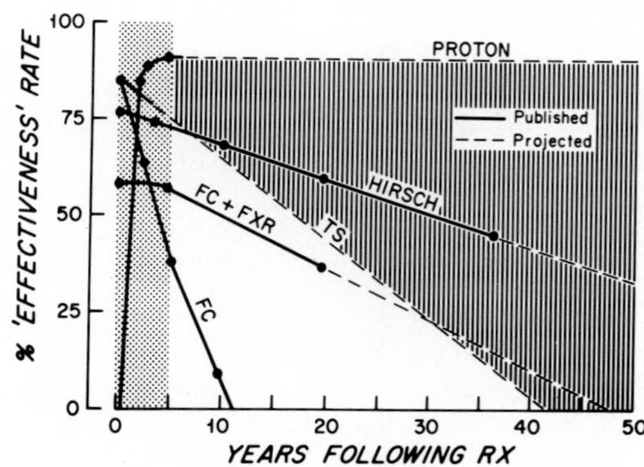

Fig. 1. Lifetime "effectiveness" of therapy for pituitary adenoma. (TS) Transsphenoidal (RNK); (FC) frontal craniotomy; (FXR) fractionated X-ray. The figure is intended to illustrate the importance of considering recurrence rates in judging the effectiveness of various forms of therapy when extrapolated to the anticipated lifetime of patients up to 50 years from the time of therapy. The vertical coordinate represents the percentage of patients "effectively" (remission and improved) treated at the time of hospitalization. The solid line for proton-treated cases is taken from Fig. 5. The vertical stippled area on the left encompasses the first 5 years following therapy, during which the comparative effectiveness of various methods is rapidly changing. It is in the period beyond 5 years that the proton method appears to be increasingly effective, but long-term follow-up is required to document this anticipation more fully.

becomes apparent that recurrence rates become of overriding importance in assessing the prospects for lifetime cure or remission of the threats of pituitary adenomas. Recurrence rates of 2% per year following excision alone guarantee that a patient surviving 50 years will require further therapy. If the recurrence rate is reduced to 1% per year, a reasonable expectation from conventional excision plus conventional X-ray, only half the proportion of pituitary adenoma patients are required to undergo further therapy at some time in their lives.

If, however, "informed consent" leads a patient to choose the lowest procedure-related mortality rate and the greatest prospect of not requiring further therapy for pituitary adenoma, it appears that Bragg-peak proton-beam hypophysectomy best fulfills these prospects.

Additionally, "informed consent," we think, includes some other considerations added in the list in Table 6. Our list begins with the necessity of the procedure. We avoid "unnecessary" procedures. The necessity of therapy varies depending on the diagnosis and other factors.

For acromegalic patients, there is the prospect of dying prematurely; 90% of acromegalic patients are dead by age 60.[11] Before they die, they become afflicted with hypertension, cardiomyopathy, diabetes mellitus, strokes, chronic pulmonary disease, carpal-tunnel syndrome, and a broad spectrum of bone and joint complaints. The disfigurement of the disease is never lethal and rarely disabling. Premature death and disability define the degree of "necessity" for therapy.

Untreated Cushing's disease is considered to lead to 50% mortality in 5 years. Hypertension, diabetes mellitus, osteoporosis, myopathy, obesity, and psychiatric disturbance contribute to disability, but disease-related mortality is often attributable to poor resistance to infection. This "necessity" for treatment is amply supported. However, alternative therapy exists, principally adrenalectomy. The risk of hypophysectomy seems to be less than that of adrenalectomy, and postoperative replacement therapy is often not necessary. The development of Nelson's syndrome is avoided. The alternative of medical therapy is being evaluated.

Hyperprolactinemia due to prolactinoma stands in some contrast to acromegaly and Cushing's disease. Hyperprolactinemia *per se* is not understood to have lethal risks. Further, the principal disability, infertility, is eagerly sought after by a significant fraction of women of childbearing age. Hyperprolactinemia alone does not dictate "necessity" of therapy. The associated tumor may become threatening by virtue of growth. However, it is not entirely

TABLE 6. Elements of "Informed Consent"

"Necessity" of therapy
Mortality risk
Disabling complications risk
Nondisabling complications risk
Alternative therapies
Late complications
Recurrence → Further treatment

clear that all these tumors grow. In the original description of the galactorrhea–amenorrhea syndrome by Forbes *et al.*,[12] 7 of their 15 patients had normal sellas up to 20 years following onset of symptoms.

Nonfunctioning adenomas develop "necessity" for therapy, usually by virtue of their mass. Mass effects are particularly threatening when the mass extends upward to affect the visual apparatus and the base of the brain. It is "necessary" to promptly decompress these important neural structures, and we normally favor and employ the open transsphenoidal method.

Nonfunctioning adenomas without suprasellar extension frequently are not productive of any disability. In the records of the Armed Forces Institute of Pathology,[13] there are 1000 pituitary adenomas, of which 51% were undetected prior to autopsy. We advise patients with asymptomatic nonfunctioning adenomas that they may be followed with annual radiographic, endocrine, and visual testing, and that if the lesion shows evidence of progress, therapy will be recommended. In some instances, other involved physicians or patients themselves prefer that therapy be provided, and this is done.

5. "Cost-Effectiveness"

Several elements contribute to "cost-effectiveness." The emphasis may vary when different persons judge the elements. We have listed in Table 7 several elements that came to mind.

Hospital costs of proton-beam therapy are about half those of our transsphenoidal cases. This cost reduction is in large measure due to the short hospital stay, usually 6 or 7 days. The patients leave the hospital the day following the procedure.

Further, proton-treated patients need not convalesce following the procedure, but are free to resume work or activities immediately.

Complications increase the cost of therapy by lengthening hospitalization and restricting a patient's life and work for short or long intervals.

The prospect of recurrence also influences "cost-effectiveness." The inherent prospect that further therapy will be required assures that the hospital costs and complication costs will be repeated.

In general, proton treatment of adenomas is "cost-effective" on all these counts.

TABLE 7. Costs of Therapy for Pituitary Adenoma

Hospitalization
Not working during hospitalization
Not working during convalescence
Transient complications
Permanent complications
Late complications
Recurrent activity of disease

6. Method

The stereotactic radiosurgical method employed has been described previously.[14–16] In summary, patients are hospitalized 7 days or less for clinical evaluation, radiography, and therapy. General medical and particular endocrine evaluation is done. Radiographic evaluation always includes pneumoencephalography for assessment of suprasellar extension and the course of the optic nerves, cavernous sinography to determine the width of the pituitary, and calibrated "marker films." From these films, the proton-beam diameter and configuration are selected; heterodensity measurements to control the disposition of the Bragg peak of the proton beam are done. We have always used the Bragg peak rather than intersecting portions of the plateau of the beam. There is no exit dose of beam passing beyond the sella. Second, the amount of radiation at the peak is 2–3 times greater than the amount along the entering plateau of the beam. Figure 2 illustrates that the pituitary target dose may be 20–25 times greater than the beam-path dose. The dose required to induce an appropriate degree of radionecrosis is determined.

The dose required varies according to the beam diameter being used and the therapeutic objective of the particular diagnostic category. Figure 3 illustrates our present schedule. Small beams (e.g., 7 mm) require much larger doses than large-diameter beams. The highest dose range is used for patients with acromegaly and Cushing's disease. Lower doses, still within the necrotizing range, are invoked for hyperprolactinemia, Nelson's syndrome, and

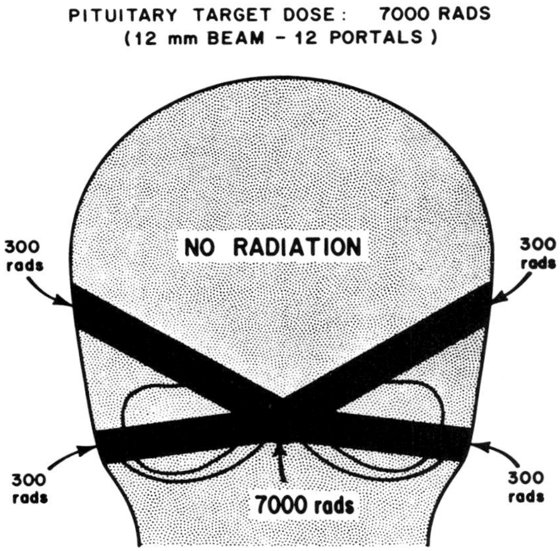

PITUITARY TARGET DOSE: 7000 RADS
(12 mm BEAM - 12 PORTALS)

NO RADIATION
300 rads
300 rads
300 rads
300 rads
7000 rads

Fig. 2. Example of proton radiation dose and distribution in the coronal plane. The diagram illustrates that by the use of multiple portals of beam entry that converge on the pituitary, the entrance dose and path dose through the brain can be kept to low levels while the pituitary target gets a high dose. Four paths are shown in the plane of the diagram; other paths (totaling 12) are in front of or behind the plane. The pituitary target dose is 23 times greater than the dose passing through skin and brain.

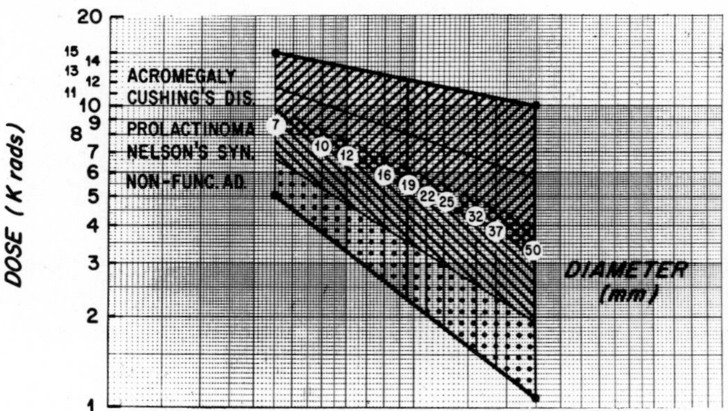

Fig. 3. Determination of radiation dose for pituitary adenomas. The diagram shows the range of doses employed for various types of pituitary adenomas. It illustrates that different dose ranges are used for different beam diameters, with smaller beams requiring larger doses.

hyperthyrotropinemia. Subnecrotizing doses are sufficient for nonfunctioning adenomas where arrest of growth of the adenoma is the therapeutic objective. Higher doses are unnecessary, and the complication rates are higher.

7. Procedures

7.1. Radiosurgical

The therapeutic radiosurgical procedure is performed at the 160 MeV Harvard cyclotron. Figure 4 shows a patient in the stereotactic instrument. Local anesthesia is provided in the ear canals for stabilization of the stereotactic instrument. Local anesthesia is applied to the malar eminences and the nuchal line region where drill rods secure skeletal fixation of the instrument. Radiographs are performed to secure precise alignment of the Bragg peak of the proton beam with the pituitary tumor. Twelve portals (six to each side) are normally used for higher doses; six portals may be used for lower doses, but the skin dose is kept below 500 rads. Depilation has rarely occurred.

In 1.5–2 hr, the patient walks away from the procedure and returns to the hospital, normally in good humor. Following overnight observation, the patient is discharged, fit for normal activities.

7.2. Microsurgical

Our microsurgical procedure is similar to that used by others. A few technical details can be mentioned.

We use a double binocular microscope, with which the assistant has access to the wound equally as facile as does the operator. The patient is positioned supine, with head extended. The viewing axis through the microscope

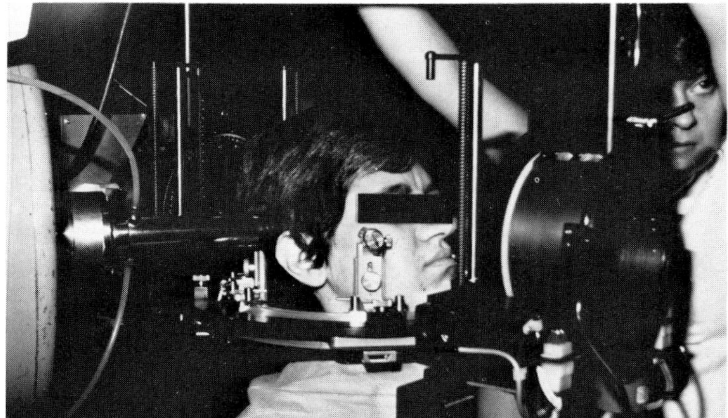

Fig. 4. An acromegalic patient in the stereotactic instrument undergoing proton radiosurgery.

is straight down. Since the head is then about 10 cm below the spinal canal, the intracranial pressure is thought to be about 300 mm of water. This helps express suprasellar tumor into the sella when the sellar contents have been removed. Normally, the diaphragmatic dome of the tumor has reversed its curvature and balloons into the sella at the end of the procedure when the tumor has been evacuated.

Our method of closure differs slightly from that usually employed. The fascia lata is dried under an infrared lamp to a parchmentlike appearance and consistency. The fascia is much easier to handle when it is stiff. A single piece is used and folded like two pages of a book. One leaf is applied to the diaphragmatic surface and the other against the anterior wall of the sella. We do not use muscle, but rather use fat in the sellar cavity to back up the fascia. The low metabolism of fat permits it to survive as fat and not shrivel down as scar. In the past, we frequently used folded gold foil to line the walls of the sellar cavity as a marker to permit early detection of recurrence by means of X-rays. This practice is less frequently employed now, since radioimmunoassy of hormones functions as a marker of pituitary function and CT scanning provides a basis of definition of mass.

8. Results

8.1. Acromegaly

Most patients begin to exhibit reversal of clinical features of acromegaly and reduction of GH 3–6 months following therapy, and clinical change and GH fall are progressive thereafter. Figure 5 shows the course of objective improvement and hormone fall indicating about 90% of patients "improved" 24 months following treatment. At this interval, 60% of patients are in remission (GH $\leq$10 ng/ml); at the 4-year interval, the remission category has risen to

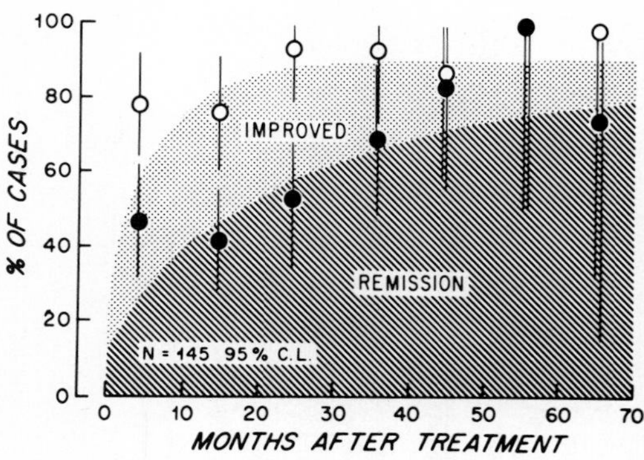

Fig. 5. Proton-beam treatment of acromegaly. The diagram shows the time course following proton treatment of acromegaly that patients enter into the categories of remission (hGH ≤10 ng/ml) or improved (objective clinical change and hGH ≤50% of preoperative). (●) Remission; (○) remission plus improved.

80%. About 10% of patients are failures, most of which receive further therapy, usually open transsphenoidal hypophysectomy.

We have not documented serious disabling complications in acromegalic patients. No patient has died as the result of therapy and no patient is known to have been blinded, although a question has been raised in two instances. Field defects have occurred, but these were largely in our early experience. Temporary or transient extraocular movement disturbance has been reduced but not really eliminated. Symptoms of diplopia or visual blurring continue to be reported in a few percent of treated patients, but are frequently not confirmed on ophthalmologic testing. About 10% of patients develop hypopituitarism and require replacement thyroid or steroid medication or both.

8.2. Cushing's Disease

In general, patients with Cushing's disease respond similarly to patients with acromegaly. Occasionally, abrupt remission is seen within weeks of treatment. Figure 6 shows pretreatment and posttreatment values in a group

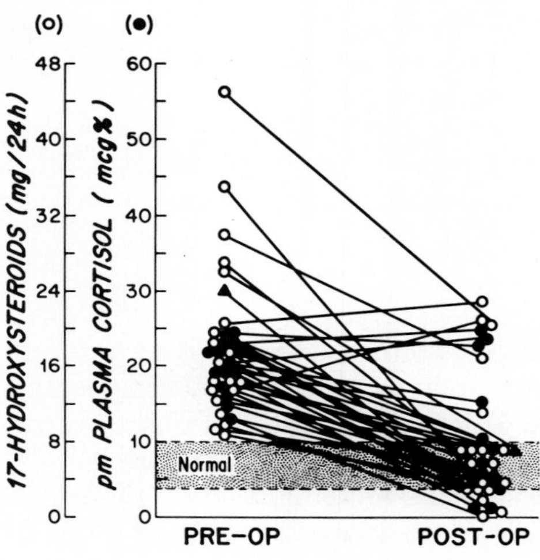

Fig. 6. Pretreatment and posttreatment corticosteroid values in patients with Cushing's disease. ▲, Values converted to 17-OH scale: urinary 17 KGS (÷2), urinary cortisol (×100).

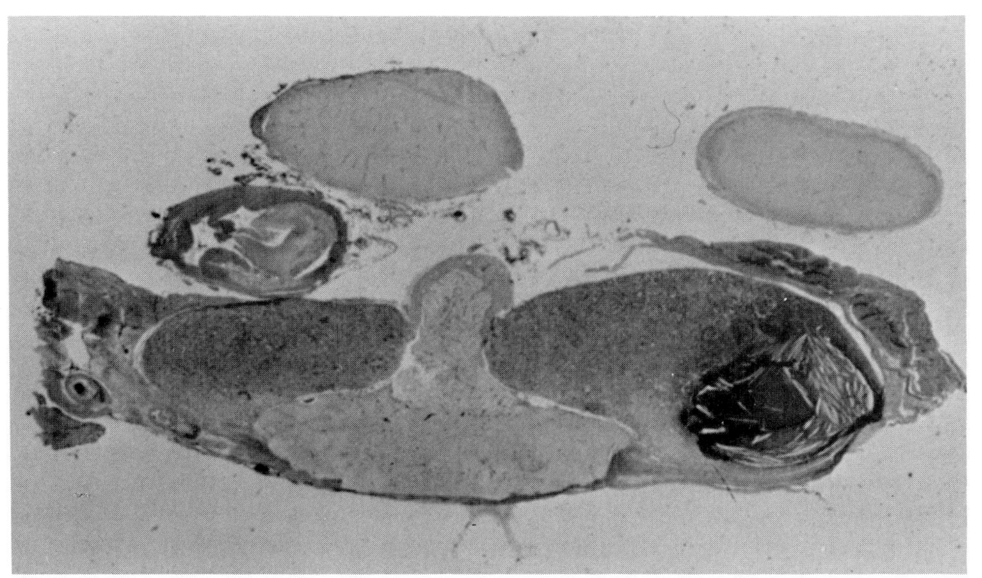

Fig. 7. Histological specimen of the pituitary from a patient who died of a heart attack 9 months following proton therapy.

of patients. About 65% of treated patients undergo complete remission with restoration of normal clinical and laboratory findings. Another 20% are improved to the extent that no further therapy is considered desirable. Of the 10–15% failures, several were operated on by adrenalectomy or open excisional hypophysectomy prior to the 24-month interval we usually consider necessary to induce a completed radiosurgical result. Nevertheless, a patient is considered a failure if further ablative therapy is invoked for any reason.

We have a histopathological specimen (Fig. 7) of a patient with Cushing's disease who was proton-treated and died 9 months later of a heart attack. The center of the tumor is amorphous due to radionecrosis. A rim of remaining tumor is visible. The normal pituitary does not exhibit change. Prior to death, the patient exhibited clinical improvement and reduction of steroid excess, but not yet to normal range.

Complications have not been serious or disabling. One early patient developed a field defect. Temporary oculomotor disturbance continues to occur in 2–4% of treated patients. In 13% of patients, replacement therapy is required, and a similar proportion of patients develop altered pituitary reserve.

8.3. Nelson's Syndrome

These patients are treated much like patients with Cushing's disease except that the dose is often lower, as shown in Fig. 3. Of 19 patients treated, follow-up was available on 14 (Table 8). Of these 14, 12 experienced more or less depigmentation following therapy. Of 11 patients with headache, the

TABLE 8. Available Data on 19 Patients with Nelson's Syndrome Treated with Proton Therapy

14/19	Follow-up available
12/14	Depigmentation
11/14	Headache
8/11	Reduced headache
0/1	Headache relieved by second operation
0/19	Fields abnormal
0/14	Fields changed
4/4	ACTH Fell
1/4	ACTH normalized
0/14	Deaths
0/14	Transient extraocular motor disturbance
1/14	Second operation for mass (invasive)
0/12	Other complications

headache was reduced or eliminated in 8. One patient with residual headache was subsequently operated on elsewhere twice by the transsphenoidal route to relieve the headache, but the headache remained unrelieved. No patients had field defects prior to proton therapy and none developed afterward. The plasma ACTH fell in 4 patients on whom data were available, but became normal in only 1 patient. One patient with a tumor widely invading the base of the skull was subsequently operated on and died due to cancer of the liver. There have been no other deaths, and no extraocular motor disturbance or other complications.

8.4. Prolactinemia

We have treated patients with amenorrhea–galactorrhea and pituitary adenoma for a decade or more. Prior to the advent of radioimmunoassay of plasma prolactin, these patients were treated according to the low-dose schedule indicated in Fig. 3 for nonfunctioning adenomas. We now treat these patients with elevated prolactin with substantially larger doses, as indicated in Fig. 8. We are satisfied from our in-flow of data (Fig. 8) that satisfactory responses are being obtained, but no systematic follow-up of these cases has been done.

8.5. Nonfunctioning Adenomas

As noted in Section 3, these patients are a nonhomogenous group and are less subject to analysis by uniform criteria that objectively document response to therapy. In any case, recurrence or need for further therapy following proton therapy in adequately treated patients has been negligible to date.

Complications have been few since we invoked a general policy of avoiding radiation of patients with suprasellar extension with generous doses of radiation. During the first 2 years of our therapeutic trials with proton therapy, three patients experienced complication outcomes in which we were con-

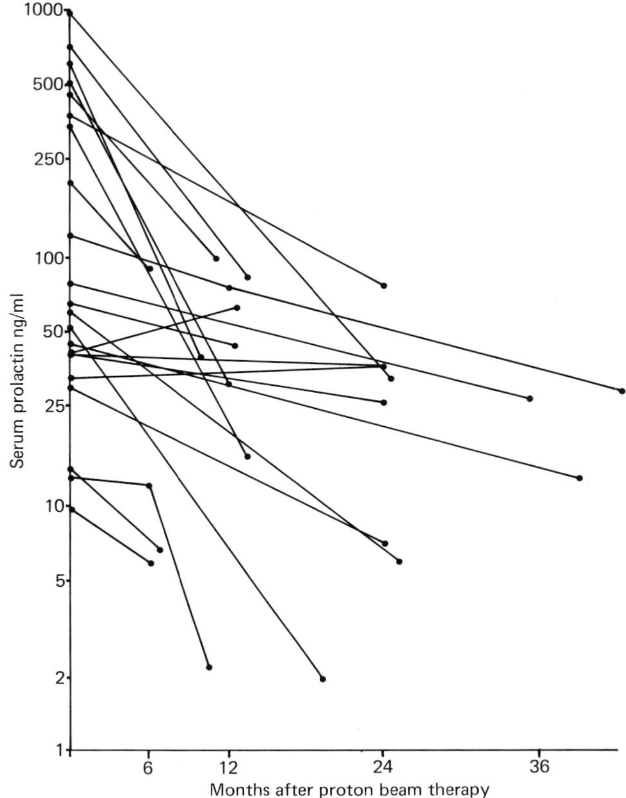

Fig. 8. Prolactin responses in prolactinoma patients. *Ordinate:* log scale of prolactin levels; *abscissa:* time in months. The pretreatment prolactin value of 14 is in error and should be 140. The two other pretreatment values of prolactin below 25 ng/ml were in women with amenorrhea, galactorrhea, and sella enlargement by tumor. The symptoms subsided about 6 months following proton therapy.

cerned that proton treatment may have contributed to an untoward result. More recently, we have treated selected patients with a "double-beam technique," an example of which is shown in Fig. 9. The larger-diameter beam delivers a dose that our data indicate is safe from injury to neural structures but capable of inducing arrest of growth of the adenoma. The smaller beam, confined to subclinoid adenoma, can be anticipated to induce radionecrossis within the adenoma. With our present dose schedule, there have been no deaths, blindness, field defects, extraocular motor disturbance, or hypopituitarism. One elderly patient with many surgical procedures has a memory disturbance of most doubtful relationship to proton therapy.

9. Radiographic Classification

In the categorization of patients, details of radiographic features are receiving increasing attention, especially since they may guide the selection of

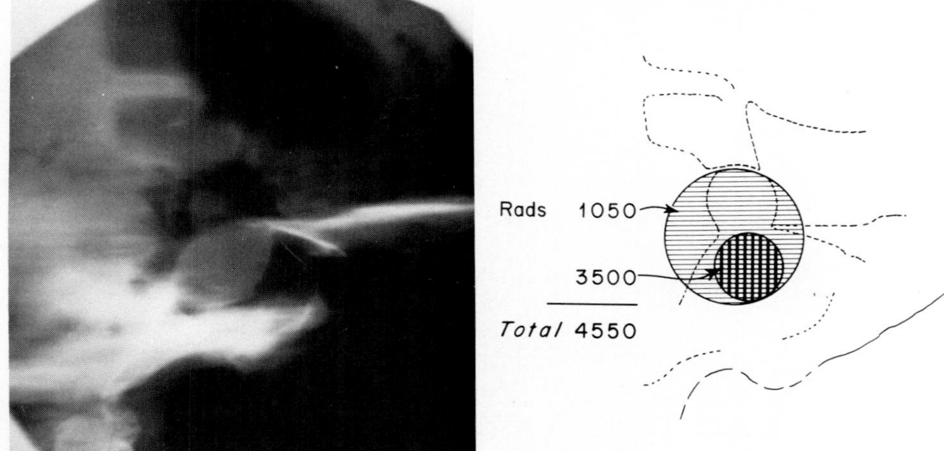

Fig. 9. Illustration of a tactic we refer to as the "double-beam technique." The larger volume that is proton-treated is directed to inducing growth arrest of adenoma without risk to visual or other neural structures. The larger infraclinoid dose can be expected to induce radionecrosis.

patients for one means of treatment or another. In general, selection by means of radiographic features is the consequence of analysis of prior therapeutic results according to such criteria.

Adenomas certainly exist in normal sellas, particularly in patients with Cushing's disease and prolactinoma. In the absence of deformity, the difficulties in locating the microadenoma are increased. The size should be computed from polytomograms using the formula of Di-Chiro and Nelson.[17] The presence or absence of suprasellar extension is relevant to sellae of any size and is established by encephalography or CT scan.

A deformed sella of normal volume typically houses a microadenoma, and the deformity leads to detection of the location, particularly the laterality.

The size of an enlarged sella is important. The prospects of cure or remission by any single procedure when the sella is modestly enlarged are different than those for one that is massive. If parasellar extension exists, prospects for cure are much modified. We avoid the use of the term "invasive" for bony change in plain X-rays because this implies a biological variant that is of uncertain relevance to a radiographic observation. Erosion of bone is, of course, seen, and this term is adequately descriptive without implications of biological character. Extension into the sphenoid sinus can be seen on polytomograms of the sella. Invasion into the cavernous sinus can be seen on CT scan and sometimes with cavernous sinography. Cavernous sinus invasion is particularly prejudicial to a good outcome for patients treated by either transsphenoidal or proton techniques. The use of the term invasion is justified in the cavernous sinus because the adenoma must clearly pass through its dural envelope to enter the sinus.

The term "invasive" as defined above may imply some biological quality similar to "malignant," but the latter term is almost never confirmed by changes recognized by light microscopy or the presence of metastases. This consideration will be discussed further below.

10. Malignancy

The optimistic outlook faced by pituitary adenoma patients is attributable to the fact that most of these tumors are benign in every sense of the word. Nevertheless, we do know that malignant tumors occur in the pituitary. We have not encountered any patient with a proven carcinoma.

Another risk of radiation is the production of sarcoma in brain following "effective" radiation therapy.[18] In the report of Waltz and Brownell,[18] 2 cases of sarcoma developed in 65 patients treated by fractionated X-ray. These and other cases reviewed were treated with 3500 rads or more. The sarcomas developed at intervals of 5 and 15 years, respectively. We have also had a single instance of sarcoma in an acromegalic patient in whom the symptoms began 7 years following proton treatment. Fractionated X-ray therapy was given without benefit. The patient died, and an autopsy was done, revealing sarcoma.

That some seemingly benign pituitary adenomas have more aggressive growth character than others was recognized by Hirsch[6] and Gordon *et al.*[19] These are not malignant in the sense of having distinguishing malignant features by light microscopy, nor do they metastasize. They have a greater tendency to recur and may transdurally invade the cavernous sinus and base of the skull.[20] They may be first recognized at postmortem. Usually, they are difficult to detect early in their course.

For a period of time, all our excised pituitary tumors were submitted to Dr. Paul Kornblith and were grown in tissue culture. Figure 10 represents the

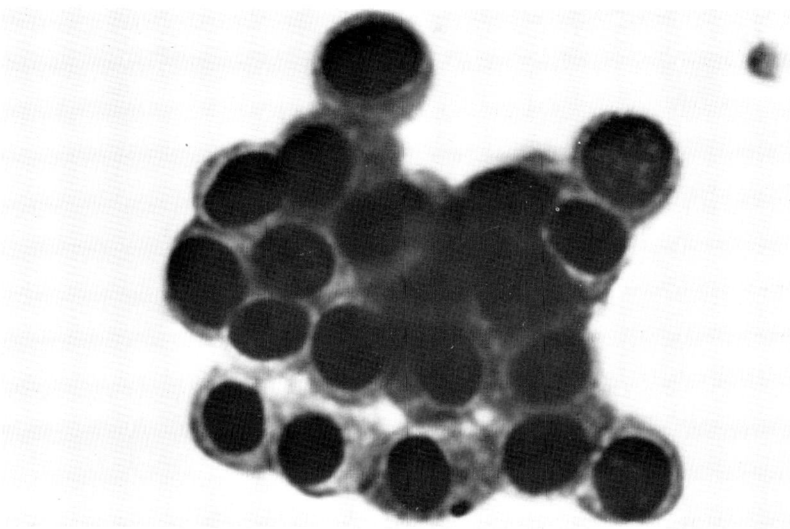

Fig. 10. Photomicrograph of typical benign pituitary cells growing in tissue culture. They float in the medium and are fairly uniform in size and staining characteristics.

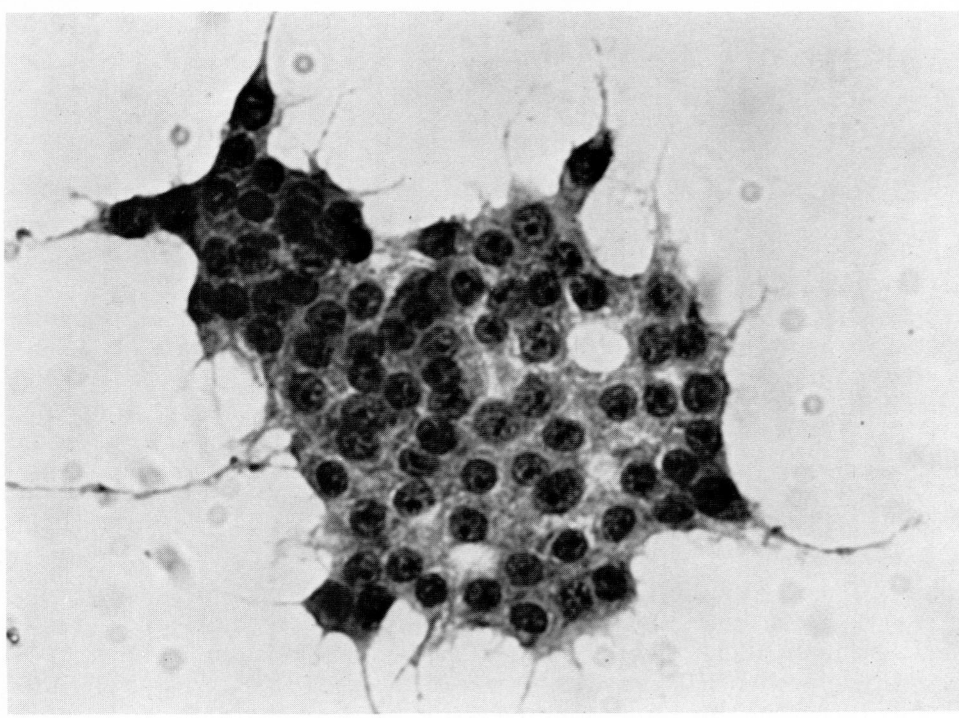

Fig. 11. Photomicrograph of pituitary cells from a recurrent acromegalic patient growing in tissue culture (compare with Fig. 10). Our specimens from recurrent acromegalic patients showed these features of adherence to the walls of the container and more variation in size and staining characteristics of the cells.

usual appearance of a typically benign tumor. Small clusters of uniform cells float about in the culture medium. Infrequently, the cells grew in a different manner (Fig. 11); they grew more rapidly, tended to adhere to container walls, and were less uniform in size and staining character—features frequently associated with malignancy in other tumors. The three acromegalic patients who were recurrent and operated on by us had all these features. Although the term "malignant" was used to describe their growth character, it is probably inappropriate to call them malignant cells for the reasons stated above, namely, that they are light-microscopically indistinguishable from benign tumors and are nonmetastasizing. However, there does appear to be a small percentage of such cases that have more biologically aggressive growth character, are not as readily brought into remission, and are invasive of surrounding structures. We, as did Gordon *et al.*,[19] currently estimate these to be 1–3% of acromegalics.

11. Summary

Bragg-peak proton-beam hypophysectomy, widely employed for over a decade, is shown to be safe, clinically effective, and cost-effective. The absence of procedure-related mortality and very low recurrence rates are desired by physicians and patients alike.

Cyclotrons providing particle-beam therapy function as area-wide resources for the provision of special therapeutic capability of specific situations.

References

1. L.T. Kurland, Geography of neural tumors, in: *Pathology of the Nervous System* (J. Minckler, ed.), pp. 2803–2808, McGraw-Hill, New York, 1968.
2. U.S. National Center for Health Statistics, International Classification of Diseases, Vol. I, Adapted for Indexing Hospital Records by Diseases and Operations, U.S. Dept. of Health, Education and Welfare, Public Health Service, Washington, D.C., 1962.
3. C.A. Fager, J.L. Poppen, and Y. Takaoka, Indications for and results of surgical treatment of pituitary tumors by the intracranial approach, in: *Diagnosis and Treatment of Pituitary Tumors* (P.O. Kohler and G.T. Ross, eds.), pp. 146–155, Excerpta Medica, Admsterdam, 1973.
4. G. Guiot, Transsphenoidal approach in surgical treatment of pituitary adenomas: General principles and indications in non-functioning adenomas, in: *Diagnosis and Treatment of Pituitary Tumors* (P.O. Kohler and G.T. Ross, eds.), pp. 159–178, Excerpta Medica, Amsterdam, 1973.
5. J. Hardy, Transsphenoidal surgery of hypersecreting pituitary tumors, in: *Diagnosis and Treatment of Pituitary Tumors* (P.O. Kohler and G.T. Ross, eds.), pp. 179–194, Excerpta Medica, Amsterdam, 1973.
6. O. Hirsch, Life-long cures and improvements after transsphenoidal operation of pituitary tumors (thirty-three patients followed-up for 20–37 years), *Acta Ophthalmol. Suppl.* **56:**5–60, 1959.
7. C.S. MacCarty, E.J. Hanson, Jr., R.V. Randall, and P.W. Scanlon, Indications for and results of surgical treatment of pituitary tumors by the transfrontal approach, in: *Diagnosis and Treatment of Pituitary Tumors* (P.O. Kohler and G.T. Ross, eds.), pp. 139–145, Excerpta Medica, Amsterdam, 1973.
8. B.S. Ray and R.H. Patterson, Jr., Surgical experience with chromophobe adenomas of the pituitary gland, *J. Neurosurg.* **34:**726–729, 1971.
9. F.P. Wirth, H.G. Schwartz, and P.R. Schwetschenau, Pituitary adenomas: Factors in treatment, in: *Clinical Neurosurgery: Proceedings of the Congress of Neurological Surgeons,* Honolulu, Hawaii, 1973 (R.H. Wilkins, ed.), pp. 8–25, Williams and Wilkins, Baltimore, 1974.
10. G.E. Sheline, Treatment of chromophobe adenomas of the pituitary gland and acromegaly, in: *Diagnosis and Treatment of Pituitary Tumors* (P.O. Kohler and G.T. Ross, eds.), pp. 201–216, Excerpta Medica, Amsterdam, 1973.
11. A.D. Wright, D.M. Hill, C. Lowy, and T.R. Fraser, Mortality in acromegaly, *Q. J. Med.* **39:**1–16, 1970.
12. A.P. Forbes, P.H. Henneman, G.C. Griswold, and F. Albright, Syndrome characterized by galactorrhea, amenorrhea and low urinary FSH: Comparison with acromegaly and normal lactation, *J. Clin. Endocrinol. Metab.* **14:**265–271, 1954.
13. K.M. Earle and S.H. Dillard, Jr., Pathology of adenomas of the pituitary gland, in: *Diagnosis and Treatment of Pituitary Tumors* (P.O. Kohler and G.T. Ross, eds.), pp. 3–16, Excerpta Medica, Amsterdam, 1973.
14. R.N. Kjellberg, A. Shintani, A.G. Frantz, and B. Kliman, Proton beam therapy in acromegaly, *N. Engl. J. Med.* **278:**689–695, 1968.
15. R.N. Kjellberg and B. Kliman, A system for therapy of pituitary tumors, in: *Diagnosis and Treatment of Pituitary Tumors* (P.O. Kohler and G.T. Ross, eds.), pp. 234–252, Excerpta Medica, Amsterdam, 1973.
16. R.N. Kjellberg and B. Kliman, Treatment of acromegaly by proton hypophysectomy, in: *Current Controversies in Neurosurgery* (T.P. Morley, ed.), pp. 392–405, W.B. Saunders, Toronto, 1976.
17. G. DiChiro and K.B. Nelson, The volume of the sella turcica, *Am. J. Roentgenol. Radium Ther. Nucl. Med.* **87:**989–1008, 1962.

18. T.A. Waltz and B. Brownell, Sarcoma: A possible late result of effective radiation therapy for pituitary adenoma, *J. Neurosurg.* **24:**901–907, 1966.
19. D.A. Gordon, F.M. Hill, and C. Ezrin, Acromegaly: A review of 100 cases, *Can. Med. Assoc. J.* **87:**1106–1109, 1962.
20. J.W. Kernohan and G.P. Sayre, *Tumors of the Pituitary Gland and Infundibulum*, Armed Forces Institute of Pathology, Washington, D.C., 1956.

23

Overview of Pituitary Tumor Treatment

PETER O. KOHLER

1. Introduction

Major advances in the diagnostic and therapeutic approaches to pituitary tumors have occurred over the past two decades. As a result of the increased capacity to detect and treat pituitary microadenomas, the goals of treatment are now often different. Several years ago, the diagnosis of pituitary tumor was most often made in patients over 40 years of age.[1] Frequently, the presenting complaints include visual defects, indicating relatively large tumors.[2] In addition, most pituitary tumors were believed to be nonfunctional because (1) no hypersecretory syndrome was clearly identified in approximately 75% of patients and (2) on histological examination, the tumor cells showed no specific chromophilic hormone granules. The therapeutic goal in patients with these so-called "chromophobe adenomas" was often to prevent expansion or control tumor growth and avoid the visual and endocrine deficiencies caused by the mass effect of the tumor. Total resection of the tumor was not necessarily recommended because of the high incidence of complete pituitary dysfunction and fatality.[3] Therapy for these tumors was usually either transfrontal surgery,[1] external irradiation,[4] or a combination of both.[5]

The recent refinements of diagnostic radiological and endocrine techniques have now resulted in the increased identification of small pituitary adenomas in younger patients.[6] The recognition that "functionless" tumors often secrete prolactin and that prolactin-secreting tumors (prolactinomas) are apparently more common than nonfunctioning tumors has occurred only in the past few years.[7,8] At the same time, advances in therapeutic approaches, such as the ability to selectively remove a microadenoma, have caused a reassessment of the optimal management of these patients. The dramatic results

PETER O. KOHLER • University of Arkansas for Medical Sciences, Little Rock, Arkansas 72205; Little Rock Arkansas University Hospital, Little Rock, Arkansas 72201.

obtained in several centers with the transsphenoidal selective removal of microadenomas have added a new dimension to the treatment of pituitary tumors, specifically the reasonable expectation that a hypersecreting microadenoma will be removed with preservation of normal pituitary function and fertility. This expectation would have been unlikely a decade ago.

With the advent of better diagnostic and therapeutic techniques, earlier diagnosis is possible, and a rational treatment plan can be individualized for each patient depending on the type (function) of tumor, the extent of tumor spread, the age and clinical condition of the patient, and the possible goals of the patient such as fertility (Table 1). The patient with a pituitary hypersecretory syndrome resulting from excess prolactin, growth hormone, or corticotropin production from a small pituitary adenoma may now have good reason to hope for a surgical cure with the retention of normal pituitary function. This felicitous result is now attained in approximately 75% of patients with small tumors and is associated with minimal morbidity and mortality in the hands of a surgeon with expertise in transsphenoidal microsurgery.

However, other therapeutic approaches (Table 2) have been successfully utilized in the treatment of pituitary tumors, and there are anatomical and other relative contraindications to transsphenoidal surgery in some patients. In addition, the natural history of the small prolactin-secreting microadenoma can only be inferred from surgical and autopsy data. The question of how often the asymptomatic pituitary microadenoma enlarges to the point of causing morbidity such as sellar erosion, visual defects, and hypopituitarism associated with a space-occupying lesion has not yet been defined by a prospective study. Another unanswered question is the incidence of recurrence of a microadenoma after successful surgical removal. Prior to therapy of any type, adequate diagnositic studies are necessary to exclude relatively benign conditions such as the empty sella syndrome, which usually requires no treatment

TABLE 1. Considerations in Plan of Therapy for Patients with Pituitary Tumors

1. Age of patient
2. General health of patient
3. Tumor size and degree of extension
   a. Visual loss
   b. Hypopituitarism
   c. Other (e.g., CSF rhinorrhea)
4. Hypersecretory status of tumor
   a. Prolactinoma
   b. Acromegaly
   c. Cushing's disease and Nelson's syndrome
   d. Miscellaneous (TSH, FSH, LH hypersecretion)
5. Therapeutic goals
   a. Preservation of vision
   b. Control of tumor growth
   c. Reversal of hypersecretory syndrome
   d. Preservation of normal pituitary function, fertility, etc.
6. Previous treatment

TABLE 2. Potential Types of Therapy for Patients with Pituitary Tumors

1. None
2. Medical
   a. Directed at pituitary tumor
   b. Directed at end organ (i.e., adrenal)
3. External irradiation of tumor
   a. Conventional supravoltage or ^{60}Co
      (i) Multiple variations in technique
   b. Heavy-particle
      (i) Proton beam with Bragg peak
      (ii) Alpha particles (helium ions)
4. Surgery
   a. Directed at pituitary
      (i) Transfrontal or intracranial hypohysectomy
      (ii) Transsphenoidal
         • Microsurgery
         • Cryohypophysectomy
         • Thermal ablation
         • Implantation of ^{90}Y or ^{198}Au in sella
   b. Directed at end organ (adrenalectomy in Cushing's disease)
5. Combined surgery and external irradiation

at all.[9] Finally, the question of retreatment of an unsuccessfully surgically treated or irradiated pituitary tumor is a rather frequent clinical problem in any referral center.

Many of these problems have no single correct answer, and controlled studies would be required for definitive results. However, management of clinical problems in patients can be considered in view of the experience to date. There are obviously multiple considerations in the planning of therapy for any specific patient. It is impossible to be dogmatic about any single form of therapy for all patients. The important concept is to use the most appropriate therapy individualized after evaluation of the problems and goals of the particular patient. Each of the types of functional pituitary tumors will be discussed separately. However, the mass effects such as visual loss in patients with the large nonfunctioning or "chromophobe adenoma" are similar to those of the large hypersecreting tumor. All large tumors will therefore be considered collectively with the understanding that special considerations must be given to the problems of hypersecretion of a specific hormone.

2. Large Nonfunctioning Tumors

The patient with a large pituitary tumor usually presents with headaches, visual disorders, or hypopituitarism, or a combination of these problems.[2] These patients are usually older and less interested in fertility than in preservation of vision and amelioration of other problems. There are no known effective medical forms of treatment for the nonfunctioning tumors. The argument could be raised that the nonfunctioning adenoma might need no treatment at all, since they are relatively slow-growing. However, Sheline[10] and Weisberg[11] have presented data indicating that untreated patients with large pituitary tumors and visual problems or hormone deficiencies frequently progress to more serious visual and other problems. Interestingly, Weisberg did not find documented progression in 13 asymptomatic patients over follow-up periods of 2–15 years.[11] Six patients had headache, but no visual or endocrine abnormalities. Of these, only one was treated after a pneumoencephalogram showed suprasellar enlargement. These data have suggested that such patients have a less ominous prognosis and may be followed without treatment. However, the period of follow-up in this series was relatively short in view of the known slow progression of these tumors. If no treatment is elected, patients must be evaluated carefully at regular intervals for the possible development of visual or endocrine deficiencies.

A particularly difficult decision arises with the patient in whom asymptomatic enlargement of the sella turcica has been found by serendipity during skull X-rays taken for other indications such as head trauma. This patient may have only the radiographic changes of sella enlargement with no visual or endocrine deficiencies. Prior to any form of treatment, it is of utmost importance to establish that the sella enlargement is the result of tumor and not the nontumorous enlargement or ballooning of the sella of the "empty sella" syndrome.[9] If the abnormal sella is the result of nontumorous enlargement and the endocrine studies are normal, no treatment is indicated in the absence of cerebrospinal fluid (CSF) rhinorrhea. If the patient has a definite mass within the sella with no visual, endocrine, or other problems, the data of Weisberg[11] would suggest that the patient might be followed closely without treatment. This approach should be followed only with a reliable patient who will return regularly for endocrine and radiographic evaluation. Otherwise, the experience reported by Sheline[10] would indicate that treatment such as conventional irradiation is indicated.

The decision to use a particular form of treatment in the patient with a large nonfunctioning pituitary lesion depends on the extent of visual loss and hypopituitarism. Also to be considered are the success and complications of any therapeutic modality to be utilized. More aggressive treatment is probably indicated in the younger patient, because although pituitary tumors grow slowly, the younger patient with a greater life expectancy is at greater risk for visual or endocrine deficiencies.

2.1. Radiation Treatment of Large Pituitary Tumors

In many centers, the strategy utilized for treatment of patients with large nonfunctioning pituitary tumors without major visual problems has been to use conventional photon irradiation alone and evaluate periodically for possible transfrontal surgery.[5] Others have combined transfrontal surgery with postoperative irradiation.[4,5] The results of these approaches have generally been good if the goals primarily included considerations such as the preservation of vision. Fager *et al.*[5] have reported improvement in 178 (65%) of 273 patients initially treated with irradiation alone. Transfrontal surgery was subsequently utilized in 88 of the 273 patients. Sheline,[4] Pistenma *et al.*,[12] and Urdaneta *et al.*[13] have also reported a good control rate with conventional radiation therapy alone or in combination with surgery for patients with large tumors. There is limited experience with heavy-particle or proton-beam therapy in patients with large tumors because of the potential for development of visual problems associated with higher doses of irradiation in tumors extending into or above the area of the optic chiasm.

Cystic tumors, which represent about 15% of pituitary adenomas, appear to respond less well than solid adenomas to most forms of radiation therapy.[4] For this reason, the question of whether pituitaries should be biopsied prior to irradiation has been raised. This appears impractical in most patients unless surgery is a planned component of the treatment regimen. However, without biopsy, it is likely that many cystic tumors have been irradiated with a poor response, and that some nontumorous lesions have been treated inadvertently and included in some series. The recent appreciation that prolactin is secreted by many tumors previously thought to be nonfunctional will, it is to be hoped, provide additional data regarding the effect of irradiation on large prolactin-producing tumors.

In general, the risks and side effects of conventional irradiation are minimal. Swelling or infarction of tumors with loss of vision rarely ever occurs. A few unusual tumors such as sarcomas and small areas of brain necrosis have been reported several years after treatment.[14–16] These complications are apparently infrequent.

2.2. Surgical Treatment of Large Pituitary Tumors

Although Cushing[17] pioneered the transsphenoidal surgical approach to the pituitary, he and others later favored the transfrontal or transcranial approach for large pituitary tumors. Several surgeons have developed an extensive experience with the transfrontal or intracranial type of operation. Ray and Patterson[18] operated on 80 patients with no operative mortality in the era after the introduction of antibiotics and cortisone in the post-operative management period. However, the mortality in the perioperative period has been greater than 3% in most series[19] and increases with size of the tumor. The transfrontal surgical approach is still indicated in the very large pituitary tumors extending well above the optic chiasm. These tumors are difficult to treat with irradiation alone because of the size and location of the tumor. The various specific advantages of the transfrontal and transsphenoidal approach are discussed elsewhere in this volume (see Chapters 18 and 19). Recently, experienced neurosurgeons have been more willing to operate on increasingly larger tumors via the transsphenoidal route.[21] However, the largest pituitary tumors are still operated on through the transfrontal approach. Unless the surgeon is confident that he has removed all the tumor, the patient should probably have postoperative irradiation with 3500–4500 rads to control regeneration of the tumor.[10]

2.3. Considerations in the Choice of Therapy for Large Tumors

There is little accumulated experience with therapy of nonfunctioning pituitary microadenomas less than 1 cm in diameter because they are usually asymptomatic, and there have been inadequate parameters for following a clinical response if the patient were treated. The relatively high (9–24%) incidence of microadenomas discovered at postmortem examination combined with the low annual occurrence rate of approximately 1:100,000 for large tumors would suggest that small nonfunctioning adenomas rarely need treatment. The reported experience with therapy of nonfunctioning tumors therefore is primarily the results with larger adenomas treated with transfrontal surgery or irradiation or both.

Large tumors do require careful follow-up examination. Both surgical and radiation therapy are more likely to result in some degree of hypopituitarism in the larger tumors. Patients with extensive surgical treatment frequently have or develop hypopituitarism and must be treated with appropriate replacement therapy. Most experienced clinicians advocate careful evaluations of these patients including visual, radiographic, and at least basal endocrine testing at not less than 12-month intervals if the patient is not on hormone-replacement therapy. If there is a question regarding the reliability of the patient, some form of treatment is probably indicated.

The hazards of each type of therapy must be considered in the decision to treat patients with pituitary tumors. Although the morbidity and mortality associated with transfrontal surgery have been reduced to low levels in larger series, they are still appreciable, particularly at institutions where this surgery is performed infrequently. The morbidity and mortality associated with transsphenoidal surgery appears generally to be less, and this approach is now being used for some of the larger tumors that previously would have been operated on by the intracranial approach. However, occasional complications such as CSF rhinorrhea, blindness, or meningitis occur with transsphenoidal surgery also.[20]

Frequently, complete surgical removal of the tumor is not possible. Conventional irradiation does provide relatively safe "control" of tumor growth and may be indicated as the primary form of therapy, particularly in the elderly patient. Sheline[10] has documented that the combination of surgery plus irradiation appears to be more successful than either approach alone in controlling tumor growth. For this reason, postoperative irradiation is probably indicated for tumor control if all tumor tissue cannot be removed at the time of surgery.

3. Acromegaly

Acromegaly is a slowly progressive disorder. Various authorities have emphasized the need for early treatment, while others[22] have suggested that the course of the disease is indolent and any form of treatment that brings the disorder under control within a few years is adequate. Several points can be raised supporting the contention that acromegaly is a disease that should be treated. The disorder not only produces progressive symptomatology, disfigurement, arthritis, and hypertension, but also is associated with increased cardiovascular disease. While the rapid symptomatic response to surgery or heavy-particle irradiation is often dramatic, the differences in overall morbidity from the disease in patients successfully treated with surgery,[20,23,24] with heavy-particle irradiation,[25,26] or with the more slowly responding forms of treatment such as conventional irradiation cannot be clearly documented.[22,27,28] It would appear that the disease rarely spontaneously "burns out" as suggested in the older literature. However, infarction is more common than one might expect, and the full-blown syndrome of pituitary apoplexy does occasionally occur.[29]

The growth hormone (GH)-secreting pituitary tumors in the acromegalic patient are usually large enough to expand the sella turcica at the time of initial diagnosis of the disease. Therefore, management should include both consideration of the mass lesion, which may produce visual-field defects and cause hypopituitarism,[30] and the excessive GH production. There are several parameters related to the GH excess that may be evaluated to document progression of the disease or response to therapy. Changes in the symptoms and soft-tissue alterations are useful, but may be difficult to quantitate accurately. Although GH probably acts in part through somatomedins, the latter are difficult to measure adequately by available assays. For these reasons, the easiest parameter to quantify accurately is the GH level. There is usually a good correlation between improvement of symptoms and signs and reduction of GH levels to less than the 5 ng/ml level. Therefore, in the acromegalic patient, the goals of treatment are the same as those for nonfunctioning tumors with the additional objective of lowering the GH level to less than 5–10 ng/ml.

The possible choices for therapy in the acromegalic patient are similar to those for other types of pituitary tumors. These include drugs, irradiation of various types discussed below, and surgery.

3.1. Medical Treatment of Acromegaly

Multiple forms of medical therapy have been tried in acromegalic patients. Treatment trials have reported variable success with estrogens, progestins, phenothiazines, and L-dopa, and limited GH suppression has occurred with corticosteroids, α-adrenergic agents, blocking agents, and antiserotonin drugs.[31–34] However, definite improvement with those drugs that have been tested has been difficult to document in subsequent series. Recently, bromocriptine has been used in the treatment of acromegaly as well as in syndromes of prolactin hypersecretion. Bromocriptine does lower the GH levels in approximately 50–80% of acromegalic patients.[35,36] However, side effects such as nausea may be troublesome,[37] and the suppressive effect appears to be temporary in that GH levels return to pretreatment values when the drug is discontinued. There is also an escape phenomenon that occurs in some patients in whom GH levels rise during the bromocriptine treatment. At present, medical therapy should be regarded as an adjunct to more definitive treatment or as a temporizing maneuver in a patient who is too ill or for other reasons unable to undergo surgery or irradiation.

3.2. Radiation Treatment of Acromegaly

Both conventional photon and heavy-particle irradiation have been successfully utilized in the treatment of acromegaly. Conventional photon radiation therapy has been used as the sole treatment or in conjunction with surgery in the management of acromegalic patients.[22,27,28] To avoid complications, conventional radiation treatment must be given slowly with multiple doses administered over several weeks regardless of the technical method such as bitemporal or multiple ports or coronal arc. The clinical response to this type of treatment occurs slowly and may take months to years to become apparent. Regression of the clinical manifestations occurs at variable intervals after treatment. However, several groups of investigators have reported effective reduction of GH levels after conventional radiation therapy in patients with acromegaly.[22,27,28] Eastman *et al.*[30] have reviewed the experience of a relatively large group of 65 acromegalic patients. Of the patients treated with conventional irradiation, 42 were followed for at least 2 years and showed 52% fall in GH levels. The cumulative fall was 77% in the 16 patients followed for 10 years. In terms of absolute GH values, 73% of 33 patients had GH levels below 10 ng/ml by 5 years after treatment. These results compare favorably to those of other forms of treatment, but are achieved after the longer period of time. These workers have made the point that this form of treatment, albeit slow to reduce GH levels, is effective and appears adequate in a slowly progressive disorder. A major virtue of this form of treatment is that it is available in most large medical centers, although experience is often variable. Side effects of conventional radiation therapy are generally minimal. However, progressive loss of other pituitary tropic hormone function does occur after radiation therapy[29,37] to the extent that about 50% of acromegalics treated in this manner are partially or completely hypopituitary as a result of either the tumor or the treatment.

The second major form of radiation therapy for acromegalic patients is with protons[25] (see Chapter 22) or alpha particles.[26] These may be given with sophisticated sterotaxic techniques utilizing the Bragg-peak phenomenon of increased energy as the protons slow down near the target. In contrast to conventional irradiation, which must be given as multiple small courses to a total of less than 5000 rads, protons or heavy particles are administered over shorter treatment periods with delivery of a greater number of rads to the target tumor tissue. The clinical response to treatment with heavy particles is also somewhat more rapid.[26] The side effects, primarily cranial nerve palsies, are probably similar to those of conventional irradiation and seem more likely to occur in patients who have previously received photon supravoltage or ^{60}Co treatment.[39] The failure of GH secretion to be adequately reduced by heavy-particle therapy in some patients often appears to be the result of irregularities of tumor shape and extension that make it difficult to effectively deliver the treatment to the tumor without risk of injury to surrounding tissue.

A third type of irradiation should be mentioned: the surgical implantation of a radioactive source such as ^{90}Y or ^{198}Au in the sella turcica. This technique has been successfully utilized in England by Fraser *et al.*[40] However, it has been generally replaced in this country by other forms of treatment.

The choice between proton-beam or conventional irradiation is often one of accessibility. The ability to utilize a brief treatment period with heavy particle–proton beam is certainly advantageous. Unfortunately, treatment centers are available in only a few areas of the country such as Boston and San Francisco. In the patient with a symmetrical tumor below the optic chiasm, the results of heavy-particle or proton-beam compare very favorably to those of other forms of treatment. However, if there are major irregularities in tumor shape or extension above the chiasm, surgical approaches may be more appropriate.

3.3. Surgical Treatment of Acromegaly

Fifty years ago, the diagnosis of acromegaly was often made only after the tumor had reached a large size. This observation is documented by the finding that 93% of patients had enlargement of the sella turcica and 62% had visual disturbances at the time of diagnosis in the large series of 100 patients reported by Davidoff[41] in 1926. Although the diagnosis is made earlier now in many instances, the pituitary tumors associated with acromegaly are still often of large size, as indicated by the finding that 90% of patients had an enlarged sella turcica in a more recent series.[42]

The surgical approach to the pituitary tumor in acromegaly is somewhat dependent on tumor size and extension. A large experience has been gained with the transfrontal surgical treatment of acromegaly, and the indications for this approach have been summarized by Post in this volume (see Chapters 16 and 19). Transfrontal surgery is still indicated in some patients with very large tumors. However, transsphenoidal microsurgery as developed by Guiot,[21] Hardy,[24] and others has now been shown to produce excellent results in acromegalic patients. The fall in GH levels to less than 5–10 ng/ml may be dramatic.[20] As with other types of transsphenoidal surgery, removal of a GH-secreting adenoma may be accomplished with retention of normal pituitary function. The success rate in a series of 120 patients reported by Hardy[43] was impressive, with normal GH levels in 94 patients and reduced GH levels in 20 additional patients. Only 6 patients did not have a significant GH reduction. Normal pituitary function was preserved in 102 patients.

Transsphenoidal surgery is usually accomplished with minimal morbidity and mortality. However, rare complications such as blindness, meningitis, and CSF rhinorrhea do occasionally occur,[20] and there is always the low risk of morbidity associated with anesthesia. Success at transsphenoidal microsurgery requires the development of surgical skills that are usually achieved only after considerable experience.

3.4. Considerations in the Choice of Therapy for Acromegaly

The decision to utilize a particular form of primary therapy for the previously untreated acromegalic patient varies from center to center. Medical treatment is primarily in the investigative stage at present. Both transsphenoidal surgery and proton-beam irradiation offer the potential for relatively rapid reduction of GH levels to less than 5–10 ng/ml. Although satisfactory results have been obtained with conventional irradiation, many clinicians have been impressed with the rapid and often dramatic results of transsphenoidal microsurgery. Therefore, the current trend is to favor the more rapid surgical treatment, but the selection of an experienced surgeon cannot be overemphasized. An advantage to the surgical approach is the rapid determination of the degree of success of the procedure. Patients who have continued GH elevation after surgery have repeat operations in a few centers. Most endocrinologists would advise postoperative irradiation for patients who do not respond to surgery.

It should be pointed out that the results with heavy-particle or proton-beam therapy are often excellent and compare favorably to the surgical results. Eccentric position or extension of the tumor is probably responsible for poor results in some cases. This is a particularly valuable form of treatment in patients who for reasons of general health are not candidates for anesthesia and surgery. Conventional irradiation also remains effective in over half of patients treated. Neurosurgeons differ in their opinion as to whether previous unsuccessful radiation treatment causes a fibrosis of the pituitary and surrounding tissue that makes surgery more difficult. However, surgical results may be good in patients who have been irradiated. Combined therapy with surgery and irradiation has often been necessary in patients with large tumors. Transfrontal surgery may be utilized and combined with conventional megavoltage irradiation in these patients. Patients with acromegaly still often have or develop associated deficiencies of other pituitary tropic hormones.[38] These deficiencies can be treated with replacement therapy.

4. Prolactinoma

The diagnosis and management of the patient with a prolactin-secreting pituitary microadenoma have been of great interest to clinicians over the past few years.[8,44,45] Identification of these small pituitary tumors in patients with galactorrhea or amenorrhea or both has occurred with increasing frequency after the development of the prolactin radioimmunoassay. This has coincided temporally with the refinements in transsphenoidal pituitary microsurgery that have permitted successful selective removal of the prolactin-secreting microadenomas with retention of normal pituitary function. Resumption of menses, restoration of fertility, and ultimately the achievement of pregnancy have been the gratifying consequence of transsphenoidal microsurgery in a large number of young women with prolactin-secreting microadenomas.[43,46,47] The development of the prolactin radioimmunoassay has also resulted in the surprising finding that a relatively large number of all pituitary adenomas, apparently 30–70% of all tumors,[7,48,49] actually secrete prolactin. Many of these tumors, particularly those in elderly patients and in men, are without endocrine manifestations. Decreased libido and infertility have been described in men with prolactinomas.[50] Several of these patients experienced a return of gonadotropic and gonadal function after removal of a pituitary adenoma or bromocriptine treatment, suggesting that prolactin played a role in the symptomatology.[50,59] Prolactin-secreting tumors in men are often larger than in women at the time of detection and produce morbidity by the mass effect of the tumor compressing normal pituitary and adjacent structures.[50] However, the major recent clinical experience has been gained in women during the reproductive years with the small prolactinomas that cause amenorrhea or galactorrhea or both. These patients frequently present initially to the obstetrician–gynecologist with complaints of amenorrhea or infertility.

The types of treatment available for prolactinoma are the same as for other types of pituitary tumors; these include drugs, surgery, and irradiation. The goals of treatment in patients with small prolactinomas should be the reversal of the clinical syndrome with retention of normal pituitary function and prevention of any mass effects of the tumor.

4.1. Medical Treatment of Prolactinomas

One of the first drugs noted to suppress prolactin levels was L-dopa.[51] This drug is thought to act by conversion to dopamine after crossing the blood–brain barrier. L-Dopa is able to reduce prolactin levels in patients with almost any type of hyperprolactinemia. However, the suppressive effect of L-dopa on prolactin levels unfortunately lasts only a few hours, and the large doses of L-dopa required for suppression of prolactin levels are associated with unpleasant side effects such as nausea. However, a dopamine agonist, the ergot derivative bromocriptine, has been found to be extremely successful in suppressing prolactin levels in essentially all patients with hyperprolactinemia, including those with prolactin-producing tumors.[52] This drug has now been extensively tested and used for the treatment of galactorrhea. Resumption of normal cyclic menses has frequently occurred after reduction of elevated prolactin levels. Usually, the effect of bromocriptine is the prompt reduction of prolactin levels to normal with return of normal cyclic hypothalamic–pituitary–gonadal function in patients with adequate pituitary function.

Pregnancy has frequently been achieved after bromocriptine in patients with pituitary tumors. However, the drug is not currently approved by the FDA as a fertility drug. One reason for caution is the normal increase in pituitary size during pregnancy that in the presence of a substantial pituitary tumor may cause compression of the optic chiasm and visual deficits.[53] Some patients have been followed through pregnancy with this visual problem.[54] Others have been treated successfully with surgery during the pregnancy for this complication. However, the consensus at present is that even if bromocriptine had FDA approval as a fertility drug, it would probably be prudent to treat surgically prior to using bromocriptine in the patient desiring pregnancy.[55] Further experience is needed to resolve this issue.

There have been recent reports that bromocriptine has specific antitumor effects, and the improvement of visual-field defects and apparent tumor regression in a previously surgically treated and irradiated patient after the drug would support this contention.[56] However, the natural history of prolactin-secreting adenomas with regard to progression, spontaneous regression, infarction, and other aspects of course is not currently known. Therefore, the potential antitumor effect will have to be evaluated carefully in the future. However, the drug is very useful in the patient with bothersome galactorrhea, in the patient who is not a candidate for other types of treatment, or as an adjunct to surgery or irradiation.

4.2. Radiation Treatment of Prolactinomas

Conventional supravoltage radiation has been utilized as the primary mode of therapy in the treatment of prolactinoma only to a limited degree after the development of the prolactin radioimmunoassay. Many prolactin-secreting adenomas were probably irradiated in the past during the treatment of so-called "chromophobe adenomas" before the development of the prolactin assay. Unfortunately, the experience for prolactinomas cannot be differentiated from that for the truly nonfunctional tumor in terms of efficacy of treatment. The limited experience reported by Kleinberg *et al.*[44] suggests that reduction of elevated prolactin secretion occurs after irradiation, although at a slower rate. Menses may resume, but the incidence of successful pregnancy has not been clearly determined in the small series available. The doses of conventional irradiation are similar to those that have been used for nonfunctional pituitary adenomas, i.e., less than 5000 rads.

Extensive experience with heavy-particle or proton-beam irradiation has not been reported with prolactinomas. However, Kjellberg and Kliman have reported in this volume (Chapter 22) that proton-beam therapy may be effective. Linfoot[57] has indicated that when alpha-particle therapy was utilized for tumor control, prolactin levels have fallen into the normal range in 12 of 29 patients with hyperprolactinemia. These patients received doses of 3200–10,000 rads and were followed for 1–2 years after treatment. However, this treatment has not been utilized routinely in patients with microadenomas, hyperprolactinemia, and infertility.

4.3. Surgical Treatment of Prolactinomas

The major advances in transsphenoidal surgery accomplished over the past two decades have had perhaps their most widespread clinical application in the treatment of prolactin-secreting microadenomas. This experience has been documented elsewhere in this volume by Post (Chapter 18). The transsphenoidal approach is well suited to the needs of the young women with a small prolactinoma, galactorrhea–amenorrhea, and infertility. In the successfully treated patient, the selective removal of the adenoma allows normalization of prolactin levels with retention of normal pituitary function, return of cyclic menses, and fertility. This approach also has the virtue of an almost immediate reduction of prolactin values in the successfully treated patient. Again, one cannot overemphasize the need for a skilled neurosurgeon. The neurosurgeon performing a rare procedure is unlikely to achieve the success rate of the surgeon who performs the procedure weekly. The success rate as indicated by reduction of prolactin to the normal range and resumption of menses in the larger series is over 75% in Grade I microadenomas.[46,47,58] The recurrence rate of these tumors is not known. In larger tumors, the success rate falls to less than 50%. This surgical approach has also been efficacious in a few men with small adenomas, but the experience is very limited.[59] Most of the prolactinomas identified in men have been larger and have been treated in the same manner as a nonfunctioning tumor. The complications of transsphenoidal surgery are fortunately infrequent,[47] but as would be expected are more common in the larger tumors.

4.4. Considerations in the Choice of Therapy for Prolactinomas

It is possible that FDA approval will be granted for the use of bromocriptine for fertility in women with prolactin-secreting adenomas, since the results of European studies have been promising and have suggested that the drug is relatively safe for use in inducing pregnancy.[59,60] However, visual problems may ensue during the course of the pregnancy. For this reason, transsphenoidal microsurgery and selective adenomectomy is probably the procedure of choice at present for the young women with a documented small prolactinoma, infertility, and the desire for pregnancy. Bromocriptine treatment frequently results in restoration of menses and fertility in the patients who have continued elevation of prolactin postoperatively. The role of the various forms of radiation therapy for small prolactinomas is not clear at present. A prospective study evaluating the success of transsphenoidal surgery vs. irradiation would be interesting but seems unlikely to be organized. Irradiation does have a role in the unsuccessfully operated patient with evidence of progressive tumor growth.

The large prolactin-producing tumor in women or men is managed in a manner analogous to the nonfunctional tumor, with the surgical approach dependent on the size and degree of extension of the tumor. Transfrontal surgery is required in the very large tumors. Irradiation may also be used for control with or without surgery.

5. Cushing's Disease

Harvey Cushing believed that the disease that now bears his name was caused by an adenoma or hyperplasia of the pituitary gland and that the proper therapeutic approach was the removal of this adenoma. Although he successfully treated several patients with transsphenoidal or transfrontal surgery, the etiology of "adrenal hyperplasia" was subsequently questioned and thought to possibly be the result of an adrenal hypersensitivity to corticotropin or possibly a lesion of the central nervous system. Bilateral adrenalectomy[61] or irradiation of the pituitary[62] was often the initial step in the therapy of a patient with a positive dexamethasone suppression test indicating Cushing's disease.[63] Both these procedures had the advantage of potentially preserving other pituitary tropic hormone function. However, the adrenalectomized patient obviously had iatrogenic adrenal insufficiency, and Nelson's syndrome could occur. Since the development of radioimmunoassays for corticotropin, it has become clear that the disease is the result of excess ACTH secretion. It is less clear whether the CNS–hypothalamus is at fault or whether the disease is the consequence of a steroid-suppressible pituitary adenoma. Nonetheless, pituitary microadenomas are now found in most of the patients with Cushing's disease who come to surgery.[64] Whether these adenomas form as the result of abnormal hypothalamic stimulation or are an independent problem is not known with certainty. However, the advances in transsphenoidal microsurgery are causing a reevaluation of the appropriate first approach to treatment of these patients.

At present, the potential methods of treatment in the patient with Cushing's disease are medical, radiotherapeutic, and surgical approaches, including pituitary surgery as well as bilateral adrenalectomy to remove the target organs. Since the glucocorticoid excess of Cushing's disease is in itself life-threatening, reduction of cortisol levels into the normal range must be a primary goal of treatment. Ideally, this could be accomplished with preservation of normal pituitary and adrenal function and prevention of Nelson's syndrome.

5.1. Medical Treatment of Cushing's Disease

Since the manifestations of Cushing's disease are usually primarily the consequence of adrenal steroid overproduction rather than the mass effect of the pituitary tumor, several drugs have been employed to block or inhibit adrenal steroid synthesis. These include metyrapone,[65] mitotane (*op'*-DDD),[62] and aminoglutethamide.[66] These drugs are generally useful only for short periods of time because of low efficacy, disagreeable side effects, or expense. However, mitotane has been used for extended periods with success in patients who are not candidates for other forms of treatment.[62] Krieger and coworkers[67,68] have found that cyproheptadine, a drug with antiserotonergic and other effects, would produce a clinical remission in approximately 50% of patients tested. These remissions are associated with lowered ACTH, reduced cortisol levels, and clearing of the signs and symptoms of Cushing's disease. Cyproheptadine treatment may therefore be useful in some patients. These findings also provide hope that a more specific drug therapy with an even higher success rate might be developed.

5.2. Radiation Treatment of Cushing's Disease

Aristizabal *et al.*[69] have recently reviewed the use of conventional irradiation in the management of Cushing's disease. The overall results from the reviewed literature indicate an improvement rate of over 50% in 149 patients. In the series of 40 patients from Vanderbilt, 10 (25%) were considered to be cured, 11 (27.5%) were improved, and 19 (47.5%) were not adequately treated by irradiation alone. None of these 40 patients developed Nelson's syndrome, although this problem has been reported in patients who have received pituitary irradiation in other series.[70] The success rate appears higher in childhood Cushing's disease, with a success rate of 80% and minimal complications.[71] In adults, the incidence of all complications of conventional radiation therapy appears related to the technique utilized for treatment. Complications are more frequent after treatment with a total dose of over 4500–5000 rads and when fraction-doses exceed 200 rads.[4,72] Aristizabal *et al.*[69] have reported a relatively high incidence of visual complications (5%) in patients with Cushing's disease, which they believe may be related to hypertension or cortisol excess. These workers also point out that complications increased when large field sizes were used.[72] When patients have been treated with a total dose of 4500 rads with fractional doses below 200 rads, complications are rare. To date, no additional therapeutic advantage has been documented for photon treatment of patients with total doses in excess of 5000 rads.[4,72] If conventional irradiation is elected as the primary form of treatment, the dose should be restricted to 4500–5000 rads except in unusual circumstances, since complications are increased above this dosage.

Alpha-particle[73] and proton-beam therapy[25] have also both been used effectively in the treatment of Cushing's disease. These have the advantage of delivering a higher dose of irradiation to the pituitary than conventional supravoltage irradiation. The remission rate is approximately 65%, with improvement in most patients.[25,73,74] The incidence of complications such as cranial nerve palsies or hypopituitarism is approximately 7–8%.[74] This form of treatment is efficacious, but is available in only a few medical centers.

5.3. Surgical Treatment of Cushing's Disease

Bilateral adrenalectomy has been utilized successfully to correct the hypercortisolism of Cushing's disease.[61] However, this procedure leaves the patient with the problems of iatrogenic adrenal insufficiency requiring lifetime replacement with medication. In addition, a few patients will develop the aggressive pituitary tumor of Nelson's syndrome. Therefore, the possibility of selective removal of a pituitary adenoma with correction of the excess ACTH secretion and retention of normal pituitary function is an extremely attractive therapeutic approach to this disorder. The recent results from Tyrrell *et al.*[64] indicate a high degree of success, with over 90% remission. The recurrence rate of adenomas appears to be low.[79] Since the adenomas are usually small and infrequently (10%) are large enough to enlarge the sella turcica, transfrontal surgery is not ordinarily considered as primary therapy in Cushing's disease, although it is often necessary in the larger tumor in Nelson's syndrome. There have been no reported cases of Nelson's syndrome after successful transsphenoidal removal of pituitary adenomas. This would appear to be another reason to suggest this form of treatment.

5.4. Considerations in the Choice of Therapy for Cushing's Disease

The decision to treat with irradiation or transsphenoidal surgery is frequently based on the availability of a skilled neurosurgeon or the willingness of the patient to travel to a center for transsphenoidal surgery or for alpha-particle or proton-beam irradiation. Drug treatment with cyproheptadine is not widely employed as definitive therapy, although it may be useful in some patients. The other drugs such as metyrapone or mitotane are used primarily to prepare patients for surgery or in patients who are not candidates for surgery or irradiation. The surgical approach can be utilized more confidently when irregularities of the sella caused by the adenoma can be identified by tomagraphy of the sella. When no radiographic abnormalities are found, the surgical approach is essentially that of an exploration, which has been successful in some centers.[64] When the radiographic studies are negative in patients with "pituitary" Cushing's disease, the use of radiotherapy appears to be a reasonable alternative. If remission does not occur after proton or conventional irradiation, transsphenoidal surgery can still be employed. At times, the reverse may be necessary; when surgery is not successful, postoperative irradiation may be utilized. There are still instances in which both surgery and conventional iradiation are unsuccessful or for other reasons the patient must finally undergo adrenalectomy. Children appear to respond well to conventional irradiation, and this would appear to be a reasonable choice for pediatric patients.

6. Miscellaneous Tumors and Lesions

Obiously, a large variety of tumors such as craniopharyngiomas or meningiomas and other lesions including cysts and granulomas may occur in the area of the sella and simulate a pituitary tumor. In general, these are treated as mass lesions.

In view of the apparent high frequency of hormone secretion by pituitary adenomas, it is of interest that the glycoprotein hormones, TSH, LH, and FSH, are not often produced in appreciable amounts by pituitary adenomas. Rarely, TSH-secreting tumors causing hyperthyroidism have been reported.[75] Pituitary tumors producing FSH or FSH and LH[76] with signs and symptoms of a space-occupying lesion have also been documented. Some of these tumors have required treatment with surgery or irradiation and hormone replacement for the mass effects.

Recently, sella enlargement as a consequence of pituitary hyperplasia secondary to end-organ failure in primary hypothyroidism has been recognized more commonly in adults as well as children.[77] An enlarged sella may also occur in patients with primary hypogonadism and elevated gonadotropin secretion such as those with Klinefelter's or Turner's syndrome.[78] In these patients, no intervention or treatment is usually needed other than replacement of the deficient hormone.

7. Summary

The therapeutic approach to pituitary tumors depends on several factors including the size and function of the tumor and the specific treatment goals for the particular patient. Medical management is possible for patients with prolactinomas, acromegaly, and Cushing's disease, although this form of treatment is not usually considered definitive therapy. Transsphenoidal microsurgery has now developed to the degree that hypersecretory small adenomas may be removed with preservation of normal pituitary function including fertility. This type of treatment appears particularly useful in prolactin- and corticotropin-secreting microadenomas and in many patients with growth-hormone-secreting tumors. Proton-beam and alpha-particle irradiation have also been effective in small tumors producing growth hormone or corticotropin. Less experience is available with prolactinomas.

Larger tumors are being resected through the transsphenoidal approach with increasing frequency as more neurosurgeons become expert at this form of surgery. However, the very large tumors extending above the optic chiasm usually still require a transfrontal approach. Conventional supravoltage irradiation is an excellent adjunct to surgery to control growth of the large pituitary tumors. Photon or conventional radiation therapy is still used as a primary form of therapy in some patients with large tumors, particularly those who are not good candidates for surgery. Conventional irradiation is also still useful in some patients with Cushing's disease, with excellent results noted in children.

Unfortunately, no single form of therapy is uniformly successful in all patients. Surgery may have to be combined with irradiation in patients with hypersecretory syndromes as well as in nonfunctioning tumors.

References

1. L. Bakay, Results of 300 pituitary tumor operations (Prof. Herbert Olivecrona's series), *J. Neurosurg.* **7**:240–255, 1950.
2. R.W. Hollenhorst and B.R. Younge, Ocular manifestations produced by adenomas of the pituitary gland: Analysis of 1000 cases, in: *Diagnosis and Treatment of Pituitary Tumors* (P.O. Kohler and G.T. Ross, eds.), pp. 53–64, Exerpta Medica, Amsterdam, 1973.
3. F.C. Grant, Pituitary tumors, *Surg. Gynecol. Obstet.* **90**:629–631, 1950.
4. G.E. Sheline, Proceedings: Treatment of nonfunctioning chromophobe adenomas of the pituitary, *Am. J. Roentgenol.* **120**:553–561, 1974.
5. C.A. Fager, J.L. Poppen, and Y. Takaoka, Indications for and results of surgical treatment of pituitary tumors by the intracranial approach, in: *Diagnosis and Treatment of Pituitary Tumors* (P.O. Kohler and G.T. Ross, eds.), pp. 146–155, Exerpta Medica, Amsterdam, 1973.
6. J.F. Annegers, C.B. Coulam, C.F. Abboud, E.R. Laws, and L.T. Kurland, Pituitary adenoma in Olmsted County, Minnesota, 1935–1977, *Mayo Clin. Proc.* **53**:641–643, 1978.
7. S. Franks, J.D.N. Nabarro, and H.S. Jacobs, Prevalence and presentation of hyperprolactinaemia in patients with "functionless" pituitary tumors, *Lancet* **1**:788–780, 1977.
8. A.G. Franz, Prolactin, *N. Engl. J. Med.* **298**:201–207, 1978.
9. B. Kaufman, The "empty" sella turcica: A manifestation of the intrasellar subarachnoid space, *Radiology* **90**:931–941, 1968.
10. G.E. Sheline, Treatment of chromophobe adenomas of the pituitary gland and acromegaly, in: *Diagnosis and Treatment of Pituitary Tumors* (P.O. Kohler and G.T. Ross, eds.), pp. 201–216, Exerpta Medica, Amsterdam, 1973.
11. L.A. Weisberg, Asymptomatic enlargement of the sella turcica, *Arch. Neurol.* **32**:483–485, 1975.
12. D.A. Pistenma, D.R. Goffinet, M.A. Bagshaw, J.W. Hanbery, and J.R. Eltringham, Treatment of chromophobe adenomas with megavoltage irradiation, *Cancer* **35**:1574–1582, 1975.
13. N. Urdaneta, H. Chessin, and J.J. Fischer, Pituitary adenomas and craniopharyngiomas: Analysis of 99 cases treated with radiation therapy, *Int. J. Radiat. Oncol. Biol. Phys.* **1**:895–902, 1976.
14. A.R.C. Amine and O. Sugar, Suprasellar osteogenic sarcome following radiation for pituitary adenoma, *J. Neurosurg.* **44**:88–91, 1976.
15. J.C. Gonzalez-Vitale, R.E. Slavin, and J.D. McQueen, Radiation-induced intracranial malignant fibrous histiocytoma, *Cancer* **37**:2960–2963, 1976.
16. A.N. Martins, J.S. Johnston, J.M. Henry, T.J. Stoffel, and G. DiChiro, Delayed radiation necrosis of the brain, *J. Neurosurg.* **47**:336–345, 1977.
17. H. Cushing, the Weir Mitchell lecture: Surgical experiences with pituitary disorders, *J. Am. Med. Assoc.* **63**:1515–1525, 1914.
18. B.S. Ray and R.H. Patterson, Jr., Surgical treatment of pituitary adenomas, *J. Neurosurg.* **19**:1–8, 1962.
19. C.S. MacCarty, E.J. Hanson, Jr., R.V. Randall, and P.W. Scanlon, Indications for and results of surgical treatment of pituitary tumors by the transfrontal approach, in: *Diagnosis and Treatment of Pituitary Tumors* (P.O. Kohler and G.T. Ross, eds.), pp. 139–145, Exerpta Medica, Amsterdam, 1973.

20. R.L. Atkinson, D.P. Becker, A.N. Martins, M. Schaaf, R.C. Dimond, L. Wartofsky, and J.M. Earll, Acromegaly: Treatment by transsphenoidal microsurgery, *J. Am. Med. Assoc.* **233:**1279–1283, 1975.
21. G. Guiot, Transsphenoidal approach in surgical treatment of pituitary adenomas: General principles and indications in non-functioning adenomas, in: *Diagnosis and Treatment of Pituitary Tumors* (P.O. Kohler and G.T. Ross, eds.), pp. 159–178, Exerpta Medica, Amsterdam, 1973.
22. J. Roth, P. Gorden, and K. Brace, Efficacy of conventional pituitary irradiation in acromegaly, *N. Engl. J. Med.* **282:**1385–1391, 1970.
23. B.S. Ray, M. Horwith, and C. Mautalen, Surgical hypophysectomy as a treatment for acromegaly, in: *Clinical Endocrinology* II (E.B. Astwood and C.E. Cassidy, eds.), pp. 93–102, Grune and Stratton, New York, 1968.
24. J. Hardy, Transsphenoidal surgery of hypersecreting pituitary tumors, in: *Diagnosis and Treatment of Pituitary Tumors* (P.O. Kohler and G.T. Ross, eds.), pp. 179–194, Exerpta Medica, Amsterdam, 1973.
25. R.N. Kjellberg and B. Kliman, A system for therapy of pituitary tumors, in: *Diagnosis and Treatment of Pituitary Tumors* (P.O. Kohler and G.T. Ross, eds.), pp. 234–252, Exerpta Medica, Amsterdam, 1973.
26. J.H. Lawrence, C.A. Tobias, J.A. Linfoot, J.L. Born, J.T. Lyman, C.Y. Chong, E. Manougian, and W.C. Wei, Successful treatment of acromegaly: Metabolic and clinical studies in 145 patients, *J. Clin. Endocrinol. Metab.* **31:**180–198, 1970.
27. A.M. Lawrence, S.M. Pinsky, and I.D. Goldfine, Conventional radiation therapy in acromegaly, *Arch. Intern. Med.* **128:**369–377, 1971.
28. D.A. Pistenma, D.R. Goffinet, M.A. Bagshaw, J.W. Hanbery, and J.R. Eltringham, Treatment of acromegaly with megavoltage radiation therapy, *Int. J. Radiat. Oncol. Biol. Phys.* **1:**885–893, 1976.
29. A.L. Taylor, J.L. Finster, P. Raskin, J.B. Field, and D.H. Mintz, Pituitary apoplexy in acromegaly, *J. Clin. Endocrinol. Metab.* **28:**1784–1792, 1968.
30. R. Eastman, P. Gorden, and J. Roth, Conventional supervoltage irradiation is effective therapy for acromegaly, *J. Clin. Endocr. Metab.* **48:**931–940, 1979.
31. A.M. Lawrence and T.C. Hagen, Alternatives to ablative therapy for pituitary tumors, in: *Diagnosis and Treatment of Pituitary Tumors* (P.O. Kohler and G.T. Ross, eds.), pp. 298–312, Exerpta Medica, Amsterdam, 1973.
32. K. Nakagawa and K. Mashimo, Suppressibility of plasma growth hormone levels in acromegaly with dexamethasone and phentolamine, *J. Clin. Endocrinol. Metab.* **37:**238–246, 1973.
33. J.M. Feldman, J.W. Plonk, and C.H. Bivins, Inhibitory effect of serotonin antagonists on growth hormone release in acromegalic patients, *Clin. Endocrinol.* **5:**71–78, 1976.
34. G. Delitala, A. Masala, S. Alagna, L. Devilla, and G. Lotti, Growth hormone and prolactin release in acromegalic patients following metergoline administration, *J. Clin. Endocrinol. Metab.* **43:**1382–1386, 1976.
35. J.A.H. Wass, M.O. Thorner, D.V. Morris, L.H. Rees, A.S. Mason, A.E. Jones, and G.M. Besser, Long-term treatment of acromegaly with bromocryptine, *Br. Med. J.* **1:**875–878, 1977.
36. G. Benker, W. Zah, K. Hackenberg, B. Hamberger, H. Gunnewig, and D. Reinwein, Long-term treatment of acromegaly with bromocryptine: Postprandial HGH levels and response to TRH and glucose administration, *Horm. Metab. Res.* **8:**291–295, 1976.
37. V.K. Summers, L.J. Hipkin, M.J. Diver, and J.C. Davis, Treatment of acromegaly with bromocryptine, *J. Clin. Endocrinol. Metab.* **40:**904–906, 1975.
38. I.D. Goldfine and A.M. Lawrence, Hypopituitarism in acromegaly, *Arch. Intern. Med.* **130:**720–723, 1972.
39. D.M. Dawson and J.F. Dingman, Hazards of proton beam pituitary irradiation, *N. Engl. J. Med.* **282:**1434, 1970.
40. R. Fraser, F. Doyle, G.F. Joplin, C.W. Burke, P. Harsoulis, M. Tunbridge, R. Arnott, and D. Child, The assessment of the endocrine effects and the effectiveness of ablative pituitary treatment by ^{90}Y or ^{198}Au implantation, in: *Diagnosis and Treatment of Pituitary Tumors* (P.O. Kohler and G.T. Ross, eds.), pp. 35–46, Exerpta Medica, Amsterdam, 1973.
41. L.M. Davidoff, Studies in acromegaly: The anamnesis and symptomatology in one hundred cases, *Endocrinology* **10:**461–483, 1926.

42. S.R. Levin, Medical Staff Conference: Manifestations of acromegaly, *Calif. Med.* **116:**57–64, 1972.
43. J. Hardy, Transsphenoidal microsurgical treatment of pituitary tumors, in: *Recent Advances in the Diagnosis and Treatment of Pituitary Tumors* (J.A. Linfoot, ed.), pp. 375–378, Raven Press, New York, 1979.
44. D.L. Kleinberg, G.L. Noel, and A.G. Frantz, Galactorrhea: A study of 235 cases including 48 with pituitary tumor, *N. Engl. J. Med.* **296:**589–600, 1977.
45. A.E. Boyd, S. Reichlin, and R.N. Turksoy, Galactorrhea–amenorrhea syndrome: Diagnosis and therapy, *Ann. Intern. Med.* **87:**165–175, 1977.
46. C.B. Wilson and L.C. Dempsey, Transsphenoidal microsurgical removal of 250 pituitary adenomas, *J. Neurosurg.* **48:**13–22, 1978.
47. K.D. Post, B.J. Biller, L.S. Adelman, M.E. Molitch, S.M. Wolpert, and S. Reichlin, Results of selective transsphenoidal adenomectomy in women with galactorrhea–amenorrhea, *J. Am. Med. Assoc.* **242:**158–162, 1979.
48. D.F. Child, S. Nader, K. Mashiter, M. Kjeld, L. Banks, and T.R. Fraser, Prolactin studies in "functionless" pituitary tumors, *Br. Med. J.* **1:**604–606, 1975.
49. N.A. Samaan, M.E. Leavens, and J.H. Jesse, Jr., Serum prolactin in patients with "functionless" chromophobe adenomas before and after therapy, *Acta Endocrinol.* **84:**449–460, 1977.
50. J.N. Carter, J.E. Tyson, G. Tolis, S. Van Vliet, C. Faiman, and H. Friesen, Prolactin-secreting tumors and hypogonadism in 22 men, *N. Engl. J. Med.* **299:**847–852, 1978.
51. W.B. Malarkey, L.S. Jacobs, and W.H. Daughaday, Levodopa suppression of prolactin in non-puerperal galactorrhea, *N. Engl. J. Med.* **285:**1160–1163, 1971.
52. E. del Pozo and I. Lancranjan, Clinical use of drugs modifying the release of anterior pituitary hormones, in: *Frontiers in Neuroendocrinology,* Vol. 5, (W.F. Ganong and L. Martini, eds.), pp. 207–247, Raven Press, New York, 1978.
53. M.O. Thorner, G.M. Besser, A. Jones, J. Dacie, and A.E. Jones, Bromocryptine treatment of female infertility: Results of 13 pregnancies, *Br. Med. J.* **4:**694–697, 1975.
54. T. Bergh, S.J. Nillius, and L. Wide, Clinical course and outcome of pregnancies in amenorrhoeic women with hyperprolactinaemia and pituitary tumors, *Br. Med. J.* **1:**875–880, 1978.
55. S. Reichlin, The prolactinoma problem (editorial), *N. Engl. J. Med.* **300:**313–315, 1979.
56. A.M. McGregor, M.F. Scanlon, K. Hall, D.B. Cook, and R. Hall, Reduction in size of a pituitary tumor by bromocryptine therapy, *N. Engl. J. Med.* **300:**291–293, 1979.
57. J.A. Linfoot, Heavy ion therapy: Alpha particle therapy of pituitary tumors, in: *Recent Advances in the Diagnosis and Treatment of Pituitary Tumors* (J.A. Linfoot, ed.), pp. 245–267, Raven Press, New York, 1979.
58. J. Hardy, H. Beauregard, and F. Robert, Prolactin-secreting pituitary adenomas: Transsphenoidal microsurgical treatment, in: *Progress in Prolactin Physiology and Pathology* (C. Robyn and M. Harter, eds.), pp. 361–369, Elsevier North-Holland, Amsterdam, 1978.
59. F.T. Murray, J. Osterman, J. Sulewski, R. Page, R. Bergland, and J.M. Hammond, Alterations in pituitary function following surgical removal of prolactin-secreting pituitary tumors, *Obstet. Gynecol.* **54:**65–73, 1979.
60. R. Mornex, J. Orgiazzi, B. Hugues, J. Gagnaire, and B. Claustrat, Normal pregnancies after treatment of hyperprolactinemia with bromergocryptine, despite suspected pituitary tumors, *J. Clin. Endocrinol. Metab.* **47:**290–295, 1978.
61. I. Ernest and H. Ekman, Adrenalectomy in Cushing's disease: A long-term follow-up, *Acta Endocrinol.* **69**(Suppl. 160):5–41, 1972.
62. D.N. Orth and G.W. Liddle, Results of treatment of 108 patients with Cushing's syndrome, *N. Engl. J. Med.* **285:**243–247, 1971.
63. G.W. Liddle, Tests of pituitary–adrenal suppressibility in the diagnosis of Cushing's syndrome, *J. Clin. Endocrinol. Metab.* **20:**1539–1560, 1960.
64. J.B. Tyrrell, R.M. Brooks, P.A. Fitzgerald, P.M. Cofoid, P.H. Forsham, and C.B. Wilson, Cushing's disease: Selective transsphenoidal resection of pituitary microadenomas, *N. Engl. J. Med.* **298:**753–758, 1978.
65. W.J. Jeffcoate, L.H. Rees, S. Tomlin, A.E. Jones, C.R.W. Edwards, and G.M. Besser, Metyrapone in long-term management of Cushing's disease, *Br. Med. J.* **2:**215–217, 1977.
66. R.I. Misbin, J. Canary, and D. Willard, Aminoglutethamide in the treatment of Cushing's syndrome, *J. Clin. Pharmacol.* **16:**645–651, 1976.

67. D.T. Krieger, L. Amorosa, and F. Linick, Cyproheptadine-induced remission of Cushing's disease, *N. Engl. J. Med.* **293:**893–896, 1975.
68. D.T. Krieger, Pharmacological therapy of Cushing's disease and Nelson's syndrome, in: *Recent Advances in Diagnosis and Treatment of Pituitary Tumors* (J.A. Linfoot, ed.), pp. 337–340, Raven Press, New York, 1979.
69. S. Aristizabal, W.L. Caldwell, J. Avila, and E.G. Mayer, Relationship of time dose factors to tumor control and complications of treatment of Cushing's disease by irradiation, *Int. J. Radiat. Oncol. Biol. Phys.* **2:**47–54, 1977.
70. T.J. Moore, R.G. Dluhy, G.H. Williams, and J.P. Cain, Nelson's syndrome: Frequency, prognosis, and effect of prior pituitary irradiation, *Ann. Intern. Med.* **85:**731–734, 1976.
71. A.S. Jennings, G.W. Liddle, and D.N. Orth, Results of treating childhood Cushing's disease with pituitary irradiation, *N. Engl. J. Med.* **297:**957–962, 1977.
72. S. Aristizabal, W.L. Caldwell, and J. Avila, The relationships of time–dose fractionation factors to complications in the treatment of pituitary tumors by irradiation, *Int. J. Radiat. Oncol. Biol. Phys.* **1:**667–673, 1977.
73. J.H. Lawrence, C.A. Tobias, J.A. Linfoot, J.L. Born, and C.Y. Chong, Heavy particle therapy in acromegaly and Cushing's disease, *J. Am. Med. Assoc.* **235:**2307–2310, 1976.
74. E.M. Gold, The Cushing's syndromes: Changing views of diagnosis and treatment, *Ann. Intern. Med.* **90:**829–844, 1979.
75. C.R. Hamilton, Jr., L.C. Adams, and F. Maloof, Hyperthyroidism due to a thyrotropin-producing pituitary chromophobe adenoma, *N. Engl. J. Med. 283:*1077–1080, 1970.
76. P.J. Snyder and F.H. Sterling, Hypersecretion of LH and FSH by a pituitary adenoma, *J. Clin. Endocrinol. Metab.* **42:**544–550, 1976.
77. A.M. Lawrence, J.F. Wilber, and T.C. Hogan, The pituitary and primary hypothyroidism, *Arch. Intern. Med.* **132:**327–333, 1973.
78. N.A. Samaan, A.V. Stepanas, J. Danziger, and J. Trujillo, Reactive pituitary abnormalities in patients with Klinefelter's and Turner's syndromes, *Arch. Intern. Med.* **139:**198–201, 1979.
79. S.T. Bigos, M. Somma, E. Rasio, R.C. Eastman, A. Lanthier, H.H. Johnson, and J. Hardy, Cushing's disease: Management by transsphenoidal pituitary microsurgery, *J. Clin. Endocrinol. Metab.* **50:**348–354, 1980.

Index